PERSISTENT BACTERIAL
INFECTIONS

PERSISTENT BACTERIAL INFECTIONS

Edited by

James P. Nataro

Center for Vaccine Development
and
Departments of Pediatrics, Medicine, and Microbiology and Immunology
University of Maryland School of Medicine
Baltimore, Maryland

Martin J. Blaser

Departments of Medicine and Microbiology
New York University School of Medicine
and
New York Harbor Veterans Affairs Medical Center
New York, New York

Susanna Cunningham-Rundles

Immunology Research Laboratory
Division of Hematology and Oncology
Department of Pediatrics
Cornell University Weill Medical College–The New York Presbyterian Hospital
New York, New York

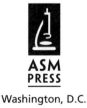

ASM
PRESS

Washington, D.C.

Copyright ©2000 ASM Press
American Society for Microbiology
1752 N St. NW
Washington, DC 20036-2804

Library of Congress Cataloging-in-Publication Data

Persistent bacterial infections / edited by James P. Nataro, Martin J. Blaser, Susanna
  Cunningham-Rundles.
   p.   cm.
  Includes bibliographical references and index.
  ISBN 1-55581-159-0
    1. Bacterial diseases.   2. Medical bacteriology.   3. Infection.
   4. Chronic diseases.   5. Host-bacteria relationships.
   I. Nataro, James P.   II. Blaser, Martin J.   III. Cunningham-Rundles, Susanna.

QR201.B34 P46 2000
616′.014—dc21

                                      00-025074

Cover photo: Laser scanning confocal microscopy image of macrophages (Nomarski differential interference contrast rendered in green) infected with *Mycobacterium bovis* BCG expressing green fluorescent protein (fluorescence rendered in red). Reprinted from L. E. Via et al., *J. Biol. Chem.* **272:**13326–13331, 1997, with permission of the publisher. Courtesy of V. Deretic (University of Michigan).

CONTENTS

CONTRIBUTORS

Ingegerd Adlerberth
Department of Clinical Immunology, Göteborg University, Guldhedsgatan 10, S-413 46
Göteborg, Sweden

Stephen W. Barthold
Center for Comparative Medicine, Schools of Medicine and Veterinary Medicine,
University of California, One Shields Avenue, Davis, California 95616

Douglas E. Berg
Departments of Molecular Microbiology and Genetics, Washington University Medical
School, St. Louis, Missouri

K. A. Bettelheim
National *Escherichia coli* Reference Laboratory, Microbiological Diagnostic Unit,
Department of Microbiology and Immunology, University of Melbourne, Melbourne,
Victoria 3010, Australia

Martin J. Blaser
Departments of Medicine and Microbiology, New York University School of Medicine,
New York, New York 10016, and New York Harbor VA Medical Center, New York,
New York 10010

Cynthia Gove Bloomquist
Department of Oral Sciences, University of Minnesota School of Dentistry,
Minneapolis, Minnesota 55455

Robert C. Brunham
University of British Columbia Centre for Disease Control, Vancouver,
British Columbia V5Z 4R4, Canada

Simon R. Carding
School of Biological Sciences, University of Leeds, Leeds LS2 9JT, England

Laurie E. Comstock
Channing Laboratory, Brigham and Women's Hospital, Harvard Medical School,
Boston, Massachusetts 02115

J. William Costerton
Center for Biofilm Engineering, Montana State University, Bozeman, Montana 59717

Susanna Cunningham-Rundles
Immunology Research Laboratory, Division of Hematology and Oncology, Department of Pediatrics, Cornell University Weill Medical College-The New York Presbyterian Hospital, New York, New York 10021

Toni Darville
Division of Pediatric Infectious Diseases, Departments of Pediatrics and of Microbiology and Immunology, University of Arkansas for Medical Sciences and Arkansas Children's Hospital, Little Rock, Arkansas 72202

V. Deretic
Department of Microbiology and Immunology, University of Michigan, Ann Arbor, Michigan 48109

Andre Dubois
Laboratory of Gastrointestinal and Liver Studies, Digestive Diseases Division, Department of Medicine, Uniformed Services University of the Health Sciences, Bethesda, Maryland 20814

Paul J. Egan
Department of Clinical Studies, School of Veterinary Medicine, University of Pennsylvania, Philadelphia, Pennsylvania 19104

Rolf Freter
Department of Microbiology and Immunology, The University of Michigan Medical School, Ann Arbor, Michigan 48109-0620

Mark C. Herzberg
Department of Preventive Sciences, School of Dentistry, University of Minnesota, Minneapolis, Minnesota 55455

Ann E. Jerse
Department of Microbiology and Immunology, Uniformed Services University of the Health Sciences, Bethesda, Maryland 20814

Howard M. Johnson
Department of Microbiology and Cell Science, University of Florida, Gainesville, Florida 32611

Denise E. Kirschner
Department of Microbiology and Immunology, The University of Michigan Medical School, Ann Arbor, Michigan 48109-0620

Jane E. Koehler
Division of Infectious Diseases, Department of Medicine, 521 Parnassus Avenue, Room C-443, University of California at San Francisco, San Francisco, California 94143-0654

Myron M. Levine
Center for Vaccine Development and Departments of Medicine and Pediatrics, University of Maryland School of Medicine, Baltimore, Maryland 21201

William F. Liljemark
Department of Oral Sciences, University of Minnesota School of Dentistry, Minneapolis, Minnesota 55455

J. T. Mader
The Marine Biomedical Institute and Division of Marine Medicine, The University of Texas Medical Branch, Galveston, Texas 77555-1115

James P. Nataro
Center for Vaccine Development and Departments of Pediatrics, Medicine, and Microbiology and Immunology, University of Maryland School of Medicine, Baltimore, Maryland 21201

Mirjana Nesin
Perinatology Center, Division of Neonatology, Department of Pediatrics, Cornell University Weill Medical College-The New York Presbyterian Hospital, New York, New York 10021

George Q. Perrin
Department of Microbiology and Cell Science, University of Florida, Gainesville, Florida 32611

Taraz Samandari
Center for Vaccine Development and Departments of Medicine and Pediatrics, University of Maryland School of Medicine, Baltimore, Maryland 21201

M. E. Shirtliff
Department of Microbiology and Immunology, The University of Texas Medical Branch, Galveston, Texas 77555-1115

Anthony P. Sinai
Department of Microbiology and Immunology, University of Kentucky College of Medicine, 800 Rose Street, Lexington, Kentucky 40536

Jeanne M. Soos
Clinical Immunology, SmithKline Beecham Pharmaceuticals, King of Prussia, Pennsylvania 19406

Philip S. Stewart
Center for Biofilm Engineering, Montana State University, Bozeman, Montana 59717

Marcelo B. Sztein
Center for Vaccine Development and Departments of Medicine and Pediatrics, University of Maryland School of Medicine, Baltimore, Maryland 21201

Barbara A. Torres
Department of Microbiology and Cell Science, University of Florida, Gainesville, Florida 32611

Michele Trucksis
Medical Service, Veterans Affairs Medical Center, and Center for Vaccine Development and Department of Medicine, University of Maryland, Baltimore, Maryland 21201

Arthur O. Tzianabos
Channing Laboratory, Brigham and Women's Hospital, Harvard Medical School, Boston, Massachusetts 02115

Anthony Welch
Laboratory of Gastrointestinal and Liver Studies, Digestive Diseases Division, Department of Medicine, Uniformed Services University of the Health Sciences, Bethesda, Maryland 20814, and Bioqual Inc., Rockville, Maryland 20850

Agnes E. Wold

Department of Clinical Immunology, Göteborg University, Guldhedsgatan 10, S-413 46
Göteborg, Sweden

John L. Wylie

Cadham Provincial Laboratory, Manitoba Health, and Department of Medical
Microbiology, University of Manitoba, Winnipeg, Manitoba, Canada

FOREWORD

Persistent Bacterial Infections attempts to place a more precise focus on the term "persistent" and broadens the concept to include our normal microbial flora—the microbes that silently accompany us throughout life. Persistence is a complex matter, since the most fundamental questions regarding microbial specialization need to be addressed. What are pathogens? How do commensal microbes differ? What are opportunistic pathogens? Why do some pathogens cause acute infection while others cause a chronic and persistent infection? At what point in evolution is the line between inapparent chronic infection and endosymbiosis crossed? In the medical sense, how long after the infective event occurs is the transition into a persistent infection made? The microbes have no difficulty in sorting all of this out; we are the ones who have difficulty thinking about these issues in evolutionary, ecological, and medical terms.

My resolution of the question of what distinguishes a pathogen from commensal and opportunistic organisms revolves around the conviction that the pathogenic way of life is a selective survival mechanism based on the microbe's ability to cross anatomic and cellular barriers of a host to attain a niche that is usually denied to other microbes. This survival mechanism assures a ready food supply and freedom from competition but is fraught with the dangers inherent in the host's immune system. Commensal organisms lack the ability to penetrate host barriers and have adapted themselves to a unique niche, often despite a limited food supply and fierce competition from other microbes. Some commensal organisms, when presented with an immunocompromised host, take advantage of the situation and can be just as aggressive and deadly as organisms that are professional pathogens, but this is not the usual case. Even in the face of a host catastrophe, such as a perforated bowel and the seeding of the extraordinarily complex microbial flora into the peritoneal cavity, only a few members of the normal flora have the ability to establish an infectious process. Faced with the opportunity to exhibit their pathogenic potential, most microbes in our normal flora fail to meet the requirements for success, i.e., the capacity to replicate and persist outside of their normal ecological compartment. Thus, organisms that have no difficulty persisting for a lifetime in the mouth or on other mucosal surfaces fail to extend beyond their defined niche. Does this reflect the individual failure of a bacterial species, or is it that most microbial species on this planet, including those within our bodies, exist as cooperative and codependent communities? Is the essential property shared by most (known) human pathogenic bacteria the ability to live independently of other microbes or the ability to live in a community of microbes? In the same vein, it is instructive to consider the many endosymbiotic relationships between microbes and their host. Interestingly, *Rickettsia*, including the agent of typhus, an acute killer, can live in a silent, persistent form in some infected hosts before reappearing in a recognizable but less-deadly form. How is the decision for persistence made? Is it the response of the host or the modulation of the microbe? It is tantalizing that the same rickettsiae are among the closest known relatives of modern-day mitochondria, which we all possess in our cells and which are necessary for life. What dictates this evolutionary sequence of events?

The chapters that follow provide the foundation for thinking about these issues, which, I suspect, will provide students and teachers of microbiology and infectious diseases with enough facts to fuel endless discussions and debates. The content of this book not only provides a view of the ecology of persistent infections and the host response to infection and a state-of-the-art portrayal of the best understood examples of persistent bacterial infections, but also engages and tempts us with the possibility that a number of clinical syndromes that appear to be noninfectious in origin might actually have an infectious etiology.

It is appropriate that *Persistent Bacterial Infections* appears at the dawn of the new millennium. It is the custom at such historical milestones to reflect on what the future will bring. I believe the study of persistent infections, at least in the context presented by the editors and authors of this book, will become the hallmark of the first decades of the new century in biology. We shall use newly available molecular and biochemical tools to probe the interactions of the host and microbe in real time. We are destined to move our studies of microbes from the confines of the laboratory flask to the real world, whether in the soil surrounding a plant, within a host cell, or within the complex biosphere of the human gingival crypt. Our ability to follow individual microbes, coupled with the techniques of genomics, brings us to a scientific era as exciting and revolutionary, in its way, as when humankind first realized that microbes, rather than swamp vapors or the curse of a witch, caused much human disease. I believe we will fully appreciate the enormity and the diversity of the microbial world, which is essential for life on this planet, and that we will face our ignorance of the other life forms that inhabit our bodies. For example, we carry numerically more bacteria, fungi, viruses, and single-celled species on us or within us than there are human cells in our bodies. Ninety-nine percent of these microbes have never been cultured in the laboratory. We know less about the extent and diversity of microbial life than about any other life form.

The subject of persistent infections has profound clinical implications for a society faced with an epidemic of human immunodeficiency virus infection and for those physicians who are not yet over the shock that some diseases, such as ulcer disease and gastric cancer, are direct and indirect manifestations of a microbial infection with *Helicobacter pylori*. Even if only a fraction of the autoimmune diseases, malignancies, and cardiovascular disorders suspected of having an infectious etiology are found to actually have one, there will be a true revolution in our view of host-parasite relationships. Perhaps the most valuable asset of this volume is that it brings together a broad representation of scientists who study population biology and ecology, immunology and immunodeficiency, and microbial genetics and human genetics, as well as those who study bacteria for the love of their biology and those who study bacteria in hopes of eradication. It is, in a way, a microcosm of all facets of contemporary biology!

STANLEY FALKOW
Department of Microbiology and Immunology
Stanford University School of Medicine
Stanford, California

INTRODUCTION

PERSISTENT BACTERIAL INFECTIONS: COMMENSALISM GONE AWRY OR ADAPTIVE NICHE?

James P. Nataro, Martin J. Blaser, and Susanna Cunningham-Rundles

I

An elderly comedian was once asked, "To what do you owe your longevity?" He quipped in response, "To the fact that I haven't died yet!" Evolution can be similarly summarized: a successful organism is one that has yet to disappear.

The perpetuation of a genome from generation to generation represents the solution to a complex mathematical problem. However, all such solutions are reached by trial and error and depend on genomic variation, which largely arises at random. Short bacterial generation times and large population sizes result in an enormous rate of variation and, ultimately, remarkably versatile solutions to the problem of genomic perpetuation (26). The ability to achieve great numbers may itself be an adaptive solution, as are the efficient metabolic pathways present in many free-living bacteria; medical bacteriologists consider only a small subset of the earth's microbiota: those whose adapted solutions occasionally or commonly cause illness in humans.

THE ECOLOGICAL PERSPECTIVE

We traditionally divide the biological relationships of equilibrium between coexisting species into three exclusive categories. The category best known to medical bacteriologists is parasitism, the biological state in which one organism benefits while the other is harmed. A second state, symbiosis, describes the situation in which both species derive benefit. The third state is commensalism, in which the host neither benefits nor is harmed. The indigenous microbiota of humans falls into the second or third category; some of these bacteria assist the host by providing resistance to colonization by pathogens and occasionally by providing important nutrients.

However, it is important to consider the fact that our indigenous microbiota are not always harmless: from time to time, coexistence with microbes carries a cost. The alpha-hemolytic streptococci, for example, are normally harmless inhabitants of the mouth, but when the opportunity arises, they can become the agents of infective endocarditis. Moreover, the violation of human mucosal and integumentary barriers can permit even the most innocuous bacteria to access spaces that are unable to resist

James P. Nataro, Center for Vaccine Development and Departments of Pediatrics, Medicine, and Microbiology and Immunology, University of Maryland School of Medicine, Baltimore, MD 21201.   *Martin J. Blaser,* Departments of Medicine and Microbiology, New York University School of Medicine, New York, NY 10016, and New York Harbor VA Medical Center, New York, NY 10010.   *Susanna Cunningham-Rundles,* Immunology Research Laboratory, Division of Hematology and Oncology, Department of Pediatrics, Cornell University Weill Medical College-The New York Presbyterian Hospital, New York, NY 10021.

Persistent Bacterial Infections, Edited by J. P. Nataro, M. J. Blaser, and S. Cunningham-Rundles, © 2000 ASM Press, Washington, D.C.

their onslaught. In acknowledgment of this potential for host injury, the term amphibiosis describes the state in which specific bacteria may be either harmless to the host or harmful, depending on the circumstances. Amphibiosis is considered from several perspectives in this book.

Recently, the spectrum of virulence has been categorized according to the ways in which the host facilitates the pathogenicity of the microbial biota (6). This approach aids our understanding of complex evolutionary relationships, yet it implies another question: which microorganisms have adapted to a pathogenic lifestyle? We will ask this critical question throughout this book.

WHAT IS A PERSISTENT INFECTION?

Since our origin, *Homo sapiens* has been besieged by infectious agents. This contest led to selection of effective defenses, which include both integumentary barriers and dynamic innate and specific immune effectors. The result of these adaptations is that the vast majority of encounters with microorganisms are either benign or represent a brief and self-limiting disturbance of homeostatic functions. The brief nature of most infections thus appears to be a triumph of the host over the pathogen. Nevertheless, pathogens may exploit even brief, acute infections as means to perpetuate their spread.

However, there also exist certain infections of humans that are not characteristically brief and self-limiting. In each of these infections, the microbe avoids early killing by the host's immune response to establish a stable existence. In some cases, this is the result of an intricate evolutionary bargain between the persistent pathogen and the host. Such organisms have developed a "balanced pathogenicity" (24), in which they must strike an equilibrium, simultaneously avoiding both eradication by and lethal damage to the host. In other cases, persistent bacterial infection represents a host-damaging amphibiotic interaction, and in still others, it represents an ecological "accident," in which an organism adapted to another host

or state finds itself introduced to an accommodating *H. sapiens* (21). We can better understand persistent infections by asking which of these contexts obtains for a given pathogen.

HOW IS PERSISTENCE ADAPTIVE?

As noted above, certain infections persist because the microbes have adapted persistence as a specific lifestyle; from these infections, we can learn much about the requirements of this arrangement. All bacterial infections require the avoidance of host defenses in order for the organism to colonize, multiply, and damage the host; for obligate parasites, it is necessary to add the need to be transmitted to another susceptible host. Even for bacteria with free-living states, human disease may provide a means of amplifying their numbers. The mathematical relationships governing the number of secondary infections (R_0) caused by each primary infection has been expressed as

$$R_0 = BN/(\alpha + b + \nu),$$

where B is the rate constant of infectious transfer of the pathogen, N is the density of the susceptible host population, α is the rate of pathogen-induced mortality, b is the rate of pathogen-independent host mortality, and ν is the rate of host recovery from infection (21). According to this equation, persistence (rather than host death or recovery) decreases both α and ν, thereby resulting in increased opportunities for pathogen transmission. Of course, persistence also requires at least a moderate degree of clinical indolence rather than fulminance; persistent infections typically result in a mildly ill (or asymptomatic) patient, perhaps with intermittently or terminally flagrant disease. Perhaps a consummate example would be chronic carriage of *Salmonella enterica* serovar Typhi. Here, the few chronically infected carriers serve as an important and efficient reservoir of infection.

The relationship described above also predicts that persistence will be favored when opportunities for transmission decrease, specifically because of a declining density of susceptible hosts, N. The story of the rabbit myxomatosis virus serves as a famous example (5). The myxomatosis virus was introduced into Australia in 1950 in an effort to control rabbit overpopulation, and initially, rabbits were infected by the millions, with a high rate of fatality. However, within 7 years, fatality rates plummeted as simultaneous selection for less susceptible rabbits and for less virulent virus supervened. An example of evolution to increased virulence may be the extraordinary influenza pandemic of 1918 and 1919 (13). Here, the remarkable host densities in the trenches of World War I are thought to have driven the equation in favor of R_0, irrespective of the values of α and v. The effect was to remove the adaptive value of host fitness in transmitting the virus from one susceptible host to another.

It may indeed be illuminating to consider persistent infections in the context of human history. Ancient human populations typically consisted of small bands of perhaps several hundred individuals who interacted with other bands and tribes for purposes of warfare, commerce, and intermarriage (8). In such a setting, highly prevalent obligate parasites tend to decrease N by eliminating susceptibles; the net effect is to increase the selective pressure toward a more indolent infection, i.e., one that would persist until the infected individual encountered a susceptible member of another tribe. The rise of civilization has provided many opportunities for infectious agents to modify their virulence (22), but pressures that favor persistence remain. The sexually transmitted diseases provide a modern example in which an otherwise healthy, persistently infected host can generate an impressive R_0.

As the following chapters illustrate, over millions of years many microorganisms have developed diverse attributes that specifically prepare them for persistence. These examples illustrate the value to microbes of persistence; but if causing mild indolent disease is adaptive, under which circumstances is it advantageous to injure the host? Although commensalism is a boon to *Bacteroides* species, examination of *Mycobacterium tuberculosis* infection provides a contrary paradigm. *M. tuberculosis* usually infects humans by the respiratory route and, in most cases, causes no illness. However, a minority of infected persons become ill. In these individuals, there is usually a persistent cough and the aerosolization of large numbers of infectious particles over a period of months to years. Although in untreated populations tuberculosis is often fatal, the dying host may propagate the pathogen to new hosts, sowing a field that will germinate as either asymptomatic, and therefore nontransmitting, individuals or as transmitting patients. The asymptomatic host may remain healthy throughout life, but in a proportion of cases (ca. 10%), *M. tuberculosis* will reactivate to cause a highly infectious pulmonary syndrome (see chapter 16). Although a minority event, reactivation-associated transmission is, presumably, the evolutionary purpose of latency. Thus, *M. tuberculosis* has two lifestyles in association with humans: an aggressive form (either primary or reactivation) that ensures transmission and a latent form that ensures survival of the microorganisms within a human population until the host encounters new susceptible persons. An examination of the pathogenetic features of *M. tuberculosis* suggests that this organism has evolved many characteristics to ensure the success of this complex strategy.

THE INCIDENTAL PERSISTENT HUMAN PATHOGEN

There are also persistent bacterial infections that result from natural accidents. We envision these in three different categories: (i) accidents of transmission; (ii) accidents of susceptibility, and (iii) accidents of response. The role of the indigenous microbiota in these accidental persistent infections is discussed throughout this book.

Accidents of transmission refer to persistent infections of humans by organisms that are not adapted to our species; i.e., humans are dead-end, incidental hosts. Lyme disease serves as an example of this phenomenon (see chapter 14). Thus, when considering *Borrelia burgdorferi*, it is important to remember that pathogenetic mechanisms have developed that allow the organism to persist in other mammalian hosts and that the human manifestations of Lyme disease are unlikely to foster genomic perpetuation.

Accidents of susceptibility are infections that occur in compromised hosts. One example is a vascular-catheter-related infection, in which a bacterial biofilm, evolved to permit the organism to persist in a free-living state, forms on the surface of the catheter and renders the pathogen refractory to immune clearance mechanisms (see chapter 23). A second, related example is the instance in which bacteria that are adapted for one body site are introduced to another, usually as a result of a local or global compromise. Nonpathogenic *Escherichia coli* normally inhabiting the colon may cause urinary tract infection due to diabetes mellitus or an indwelling catheter (21).

The third type of accidental persistent infection is the accident of response. We have considered how primary and reactivation pulmonary syndromes enable the transmission of *M. tuberculosis*; diarrhea, rhinorrhea, and pyoderma may be similar means of facilitating the propagation of other pathogens (24). However, not all symptoms of infection are highly adaptive for the bacterium. For example, meningitis does not serve to perpetuate the genome of the meningococcus. Indeed, infectious diseases frequently result from an overly vigorous host response to an offending pathogen. The response, intended to eradicate the pathogen, may be a stereotyped attempt to respond to a perceived threat, but it may contribute simultaneously to the disease.

When considering the question of whether disease signs and symptoms are adaptive or accidental manifestations of infection, it can be useful to examine differences between the current presentations of these infections and those observed in the populations in which these infections initially evolved. Thus, it is possible that *Helicobacter* virulence reflects its proximity to humans at a time when the human age distribution was substantially younger and when humans were exposed to fewer of the stresses that increase the likelihood of peptic ulcer disease. In such a setting, perhaps nearly all infected persons experienced only an asymptomatic host response. Moreover, the association of *Helicobacter* with gastric carcinoma also may be an inadvertent outcome or it may serve as a means of "thinning" of the aged populations in ancestral human communities, for whom the supplies of food and other required resources were often marginal (4).

According to this line of reasoning, so-called opportunistic pathogens may have evolved as such in ancestral populations. One example is *Pseudomonas aeruginosa*, long considered a prototypic opportunistic pathogen (see chapter 15). Ongoing studies reveal a substantial number of factors that injure human tissues (12, 15, 19, 30), suggesting that the organism is indeed adapted to virulence. *P. aeruginosa* is therefore well equipped to cause disease in debilitated humans (the elderly, the malnourished, or those weakened by other infections), who are common in populations living under the primitive conditions long relevant to human evolution. *Staphylococcus aureus* may be another example. This organism is a common and successful commensal of the human pharynx and, to a lesser extent, the skin. But in primitive populations there are dramatic and persistent cases of pyoderma, often in the setting of scabies or other integumentary insults. Indeed, molecular studies now reveal that *S. aureus* has finely adapted mechanisms for avoidance of the immune response and for the establishment of localized and persistent pyogenic infections (33). Presumably, such superficial infections provide the same advantages for multiplication and dissemination present in the more familiar pneumonic and enteric bacterial infections.

WHAT MECHANISMS HAVE EVOLVED TO PROMOTE PERSISTENCE?

Life forms have developed a seemingly infinite number of solutions to the problem of genomic persistence. The fact that we are as yet unable to predict how a microorganism will evolve indicates the complexity of these issues. Never-

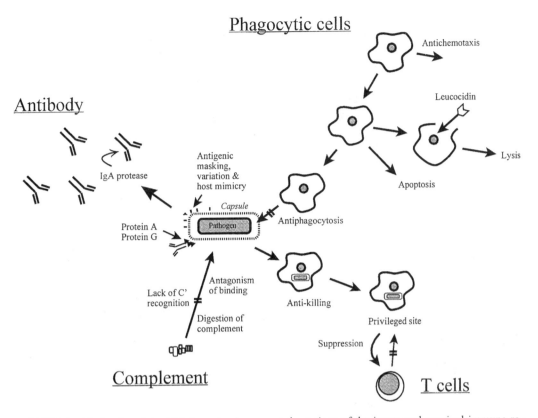

FIGURE 1 Mechanisms by which bacteria circumvent the actions of the innate and acquired immune responses. The major immune effectors comprise phagocytic cells, T-cell lineages, complement and other soluble antibacterial factors, and specific antibodies. Bacterial pathogens have evolved means to avoid these mechanisms. Since the immune system works in concert, persistent bacterial pathogens must deploy a variety of host avoidance approaches simultaneously. Examples of the various host avoidance mechanisms are presented in Tables 1 and 2.

theless, there are constraints on microbial evolution dictated by the host-imposed obstacles that the organism must overcome.

Host antibacterial weapons can be classified as follows (see chapter 8): (i) physical mechanisms, such as peristalsis and the flushing of secretions; (ii) innate immune mechanisms, such as polymorphonuclear cells and complement; and (iii) specific (adaptive) antibacterial immunity, such as cytotoxic T cells and antibodies. Persistent pathogens are exposed simultaneously and sequentially to multiple aspects of the host's defenses. In response, the pathogen employs a panoply of feints and deceptions. For example, *Neisseria gonorrhoeae* (see chapter 11)

modifies its lipooligosaccharide to mask the structure from recognition by the humoral response and by the alternative complement pathway. If effective antibodies are formed against the gonococcus, their effects are thwarted by antigenic variation of the major exposed virulence proteins. If the organism is engulfed by a phagocytic cell, the P1 outer membrane protein prevents fusion of the phagosome with lysosomes, permitting intracellular persistence.

We have classified the strategies used by the pathogen to circumvent complex host defenses as (i) sequestration, (ii) humoral evasion, and (iii) cellular evasion strategies (Fig. 1).

Sequestration

Certain persistent bacterial infections are characterized by the presence of a physical barrier between the microbe and the host, and important examples are described in this volume. One common mechanism is the establishment of a biofilm of bacterial and/or host origin. Examples include dental plaque (chapter 21), vegetations on heart valves in endocarditis (see chapter 19), the growth of *P. aeruginosa* in the lungs of cystic fibrosis patients (chapter 15), and the growth of a variety of bacteria on vascular devices (see chapter 23). Alternatively, some bacteria are sequestered in abscesses or in fibrinous, hypoperfused sanctuaries within body sites, such as the cortex of bone (see chapters 19 and 20). Such physical structures present a barrier to the penetration of the humoral defenses, including antibody and complement, as well as an obstacle to effective interaction with phagocytic cells and lymphocytes (cellular defenses).

Humoral Evasion

Extracellular bacteria must avoid the actions of complement and antibodies, including inhibition of bacterial binding to host cells, opsonization, complement-mediated lysis, and antibody-dependent cell-mediated cytotoxicity (see chapters 2 and 4). The mechanisms by which bacteria avoid antibody functions are varied (Table 1); however, bacterial pathogens adapted for persistence commonly express more than one mechanism. Evasion of the humoral response is considered in greater detail in chapter 4.

Cellular Evasion

Persistent infection exposes the microbe to a variety of leukocyte-dependent antibacterial mechanisms, including activation of macrophages/monocytes, polymorphonuclear phagocytes, NK cells, and lymphocytes. All pathogens, particularly those that are intracellular, must avoid these agents of destruction. The principal means of avoiding these cellular defenses are listed in Table 2. Further discussion of these issues can be found in chapters 3 and 4.

DEVELOPMENT OF EQUILIBRIA

What is the metabolic state of pathogens that permits them to remain viable in the host for extended periods? In most cases, this question has not been addressed in sufficient detail. Persistent viral pathogens may adopt a truly latent state, in which replication is minimal or nonexistent. However, it is unlikely that many bacterial pathogens are capable of establishing true latency (see chapter 16). Most likely, the bacteria survive in an equilibrium of multiplication and death, presumably analogous to the sta-

TABLE 1 Bacterial defenses against humoral immunity

Mechanism	Example(s)	Reference
Expression of poorly immunogenic antigens	*Treponema pallidum*	27
Antigenic variation	*Borrelia recurrentis*	34
	Campylobacter fetus	9
	N. gonorrhoeae	29
Antigenic mimicry	*E. coli* K1	3
	Neisseria meningitidis group B	3
	H. pylori	35
Antigenic masking	*N. gonorrhoeae*	23
	S. aureus	10
Expression of antibody-cleaving proteases	*Haemophilus influenzae*	28
	N. meningitidis	31
Expression of antibody-adsorbing molecules	*Streptococcus pyogenes* protein G	20
	S. aureus protein A	16

TABLE 2 Defenses against cell-mediated host mechanisms

Mechanism	Example	Reference
Killing of phagocytes	*S. aureus*	25
Inhibition of chemotaxis	*Yersinia pestis*	32
Inhibition of phagocytosis	*M. tuberculosis*	14
Occupation of a "safe" intracellular site	*M. tuberculosis*	7
	Rickettsia spp.	17
	Chlamydia spp.	18
Resistance to intravacuolar killing	*Salmonella* spp.	11
Suppression of cellular responses (cytokine manipulation)	*Yersinia* spp.	1

tionary phase of in vitro cultures. The amplitude of the equilibrium may vary from low grade (e.g., latent *M. tuberculosis* in granulomata) to high grade (e.g., *Helicobacter pylori*; on the order of 10^7 to 10^{10} bacteria in the stomach present for the life of the individual) (2). Over years, the opportunities for disruption of this equilibrium are many, and it is likely that persistent pathogens must at least intermittently expend energy to manipulate host defenses, thereby reestablishing a favorable balance.

Persistent infections are clinical problems. However, they clearly occur in a biological context. Careful analysis of the biology of persistence will permit new insights that can be broadly useful to science and ultimately to clinicians. It is in this spirit that this volume was conceived and has been prepared. We have sought to provide analyses of the most important organisms and mechanisms in the context of current research. Several chapters on the basis of persistence have been included, especially focusing on the most active fields of study. We hope to generate both questions and themes that will stimulate further advances in this field.

REFERENCES

1. **Aepfelbacher, M., R. Zumbihl, K. Ruckdeschel, C. A. Jacobi, C. Barz, and J. Heesemann.** 1999. The tranquilizing injection of Yersinia proteins: a pathogen's strategy to resist host defense. *J. Biol. Chem.* **380:**795–802.
2. **Atherton, J. C., K. T. Tham, R. M. Peek, Jr.,** T. L. Cover, and M. J. Blaser. 1996. Density of *Helicobacter pylori* infection in vivo as assessed by quantitative culture and histology. *J. Infect. Dis.* **174:**552–556.
3. **Azmi, F. H., A. H. Lucas, H. V. Raff, and D. M. Granoff.** 1994. Variable region sequences and idiotypic expression of a protective human immunoglobulin M antibody to capsular polysaccharides of *Neisseria meningitidis* group B and *Escherichia coli* K1. *Infect. Immun.* **62:**1776–1786.
4. **Blaser, M. J.** 1997. Ecology of *Helicobacter pylori* in the human stomach. *J. Clin. Invest.* **100:** 759–762.
5. **Burnet, M., and D. O. White.** 1972. *Natural History of Infectious Disease,* 4th ed. Cambridge University Press, Cambridge, United Kingdom.
6. **Casadevall, A., and L. Pirofski.** 1999. Host-pathogen interactions: redefining the basic concepts of virulence and pathogenicity. *Infect. Immun.* **67:**3703–3713.
7. **Deretic, V., and R. A. Fratti.** 1999. *Mycobacterium tuberculosis* phagosome. *Mol. Microbiol.* **31:** 1603–1609.
8. **Diamond, J.** 1999. *Guns, Germs, and Steel: the Fates of Human Societies.* W. W. Norton & Co., New York, N.Y.
9. **Dworkin, J., and M. J. Blaser.** 1997. Molecular mechanisms of *Campylobacter fetus* surface layer protein expression. *Mol. Microbiol.* **26:**433–440.
10. **Dziewanowska, K., J. M. Patti, C. F. Deobald, K. W. Bayles, W. R. Trumble, and G. A. Bohach.** 1999. Fibronectin binding protein and host cell tyrosine kinase are required for internalization of *Staphylococcus aureus* by epithelial cells. *Infect. Immun.* **67:**4673–4678.
11. **Ernst, R. K., T. Guina, and S. I. Miller.** 1999. How intracellular bacteria survive: surface modifications that promote resistance to host innate immune responses. *J. Infect. Dis.* **179**(Suppl. 2): S326–S330.
12. **Evans, D. J., D. W. Frank, V. Finck-Barbancon, C. Wu, and S. M. Fleiszig.** 1998. *Pseudo-*

monas aeruginosa invasion and cytotoxicity are independent events, both of which involve protein tyrosine kinase activity. *Infect. Immun.* **66:** 1453–1459.

13. **Ewald, P. W.** 1994. *Evolution of Infectious Disease.* Oxford University Press, Oxford, United Kingdom.

14. **Ferguson, J. S., D. R. Voelker, F. X. McCormack, and L. S. Schlesinger.** 1999. Surfactant protein D binds to *Mycobacterium tuberculosis* bacilli and lipoarabinomannan via carbohydrate-lectin interactions resulting in reduced phagocytosis of the bacteria by macrophages. *J. Immunol.* **163:** 312–321.

15. **Frank, D. W.** 1997. The exoenzyme S regulon of *Pseudomonas aeruginosa. Mol. Microbiol.* **26:** 621–629.

16. **Gemmell, C. G., S. C. Goutcher, R. Reid, and R. D. Sturrock.** 1997. Role of certain virulence factors in a murine model of *Staphylococcus aureus* arthritis. *J. Med. Microbiol.* **46:**208–213.

17. **Hackstadt, T.** 1998. The diverse habitats of obligate intracellular parasites. *Curr. Opin. Microbiol.* **1:**82–87.

18. **Hackstadt, T., E. R. Fischer, M. A. Scidmore, D. D. Rockey, and R. A. Heinzen.** 1997. Origins and functions of the chlamydial inclusion. *Trends Microbiol.* **5:**288–293.

19. **Hahn, H. P.** 1997. The type-4 pilus is the major virulence-associated adhesin of *Pseudomonas aeruginosa*—a review. *Gene* **192:**99–108.

20. **Leonetti, M., J. Galon, R. Thai, C. Sautes-Fridman, G. Moine, and A. Menez.** 1999. Presentation of antigen in immune complexes is boosted by soluble bacterial immunoglobulin binding proteins. *J. Exp. Med.* **189:**1217–1228.

21. **Levin, B. R.** 1996. The evolution and maintenance of virulence in microparasites. *Emerg. Infect. Dis.* **2:**93–102.

22. **Levin, B. R., M. Lipsitch, and S. Bonhoeffer.** 1999. Population biology, evolution, and infectious disease: convergence and synthesis. *Science* **283:**806–809.

23. **McQuillen, D. P., S. Gulati, S. Ram, A. K. Turner, D. B. Jani, T. C. Heeren, and P. A. Rice.** 1999. Complement processing and immunoglobulin binding to *Neisseria gonorrhoeae* determined in vitro simulates in vivo effects. *J. Infect. Dis.* **179:**124–135.

24. **Mims, C., N. Dimmock, A. Nash, and J. Stephen.** 1995. *Mims' Pathogenesis of Infectious Disease,* 4th ed. Academic Press Ltd., London, United Kingdom.

25. **Olson, R., H. Nariya, K. Yokota, Y. Kamio, and E. Gouaux.** 1999. Crystal structure of staphylococcal LukF delineates conformational changes accompanying formation of a transmembrane channel. *Nat. Struct. Biol.* **6:**134–140.

26. **Pace, N. R.** 1997. A molecular view of microbial diversity and the biosphere. *Science* **276:**734–740.

27. **Radolf, J. D., T. E. Fehniger, F. J. Silverblatt, J. N. Miller, and M. A. Lovett.** 1986. The surface of virulent *Treponema pallidum:* resistance to antibody binding in the absence of complement and surface association of recombinant antigen 4D. *Infect. Immun.* **52:**579–585.

28. **Rao, V. K., G. P. Krasan, D. R. Hendrixson, S. Dawid, and J. W. St. Geme.** 1999. Molecular determinants of the pathogenesis of disease due to non-typeable *Haemophilus influenzae. FEMS Microbiol. Rev.* **23:**99–129.

29. **Seifert, H. S., C. J. Wright, A. E. Jerse, M. S. Cohen, and J. G. Cannon.** 1994. Multiple gonococcal pilin antigenic variants are produced during experimental human infections. *J. Clin. Investig.* **93:**2744–2749.

30. **Van Delden, C., and B. H. Iglewski.** 1998. Cell-to-cell signaling and *Pseudomonas aeruginosa* infections. *Emerg. Infect. Dis.* **4:**551–560.

31. **Vitovski, S., R. C. Read, and J. R. Sayers.** 1999. Invasive isolates of *Neisseria meningitidis* possess enhanced immunoglobulin A1 protease activity compared to colonizing strains. *FASEB J.* **13:** 331–337.

32. **Welkos, S., A. Friedlander, D. McDowell, J. Weeks, and S. Tobery.** 1998. V antigen of *Yersinia pestis* inhibits neutrophil chemotaxis. *Microb. Pathog.* **24:**185–196.

33. **Wesson, C. A., L. E. Liou, K. M. Todd, G. A. Bohach, W. R. Trumble, and K. W. Bayles.** 1998. *Staphylococcus aureus* Agr and Sar global regulators influence internalization and induction of apoptosis. *Infect. Immun.* **66:**5238–5243.

34. **Wilske, B., A. G. Barbour, S. Bergstrom, N. Burman, B. I. Restrepo, P. A. Rosa, T. Schwan, E. Soutschek, and R. Wallich.** 1992. Antigenic variation and strain heterogeneity in *Borrelia* spp. *Res. Microbiol.* **143:**583–596.

35. **Wirth, H. P., M. Yang, R. M. Peek, Jr., K. T. Tham, and M. J. Blaser.** 1997. *Helicobacter pylori* Lewis expression is related to the host Lewis phenotype. *Gastroenterology* **113:**1091–1098.

THE BIOLOGY OF
PERSISTENT
INFECTION

ANTIGENIC VARIATION AND THE PERSISTENCE OF EXTRACELLULAR BACTERIA IN VERTEBRATE HOSTS

John L. Wylie and Robert C. Brunham

2

Higher-eukaryotic multicellular organisms act as microenvironments for numerous species of prokaryotic and eukaryotic microorganisms. The successful reproduction of a microbial species within such microenvironments entails competition for limited space and nutrients and evasion of host defense mechanisms. Additionally, from a microbial perspective, higher organisms constitute noncontiguous "island" habitats, necessitating between-host transmission strategies to ensure long-term survival of the species. Although faced with common environments and common environmental variables, the microbial species typically found within any given host have evolved numerous types of symbiotic relationships, ranging from mutualistic and commensalistic to parasitic. Parasitic life cycles are highly diverse, encompassing both acute (short-lived) and persistent infections. Additionally, opportunistic pathogens can cross the boundary from one symbiotic relationship to another as they take advantage of changes in the host environment, such as host defense mechanisms.

Despite the evolution of these different life cycles, each member of the microbial flora within a host is selected for a common evolutionary goal: the persistence over time within and between hosts. This evolutionary goal is encapsulated in the concept of the basic reproductive number (R_o) (60). Phenotypic-genotypic changes which act to maximize R_o for a given bacterial species will be selected for. Pathophysiologic sequelae of infectious disease can increase R_o for a pathogen by enhancing transmission to the next host; however, within- and between-host factors must be balanced, as persistence within a host must be sufficiently long to ensure between-host transmission. Genetic changes which enhance the within-host growth rates of a pathogen may be counterproductive if the premature death of the host reduces or eliminates the opportunity for between-host transmission. Although both commensals and pathogens may be driven by common ecological goals, there has been an understandable bias within medical microbiology to focus on pathogens and their virulence factors. A greater understanding of the mechanisms for microbial persistence within a host may aid in understanding the unique pathogenic mechanisms which acute and persistent pathogens have evolved de novo or have modified from mechanisms found in commensal or-

John L. Wylie, Cadham Provincial Laboratory, Manitoba Health, and Department of Medical Microbiology, University of Manitoba, Winnipeg, Manitoba, Canada. *Robert C. Brunham*, University of British Columbia Centre for Disease Control, Vancouver, British Columbia V5Z 4R4, Canada.

Persistent Bacterial Infections, Edited by J. P. Nataro, M. J. Blaser, and S. Cunningham-Rundles, © 2000 ASM Press, Washington, D.C.

ganisms and also the manner in which these changes affect the reproductive number of pathogens versus commensals.

Evolutionary ecology encompasses both "functional" and "evolutionary" approaches to biology. The functional approach to ecological questions addresses underlying mechanisms (e.g., the genetic basis of antigenic variation in bacteria), while the evolutionary approach addresses the significance of the phenomenon in terms of the ecological success of an organism (the selective advantage of developing antigenic-variation mechanisms). Functional studies are more frequently conducted, as hypotheses addressing functionality are often more readily tested. In contrast, evolutionary questions can be hampered by the time scale and the frequently circular nature of "cause and effect" interpretations. Although more difficult to address, evolutionary approaches to pathogenicity are necessary not only to provide a greater understanding of microbial pathogenicity but also to understand how microbes will react and evolve in response to human influences, such as the introduction of antibiotics and vaccines.

The goal of this chapter is to examine persistent bacterial pathogens within the context of evolutionary ecology by addressing the functional and evolutionary aspects of the mechanisms that bacteria have developed to persist in mammalian hosts. The first section will address functionality: the genetic mechanisms bacterial pathogens possess for establishing and maintaining persistence within a host. The remaining sections, necessarily more speculative than the first, will deal with the evolutionary origin and control of these mechanisms with respect to the natural selection of persistent pathogenic life styles. The focus will be on antigenic variation, as this is one of the most widely studied aspects of persistence and also one of the most variable in terms of the extent to which extracellular pathogens have developed genetic mechanisms to enable variation to occur. A recent paper has provided an overview of the significance of antigenic variation in terms of the evolutionary forces driving host-pathogen

coevolution (8). In this chapter we intend to expand on this theme by comparing the interrelatedness of antigenic variation and pathogen life cycles, including both persistent opportunistic pathogens and persistent primary pathogens. Variation within an antigen is now widely accepted as providing a mechanism for evasion of the host immune system and is selected for as such in many species of bacteria, viruses, and parasites (8, 20, 51). Yet in terms of the population biologies of persistent bacterial infections, the relative significance of a point mutation in an outer membrane protein of *Haemophilus* or *Streptococcus* compared to the elaborate gene switching evolved by *Borrelia* spp. should be considered.

This chapter will present information on extracellular bacteria, as an accompanying chapter deals primarily with intracellular pathogens. Extensive development of antigenic variation is uncommon in intracellular pathogens, since they interact with different components of the host immune response. In contrast to the relatively restricted targeting of antibodies to surface and secreted antigens of extracellular pathogens, intracellular pathogens are subjected to cell-mediated immunity in which antigenic variation plays a less prominent role. Antigenic variation may be more prominent among extracellular pathogens because of the bimolecular interaction that occurs between antigenic epitopes and immunoglobulin (Ig) complementarity-determining regions. Antigen recognition by T lymphocytes depends on a trimolecular interaction among antigen-presenting molecules, antigenic peptide, and a T-cell antigen receptor. Because of this, constraints on the evolution of T-cell antigenic peptides are likely more severe than those on the evolution of B-cell antigenic epitopes.

Although the focus of this chapter will be on persistent bacterial infections, some reference will be made to the literature on protozoan and metazoan pathogens where appropriate. Attempts will also be made to examine the population biology of organisms in a commensal state to provide insights into the evolution of pathogens and their distinctive lifestyles. It should be noted that in terms of medical intervention and treatment, persistence of a bacterial infection within an individual patient can largely be considered in isolation. From a microbial perspective, however, considering only within-host persistence provides a restricted view of the ecological success of a species. Persistence within a host is a means to an end, as it provides enhanced opportunities for between-host transmission and ensures long-term survival and persistence of bacteria within the host populations. As this chapter is intended to focus on persistence from a microbial perspective, the discussions will include both within- and between-host factors. Overall, we intend to highlight both the common themes of antigenic variation and the subtle differences which have arisen among species as they adapt to their respective environmental niches.

MECHANISMS GENERATING VARIABLE ANTIGENS IN BACTERIAL POPULATIONS

Bacterial populations are currently viewed as consisting of distinct clonal groups. In the absence of sexual reproduction, prokaryotic organisms have developed alternative mechanisms for the divergence of genetic material. The genetic basis driving these processes can be broadly grouped into intergenomic (DNA translocation between cells) and intragenomic (DNA replication errors and chromosomal rearrangements) mechanisms. Although the divergence of bacterial clonal populations is critical for maintaining the fitness of prokaryotic organisms, the extensive development of intracellular genetic mechanisms for the rapid generation of diversity within clonal populations of extracellular pathogens underscores the importance of a flexible genome for the successful evolution of, and adaptation to, a pathogenic life cycle in vertebrate hosts. The following sections summarize the genetic basis of antigenic variation, focusing on common themes present in diverse groups of pathogens.

Intergenomic Mechanisms of Antigenic Variation

Three distinct mechanisms contribute to the translocation of DNA between bacterial cells:

transduction, conjugation, and transformation (reviewed in references 22, 57, 76). Transduction is a DNA translocation process mediated by bacteriophage introduction of DNA into a bacterial cell. Bacterial conjugation is a plasmid-mediated process involving the direct transfer of DNA from a donor to a recipient cell. Transformation describes the uptake by a bacterial cell of free DNA from the surrounding medium.

Any of the three DNA translocation processes can introduce either novel genetic traits or new alleles of existing genes. Recently, an emerging paradigm for the evolution of pathogenicity in bacteria has focused on the interspecific transfer of pathogenicity islands, which are large transmissible genetic elements encoding novel toxins, adhesins, and/or invasins (36). Although relevant to the emergence of bacterial pathogenicity, the acquisition of novel traits is of less significance to a discussion of immune evasion than is the transfer of homologous DNA fragments. The latter event generates novel immunogenic alleles which contribute to the evasion of an adaptive immune response during the course of an infection or to the evasion of host immune memory in subsequent infections.

A distinction among conjugation, transduction, and transformation is that the first two processes are largely driven by factors external to the cell receiving the DNA while transformation is largely under the control of the recipient cell. As such, elaborate genetic mechanisms have evolved to regulate and control the extent to which a cell is competent for transformation. DNA recognition and uptake are largely species specific, mediated by intraspecific cell-cell signaling via peptide messengers (e.g., in *Streptococcus pneumoniae* and *Bacillus subtilis* [37, 76]) or recognition of specific oligonucleotide sequences on double-stranded extracellular DNA (e.g., in *Haemophilus influenzae* and *Neisseria gonorrhoeae* [31, 57]). This specificity reflects the importance of transformation as a means of intraspecific genetic communication. However, the significance of transformation in relation to the population biology of a

16

given species and the extent to which it drives antigenic variation are not completely understood. In *Escherichia coli*, intercellular DNA exchange has been alternately viewed as the main source of clonal divergence (23, 35) or as insignificant in comparison to intracellular DNA mutation events (74, 75). The ability to take up free DNA is widespread in many bacterial genera, suggesting that DNA exchange may be important for the adaptive evolution of many species of bacteria.

Intragenomic Mechanisms Generating Antigenic Variation

In reviewing the adaptive evolution of pathogenic bacteria, Moxon et al. (63) differentiated intragenomic mutational processes into indiscriminate and discriminate processes. Indiscriminate processes include classical mutational processes resulting from the imperfect nature of DNA replication and are expected to occur at fairly equal rates across all loci. Although these mutational processes are not directed at specific loci, minor mutational events of this type can play a role in immune evasion (88). Discriminate processes are mutational processes occurring at specific loci at unusually high frequency. Moxon et al. (63) coined the term "contingency loci" to describe the genes affected by these discriminate processes.

Phase variation and gene switching are the two primary processes involved in discriminate mutational processes (20, 28). Phase variation alters gene expression through on–off switching of a given gene product or by quantitative changes in the level of gene transcription or translation. At the molecular level, a main determinant of phase variation is the presence of repeating DNA units, primarily in the form of short homopolymeric tracts or oligonucleotide repeats at the 5′ end of an open reading frame. Slipped-strand mispairing alters the translational frame of a gene by changing the number of nucleotides present in the repeat region. The same process acting on oligonucleotide repeats between the −10 and −35 regions quantitatively alters the transcriptional level of a gene (85). Oligonucleotide repeats have been iden-

tified in numerous pathogens, including *Neisseria meningitidis*, *N. gonorrhoeae*, *H. influenzae*, and *Mycobacterium* spp., but were largely absent from commensal (*E. coli*) and free-living (*Methanococcus jannaschii*) organisms (40). Their presence is not universal in extracellular pathogens, however, as tetranucleotide repeats are not present in significant numbers in *Mycoplasma genitalium* (40). On–off phase variation of antigens can also result from DNA inversion events, as seen in flagellar-antigen expression in *Salmonella* (73) and pilin expression in *Moraxella* (59).

In contrast to the on–off characteristics of most phase variation events, the continuous sequential production of antigenic variants of a single protein may result from gene switching. The underlying basis of the process is the presence of multiple duplicate copies of a given gene product. Expression of new variant proteins results from the nonreciprocal recombination of a silent gene into a functional expression site. An exception to this mechanism is the *opa* gene of *N. meningitidis* and *N. gonorrhoeae* (79). Oligonucleotide repeats are present at the 5′ end of each *opa* gene. Slipped-strand mispairing within these repeats independently turns the *opa* gene repertoire of these bacteria on and off.

ECOLOGICAL ASPECTS OF ANTIGENIC VARIATION

The previous section summarized the mechanisms which generate antigenic variation in diverse groups of microorganisms. The underlying similarity of these mechanisms largely reflects the common and finite molecular processes upon which natural selection can act and the common environmental variables that microorganisms encounter within a vertebrate host. Convergent evolution of pathogenicity has been the subject of several recent reviews (20, 28).

Examining the differences among organisms with respect to antigenic variation, however, is equally revealing in terms of the elaborate fine-tuning which can occur in response to (or potentially result in) adaptation of a given pathogen to a specific microhabitat within vertebrate hosts. Antigenic variation has been described as an immune evasion strategy for many pathogens, yet its significance in the life cycle of a given pathogen can vary widely. This section will highlight the genetic differences among pathogens in relation to the different environmental niches they occupy. Several model organisms will be considered in order to highlight the extent to which antigenic-variation mechanisms have been fine-tuned in response to the specific environmental problems faced by these organisms and the insights into their lifestyles that comparative studies can provide.

H. influenzae

H. influenzae is an obligate colonizer and a pathogen of human mucosal surfaces. As a pathogen, H. influenzae is associated with upper and lower respiratory tract infections. Among weakly virulent, nonencapsulated H. influenzae organisms, which spend more of their time colonizing than infecting, outer surface antigens come into direct contact with, and are vulnerable to, components of the humoral immune response. Antigenic drift, consisting primarily of point mutations within externally exposed surfaces of outer membrane proteins, is considered to be a mechanism for evasion of the humoral response in these organisms (29). And to be sure, the emergence of variants in vivo in animal models (88), and in human patients suffering from chronic obstructive pulmonary disease (33), demonstrates the potent selective effects of the immune system on H. influenzae.

Yet although immune selection of antigenic variants in this relatively opportunistic pathogen does occur, in terms of long-term survival within the host, it is not as significant as other persistence mechanisms. Spontaneous outer membrane protein variants emerge in vitro at a rate of 10^{-9} to 10^{-11} (84) compared to rates of antigenic variation of 10^{-3} observed in some extracellular pathogens (8). The lower rate at which mutants are generated reflects the stochastic, indiscriminate nature of the process in these bacteria compared to the discriminate

processes altering contingency loci in more virulent primary pathogens. Strains of H. influenzae can persist in vivo for several months with no apparent change in the genotype or phenotype of the infecting strain (32). This long-term stability reflects the defensive mode of growth adopted by many opportunistic or occasional pathogens within the host environment (43). The secretion of IgA proteases or the sequestration of organisms in sites protected from humoral defense mechanisms would largely negate the need for antigenic variability. Rare escape mutants of H. influenzae, nonreactive with circulating antibodies, can contribute to exacerbations within infected patients (32); however, from a microbial perspective, within-host persistence does not depend entirely on this process. Escape mutants may be of greater significance to the pathogen in facilitating between-host persistence, as antigenic differences in strains appear to be a necessary prerequisite for evading primed humoral defenses in previously colonized patients (46).

N. gonorrhoeae

Like H. influenzae, the only environmental niche for N. gonorrhoeae is within human hosts. In contrast to H. influenzae, however, N. gonorrhoeae acts as a primary pathogen infecting otherwise healthy individuals and is dependent on sexual contact for between-host transmission. Reflecting its route of transmission, N. gonorrhoeae primarily occupies the urogenital tract, although it can adhere to mucosal surfaces in the pharynx, rectum, and conjunctiva.

Antigenic variation has been described for the loci encoding the pilin and opacity proteins of N. gonorrhoeae (30, 80). Multiple copies of the genes encoding these proteins are present throughout the chromosome (61, 80). Pilin protein is expressed from one active pilE expression site, while the silent pilS loci are not transcribed. Gene switching occurs following the transposition of silent pilS into the pilE locus through a nonreciprocal recombination process (gene conversion). Pilin phase variation producing Pil⁻ variants arises following the transposition of pilS loci incapable of producing functional pilin protein. Additional control of pilin production is mediated by the *pilC* gene product (42). The PilC protein, an adhesin located at the pilus tip, is preceded by a homopolymeric (G) tract and is subject to phase variation. Opa variation differs from that of pilin in that transcription of each of the *opa* loci is controlled independently. Tandem CTCTT oligonucleotide repeats at the 5′ end of each *opa* locus allow on-off phase variation to occur through a slipped-strand mispairing process. A given gonococcal cell can be Opa$^+$ or Opa$^-$. Opa$^+$ cells can produce either a single Opa type or multiple Opa variants. Pilin and Opa can appropriately be considered contingency loci, given the emergence of variants at rates of approximately 10^{-3}. The identification of phase variation in *N. gonorrhoeae* lipooligosaccharides (19, 71), and in the ability of *N. gonorrhoeae* to use human hemoglobin as a source of iron (17), suggests that other variable loci also exist.

With respect to the evolution of antigenic variation and its primary function in gonococcal infections, definitive cause and effect arguments are difficult to prove. Opa and pilin variations have been proposed as both a means of evading host defenses (28) and a mechanism to alter the tissue tropism of individual gonococcal cells through the variation in adherence properties of different pilin and Opa variants (20, 49). These mechanisms are closely intertwined, as antigenic variation in extracellular pathogens would ensure continual exposure of essential virulence factors on the cell surface in the presence of a host humoral response.

Examining the pace and qualitative characteristics of antigenic variation can help to decipher the primary roles the process plays in the life history of a given pathogen. Multiple Opa protein variants are expressed simultaneously during the course of an *N. gonorrhoeae* infection (41), in comparison to the sequential appearance of variant cell types in relapsing fever borreliae and eukaryotic trypanosome parasites (see below). Multiple, random expression of epitopes would appear to be disadvantageous to the pathogen, as it would provide the host with the opportunity to simultaneously mount an immune response to many of the Opa and pilin proteins within a gonococcal cell. This strategy may be beneficial, however, for a sexually transmitted pathogen to ensure successful between-host transmission. In contrast to the high densities characterizing human populations today, the evolution of *N. gonorrhoeae* pathogenicity occurred during periods in which humans existed in relatively small, geographically isolated population clusters. Potential opportunities for sexual transmission would have been limited, and many of the potential hosts would have experienced previous gonococcal infections. Since current evidence suggests short-term immunity to a given gonococcal strain exists (67), rapidly producing several pilin and Opa proteins may increase the likelihood that at least one of the variants will be able to successfully establish an infection. Production of one main variant type, as occurs in trypanosomes, may be counterproductive in situations where the numbers of potential hosts are small and immunologic memory is common.

Although between-host transmission may be a critical factor in the evolution of antigenic variation in *N. gonorrhoeae*, the protein species that undergo variation may not be equally important in this respect. Pili contribute to the initial attachment of gonococcal cells to host cells, and rapid variation of these proteins may be critical for host-to-host transmission. In contrast, an increase in the number of antibodies that recognize Opa variants does not correlate with an increased protection against infection (66). An inverse correlation is present, however, between antibodies to an increasing number of Opa proteins and the risk of salpingitis, suggesting that Opa variation may play a greater role in within-host persistence and dissemination of disease into the upper genital tract. Upper genital tract infection can cause infertility, and this virulence effect of gonococci may contribute to its ecological success by slowing population growth rates. Slowing the growth rate of its host population ensures that the rate of transmission between hosts is not greatly exceeded by the rate at which the host population grows (5). These observations reflect the underlying importance of the small populations within which *N. gonorrhoeae* has evolved and the increased likelihood that hosts within a small population will present with antibodies from a previous infection.

Borrelia spp.

All *Borrelia* spp. are arthropod borne and rely on these vectors as intermediates for between-host transmission to their respective vertebrate hosts. Individual *Borrelia* spp. differ in the arthropod species they parasitize and in their primary host reservoirs (rodent species are the most common mammalian hosts). Many *Borrelia* spp. produce a relapsing fever, characterized by recurring waves of spirochetemia, similar to the relapsing nature of trypanosome infection.

A well-characterized antigenic variation mechanism is present in relapsing fever *Borrelia* (21). *Borrelia hermsii* contains up to 40 complete copies of *vmp*, the product of which is a surface-exposed lipoprotein (the products of this gene family have recently been split into various small and large proteins, but for simplicity it will be referred to here as *vmp*). Expression originates from specific *vmp* expression loci located near the telomere of a linear plasmid. Silent copies are translocated to the expression site following a nonreciprocal recombination process. The location of the expression site near a telomere may facilitate gene recombination (45) and/or gene expression (2). The presence of silent copies of *vmp* is analogous to the mechanism of *vsg* variation in trypanosomes, although in the latter genera as many as 1,000 copies of *vsg* alleles are maintained within a cell (86).

At the molecular level, *Borrelia burgdorferi*, the agent of Lyme disease, appears to have a reduced capacity for antigenic variation in comparison to *B. hermsii* or *Borrelia recurrentis*. One expression gene (*vlp*), homologous to *vmp-33* of *B. hermsii*, exists near the telomere of a linear plasmid (91). Arranged head to tail with respect to this expression site are 15 tan-

dem repeats corresponding to a small hypervariable region of *vlp*. Oligonucleotide repeats at both the 5′ and 3′ ends of each hypervariable gene fragment match nucleotide sequences within the *vlp* gene and act as initiation sites for reciprocal recombination. Although *vlp* appears somewhat limited in potential variants, expression of a new *vlp* variant in *B. burgdorferi* results from multiple recombination events, and therefore, the antigenic-variation capacity of *B. burgdorferi* is almost unlimited (90, 91).

B. burgdorferi differs significantly from relapsing fever *Borrelia* in the characteristics of its spirochetemia within the vertebrate host. Relapsing fever is characterized by the sudden onset of febrile disease concurrent with maximum levels of spirochetes within the blood. Current evidence suggests that a humoral immune response reduces the first spirochete cycle, followed by multiple relapses separated by days to weeks (2, 81). The spirochete population at the height of any single cycle is dominated by one or a few clonal populations, each expressing a specific *vmp* gene (81). Each subsequent wave occurs as the previous clonal population is cleared by the immune system. *B. burgdorferi* infection of a vertebrate host differs in that clear waves of spirochetemia do not occur, numerous *vlp* variants are simultaneously isolated from the same host (90, 91), the onset of peak spirochetemia is slow compared to the rapid onset of the relapsing fever spirochetemia (11), and the humoral immune response is correspondingly slower than that observed for *B. hermsii* and *B. recurrentis* (11).

The characteristics of antigenic variation and the distinct within-host population dynamics of these two groups of spirochetes correlate with the different life cycles and behaviors of their respective arthropod vectors. *Ornithodoros* ticks (relapsing fever vectors) do not disperse widely, instead spending their entire lives in microhabitats closely associated with the nests of their mammalian (rodent) hosts (72). The ticks feed quickly, often remaining on the host for only 30 to 45 min. High spirochete levels in the blood may facilitate transmission of relapsing fever *Borrelia* during the short time during which *Ornithodoros* ticks feed. The relatively rapid onset of spirochetemia correlates with the constant association between tick and host and, therefore, the relative ease with which ticks find their next host. The cyclical waves of spirochetemia would be advantageous to the pathogen, since constant debilitating febrile illness may reduce normal host activities and negatively affect the ecological success of *Borrelia*. In contrast, *Ixodes* ticks feed on different mammalian species at different stages in their life cycle (72). While the larvae and nymphs feed primarily on rodents, adults feed on several species of large mammals (deer, racoons, carnivores, and large domestic mammals). *Ixodes* ticks feed for long periods and become widely dispersed in association with their hosts' movements. The relatively low spirochete levels attained by *B. burgdorferi* may be sufficient for transmission, as the long feeding periods of *Ixodes* provide extended opportunities for tick infection. The noncycling nature of spirochetemia in Lyme disease would provide a constant state of readiness for the rarer occasions when an infected vertebrate host encounters an *Ixodes* tick.

Although the contribution of antigenic variation to spirochete cycling in relapsing fever seems intuitively clear, the mechanisms driving the systematic appearance of only a few clonal types is not well understood. Gene switching of *vmp* in *B. hermsii* has been estimated at a rate of 10^{-3} (81). With spirochete levels greater than 10^7 per ml of serum (3, 64), it is not clear how these pathogens prevent the majority of their variant repertoire from being expressed in the first spirochete cycle and why only a few clonal populations dominate throughout the host in any given cycle.

Cyclical parasitemia also occurs in trypanosome infections, and considerably greater research effort has been directed at addressing this phenomenon in the parasitological literature. Initial estimates of gene switching in trypanosomes were on the order of 10^{-6} to 10^{-9} (approaching the mutational rates of indiscriminate processes seen in most cell types); however, even these rates were seen as too high to allow for the expansion of single clones (87).

This problem was compounded by updated estimates of 10^{-3} (87), indicating discriminate genetic processes equal to those seen in bacterial pathogens. Explanations offered for the emergence of single clones have included differential growth rates of different VSG variants (50), protein-protein interactions in the cell membrane preventing or favoring specific switch events (following gene switching, two protein species would temporarily be present in the cell membrane) (6, 87), and different protein functions favoring the appearance of specific protein variants at specific points in the infectious process (87).

Mathematical modeling of trypanosome within-host population dynamics suggests that protein-protein interactions within the cell membrane may be the critical factor in both the ordered appearance of variants and the cyclical nature of parasitemia (1). The key determinant in these models was the transient presence of double expressor cells expressing two variants of the VSG protein immediately after the gene switch event. Differential susceptibility of these cells to both humoral and innate host defenses was sufficient to produce cyclical clonal populations. Comparable attempts to model *Borrelia* dynamics must also incorporate the cyclical nature of *Borrelia* relapsing fever versus noncyclical *B. burgdorferi* infections.

ANTIGENIC VARIATION AND THE EVOLUTION OF HOST-PARASITE INTERACTIONS

The previous section focused on the differences among antigenic-variation mechanisms and their correlation with the population biologies and the ecological success of pathogens within their niches. Therefore, we mainly addressed the extent to which superficially similar antigenic-variation mechanisms have diverged but we did not address the de novo evolution of these mechanisms. The evolution of well-developed antigenic-variation mechanisms could be a prerequisite for enabling potential pathogens to engage in naive explorations of novel microhabitats in the host, or they may only arise in response to the considerable repertoire of host defenses potential pathogens encounter after crossing the physical anatomical barriers of the host. Resolving alternate hypotheses of this type is problematic given the difficulty in discerning the course of past evolutionary events. Some insight can be gained by examining and comparing the population biologies of commensal organisms or pathogens occupying a commensal niche (see chapter 8). This approach is limited, however, by the relative scarcity of information available on commensal bacterial species. Thus, this section raises more questions than answers and serves primarily to highlight areas where additional research effort could be directed to provide a more complete understanding of the evolution of pathogenicity.

The current paradigm describing the evolution of pathogens is one in which virulence develops abruptly, frequently following the introduction of foreign DNA into bacterial cells, and results in evolution through quantal discontinuities as a form of punctuated equilibrium. This paradigm should be differentiated from the more classical Darwinian evolution of phyletic gradualism, which reflects single-gene evolution within the context of a stable genome (epistatic restraint). Pathogenicity islands, consisting of large blocks of DNA encoding multiple, and frequently related, gene products, have been identified in some bacterial populations (28, 36). The incorporation of these DNA blocks can create or expand the pathogenic potential of a cell by providing novel adhesins, invasins, or toxins. Bacteria could acquire the ability to vary a surface antigen via this process by incorporating blocks of DNA containing multiple copies of a gene encoding a novel protein; however, within the genus *Neisseria*, comparisons of commensal species with *N. meningitidis* and *N. gonorrhoeae* suggest that gene duplication was an intraspecific event. Commensal *Neisseria* spp. contain single copies of *pil* and *opa*, in contrast to the multiple copies found in pathogenic *Neisseria* spp. (89). The scattered occurrence of these loci around the chromosomes of these bacteria (61, 80) also implies intracellular events leading to the duplication of genes present in ancestral commensal species rather than the extracellular acquisition of multiple loci on a single DNA fragment.

Although the presence of contingency loci in *N. meningitidis* and *N. gonorrhoeae* and their apparent absence in commensals correlate with pathogenicity, it is worth noting that *N. meningitidis* occurs as an asymptomatic commensal in 5 to 15% of the population. Given the genetic investment necessary to carry multiple gene copies and the relatively rare occasions on which the organism becomes pathogenic, questions remain as to whether this bacterium relies on gene switching for invasive infection alone or whether antigenic variation of surface epitopes is advantageous for its existence in a commensal state. If the latter were true, this would suggest that some bacterial species are preadapted to pathogenicity by possessing some of the requisite genetic mechanisms for survival as a commensal despite the presence of adaptive immune responses in the host. Antigenic variation within commensal species may be advantageous for evading the host secretory IgA response or may assist in interspecific interactions. Although research efforts are directed towards *N. meningitidis* due to its pathogenic potential, from a microbial perspective, some of the commensal *Neisseria* spp. could be considered competitively and ecologically superior to *N. meningitidis* within the microenvironment of the oropharynx. Commensal *Neisseria* spp. are more common than *N. meningitidis* in healthy individuals (48). The relative infrequency of *N. meningitidis* does not reflect medical treatment, since the asymptomatic presence of *N. meningitidis* is not normally screened for or treated. Although it is not known whether interspecific *Neisseria* competition occurs within the oropharynx, variable surface antigens in *N. meningitidis* may have evolved as a countermeasure in response to the apparent ecological success of the nonpathogenic *Neisseria* spp. The common occurrence of commensal *Neisseria* spp., coupled with the observed fact that their presence induces antibodies which cross-react with *N. meningitidis*

(12), may have selected for the evolution of variable surface antigens in the latter species. In turn, the potential to alter its surface properties may have provided *N. meningitidis* with the ability to explore other habitats, including the successful occupation of the urogenital tract and its subsequent speciation as *N. gonorrhoeae*.

These observations are speculative and are intended primarily to highlight the potential shortcomings of focusing on bacterial pathogens in isolation. In comparison to the relatively small number of bacterial pathogens, the evolution of bacterial commensal associations with vertebrate hosts is common. Over 700 species of commensal bacteria have been identified in the upper respiratory and digestive tracts of humans (9, 25, 27). This observation is significant in a discussion of bacterial pathogenicity for two reasons. First, although antigenic variation of pathogenic organisms is almost universally accepted as a means of immune evasion, and therefore as a means of extending the within-host persistence time of these pathogens, many commensal organisms appear to persist for the lifetime of the host in the presence of a secretory IgA response (39). Antigenic variation could have arisen as one of the mechanisms bacteria use to develop commensal relationships with the host. Second, as alluded to above, the large number of successful commensal organisms potentially places some pathogenic species at a competitive disadvantage. Many viral and bacterial pathogens have only emerged in humans following the widespread domestication of animals within the last 10,000 years. Many emerging pathogens would encounter analogous commensal organisms in new hosts, and the evolution of virulence traits may have emerged as much in response to competition from their bacterial counterparts as to the defense mechanisms of the host itself. Li et al. (52) suggest that the emergence of *Salmonella* as a pathogen in mammals following its jump from a reptile reservoir may partially be in response to *E. coli* occupying the commensal enteric niche within mammals. The earlier occupation of this habitat by *E. coli* was favored by the ability of that bacterium to obtain energy by the fermentation of lactose in mammalian milk, a biochemical pathway missing in *Salmonella*.

Examination of the means by which commensal organisms persist in the host may contribute to an understanding of the relationship between antigenic variation, commensalism, and pathogenicity. Limited experimental evidence is available on the population biologies of commensal organisms; however, the available evidence suggests that they persist by different mechanisms. Longitudinal studies of *Streptococcus mutans* and *Actinomyces* spp. in the oral cavity indicate long-term survival of individual clones of these species (4, 14). Long-term clonal persistence could correlate with the hypo- or nonresponsiveness of the human mucosal antibody response to some commensal organisms, as has been observed for *Streptococcus sanguis* and *Streptococcus oralis* (44). In contrast, *E. coli* undergoes continual clonal replacement over time (16). This is also true for *H. influenzae* (77, 83), *Staphylococcus aureus* (47), and *N. meningitidis* (15) when they are present as commensal organisms in healthy individuals. Bos et al. (7) have suggested that within the gut, commensals and pathogens may encounter different selective pressures from the host's mucosal immune response. Species which elicit a strong IgA response from the host may benefit from the evolution of antigenic-variation mechanisms.

Analysis of *H. influenzae* isolates from healthy children indicates that a key difference between sequential clonal types is the immunogenicity of the IgA1 protease produced by each successive clonal population (56). *H. influenzae* IgA1 protease elicits an IgA response in humans. Newly colonizing *H. influenzae* produces an IgA1 protease which does not cross-react with the IgA1 raised against the previous clonal group. Therefore, antigenic variation in IgA1 protease, driven by a mucosal immune response, may be an important determinant of successful colonization of a commensal niche in healthy children. Detailed analysis of other organisms has not been conducted; however, Gupta et al. (34) have gathered empirical evidence that antigenic polymorphism within the *porA* gene of *N. meningitidis* is nonrandom and is driven by immune selection. These observations suggest that polymorphic epitopes are necessary for the successful long-term persistence of some bacterial species that occupy commensal niches in vertebrate hosts. In many cases, long-term persistence of organisms in a commensal state is correctly seen as continuous clonal exchange (i.e., cycles of infection and reinfection) in response to bacterium-host interactions.

The factors governing successful clonal establishment in a host will likely prove more complex than the above observations imply. Successful establishment of a clonal population producing a given IgA1 protease is a multifactorial process including not only the cross-reactive potential of IgA1 antibodies produced by previous clones of the same species but also the cross-reactive potential of antibodies raised by other species, the presence of glycosidases which increase or decrease the susceptibility of IgA1 to protease action, the persistence of a given IgA immune response, and the possibility that the presence of other strong IgA1 protease-producing species could allow IgA1 protease nonproducers to increase in numbers and consequently increase interspecific competition (18, 44, 53, 54, 68). Additionally, some clonal replacement may be based strictly on bacterial interactions. Intraspecific competition within *E. coli* may result from bacteriocin-mediated interclonal competition (70, 82). Therefore, the antigenic polymorphism seen across bacterial populations contributes to the ecological success of bacteria but should be viewed within a broader perspective that includes both the host response to a given bacterium and interspecific bacterial interactions.

Although polymorphic loci are frequently necessary for bacteria to persist in a population, intracellular gene-switching mechanisms for these loci have not been described. In contrast to the *opa* and *pil* loci of *N. meningitidis*, the IgA1 protease gene of *H. influenzae* and *N. meningitidis* and the *por* gene of *N. meningitidis* exist as single copies. In many cases, therefore,

the antigenic polymorphism required for successful bacterial transfer between hosts is only observed as antigenic differences at the clonal level. Examination of the IgA1 protease gene of *H. influenzae* clones indicates that the antigenic differences of IgA1 protease result from intergenomic transfer of DNA between cells and recombination between homologous gene fragments (55). Therefore, genetic communication between clonal populations is critical for generating clonal divergence and, in turn, ensuring the ecological success of the species. The intercellular exchange of DNA has been identified in numerous bacterial species and represents a common mechanism adopted by bacteria to ensure the long-term presence of a species through sequential clonal replacement.

Although the above observations suggest that genetic transformation is important for successive establishment of clonal populations, it does not address the evolution of contingency loci enabling single cells to vary their surface antigens. Evidence exists to suggest that between-host factors provide a selective force for the evolution of rapid intracellular switching mechanisms. Madoff et al. (58) identified size variability in the alpha C protein of group B streptococci mediated by deletion of intragenic repeat units within the *bca* gene encoding alpha C. Deletion of the repeating units shortened the protein, making it less susceptible to maternal antibodies and contributing to successful vertical transmission from mother to neonate. Stäger et al. (78) also demonstrated that antigenic variation of the variant surface proteins of *Giardia lamblia* is driven by maternal IgA antibodies and determines the early course of parasite infection. Therefore, the vertical transfer of organisms concurrently with reactive antibodies selects for intracellular genetic variation. Similarly, as outlined above for *N. gonorrhoeae*, small population sizes coupled with a dependence on low-frequency horizontal transmission between hosts (i.e., sexual transmission) also provide conditions favoring intracellular antigenic-variation capabilities.

The direction of transmission that a pathogenic microbe exploits (vertical or horizontal) and the ease with which transmission occurs between hosts have been identified as key epidemiological factors in the evolution of virulence mechanisms. The traditional view that pathogens evolve towards lesser virulence has been challenged by the concept that virulence is a dynamic process moving along a gradient in response to changes in the transmission opportunities within host populations. At one extreme, pathogens that are absolutely dependent on vertical transmission (i.e., mother to offspring) often produce little host damage, are markedly attenuated in virulence, and persist for extended periods of time in the host. Microbes which exploit horizontal transmission set virulence at a level which maximizes transmission. Virulence is maximized when horizontal transmission is largely independent of the infected host's health and mobility. These conditions occur when transmission is dependent on intermediate vectors, including environmental, arthropod, or human vectors (e.g., waterborne diarrheal pathogens, arthropod-borne *Trypanosoma*, and hospital attendant-borne nosocomial pathogens [26]).

Within a given host, descendants of a pathogen are usually clonally related if superinfection has not occurred. When opportunities exist for the same host to be concurrently infected with different strains of a given pathogen, competition among the strains for growth in the host occurs. This competition can lead to selection for higher growth rates and greater virulence. Thus, under circumstances of frequent infection, with individual hosts exposed to multiple strains of a pathogen, virulence characteristics in the pathogen are strongly selected for (65). This feature explains why the severity of illness often accelerates as an epidemic spreads in a population.

As the opportunities for, or direction of, transmission change within a host population, the response of a parasite population can be inter- or intraspecific. Interspecific responses are manifested in the form of species displacement as external factors differentially affect the ecological success of the microbial species within an ecosystem. Ewald (26) cites several examples, including the introduction of uncontaminated water supplies correlating with the displacement of virulent pathogens (*Shigella dysenteriae* or classic *Vibrio cholerae*) by closely related, less virulent species (*Shigella sonnei* and El Tor *V. cholerae*) and the differential evolution of human immunodeficiency virus types in populations characterized by different sexual mixing patterns. Intraspecific responses encompass evolutionary change within a species. Experimental evidence for a wide range of viral, bacterial, protozoan, and metazoan parasites indicates that conditions which favor horizontal over vertical transmission or which increase the rate of horizontal transmission drive pathogen evolution towards increased virulence. This has been directly observed in experimental systems or inferred from empirical observations of past evolutionary events (10, 24, 38, 69).

Evolution, like transmission, occurs in either a vertical or horizontal direction. Horizontal evolution describes the intercellular transfer of genetic material (e.g., pathogenicity islands and plasmids) between two unrelated cells. Discontinuous evolution of this type can be depicted as occurring between the terminal branches of evolutionary trees. Vertical evolution refers to classic Darwinian evolution based on mutational events within a cell resulting from intracellular DNA metabolic processes. This form of evolution may be inherently more stable than horizontal evolution, as host and pathogen coevolve and gradually accumulate changes in their genomes which continually link the pathogen to its host.

Although Darwinian evolution is traditionally viewed as a gradual process involving the random accumulation of favorable mutations, recent evidence suggests that vertical evolution in some organisms may occur in a discontinuous manner. Experimental and theoretical studies suggest that mutator alleles (i.e., mutations in genes involved in DNA metabolism, which in turn can accelerate the overall rate at which mutations occur in the rest of the genome) result in temporal fluctuations in the rate at which fit individuals appear in a population. Moxon and Thaler (62) describe a process in which mutator alleles predispose other genes to beneficial or deleterious mutations. Mutator alleles remain associated with beneficial mutations by hitchhiking within the genomes of successful cells. In turn, the presence of the mutator allele can contribute to the rapid appearance of other beneficial mutations. Central to this concept is the requirement that the mutator allele be capable of reversion to a nonmutator. Otherwise, detrimental mutations within the genome would be inevitable, leading to extinction of the cell line and loss of the beneficial mutations.

Ultimately, the evolution and the ecological success of pathogens may be optimized if cells direct mutations towards specific parts of the genome. Moxon and Thaler (62) argue that combining contingency loci with physiological modulation of the mutation rate in a cell could provide a pathogen with a form of "directed mutation." In conjunction with the genetic processes discussed above (allelic duplication of genes and DNA repeats promoting slipped-strand mispairing), heightened DNA metabolic processes in the vicinity of virulence genes (e.g., gyrase binding sites and site-specific recombination sites) would contribute to the rapid generation of novel virulence alleles.

With respect to the evolution of antigenic variation, the above discussion serves to stimulate the formation of questions regarding pathogen evolution. Population genetic studies of several human pathogens (e.g., *S. aureus*, *H. influenzae*, and *N. meningitidis*) demonstrate continual clonal replacement of these organisms, suggesting that each exploits horizontal transmission. Conversely, some microbes persist for long periods in their human hosts and appear to exploit vertical transmission (14). Conceivably, a switch from vertical to horizontal transmission may either favor or be favored by the acquisition of genetic flexibility, allowing cells to rapidly adapt following their continued exposure to genetically diverse host environments. In turn, exploiting horizontal transmission may preadapt microbes for pathogenicity by providing them with genetic mech-

anisms necessary for engaging in invasive exploration of novel host environments. Antigenic variation is most frequently cited as a means of persisting within a host in the presence of a humoral immune response; however, evolutionary snapshots of the current function of a virulence trait do not necessarily provide information on the selective forces driving the initial emergence of that trait or the mechanism by which it arose. An understanding of the forces driving the evolution of intracellular antigenic variation would be assisted by analysis of knockout mutations within the contingency loci of pathogenic organisms and their effect on all stages of the infectious cycle, including between-host transfer, colonization, and existence as a commensal.

CONCLUSIONS

Antigenic variation is almost universally accepted as providing a means for pathogens to persist within a vertebrate host by evading host immune responses. The goal of this paper has been to broaden this perspective by considering the coevolution of antigenic-variation mechanisms and distinct pathogen life cycles and the role of polymorphic antigens in the population biologies of organisms in both commensal and pathogenic states. Antigenic-variation mechanisms have been identified in some free-living protozoa (13), and the humoral immune system that invasive pathogens encounter may be only one of the selective forces driving the evolution of variable surface antigens. Additional efforts directed at understanding commensal persistence in vertebrate hosts may expand our understanding of the evolution of antigenic variation. The emergence of intracellular antigenic variation may be a multifactorial process, governed by the population biology of the organism, the response of the vertebrate host, and the specific bacterial interactions encountered within the host environment.

Understanding the evolution of bacteria within human hosts is critical for maintaining our ability to control infectious disease. In contrast to other diseases, infectious diseases are unique in being moving targets, able to adapt and change in response to human control efforts. Human evolution has created three distinct phases of bacterial evolution. Prior to the domestication of plants and animals, humans existed in small isolated populations, effectively preventing the emergence of numerous communicable human pathogens that are density dependent. The domestication of animals coupled with the aggregation of human communities provided opportunities for several viral and bacterial species to move into human hosts and provided enhanced opportunities for horizontal transmission between human hosts. The third, and most recent, phase began within the last 100 years as effective treatments for infectious diseases were developed and widely implemented. Presently, the classification of any microorganism as a pathogen immediately places it under new selection pressures as it becomes the subject of human efforts at control and eradication. These efforts could drive pathogen evolution in multiple directions by contributing either to the emergence of asymptomatic infections or of heightened virulence to ensure rapid between-host transmission. Analysis of the mechanisms and population biologies of bacterial persistence within and between hosts is only one area in which a greater understanding of microbial evolution will facilitate proactive approaches for the control of infectious disease.

REFERENCES

1. **Agur, Z., D. Abiri, and L. H. T. Van der Ploeg.** 1989. Ordered appearance of antigenic variants of African trypanosomes explained in a mathematical model based on a stochastic switch process and immune-selection against putative switch intermediates. *Proc. Natl. Acad. Sci. USA* **86:**9626–9630.
2. **Barbour, A. G.** 1990. Antigenic variation of a relapsing fever *Borrelia* species. *Annu. Rev. Microbiol.* **44:**155–171.
3. **Barbour, A. G., and S. F. Hayes.** 1986. Biology of *Borrelia* species. *Microbiol. Rev.* **50:**381–400.
4. **Barsotti, O., J. J. Morrier, D. Decoret, G. Benay, and J. P. Rocca.** 1993. An investigation into the use of restriction endonuclease analysis for the study of transmission of *Actinomyces. J. Clin. Periodontol.* **20:**436–442.
5. **Boily, M., and R. C. Brunham.** 1993. The impact of HIV and other STDs on human populations. *Infect. Dis. Clin. N. Am.* **7:**771–792.
6. **Borst, P.** 1991. Molecular genetics of antigenic variation. *Immunol. Today* **12:**A29–A33.
7. **Bos, N. A., J. C. A. M. Bun, S. H. Popma, E. R. Cebra, G. J. Deenen, M. J. F. van der Cammen, F. G. M. Kroese, and J. J. Cebra.** 1996. Monoclonal immunoglobulin A derived from peritoneal B cells is encoded by both germ line and somatically mutated V$_H$ genes and is reactive with commensal bacteria. *Infect. Immun.* **64:**616–623.
8. **Brunham, R. C., F. A. Plummer, and R. S. Stephens.** 1993. Bacterial antigenic variation, host immune response, and pathogen-host coevolution. *Infect. Immun.* **61:**2273–2276.
9. **Bry, L., P. G. Falk, T. Midtvedt, and J. I. Gordon.** 1996. A model of host-microbial interactions in an open mammalian ecosystem. *Science* **273:**1380–1383.
10. **Bull, J. J., I. J. Molineux, and W. R. Rice.** 1991. Selection of benevolence in a host-parasite system. *Evolution* **45:**875–882.
11. **Cadavid, D., and A. G. Barbour.** 1998. Neuroborreliosis during relapsing fever: review of the clinical manifestations, pathology, and treatment of infections in humans and experimental animals. *Clin. Infect. Dis.* **26:**151–164.
12. **Cann, K. J., and T. R. Rogers.** 1989. Detection of antibodies to common antigens of pathogenic and commensal Neisseria species. *J. Med. Microbiol.* **30:**23–30.
13. **Caron, F., and E. Meyer.** 1989. Molecular basis of surface antigen variation in *Paramecia. Annu. Rev. Microbiol.* **43:**23–42.
14. **Caufield, P. W., and T. M. Walker.** 1989. Genetic diversity within *Streptococcus mutans* evident from chromosomal DNA restriction fragment polymorphism. *J. Clin. Microbiol.* **27:**274–278.
15. **Caugant, D. A., B. Kristiansen, L. O. Froholm, K. Bovre, and R. K. Selander.** 1988. Clonal diversity of *Neisseria meningitidis* from a population of asymptomatic carriers. *Infect. Immun.* **56:**2060–2068.
16. **Caugant, D. A., B. R. Levin, and R. K. Selander.** 1981. Genetic diversity and temporal variation in the *Escherichia coli* population of a human host. *Genetics* **98:**377–384.
17. **Chen, C., C. Elkins, and P. F. Sparling.** 1998. Phase variation of hemoglobin utilization in *Neisseria gonorrhoeae. Infect. Immun.* **66:**987–993.
18. **Cole, M. F., M. Evans, S. Fitzsimmons, J. Johnson, C. Pearce, M. J. Sheridan, R. Wientzen, and G. Bowden.** 1994. Pioneer oral streptococci produce immunoglobulin A1 protease. *Infect. Immun.* **62:**2165–2168.

19. **Danaher, R. J., J. C. Levin, D. Arking, C. L. Burch, R. Sandlin, and D. C. Stein.** 1995. Genetic basis of *Neisseria gonorrhoeae* lipooligosaccharide antigenic variation. *J. Bacteriol.* **177:** 7275–7279.

20. **Deitsch, K. W., E. R. Moxon, and T. E. Wellems.** 1997. Shared themes of antigenic variation and virulence in bacterial, protozoal, and fungal infections. *Microbiol. Mol. Biol. Rev.* **61:**281–293.

21. **Donelson, J. E.** 1995. Mechanisms of antigenic variation in *Borrelia hermsii* and African trypanosomes. *J. Biol. Chem.* **270:**7783–7786.

22. **Dreiseikelmann, B.** 1994. Translocation of DNA across bacterial membranes. *Microbiol. Rev.* **58:**293–316.

23. **Dykhuizen, D. E., and L. Green.** 1991. Recombination in *Escherichia coli* and the definition of biological species. *J. Bacteriol.* **173:**7257–7268.

24. **Ebert, D.** 1998. Experimental evolution of parasites. *Science* **282:**1432–1435.

25. **Evaldson, G., A. Heimdahl, L. Kager, and C. E. Nord.** 1982. The normal human anaerobic microflora. *Scand. J. Infect. Dis. Suppl.* **35:**9–15.

26. **Ewald, P. W.** 1993. The evolution of virulence. *Sci. Am.* **268**(4):86–93.

27. **Falkow, S.** 1998. The microbe's view of infection. *Ann. Intern. Med.* **129:**247–248.

28. **Finlay, B. B., and S. Falkow.** 1997. Common themes in microbial pathogenicity revisited. *Microbiol. Mol. Biol. Rev.* **61:**136–169.

29. **Foxwell, A. R., J. M. Kyd, and A. W. Cripps.** 1998. Nontypable *Haemophilus influenzae*: pathogenesis and prevention. *Microbiol. Mol. Biol. Rev.* **62:**294–308.

30. **Gibbs, C. P., B. Y. Reimann, E. Schultz, A. Kaufmann, R. Haas, and T. F. Meyer.** 1989. Reassortment of pilin genes in *Neisseria gonorrhoeae* occurs by two distinct mechanisms. *Nature* **338:** 651–652.

31. **Goodman, S. D., and J. J. Scocca.** 1988. Identification and arrangement of the DNA sequence recognized in specific transformation of *Neisseria gonorrhoeae*. *Proc. Natl. Acad. Sci. USA* **85:** 6982–6986.

32. **Groeneveld, K., L. van Alphen, P. P. Eijk, G. Visschen, H. M. Jansen, and H. C. Zanen.** 1990. Endogenous and exogenous reinfection by *Haemophilus influenzae* in patients with chronic obstructive pulmonary disease: the effect of antibiotic treatment on persistence. *J. Infect. Dis.* **161:** 512–517.

33. **Groeneveld, K., L. van Alphen, C. Voorter, P. P. Eijk, H. M. Jansen, and H. C. Zanen.** 1989. Antigenic drift of *Haemophilus influenzae* in patients with chronic obstructive pulmonary disease. *Infect. Immun.* **57:**3038–3044.

34. **Gupta, S., M. C. J. Maiden, I. M. Feavers, S.** Nee, R. M. May, and R. M. Anderson. 1996. The maintenance of strain structure in populations of recombining infectious agents. *Nat. Med.* **2:** 437–442.

35. **Guttman, D. S., and D. E. Dykhuizen.** 1994. Clonal divergence in *Escherichia coli* as a result of recombination, not mutation. *Science* **266:** 1380–1383.

36. **Hacker, J., G. Blum-Oehler, I. Muhldorfer, and H. Tschape.** 1997. Pathogenicity islands of virulent bacteria: structure, function, and impact on microbial evolution. *Mol. Microbiol.* **23:** 1089–1097.

37. **Håvarstein, L. S., R. Hakenbeck, and P. Gaustad.** 1997. Natural competence in the genus *Streptococcus*: evidence that streptococci can change pherotype by interspecies recombinational exchanges. *J. Bacteriol.* **179:**6589–6594.

38. **Herre, E. A.** 1993. Population structure and the evolution of virulence in nematode parasites of fig wasps. *Science* **259:**1442–1445.

39. **Hohwy, J., and M. Kilian.** 1995. Clonal diversity of the *Streptococcus mitis* biovar 1 population in the human oral cavity and pharynx. *Oral Microbiol. Immunol.* **10:**19–25.

40. **Hood, D. W., M. E. Deadman, M. P. Jennings, M. Bisercic, R. D. Fleischmann, J. C. Venter, and E. R. Moxon.** 1996. DNA repeats identify novel virulence genes in *Haemophilus influenzae*. *Proc. Natl. Acad. Sci. USA* **93:**11121–11125.

41. **Jerse, A. E., M. S. Cohen, P. M. Drown, L. G. Whicker, S. F. Isbey, H. S. Seifert, and J. G. Cannon.** 1994. Multiple gonococcal opacity proteins are expressed during experimental urethral infection in the male. *J. Exp. Med.* **179:** 911–920.

42. **Jonsson, A. B., G. Nyberg, and S. Normark.** 1991. Phase variation of gonococcal pili by frameshift mutation in *pilC*, a novel gene for pilus assembly. *EMBO J.* **10:**477–488.

43. **Kharazmi, A.** 1991. Mechanisms involved in the evasion of the host defense by *Pseudomonas aeruginosa*. *Immunol. Lett.* **30:**201–206.

44. **Kilian, M., J. Reinholdt, H. Lomholt, K. Poulsen, and E. V. G. Frandsen.** 1996. Biological significance of IgA1 proteases in bacterial colonization and pathogenesis: critical evaluation of experimental evidence. *APMIS* **104:**321–338.

45. **Kitten, T., A. V. Barrera, and A. G. Barbour.** 1993. Intragenic recombination and a chimeric outer membrane protein in the relapsing fever agent *Borrelia hermsii*. *J. Bacteriol.* **175:**2516–2522.

46. **Klein, J.** 1994. Otitis media. *Clin. Infect. Dis.* **19:** 823–833.

47. **Kluytmans, J., A. van Belkum, and H. Verbrugh.** 1997. Nasal carriage of *Staphylococcus au-*

reus: epidemiology, underlying mechanisms, and associated risks. *Clin. Microbiol. Rev.* **10**:505–520.

48. **Knapp, J. S., and E. W. Hook III.** 1988. Prevalence and persistence of *Neisseria cinerea* and other *Neisseria* spp. in adults. *J. Clin. Microbiol.* **26**: 896–900.

49. **Knepper, B., I. Heuer, T. F. Meyer, and J. P. M. Putten.** 1997. Differential response of human monocytes to *Neisseria gonorrhoeae* variants expressing pili and opacity proteins. *Infect. Immun.* **65**: 4122–4129.

50. **Kosinki, R. J.** 1980. Antigenic variation in trypanosomes: a computer analysis of variant order. *Parasitology* **80**:343–357.

51. **Kotwal, G. J.** 1997. Microorganisms and their interaction with the immune system. *J. Leukoc. Biol.* **62**:415–429.

52. **Li, J., H. Ochman, E. A. Groisman, E. F. Boyd, F. Solomon, K. Nelson, and R. K. Selander.** 1995. Relationship between evolutionary rate and cellular location among the Inv/Spa invasion proteins of *Salmonella enterica*. *Proc. Natl. Acad. Sci. USA* **92**:7252–7256.

53. **Lomholt, H.** 1996. Molecular biology and vaccine aspects of bacterial immunoglobulin A1 proteases. *APMIS* **104**(Suppl. 62):5–28.

54. **Lomholt, H., and M. Kilian.** 1994. Antigenic relationships among immunoglobulin A1 proteases from *Haemophilus*, *Neisseria*, and *Streptococcus* species. *Infect. Immun.* **62**:3178–3183.

55. **Lomholt, H., K. Poulsen, and M. Kilian.** 1995. Antigenic and genetic heterogeneity among Haemophilus influenzae and Neisseria IgA1 proteases. *Adv. Exp. Med. Biol.* **371A**:599–603.

56. **Lomholt, H., L. van Alphen, and M. Kilian.** 1993. Antigenic variation of immunoglobulin A1 proteases among sequential isolates of *Haemophilus influenzae* from healthy children and patients with chronic obstructive pulmonary disease. *Infect. Immun.* **61**:4575–4581.

57. **Lorenz, M. G., and W. Wackernagel.** 1994. Bacterial gene transfer by natural genetic transformation in the environment. *Microbiol. Rev.* **58**: 563–602.

58. **Madoff, L. C., J. L. Michel, E. W. Gong, D. E. Kling, and D. L. Kasper.** 1996. Group B streptococci escape host immunity by deletion of tandem repeat elements of the alpha C protein. *Proc. Natl. Acad. Sci. USA* **93**:4131–4136.

59. **Marrs, C. F., W. W. Ruehl, G. K. Schoolnik, and S. Falkow.** 1988. Pilin gene phase variation of *Moraxella bovis* is caused by an inversion of the pilin gene. *J. Bacteriol.* **170**:3032–3039.

60. **May, R. M., and R. M. Anderson.** 1990. Parasite-host coevolution. *Parasitology* **100**(Suppl.): S89–S101.

61. **Meyer, T. F., E. Billgard, R. Haas, S. Story-**

book, and M. So. 1984. Pilin genes of *Neisseria gonorrhoeae*: chromosomal organization and DNA sequence. *Proc. Natl. Acad. Sci. USA* **81**:6110–6114.

62. **Moxon, E. R., and D. S. Thaler.** 1997. Microbial genetics. The tinkerer's evolving tool-box. *Nature* **357**:659, 661–662.

63. **Moxon, E. R., P. B. Rainey, M. A. Nowak, and R. E. Lenski.** 1994. Adaptive evolution of highly mutable loci in pathogenic bacteria. *Curr. Biol.* **4**:24–33.

64. **Newman, K., Jr., and R. C. Johnson.** 1981. T-cell-independent elimination of *Borrelia turicatae*. *Infect. Immun.* **31**:465–469.

65. **Nowak, M. A., and R. M. May.** 1994. Superinfection and the evolution of parasite virulence. *Proc. R. Soc. Lond. Ser. B* **255**:81–89.

66. **Plummer, F. A., H. Chubb, J. N. Simonsen, M. Bosire, L. Slaney, N. J. D. Nagelkerke, I. Maclean, J. O. Ndinya-Achola, P. Waiyaki, and R. C. Brunham.** 1994. Antibodies to opacity proteins (Opa) correlate with a reduced risk of gonococcal salpingitis. *J. Clin. Investig.* **93**: 1748–1755.

67. **Plummer, F. A., J. N. Simonsen, H. Chubb, L. Slaney, J. Kimata, M. Bosire, J. O. Ndinya-Achola, and E. N. Ngugi.** 1989. Epidemiologic evidence for the development of serovar-specific immunity after gonococcal infection. *J. Clin. Investig.* **83**:1472–1476.

68. **Reinholdt, J., and M. Kilian.** 1997. Comparative analysis of immunoglobulin A1 protease activity among bacteria representing different genera, species, and strains. *Infect. Immun.* **65**:4452–4459.

69. **Rennie, J.** 1992. Trends in parasitology. Living together. *Sci. Am.* **266**:122–123, 126–133.

70. **Riley, M. A., Y. Tan, and J. Wang.** 1994. Nucleotide polymorphism in colicin E1 and Ia plasmids from natural isolates of *Escherichia coli*. *Proc. Natl. Acad. Sci. USA* **91**:11276–11280.

71. **Schneider, H., C. A. Hammack, M. A. Apicella, and J. M. Griffiss.** 1988. Instability of expression of lipooligosaccharides and their epitopes in *Neisseria gonorrhoeae*. *Infect. Immun.* **56**: 942–946.

72. **Schwan, T. G., W. Burgdorfer, and P. A. Rosa.** 1995. Borrelia, p. 626–635. *In* P. R. Murray, E. J. Baron, M. A. Pfaller, F. C. Tenover, and R. H. Yolken (ed.), *Manual of Clinical Microbiology*, 6th ed. American Society for Microbiology, Washington, D.C.

73. **Simon, M., J. Zieg, M. Silverman, G. Mandel, and R. Doolittle.** 1980. Phase variation: evolution of a controlling element. *Science* **209**: 1370–1374.

74. **Smith, J. M., C. G. Dowson, and B. G.**

Spratt. 1991. Localized sex in bacteria. *Nature* **349**:29–31.

75. **Smith, J. M., N. H. Smith, M. O'Rourke, and B. G. Spratt.** 1993. How clonal are bacteria? *Proc. Natl. Acad. Sci. USA* **90**:4384–4388.

76. **Solomon, J. M., and A. D. Grossman.** 1996. Who's competent and when: regulation of natural genetic competence in bacteria. *Trends Genet.* **12:** 150–155.

77. **Spinola, S. M., J. Peacock, F. W. Denny, D. L. Smith, and J. G. Cannon.** 1986. Epidemiology of colonization by nontypable *Haemophilus influenzae* in children: a longitudinal study. *J. Infect. Dis.* **154**:100–109.

78. **Stäger, S., B. Gottstein, H. Sager, T. W. Jungi, and N. Müller.** 1998. Influence of antibodies in mother's milk on antigenic variation of *Giardia lamblia* in the murine mother-offspring model of infection. *Infect. Immun.* **66**:1287–1292.

79. **Stern, A., and T. F. Meyer.** 1987. Common mechanism controlling phase and antigenic variation in pathogenic Neisseriae. *Mol. Microbiol.* **1:** 5–12.

80. **Stern, A., M. Brown, P. Nickel, and T. F. Meyer.** 1986. Opacity genes in *Neisseria gonorrhoeae*: control of phase and antigenic variation. *Cell* **47**:61–71.

81. **Stoenner, H. G., T. Dodd, and C. Larsen.** 1982. Antigenic variation of *Borrelia hermsii*. *J. Exp. Med.* **156**:1297–1311.

82. **Tan, Y., and M. A. Riley.** 1996. Rapid invasion by colicinogenic *Escherichia coli* with novel immunity functions. *Microbiology* **142**:175–180.

83. **Trottier, S., K. Stenberg, and C. Svanborg-Edén.** 1989. Turnover of nontypeable *Haemophilus influenzae* in the nasopharynges of healthy children. *J. Clin. Microbiol.* **27**:2175–2179.

84. **Van Alphen, L., P. Eijk, L. Geelen-van den Broek, and J. Dankert.** 1991. Immunochemical characterization of variable epitopes of outer membrane protein P2 of nontypeable *Haemophilus influenzae*. *Infect. Immun.* **59**:247–252.

85. **Van der Ende, A., C. T. P. Hopman, S. Zaat, B. B. Oude Essink, B. Berkhout, and J. Dankert.** 1995. Variable expression of class 1 outer membrane protein in *Neisseria meningitidis* is caused by variation in the spacing between the −10 and −35 regions of the promoter. *J. Bacteriol.* **177**:2475–2480.

86. **Van der Ploeg, L. H. T., D. Valerio, T. de Lange, A. Bernards, P. Borst, and F. G. Grosveld.** 1982. An analysis of cosmid clones of nuclear DNA from *Trypanosoma brucei* shows that the genes for variant surface glycoproteins are clustered in the genome. *Nucleic Acids Res.* **10:** 5905–5923.

87. **Vickerman, K.** 1989. Trypanosome sociology and antigenic variation. *Parasitology* **99**:S37–S47.

88. **Vogel, L., B. Duim, F. Geluk, P. Eijk, H. Jansen, J. Dankert, and L. van Alphen.** 1996. Immune selection for antigenic drift of major outer membrane protein P2 of *Haemophilus influenzae* during persistence in subcutaneous tissue cages in rabbits. *Infect. Immun.* **64**:980–986.

89. **Wolff, K., and A. Stern.** 1995. Identification and characterization of specific sequences encoding pathogenicity associated proteins in the genome of commensal *Neisseria* species. *FEMS Microbiol. Lett.* **125**:255–264.

90. **Zhang, J., and S. J. Norris.** 1998. Genetic variation of the *Borrelia burgdorferi* gene *vlsE* involves cassette-specific, segmental gene conversion. *Infect. Immun.* **66**:3698–3704.

91. **Zhang, J., J. M. Hardham, A. G. Barbour, and S. J. Norris.** 1997. Antigenic variation in Lyme disease Borreliae by promiscuous recombination of Vmp-like sequence cassettes. *Cell* **89:** 275–285.

LIFE ON THE INSIDE: MICROBIAL STRATEGIES FOR INTRACELLULAR SURVIVAL AND PERSISTENCE

Anthony P. Sinai

3

A group of microorganisms have evolved mechanisms to invade or be taken up by host cells and then to survive and propagate within them (51, 52, 101). The strategies utilized by intracellular pathogens to propagate their genomes will be discussed in this chapter in the context of recent developments in our understanding of cell biology.

From an ecological perspective, the relationship between intracellular pathogens and the host cell is generally considered to represent parasitism. Despite this negative connotation, we owe our very existence to the parasitization of the ancestral eukaryote by a bacterium that has evolved into the mitochondrion. This event established a mutualistic relationship, as a potentially unwelcome visitor has now become an indispensable "endosymbiont," requiring residence in the host cell for its and the host's survival (63). The recent sequencing of the genome of the obligately intracellular bacterium *Rickettsia prowazekii* suggests that this bacterium may be moving toward mutualism (8). The *R. prowazekii* genome appears to be rapidly degenerating, cementing its relationship with the host cell (8). Can the mutualism between an intracellular endosymbiont and the host cell go to the extreme of the loss of the former's genome altogether? Exactly that appears to have happened with the hydrogenosome, a unique energy-producing organelle in protists (92, 103). Recent evidence, based on the analysis of nuclear genes, indicates that extant mitochondria and hydrogenosomes share a common ancestor (28). The recent discovery of a hydrogenosomal genome in that organelle of a ciliate (3) and the identification of eubacterial genes in *Entamoeba histolytica* (which has no energy-producing organelle) (30) support the conclusion that the progressive degeneration of the "pathogen" genome, in response to adaptation to the intracellular lifestyle, may indeed be an evolutionary trend in these intimate interactions.

Unfortunately for us, many interactions between intracellular organisms and the host are not so amicable. Intracellular parasitism itself can be broadly divided into two groups, facultative and obligate (52, 101). The distinction between them is that the facultative intracellular pathogens are capable of a free-living existence either as extracellular organisms or within the environment (101). In contrast, obligately intracellular pathogens are unable to propagate extracellularly or in the environment, making their relationship with the

Anthony P. Sinai, Department of Microbiology and Immunology, University of Kentucky College of Medicine, 800 Rose St., Lexington, KY 40536.

Persistent Bacterial Infections, Edited by J. P. Nataro, M. J. Blaser, and S. Cunningham-Rundles, © 2000 ASM Press, Washington, D.C.

host cell absolutely essential (101). As with the facultative intracellular organisms, once within the cell, obligate intracellular pathogens must survive the host cell defenses and acquire the nutrients necessary for replication (101, 142).

Conventional wisdom has argued that the selective advantage promoting the lifestyle of intracellular parasitism is shelter from the humoral immune system. Without a doubt, intracellular parasitism offers some distinct advantages: the intracellular environment is relatively constant and nutrient rich, is generally free of competition, and potentially provides a "free ride" to tissue sites away from the site of infection (52). But these advantages come at a cost. By being intracellular, these pathogens are in the line of fire of the cell-mediated immune system (69) and must evolve and maintain the means to neutralize cellular defenses and access cellular nutrient pools (52, 69, 101, 142).

All intracellular pathogens gain access to the cell within a membrane-bound compartment (86). The internalization of cells by pathogens can be passive and directed by the host cell (phagocytosis) (52, 59), triggered by the induction of membrane ruffling and macropinocytosis (52, 59), or can be active, as exhibited by protozoan parasites of the phylum *Apicomplexa*, such as *Toxoplasma gondii* (42) and *Plasmodium* spp. (109). The mechanism of invasion by bacterial pathogens has been covered extensively in several recent reviews (37, 52, 57, 157) and will not be discussed further unless it is germane to downstream events.

Uptake of particulate matter, generally by a phagocytic or macropinocytic event, triggers a series of membrane-trafficking events that have been extensively studied for inert particles (reviewed in references 64 and 148). These studies provide a framework within which to examine how pathogenic bacteria have adapted to, escaped from, or modulated the endocytic-lysosomal cascade to establish their respective replication-permissive niches (64, 85, 142). In the next section I will briefly cover salient features of the endosomal-phagosomal pathways in mammalian cells, using inert particles as a model.

The fate of an inert particle following uptake by phagocytosis terminates with the formation of a phagolysosome (148). The events surrounding the maturation of a phagosome closely parallel those for an endosome (uptake by receptor-mediated endocytosis) (111). The stages in this maturation are characterized by a series of highly dynamic and specific membrane fusion and remodeling events (148). These events, defined by the presence or absence of both soluble and fixed (membrane-associated) markers within a temporal framework, provide molecular milestones for the progression to a phagolysosome (41). Key markers associated with the progression of an inert particle along the phagocytic pathway are presented in Fig. 1. A comprehensive treatment of markers defining phagosome maturation can be found in a review by Haas (64).

Typically, plasma membrane markers, predominantly surface receptors, are rapidly removed or recycled (105, 110, 111). The nascent compartment, the "early endosome," begins to acquire annexins, immature cathepsins, and the Rab5 GTPases (21, 22, 64). The Rab family of GTPases act as highly stage-specific switches regulating both the timing and fidelity of vesicle fusion events that govern membrane traffic in eukaryotes (106). These proteins are central players in the regulation of vesicle docking and fusion as defined by the SNARE hypothesis (see below) (108, 127). The progression from an early to a late endosome is accompanied by the acquisition of Rab7 (49, 98) at the expense of Rab5. In addition, there is an increase in vacuolar acidification due to the delivery of the vacuolar-type proton ATPase (62). This coincides with the arrival of the mannose-6-phosphate receptor (M6PR), lysosomal glycoproteins (LAMPs and lgp), cathepsins, and lysosomal acid phosphatases (reviewed in references 21 and 64). The increasing acidification is accompanied by the processing of cathepsins, which can now be found both in the immature and mature forms. The late endosome serves additionally as a crossover point for traffic from the Golgi bodies to lysosomes

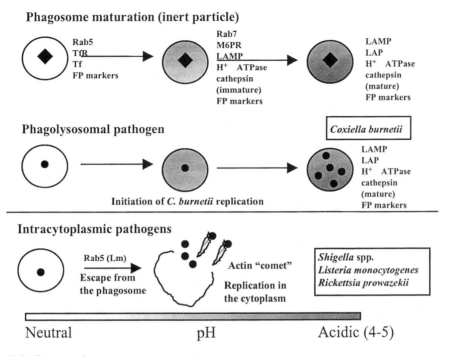

FIGURE 1 Schematic representation of phagosomal maturation and the establishment of the phagolysosomal and cytoplasmic compartments as replication-permissive niches. FP, fluid phase; Lm, *L. monocytogenes*. See the text for a detailed description of these and other markers.

(84). The culmination of this pathway is the formation of the phagolysosome, an acidic compartment (pH 4.5 to 5) rich in hydrolytic enzymes and defined by lysosomal markers (Fig. 1). Notably, the phagolysosome is completely negative for the M6PR, Rab5, and Rab7 (reviewed in reference 64). This complex series of events can be completed within 15 to 30 min, depending on the cell type examined (reviewed in references 21 and 64). The mature phagolysosome and each of the stages leading to its formation are fundamentally distinct. These differences manifest themselves both in the biochemical properties (41) and the composition (39, 40). Phagosomes, in addition to being dynamic, are also complex, as latex bead phagosomes contain at least 200 distinct proteins (39). Interestingly, even "inert" particles are able to exert an influence on the progression of the endocytic cascade (105), suggesting that complex biotic

cargoes (bacteria or parasites) can and do have dramatic effects (see below).

It is clear that the orchestration of such a dynamic sequence of events requires a mechanism to ensure both its efficiency and fidelity. The molecular basis of these events is defined by the SNARE hypothesis. The SNARE hypothesis, defining the molecular events surrounding the efficiency and fidelity of vesicle fusion events, is now widely accepted and has been extensively reviewed (108, 126). In its most basic form, the hypothesis posits that high-affinity, highly specific interactions between integral membrane proteins on the "target" membrane (t-SNARE) and the vesicle (v-SNARE) define the specificity of a given interaction. The vesicles containing these signals will ultimately fuse, as a consequence of the assembly of cytosolic proteins, including NSF (*N*-ethylmaleimide-sensitive factor) and the soluble NSF attachment proteins (SNAPs), into the 20S complex (145). The formation of the complex, in conjunction with coating-un-coating reactions and activation by GTP hydrolysis by the specific Rab-GTPase catalyzing that interaction, will culminate in fusion (106, 108). Following vesicle fusion, the luminal and membrane contents mix (108).

The SNARE hypothesis can be extended to pathogen-containing vacuoles (85), with the proviso that the presence of a biotic cargo may (particularly in the case of intravacuolar pathogens) affect the behavior of the compartment, causing it to deviate from its preordained maturation pathway (64, 85, 142). While the precise mechanisms by which pathogens modulate their interactions with the pathways of membrane traffic in the infected cell remain to be elucidated, a cell biological perspective provides an excellent framework to define and address these questions.

Bacteria gain access to the intracellular environment either passively (by conventional phagocytosis or receptor-mediated endocytosis) or by a trigger mechanism (membrane-ruffling and macropinocytosis) (reviewed in references 37, 52, 57, and 157). These events are characterized by changes in the organization of the host cytoskeleton and result in the bacterium localizing intracellularly within a membrane-bound compartment (37, 52, 57, 157). Notably, bacterial type III secretion systems and their effector molecules play a critical role in triggering the uptake of several invasive pathogens by modulating the activities of host components (81).

The presence of a viable intracellular pathogen within the nascent vacuole generally alters the fate of the compartment as it progresses through (or exits) the preordained pathway to the phagolysosome (85). Earlier studies, which had focused on either the detection or the absence of phagosome-lysosome fusion, have been considerably refined in the context of advances in cell biology (85, 130, 142). These advances point to a myriad of strategies employed by intracellular bacteria to arrive at and propagate within their respective replication-permissive niches (85, 130, 142). The strategies

employed by intracellular bacteria, defined by the establishment of replication-permissive niches, include (i) survival and replication within a phagolysosome (Fig. 1), (ii) escape from the phagosome and replication within the cytoplasm (Fig. 1), (iii) modulation of progression along the endocytic cascade (Fig. 2), and (iv) exit from the endocytic cascade by entry into alternative pathways of membrane traffic within the host cell (Fig. 3). Each of these scenarios is discussed using examples of pathogens that employ them, with particular emphasis on the host cell components that define the replication-permissive niche.

SURVIVAL WITHIN THE PHAGOLYSOSOME

Coxiella burnetii is an obligately intracellular pathogen that requires the conditions of the phagolysosome to replicate (Fig. 1) (11, 12). Following infection of a cell, the *C. burnetii*-containing vacuoles display promiscuous homotypic and heterotypic fusion with organelles in the endocytic pathway (11, 116). Thus, the contents of all phagocytic vesicles finally colocalize with the *C. burnetii* cells (116, 162). As the bacterium replicates, so does the vacuole, eventually incorporating all membranes of the endosomal-phagolysosomal pathway within it (116, 162). Interestingly, pathogen vacuoles that are divorced from the endocytic pathway (*Toxoplasma* and *Chlamydia*) are refractory to the hyperfusogenic nature of the *Coxiella* phagosome (73, 142a). This is in keeping with the tenets of the SNARE hypothesis, which posits that specific signals in both interacting compartments are required to maintain the fidelity of membrane fusion events (108, 142a). In contrast, coinfection by *Coxiella* and the intraphagolysosomal protozoan *Leishmania mexicana* (129) results in the cohabitation of these organisms within a compartment within which both replicate (116, 163). Predictably, inert particles which are destined to be digested in phagolysosomes also colocalize with intracellular *C. burnetii* (162). It appears that unlike the pathogens discussed below, *C. burnetii* modulates the endocytic pathway by accelerating its

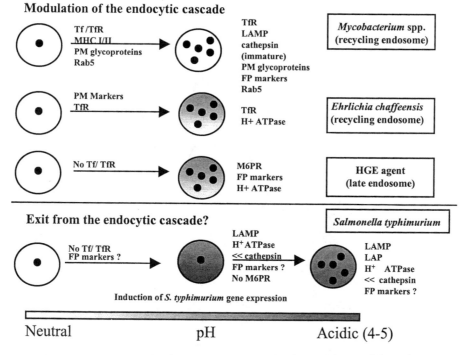

FIGURE 2 Establishment of replication-permissive niches by modulation of the endocytic cascade. PM, plasma membrane; FP, fluid phase. See the text for a detailed description of these and other markers.

inevitable maturation into a phagolysosome (116).

ESCAPE FROM THE PHAGOSOME

It may be argued that the best way to prevent phagolysosome formation is to escape from the phagocyte vacuole into the cytoplasm. This strategy has been employed by several intracellular pathogens, including the obligately intracellular *Rickettsia* spp. (169) and the facultatively intracellular pathogens of the genus *Shigella*, the *Shigella*-like enteroinvasive *Escherichia coli* (68), and the gram-positive bacterium *Listeria monocytogenes* (37). Escape from the phagosome is essential for these bacteria to replicate (reviewed in reference 52). Mutants of both *Shigella* and *L. monocytogenes* that fail to escape the vacuole may or may not progress to a lysosomal compartment but fail to replicate (reviewed in references 10 and 52). Work by

the Stahl group has shown that listeriolysin-deficient *Listeria* resides in a compartment that actively recruits the early endosomal marker Rab5 (6, 7). As a consequence, the *Listeria*-containing vacuole fails to follow the progression to the phagolysosome (6, 7).

It should be noted, however, that the mere ability to escape from a phagosome into the cytoplasm may serve functions other than the avoidance of phagolysosomal fusion. This is clearly the case for the protozoan parasite *Trypanosoma cruzi*, which actually recruits lysosomes to fuse with the plasma membrane as its mechanism to enter cells and escapes from the resultant vacuole into the cytoplasm to differentiate and divide intracellularly (10, 154).

Listeria and *Shigella* move within the infected cell and infect neighboring cells by polymerizing host actin into distinctive "comets" (20, 37, 158). This allows cell-to-cell spread

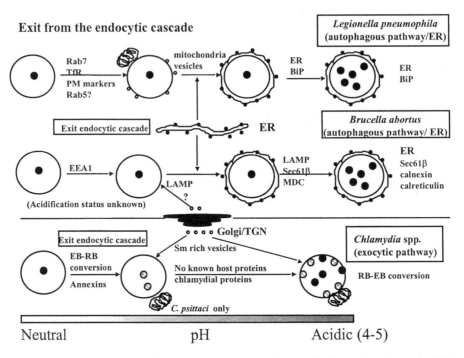

FIGURE 3 Establishment of replication-permissive niches outside the endocytic cascade. PM, plasma membrane; Sm, sphingomyelin. See the text for a detailed description of these and other markers.

without exiting the originally infected cell (20, 37, 158). Indeed, the response of the host cell to infection is governed to some extent by the bacterium. In the case of *Shigella*, infection of macrophages triggers apoptosis in those cells, while fibroblasts are necrotized (29, 174). The environment of the mammalian cytoplasm is nutrionally rich, as demonstrated by the fact that the expression of *L. monocytogenes* listeriolysin in the nonpathogenic *Bacillus subtilis* allows those bacteria to escape from the vacuole and then replicate efficiently (23).

MODULATION OF THE ENDOCYTIC CASCADE

Several intracellular pathogens have evolved the ability to modulate maturation of the endocytic cascade, thereby establishing a unique niche best suited for their replication (52, 142). The molecular mechanisms by which these intravacuolar pathogens modulate the progression along the endosomal-phagosomal cascade

are arguably the most exciting area of cellular microbiology (142). This area has blossomed as a consequence of the convergence of mutational and genetic studies of pathogens and an explosion in our understanding of the molecular basis and regulation of membrane traffic in mammalian cells (52, 64, 142).

How pathogens derail or retard the endocytic cascade at the molecular level is not known. The presence or absence of host cell markers within the lumen or membrane of the pathogen vacuole acts as a milestone for progression along the endocytic cascade (64). While the cargo does influence the endocytic cascade, comparison with phagosomes containing abiotic cargoes provides an excellent set of molecular milestones (64, 85, 142). However, use of these milestones is often complicated by the fact that pathogens often establish themselves in compartments with markers associated with more than one stop on the endocytic cascade, or even outside of it (see below).

Mycobacterium **spp.**

In recent years, our understanding of the molecular and cell biological basis of mycobacterial pathogenicity has increased tremendously. We now have a significantly more refined understanding of the mechanism by which mycobacteria survive within the susceptible cell (Fig. 2) (reviewed in reference 142). These studies will undoubtedly be accelerated by the recent sequencing of the genome of *Mycobacterium tuberculosis* (35). This resource not only provides insight into the basic biology of the organism but will also facilitate a more targeted approach to defining the pathogenic personality of *M. tuberculosis* and other pathogenic mycobacteria (35).

Early studies had suggested that upon interaction with macrophages, virulent mycobacteria "blocked" phagolysosome formation by residing in a nonfusogenic vacuole (reviewed in reference 142). This conclusion was based on a series of studies that showed that live mycobacteria failed to colocalize with both endogenous and exogenous markers of lysosomes (in contrast, these same markers colocalized with killed bacteria and inert particles) (142). This conclusion was reached when the prevailing wisdom dictated that the interactions of microorganisms and the cells they infected could be analyzed simply on the basis of the detection, or lack thereof, of lysosome fusion (130). We now know that this is overly simplistic: the interaction between *Mycobacterium*-containing phagosomes and the endocytic cascade is considerably more complicated (130, 142).

Recent evidence indicates that the mycobacterial phagosome is a highly dynamic fusogenic compartment (32–34, 131, 149, 150). These investigations have employed cell biological criteria, based on the detection of endogenous and exogenous fixed and soluble markers, as milestones for progression along the endocytic cascade. The data suggest that vacuoles containing live mycobacteria are "arrested" in their maturation at the recycling or sorting endosomal compartment of the cell (reviewed in reference 142). The early mycobacterium-containing phagosome (up to 24 h) contains markers of the plasma membrane and early endosomes (32, 33); upon maturation, the transferrin receptor (TfR), a marker for the recycling-sorting endosome, is retained while late endosomal lysosomal markers like LAMP and CD63 are present but at lower levels than are observed with latex bead phagosomes or dead bacteria (33). Notably, the mycobacterial phagosome fails to acidify, a property believed to be the consequence of the exclusion of the vacuolar proton ATPase from the phagosomal membrane (150). This failure to acidify has been shown to be responsible for the observation that cathepsin D, a soluble late-endosomal-lysosomal protease, is not processed within mycobacterial phagosomes (149).

While inaccessible to certain lysosomal markers, *Mycobacterium*-containing vacuoles are accessible to plasma membrane markers and exogenous fluid phase markers, supporting their residence in the transferrin-recycling compartment (31, 38, 54, 131). It is interesting to note that the membranes of *Mycobacterium*-containing vacuoles retain Rab5 GTPase (106, 164). Rab5 is generally associated with regulating homotypic fusion between early endosomal compartments. The retention of Rab5 may lock mycobacterial vacuoles at the early-endosome stage or alternatively may prevent the acquisition of signals required to progress along the endocytic cascade. The failure of the mycobacterial vacuole to acquire the late-endosomal marker Rab7 suggests that the latter scenario may be at work (164).

Much like an inert particle, killed mycobacteria induce true phagolysosomes (reviewed in reference 142). This indicates that bacterial viability is essential for the maintenance of the vacuole in the recycling compartment (reviewed in reference 142). However, within the infected cell, the phagosomes containing mycobacteria, but not those containing inert particles, are altered in their maturation properties (70, 164). Early work by Hart and colleagues had shown that ammonium ions inhibited the saltatory motion of lysosomes (70, 71). Ammonia produced by some mycobacteria (60), perhaps as a consequence of mycobacterial glutamine synthase activity (72), could potentially retard lysosomal function. In addition, products secreted or released from growing mycobacteria, most notably sulfatides, may or may not inhibit lysosomal activity (61, 100).

Both survival within the host cell and the ability to replicate have been strong selective pressures in the evolution of intracellular parasitism (51, 52, 142). While the specific nutrient status of the mycobacterial phagosome is not known, its residence in the transferrin-rich recycling compartment (reviewed in reference 142), coupled with the ability of the bacteria to scavenge this micronutrient (74, 95, 173), may play a role in establishing their replication-permissive niche. Deviation from this compartment, as observed in activated macrophages (107) infected with *Mycobacterium avium*, results in the failure to be localized in the transferrin-recycling compartment, the acquisition of proton ATPase, acidification, and the establishment of a lysosomal environment (135). Within this compartment, mycobacteria fail to replicate and are eventually killed (135).

The notoriously slow growth of mycobacteria has prompted the study of "fast-growing" mycobacteria, including *Mycobacterium marinum*, an amphibian pathogen that can infect mammalian macrophages in vitro (117) and cause human disease (118). One study indicates that *M. marinum* replicates in an intracellular compartment which is prelysosomal and is not acidified (13). The lack of acidification correlates with the inability to detect the V-H^+ ATPase in the phagosomal membrane (13). Whether *M. marinum* resides in a recycling TfR-positive compartment was not examined.

The use of fast-growing mycobacteria in such studies, combined with genetic (83) and cell biological techniques to screen for bacterial mutants with altered intracellular behavior (160, 161), could provide information regarding the molecular basis of intracellular survival and replication by the slow-growing mycobacteria. Such studies, combined with the sequence of *M. tuberculosis*, promise to accelerate the process of discovery with this important group of pathogens (35).

Ehrlichia spp.

The genus *Ehrlichia*, within the family *Rickettsiaceae*, includes a group of obligately intracellular bacteria that reside within membrane-bound inclusions within phagocytic cells (121). The study of the cell biology of *Ehrlichia*-containing vacuoles is in its infancy, but it does suggest differences among species (see below).

Based on the distribution of fixed cell markers, it has been suggested that vacuoles containing *Ehrlichia chaffeensis* reside in a TfR-positive early-endosomal compartment (14). Similar to what is observed with mycobacterial vacuoles, the *E. chaffeensis* vacuoles display a delayed clearance of plasma membrane markers (14). Unlike those of mycobacteria, however, the *E. chaffeensis* vacuole is slightly acidified and possesses detectable levels of the vacuolar proton ATPase (14). Furthermore, in contrast to mycobacterial vacuoles, the *E. chaffeensis* compartment fails to colocalize with the late-endosomal–lysosomal marker LAMP-1 (14). The role of the concentration of TfR in the *E. chaffeensis* vacuole is potentially related to iron scavenging, as the growth of these bacteria is exquisitely sensitive to the iron chelator deferoxamine (14).

The agent of human granulocytic ehrlichiosis (HGE) appears to behave somewhat differently in infected neutrophils (167). Based on immunoelectron microscopic data, Webster and colleagues suggest that the compartment containing the HGE agent is somewhat accessible to a fluid phase tracer (BSA-gold) added to infected cells (167). This indicates that at least a population of *Ehrlichia* vacuoles is on the endocytic pathway (167). These authors were unable to detect the TfR in the membranes of HGE vacuoles, unlike for *E. chaffeensis* (167). The difference in the apparent intracellular lifestyles of these closely related organisms is supported by other data. Examination of markers indicates HGE-containing vacuoles are positive for the M6PR but not LAMP1 and are not significantly acidified (167). Taken together, these data suggest the HGE agent is connected to the endocytic pathway, possibly in a late-endosomal compartment (167).

Salmonella enterica Serovar Typhimurium

Considerably more is known about the molecular and cellular bases of host cell invasion by *Salmonella* serovar Typhimurium than about the events downstream of entry (reviewed in references 52 and 57). What is clear, despite a body of seemingly contradictory results, is that the *Salmonella*-containing phagosome is a dynamic and privileged compartment that may (104) or may not (58, 119) reside within the endocytic cascade. Interpretation of the literature is complicated by the differences in host cells, bacterial strains, and experimental protocols used. These are discussed in greater detail by Rathman and colleagues (119).

Serovar Typhimurium resides within a specialized compartment within both phagocytic and nonphagocytic cells (52) (Fig. 2). Entry by wild-type *Salmonella* occurs by the triggering of localized membrane ruffling at the point of bacterial contact, which precedes macropinocytosis (4, 53). The macropinocytic event results in the internalization of the bacterium within a spacious vacuole (unlike a tightly fitting phagosome) (4, 53) and is triggered by effectors secreted by the bacterium via a Type III secretion pathway (57, 81). The determinants involved in invasion do not appear to significantly alter downstream events (119). Bacteria with specific defects in triggering uptake by macropinocytosis are still taken up by professional phagocytes and are not altered in their intracellular trafficking (119).

The newly formed *Salmonella*-containing vacuole expresses host surface markers, which are selectively recycled and/or maintained (104). Maturation of the vacuole proceeds with the loss of surface markers and acquisition of lysosomal markers (104, 119). However, the delivery of lysosomal markers may not be associated with endocytic lysosomes, as they appear to bypass the mannose 6-phosphate compartment (58, 119).

The origin of lysosomal markers within the *Salmonella* vacuole has been the cause of much debate concerning whether the bacterium does (27, 82) or does not inhibit phagolysosome formation (5, 104, 120). Contributing to the debate has been the observation that the *Salmonella* vacuole is acidified to a pH of 4.5 to 5.0 (5, 120). Recent studies indicate that this acidification occurs within 30 min of bacterial entry and is a necessary event for the establishment of the replication-permissive niche (5, 120).

The acidified conditions have been shown to be essential for the activation of the *Salmonella* PhoP-PhoQ sensor-regulator system (99). Activation of this pathway results in the induction of a series of *Salmonella* genes (the *pag* genes [for PhoP-PhoQ-activated gene]) and repression of another set (the *prg* genes [for PhoP-PhoQ-repressed genes]) (99). Genetic screens have identified several PhoP-PhoQ-regulated genes that are specifically induced in macrophages (5, 17). These events are essential in priming the bacteria, which, following a roughly 4-h lag, enter a phase of intracellular multiplication (88). The phase of intracellular multiplication is accompanied by the formation of a novel set of stable filamentous structures that contain lysosomal glycoproteins and are connected to the replication-permissive vacuole (58). It has been suggested that these filaments may form a mechanism to access host nutrient pools (58).

In summary, the *Salmonella* vacuole, while containing markers for lysosomes, resides in a distinct compartment that may or may not be on the endocytic cascade. The characterization of mutants with distinct intracellular trafficking defects will undoubtedly bring the power of *Salmonella* genetics to bear on defining cellular functions.

AN ALTERNATIVE LIFESTYLE: OUTSIDE THE ENDOCYTIC CASCADE

An alternative strategy employed by intracellular pathogens to avoid being killed by phagolysosomes is to remain within a vacuolar compartment but to exit the endocytic cascade (52,

64, 142). This property is exhibited by *Legionella pneumophila* (142) and *Brucella abortus* (112), both of which interact with the autophagous pathway, replicating in an endoplasmic reticulum (ER)-associated compartment, and *Chlamydia* spp., which reside on the exocytic cascade (65, 142). Exit from the endocytic cascade not only ensures survival but also establishes these pathogens in a replication-permissive niche (112, 142). Interestingly, while avoiding interactions with the endocytic cascade, *L. pneumophila*, *B. abortus*, and some strains of *Chlamydia psittaci* display intimate interactions with other organelle systems, most notably the ER (112, 142) and mitochondria (94). Such interactions have been characterized for the parasite *T. gondii*, where the vacuolar membranes are likely to be involved in nutrient scavenging (143).

L. pneumophila

Generally resident as a pathogen of free-living amebae (1, 25), *L. pneumophila* has entered human populations in ameba-contaminated aerosols generated by human conveniences, such as shower heads, air conditioning systems, and whirlpool baths (2, 48). These bacteria cause a severe and debilitating pneumonia that can be fatal (97).

There are many morphological and other similarities between the progression of infection in free-living protozoa and mammalian macrophages (50). Bacterial internalization in macrophages can occur both by conventional phagocytosis and by an unusual mechanism termed coiling phagocytosis (79, 142). Coiling phagocytosis is a slower process than conventional phagocytosis (79, 123), a fact that may contribute to more extensive and efficient sorting of several plasma membrane proteins (79, 123). Despite these differences, the progression of the nascent vacuole to a replication-permissive compartment is unaffected (79).

The establishment of the replication-permissive vacuole occurs by a series of morphologically distinct events. The nascent vacuole, established by either conventional or coiling phagocytosis, exhibits transient interactions with smooth vesicles and host mitochondria, which give way to a stable interaction with the host ER (78, 151) (Fig. 3). It is in this ribosome-studded compartment that *Legionella* replication is initiated (78, 151). The formation of the replicative phagosome is dependent on bacterial viability (76, 79) and the orchestrated effects of several bacterial gene products (see below).

Much of our understanding of the cell biology of *Legionella* stems from the analysis of mutants in which various stages of this pathway are affected (reviewed in references 52, 64, and 142). The analysis of mutants indicates that the ability to form a replication-permissive compartment is dependent on multiple gene products. The strategy of identifying mutants with defects in intracellular growth led to the isolation of strain 25D, which entered cells efficiently but failed to recruit host organelles (mitochondria and ER) and to establish a replicative phagosome (75). This mutant entered cells by coiling phagocytosis but failed to progress through the downstream events (75). The importance of organelle recruitment to *Legionella* is underscored by the avirulence of this mutant in a guinea pig model (24). The defect was complemented by a clone encoding the operon *icmWXYZ* (*icm* for intracellular multiplication) and the gene *dotA* (*dot* for defective in organelle trafficking) (18, 26, 91). The *dotA* locus had been identified in a thymineless death screen for mutants defective in intracellular replication (18, 19). This analysis revealed two classes of mutants: one exhibited defects in organelle recruitment and the inhibition of phagolysosome fusion; the other class was defective in recruitment only. Both classes were complemented by the *dotA* locus (18, 19). Transposon mutagenesis also yielded mutations in these genes based on their ability to enter but not kill macrophages (132). Interestingly, mutations in the *icm* and *dot* loci were found to confer sensitivity to high salt concentration in the medium (132).

Using both defects in intracellular multiplication and salt sensitivity, an additional unlinked region comprising 16 genes (*icmTSRO-*

POMLKEGCDJBF) has been identified (9, 115, 139, 140, 165). These mutants have led to the identification of a functional DNA conjugative transport system (140, 165), which is believed to transport an unidentified factor into the replicative phagosome (140, 165).

As noted, the *Legionella* phagosome does not fuse with lysosomes (77, 78), and traffic along the endocytic pathway is aborted soon after infection (128, 168). The role of the DotA protein in this process appears to be temporal (128, 168). Expression of the protein is required before uptake by macrophages, supporting its essential role in exiting the endocytic cascade early in the course of *Legionella's* interaction with cells (128, 168). The inability of *Legionella*-containing vacuoles to associate with the late-endosomal markers Rab7 and LAMP-1 while not retaining early-endosomal markers further supports an early exit from the progression of the endocytic cascade (128). Notably, some differences exist in the kinetics with which *icm-dotA* mutants acquire endocytic markers, suggesting subtle differences in the robustness of the mutations (128, 168).

The interaction of *Legionella* vacuoles with lysosomes has been examined using both fluid phase and fixed markers (33, 152). Vacuoles containing wild-type *Legionella* are significantly less likely to colocalize with the lysosomal markers LAMP and cathepsin D or exogenous fluid phase markers, as shown by both immunofluorescence and immunoelectron microscopy (33, 152). Colocalization was observed with high frequency when mutants defective in intracellular growth were examined (152). Furthermore, the *Legionella* vacuole fails to significantly acidify, reaching a pH of only 5.7 to 6.5 (77).

Upon exit from the endocytic cascade, the *Legionella* phagosome exhibits transient interactions with host vesicles and mitochondria, which give way to a vacuole that is observed morphologically as a ribosome-studded phagosome (75, 76, 151) and immunocytochemically by staining for the ER luminal marker BiP (151). Progression along this pathway is required for intracellular growth (75, 76, 151).

Morphologically, the engulfment of cytoplasmic and organellar components by the ER is an indication of the induction of autophagy, a pathway used by cells to recycle components (43, 44). The autophagous pathway is known to intersect the endocytic pathway, as autophagous vacuoles generally fuse with lysosomes, promoting the degradation of their contents (43, 89). This final step is clearly not occurring with the *Legionella* phagosome, as the mature compartment does not acquire lysosomal markers (76, 77, 142).

A clue to the reason for entering the autophagous pathway may be found in the basic physiology of extracellular *Legionella* in vitro (reviewed in reference 142). The amino acids serine and threonine appear to be the primary substrates for energy production in these bacteria and can serve as the sole carbon and nitrogen sources in defined media (122, 156, 166). While able to synthesize most amino acids de novo, legionellae are auxotrophic for serine and threonine (122, 156, 166). Notably, upon infection of host cells starved for serum, a condition known to trigger autophagy, legionellae exhibit a shorter lag time before the initiation of replication (151). Whether or not this is due to increased pools of amino acids as a result of cytoplasmic degradation is not known, but it may define the basis of this unique compartment (151).

B. abortus

B. abortus is a pathogen of both clinical and veterinary importance (47). In a natural infection, the organism grows within professional phagocytes and has been proposed to avoid destruction by inhibiting phagolysosome formation (55). Recent evidence, outlined below, suggests that this is achieved by *B. abortus*-containing phagosomes exiting the endocytic pathway and transiting through the autophagous pathway in a manner somewhat different from *Legionella* (Fig. 3) (112, 113).

Soon after infection, the *B. abortus* phagosome is found to colocalize with the early-endosomal antigen (EEA1), which is followed by the acquisition of the lysosomal membrane marker LAMP1 (112) but not the soluble ca-thepsin D (113). Notably, neither wild-type nor attenuated organisms were found to colo-calize with the late-endosomal markers, cation-independent or cation-dependent M6PRs, or Rab7 (112). In contrast, these markers were acquired readily by latex bead phagosomes (112). The acquisition of the lysosomal marker LAMP (112), while bypassing the late-endoso-mal compartment, is explained by the localiza-tion of brucellae within vacuoles surrounded by the ER, identified by staining with Sec61β (112). This marker was never observed with latex bead phagosomes (112). Of note, unlike late *Legionella* phagosomes, the luminal marker BiP was not detected (112). The presence of LAMP1 and Sec61β, along with the accumula-tion of monodansylcadaverine, suggests entry into an autophagous pathway (43, 112). Up to this point in the intracellular progression, wild-type and attenuated *B. abortus* cells behave very similarly (112).

The ability to enter the autophagous path-way appears to involve the *Brucella* BvrS-BvrR two-component regulatory system, as mutants in this sensor-signaling pathway rapidly enter cathepsin D-positive lysosomal compartments and are killed (144). These mutants do not enter the autophagous pathway (144). In con-trast, an attenuated strain, S19, which is unable to efficiently replicate intracellularly and ex-hibits delayed targeting to lysosomes, does pas-sage through the autophagosomal stage (113).

Virulent wild-type *B. abortus* cells progress beyond the autophagosome to replicate within the ER in a compartment which is devoid of LAMP1 (112), suggesting that entry into the autophagosomal pathway does not define the final replication-permissive niche for *B. abortus* (112). The actual replication-permissive niche for brucellae appears to be the ER on the basis of (i) the localization of several ER markers, (ii) the redistribution of Golgi markers to *Brucella*-containing compartments following treatment with brefeldin A, and finally (iii) the vacuoliza-tion of the *Brucella*-containing compartments following treatment of infected cells with aero-

lysin, a toxin known to cause ER vacuolization (112).

In summary, the data suggest that *B. abortus*-containing phagosomes exit the endocytic pathway and transit through the autophagous pathway en route to their replication-permis-sive niche, the ER (112). Transit through auto-phagosomes has been postulated to be impor-tant for the induction of specific genes which are required to fully exploit the resources within the infected cell, resulting in bacterial proliferation and the death of the host cell (112, 144).

Chlamydia spp.

Members of the genus *Chlamydia* are responsi-ble for a wide range of human and animal dis-eases (134). These obligately intracellular pathogens exhibit a developmental cycle alter-nating between the relatively metabolically inert but infectious extracellular form, the ele-mentary body (EB), and the replicating nonin-fectious intracellular form, the reticulate body (RB) (102, 133) (see also chapter 18). Follow-ing internalization by phagocytosis, receptor-mediated endocytosis, or pinocytosis, the EB establishes itself in a vacuole traditionally re-ferred to as an inclusion (reviewed in references 102 and 142). Within the inclusion, the highly disulfide-cross-linked outer membrane pro-teins of the EB are reduced (16) and the de-velopmental sequence giving rise to the RB is initiated (96). The cell biology of the estab-lishment of the replication-permissive chla-mydial vacuole (Fig. 3) defines a fascinating, if poorly understood, problem (reviewed in ref-erences 65 and 142).

The pioneering work of Friis showed by subcellular fractionation that inclusions con-taining *C. psittaci* banded in density gradients at a position distinct from lysosomes (56). This property was lost following heat treatment of the EBs (56). In an extension of these studies, Zeichner showed that while live EBs formed true inclusions, distinct from phagolysosomes, heat-killed organisms terminated as phagolyso-somes (172). Examination of the protein pro-files of the vacuoles revealed that they had some similar but many different proteins, providing a molecular clue to the existence of differences in the biogenesis and/or maturation of a viable inclusion as opposed to a phagolysosome (171, 172).

More recent studies confirm morphologically the lack of endogenous lysosomal markers (LAMP and lysosomal acid phosphatase) or exogenous fluid phase markers (fluorescent markers, thorotrast, and ferretin) in inclusions containing viable bacteria (73, 87, 114, 153, 155, 170). The ability to avoid interaction with lysosomes may be an intrinsic property of the relatively inert EB, as UV irradiation, antibiotic treatment, and even EB outer membrane ghosts do not fuse with lysosomes upon uptake (46, 56, 159). The failure of EB ghosts to fuse with lysosomes may be a consequence of the relatively short incubation times used in these experiments (138). In contrast, as shown biochemically by Friis and Zeichner (56, 172), heat treatment does increase colocalization of lysosomal markers (46).

The chlamydial inclusion is fundamentally different from that of the phagolysosomal pathogen C. burnetii (73). The inclusion fails to acquire fluid phase markers over a relatively long (up to 12-h) time period (73). Accordingly, TfR and exogenously labeled transferrin do not accumulate (73). Unlike an inert particle, or vacuoles containing C. burnetii, the chlamydial inclusion does not acidify and maintains a pH above 6 (136). In contrast, heat-killed bacteria enter an acidified lysosomal compartment (136). This, coupled with the inability to detect lysosomal markers, suggests that the chlamydial inclusion is truly divorced from the endocytic pathway (reviewed in references 73 and 142).

Much of the morphological and biochemical data has implicated a component(s) on the EB surface in blocking traffic to lysosomes (45, 46). This is in conflict with more recent evidence suggesting that protein synthesis closely following internalization plays a role in delivering the inclusion to a perinuclear location and to its replication-permissive niche (138). This replication-permissive niche, while divorced

from the endocytic cascade, appears to lie on the exocytic (secretory) pathway of the host cell (reviewed in references 65 and 142).

Membrane traffic in eukaryotic cells, paradoxically, has been studied predominantly by examining the behavior and distribution of proteins rather than lipid markers (127). The introduction of fluorescent lipid analogs, particularly for lipids that accumulate in specific compartments, has made it possible to trace the fate and behavior of lipids within membranes (90). Over the past several years, Hackstadt et al. have exploited the properties of fluorescent lipids, in particular derivatives of ceramide (C6-NDB-ceramide and Bodipy-ceramide) to define the location of the chlamydial inclusion in the sequence of membrane traffic (66, 137). Ceramide and its fluorescent analogs serve as markers for the Golgi apparatus, where they are concentrated and converted to sphingomyelin and/or glucocerebrosides (90). The traffic of these fluorescent sphingolipids to the cell surface serves as an excellent marker of the exocytic pathway (90).

Hackstadt and colleagues found that in Chlamydia-infected cells, roughly half of the C6-NDB-ceramide label is directed to the inclusion and incorporated as sphingomyelin in the chlamydial envelope (66, 137). The ability to hijack exocytic traffic is specific to the chlamydial inclusion and was not observed in C. burnetii-infected cells (73). Other fluorescent lipid analogs are directed to the inclusion, although only ceramide derivatives (sphingomyelin) are retained in the RB envelope (66, 67).

The delivery of fluorescent ceramide into the inclusion does not occur directly from the host plasma membrane and must transit through the Golgi (66, 137). Treatments that affect the organization of and traffic out of the Golgi (brefeldin A and monensin) were found to inhibit accumulation of sphingomyelin in the inclusion (66, 137). While receiving labeled sphingolipids from the Golgi, the chlamydial inclusion does not interact with the trafficking pathways from the ER and Golgi or that for glycoprotein traffic to the cell surface or lysosomes (66, 137). The inclusion fails to acquire or retain protein markers from any of these compartments, including the *trans*-Golgi network (*trans*-Golgi network marker AP-1 and the Golgi body markers p58, mannosidase II, and β-COP), or clathrin as a marker for Golgi-lysosome traffic (66, 137). Furthermore, model glycoproteins targeted to the plasma membrane are not incorporated in the chlamydial inclusion either from the Golgi or plasma membrane, nor is TfR a marker for early endosomes (137, 153).

Taken together, these data suggest that the chlamydial inclusion lies in an aberrant compartment (with properties resembling the *trans*-Golgi network) which is defined by selectively fusing with sphingolipid-rich vesicles but little else (reviewed in references 65 and 142). This points to the existence of different classes of exocytic vesicles which may define the sorting and delivery of protein cargoes within the cell (141).

While host protein markers have not been identified within the chlamydial inclusion, several pathogen proteins have (reviewed in references 65 and 142). These include the IncA and -B proteins, which are known to be exposed to the host cytoplasm, where they likely interact with host components (125). In fact, IncA is phosphorylated by a host kinase(s), although neither the enzyme(s) nor the role of phosphorylation is known (124). The identification of a predicted type III secretion system (80), coupled with the reinterpretation of older morphological data (93), suggests that chlamydiae may inject proteins directly into the host cytoplasm or associated organelles (in the case of *C. psittaci*) (15). Such putative effectors likely play a significant role in the intracellular growth and survival of these organisms.

A major impediment to the study of chlamydiae has been the lack of a well-developed genetic system (147). A major impetus to the

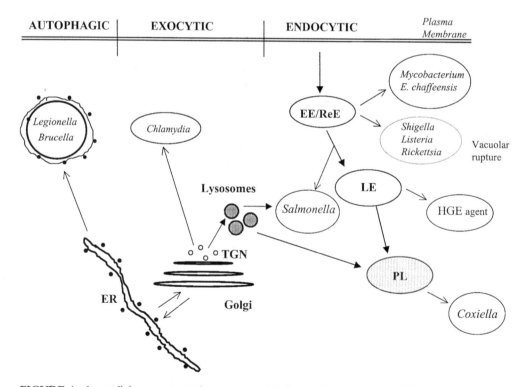

FIGURE 4 Intracellular transport pathways coopted by bacterial pathogens. EE/ReE, early and recycling endosomes; LE, late endosome; PL, phagolysosome; TGN, *trans*-Golgi network. See the text for a discussion.

field will undoubtedly come from the recent sequencing of the genome of *Chlamydia trachomatis* (146). This project has already revolutionized our views on the physiology of the bacterium and will greatly advance our understanding of the fascinating biology surrounding its pathogenesis (146).

CONCLUSIONS

The new discipline of cellular microbiology has emerged at the confluence of microbiology and cell biology (36). This new discipline presents exciting opportunities to address questions of both basic and clinical importance. Intracellular pathogens have evolved complex relationships with the host cell, which we are just beginning to appreciate (Fig. 4). The study of the mechanisms by which these pathogens infect mammalian cells will undoubtedly yield fascinating insights into both microbiology and cell biology at the most intimate interface between the pathogen and host.

ACKNOWLEDGMENTS

I thank Keith Joiner (Infectious Diseases Section, Yale University School of Medicine) for his support during the preparation of this chapter.

The author is a recipient of an Affiliate Fellowship from the American Heart Association.

REFERENCES

1. **Abu Kwaik, Y.** 1996. The phagosome containing *Legionella pneumophila* within the protozoan *Hartmannella vermiformis* is surrounded by the rough endoplasmic reticulum. *Appl. Environ. Microbiol.* **62:**2022–2028.

2. **Abu Kwaik, Y., L.-Y. Gao, B. J. Stone, C. Venkataraman, and O. Harb.** 1998. Invasion of protozoa by *Legionella pneumophila* and its role in bacterial ecology and pathogenesis. *Appl. Environ. Microbiol.* **64:**3134–3139.

3. **Akhamova, A., F. Voncken, T. van Alen, A. van Hoek, B. Boxma, G. Vogels, M. Veenhuis, and J. Hackstein.** 1998. A hydrogenosome with a genome. *Nature* **396:**527–528.

4. **Alpuche-Aranda, C. M., E. L. Racoosin, J. A. Swanson, and S. I. Miller.** 1994. *Salmonella* stimulate macrophage macropinocytosis and persist within spacious phagosomes. *J. Exp. Med.* **179:**601–608.

5. **Alpuche-Aranda, C. M., J. A. Swanson, W. P. Loomis, and S. I. Miller.** 1992. *Salmonella typhimurium* activates virulence gene transcription within acidified macrophage phagosomes. *Proc. Natl. Acad. Sci. USA* **89:**10079–10083.

6. **Alvarez-Dominguez, C., A. M. Barbieri, W. Beron, A. Wandinger-Ness, and P. D. Stahl.** 1996. Phagocytosed live *Listeria monocytogenes* influences Rab 5 regulated in vitro phagosome-endosome fusion. *J. Biol. Chem.* **271:**13834–13843.

7. **Alvarez-Dominguez, C., R. Roberts, and P. Stahl.** 1997. Internalized *Listeria monocytogenes* modulates intracellular trafficking and delays maturation of the phagosome. *J. Cell Sci.* **110:** 731–743.

8. **Andersson, S., A. Zomorodipour, J. Andersson, T. Sicheritz-Ponten, U. Alsmark, R. Podowski, A. Naslund, A.-S. Eriksson, H. Winkler, and C. Kurland.** 1998. The genome sequence of *Rickettsia prowazekii* and the origin of mitochondria. *Nature* **396:**133–140.

9. **Andrews, H., J. Vogel, and R. Isberg.** 1998. Identification of linked *Legionella pneumophila* genes essential for intracellular growth and evasion of the endocytic pathway. *Infect. Immun.* **66:** 950–958.

10. **Andrews, N. W., and P. Webster.** 1991. Phagolysosomal escape by intracellular pathogens. *Parasitol. Today* **7:**335–340.

11. **Baca, O., Y. Li, and H. Kumar.** 1994. Survival of the Q-fever agent *Coxiella burnetii* in the phagolysosome. *Trends Microbiol.* **2:**476–480.

12. **Baca, O., and D. Paretsky.** 1983. Q-fever and *Coxiella burnetii*: a model for host-parasite interactions. *Microbiol. Rev.* **47:**127–149.

13. **Barker, L., K. George, S. Falkow, and P. Small.** 1997. Differential trafficking of live and dead *Mycobacterium marinum* organisms in macrophages. *Infect. Immun.* **65:**1497–1502.

14. **Barnewall, R., Y. Rikihisa, and E. Lee.** 1997. *Ehrlichia chaffeensis* inclusions are early endosomes which selectively accumulate transferrin receptor. *Infect. Immun.* **65:**1455–1461.

15. **Bavoil, P., and R.-C. Hsia.** 1998. Type III secretion in *Chlamydia*: a case for deja vu? *Mol. Microbiol.* **28:**860–862.

16. **Bavoil, P., O. Ohlin, and J. Schachter.** 1984. Role of disulfide bonding in outer membrane structure and permeability of *Chlamydia trachomatis*. *Infect. Immun.* **44:**479–485.

17. **Belden, W., and S. Miller.** 1994. Further characterization of the PhoP regulon: identification of new PhoP-activated virulence loci. *Infect. Immun.* **62:**5095–5101.

18. **Berger, K. H., and R. R. Isberg.** 1993. Two distinct defects in intracellular growth complemented by a single genetic locus in *Legionella pneumophila*. *Mol. Microbiol.* **7:**7–19.

19. **Berger, K. H., J. J. Merriam, and R. R. Isberg.** 1994. Altered intracellular targeting proper-

ties associated with mutations in the *Legionella pneumophila dotA* gene. *Mol. Microbiol.* **14:** 809–822.

20. **Bernardini, M. L., J. Mounier, H. D'Hauteville, M. Coquis-Rondon, and P. J. Sansonetti.** 1989. Identification of *icsA*, a plasmid locus of *Shigella flexneri* that governs bacterial intra- and intercellular spread through interaction with F-actin. *Proc. Natl. Acad. Sci. USA* **86:**3867–3871.

21. **Beron, W., C. Alvarez-Dominguez, L. Mayorga, and P. Stahl.** 1995. Membrane traffic along the phagocytic pathway. *Trends Cell Biol.* **5:** 100–104.

22. **Beron, W., M. Colombo, L. Mayorga, and P. Stahl.** 1995. In-vitro reconstitution of phagosome-endosome fusion: evidence for regulation by heterotrimeric GTPases. *Arch. Biochem. Biophys.* **317:**337–342.

23. **Bielecki, J., P. Youngman, P. Connelly, and D. A. Portnoy.** 1990. *Bacillus subtilis* expressing a haemolysin gene from *Listeria monocytogenes* can grow in mammalian cells. *Nature* **345:**175–176.

24. **Blander, S. J., R. F. Breiman, and M. A. Horwitz.** 1989. A live avirulent mutant *Legionella* vaccine induces protective immunity against lethal aerosol challenge. *J. Clin. Investig.* **83:**810–815.

25. **Bozue, J. A., and W. Johnson.** 1996. Interaction of *Legionella pneumophila* with *Acanthamoeba castellani*: uptake by coiling phagocytosis and inhibition of phagosome-lysosome fusion. *Infect. Immun.* **64:**668–673.

26. **Brand, B. C., A. B. Sadosky, and H. Shuman.** 1994. The *Legionella pneumophila icm* locus: a set of genes required for intracellular multiplication in human macrophages. *Mol. Microbiol.* **14:** 797–808.

27. **Buchmeier, N. A., and F. Heffron.** 1991. Inhibition of macrophage phagosome-lysosome fusion by *Salmonella typhimurium*. *Infect. Immun.* **59:** 2232–2238.

28. **Bui, E., P. Bradley, and P. Johnson.** 1996. A common evolutionary origin for mitochondria and hydrogenosomes. *Proc. Natl. Acad. Sci. USA* **93:**9651–9656.

29. **Chen, Y., and A. Zychlinsky.** 1994. Apoptosis induced by bacterial pathogens. *Microb. Pathog.* **17:** 203–212.

30. **Clark, C., and A. Roger.** 1995. Direct evidence for the secondary loss of mitochondria in *Entamoeba histolytica*. *Proc. Natl. Acad. Sci. USA* **92:** 6518–6521.

31. **Clemens, D., and M. Horwitz.** 1996. The *Mycobacterium tuberculosis* phagosome interacts with early endosomes and is accesible to exogenously administered transferrin. *J. Exp. Med.* **184:** 1349–1355.

32. **Clemens, D. L.** 1996. Characterization of the *Mycobacterium tuberculosis* phagosome. *Trends Microbiol.* **4:**113–118.

33. **Clemens, D. L., and M. A. Horwitz.** 1995. Characterization of the *Mycobacterium tuberculosis* phagosome and evidence that phagosome maturation is inhibited. *J. Exp. Med.* **181:**257–270.

34. **Clemens, D. L., and M. A. Horwitz.** 1996. The *Mycobacterium tuberculosis* phagosome interacts with early endosomes and is accessible to exogenously administered transferrin. *J. Exp. Med.* **184:** 1349–1355.

35. **Cole, S., R. Brosch, J. Parkhill, T. Garnier, C. Churcher, D. Harris, S. Gordon, K. Eiglmeier, S. Gas, C. I. Barry, F. Tekaia, K. Badcock, D. Basham, D. Brown, T. Chillingworth, R. Connor, R. Davies, K. Devlin, T. Feltwell, S. Gentles, N. Hamlin, S. Holroyd, T. Hornsby, K. Jagels, and B. Barrell.** 1998. Deciphering the biology of *Mycobacterium tuberculosis* from the complete genome sequence. *Nature* **393:**537–544.

36. **Cossart, P., P. Boquet, S. Normark, and R. Rappuoli.** 1996. Cellular microbiology emerging. *Science* **121:**315–316.

37. **Cossart, P., and M. Lecuit.** 1998. Interactions of *Listeria monocytogenes* with mammalian cells during entry and actin based movement: bacteria factors, cellular ligands and signaling. *EMBO J.* **17:** 3797–3806.

38. **DeChastellier, C., T. Lang, and T. Thilo.** 1995. Phagocytic processing of the macrophage endoparasite, *Mycobacterium avium*, in comparison to phagosomes which contain *Bacillus subtilis* or latex beads. *Eur. J. Cell Biol.* **68:**167–182.

39. **Desjardins, M., J. E. Celis, G. van Meer, H. Dieplinger, A. Jahraus, G. Griffiths, and L. A. Huber.** 1994. Molecular characterization of phagosomes. *J. Biol. Chem.* **269:**32194–32200.

40. **Desjardins, M., L. Huber, R. Parton, and G. Griffiths.** 1994. Biogenesis of phagolysosomes proceeds through a sequential series of interactions with the endocytic apparatus. *J. Cell Biol.* **124:** 677–688.

41. **Desjardins, M., N. Nzala, R. Corsini, and C. Rondeau.** 1997. Maturation of phagosomes is accompanied by changes in their fusion properties and size selective acquisition of solute materials from endosomes. *J. Cell. Sci.* **110:**2303–2314.

42. **Doborowski, J. M., and L. D. Sibley.** 1996. *Toxoplasma* invasion of mammalian cells is powered by the actin cytoskeleton. *Cell* **84:**933–939.

43. **Dunn, W.** 1994. Autophagy and related mechanisms of lysosome-mediated protein degradation. *Trends Cell Biol.* **4:**139–143.

44. **Dunn, W.** 1990. Studies on the mechanism of autophagy: formation of the autophagic vacuole. *J. Cell. Biol.* **110:**1923–1933.

45. **Eissenberg, L. G., and P. B. Wyrick.** 1981. Inhibition of phagolysosomal fusion is localized to the *Chlamydia psittaci*-laden vacuoles. *Infect. Immun.* **32**:880–896.

46. **Eissenberg, L. G., P. B. Wyrick, C. H. Davis, and J. W. Rumpp.** 1983. *Chlamydia psittaci* elementary body envelopes: ingestion and inhibition of lysosomal fusion. *Infect. Immun.* **40**:741–751.

47. **Enright, F.** 1990. *The Pathogenesis and Pathobiology of Brucella Infection in Domestic Animals.* CRC Press, Boca Raton, Fla.

48. **Falkow, S.** 1998. Who speaks for the microbes? *Emerg. Infect. Dis.* **4**:495–497.

49. **Feng, Y., B. Press, and A. Wandlinder-Ness.** 1995. Rab7: an important regulator of late endocytic membrane traffic. *J. Cell Biol.* **131**:1435–1452.

50. **Fields, B. S.** 1993. Interaction of a pathogen and its natural host. *In* J. M. Barbaree, R. F. Breiman, and A. P. Doufour (ed.), *Legionella: Current Status and Emerging Perspectives.* ASM Press, Washington, D.C.

51. **Finlay, B., and P. Cossart.** 1997. Exploitation of mammalian host cell functions by bacterial pathogens. *Science* **276**:718–725.

52. **Finlay, B., and S. Falkow.** 1997. Common themes in microbial pathogenesis revisited. *Microbiol. Mol. Biol. Rev.* **61**:136–139.

53. **Francis, C. L., T. A. Ryan, B. D. Jones, S. J. Smith, and S. Falkow.** 1993. Ruffles induced by *Salmonella* and other stimuli direct macropinocytosis of bacteria. *Nature* **364**:639–642.

54. **Frehel, C., C. de Chastellier, T. Lang, and N. Rastogi.** 1986. Evidence for inhibition of fusion of lysosomal and prelysosome compartments with phagosomes in macrophages infected with pathogenic *Mycobacterium avium. Infect. Immun.* **52**:252–262.

55. **Frenchick, P., R. Markham, and A. Cochrane.** 1985. Inhibition of phagosome-lysosome fusion in macrophages by soluble extracts of virulent *Brucella abortus. Am. J. Vet. Res.* **46**:332–335.

56. **Friis, R. R.** 1972. Interactions of L cells and *Chlamydia psittaci*: entry of the parasite and host responses to its development. *J. Bacteriol.* **110**:706–721.

57. **Galan, J.** 1996. Molecular genetic basis of *Salmonella* entry into host cells. *Mol. Microbiol.* **20**:263–271.

58. **Garcia-del Portillo, F., and B. B. Finlay.** 1995. Targeting of *Salmonella typhimurium* to vesicles containing lysosomal membrane glycoproteins bypasses compartments with mannose 6 phosphate receptors. *J. Cell Biol.* **129**:81–97.

59. **Garcia-del Portillo, F., and B. B. Finlay.** 1995. The varied lifestyles of intracellular pathogens within eukaryotic vacuolar compartments. *Trends Microbiol.* **3**:373–380.

60. **Gordon, A. H., P. D. Hart, and M. R. Young.** 1980. Ammonia inhibits phagosome-lysosome fusion in macrophages. *Nature* **286**:79–80.

61. **Goren, M., P. Hart, M. Young, and J. Armstrong.** 1976. Prevention of phagosome-lysosome fusion in cultured macrophages by sulfatides of *Mycobacterium tuberculosis. Proc. Natl. Acad. Sci. USA* **73**:2510–2514.

62. **Grinstein, S., A. Nanda, G. Lukacs, and O. Rotstein.** 1992. V-ATPases in phagocytic cells. *J. Exp. Biol.* **172**:179–192.

63. **Gupta, R., and G. Golding.** 1996. The origin of the eukaryotic cell. *Trends Biochem. Sci.* **21**:166–171.

64. **Haas, A.** 1998. Reprogramming the phagocytic pathway—intracellular pathogens and their vacuoles. *Mol. Membr. Biol.* **15**:103–121.

65. **Hackstadt, T., E. Fischer, M. Scidmore, D. Rockey, and R. Heizen.** 1997. Origins and functions of the chlamydial inclusion. *Trends Microbiol.* **5**:288–293.

66. **Hackstadt, T., D. D. Rockey, R. A. Heizen, and M. A. Scidmore.** 1996. *Chlamydia trachomatis* interrupts an exocytic pathway to acquire endogenously synthesized sphingomyelin in transit from the Golgi apparatus to the plasma membrane. *EMBO J.* **15**:964–977.

67. **Hackstadt, T., M. Scidmore, and D. Rockey.** 1995. Lipid metabolism in *Chlamydia trachomatis*-infected cells: directed trafficking of Golgi-derived sphingolipids to the chlamydial inclusion. *Proc. Natl. Acad. Sci. USA* **92**:4877–4881.

68. **Hale, T. L.** 1991. Genetic basis of virulence in *Shigella* species. *Microbiol. Rev.* **55**:206–224.

69. **Harding, C., R. Song, J. Griffin, J. France, M. Wick, J. Pfeifer, and H. Geuze.** 1995. Processing of bacterial antigens for presentation to class I and II MHC-restricted T lymphocytes. *Infect. Agents Dis.* **4**:1–12.

70. **Hart, P., and M. Young.** 1991. Ammonium chloride, an inhibitor of phagosome-lysosome fusion in macrophages, concurrently induces phagosome-endosome fusion, and opens a novel pathway: studies of a pathogenic *Mycobacterium* and a nonpathogenic yeast. *J. Exp. Med.* **174**:881–889.

71. **Hart, P., M. Young, M. Jordan, W. Perkins, and M. Geisow.** 1983. Chemical inhibitors of phagosome-lysosome fusion in cultured macrophages also inhibit saltatory lysosomal movements. *J. Exp. Med.* **158**:477–492.

72. **Harth, G., D. L. Clemens, and M. A. Horwitz.** 1994. Glutamine synthetase of *Mycobacterium tuberculosis*: extracellular release and characterization of its enzymatic activity. *Proc. Natl. Acad. Sci. USA* **91**:9342–9346.

73. **Heizen, R. A., M. A. Scidmore, D. D. Rockey, and T. Hackstadt.** 1996. Differential interactions with the endocytic and exocytic pathways distinguish the parasitophorous vacuoles of *Coxiella burnetii* and *Chlamydia trachomatis. Infect. Immun.* **64:**796–809.

74. **Homuth, M., P. Valentin-Weigand, M. Rohde, and G. Gerlach.** 1998. Identification and characterization of a novel extracellular ferric reductase from *Mycobacterium paratuberculosis. Infect. Immun.* **66:**710–716.

75. **Horwitz, M. A.** 1987. Characterization of avirulent mutant *Legionella pneumophila* that survive but do not multiply within human monocytes. *J. Exp. Med.* **166:**1310–1328.

76. **Horwitz, M. A.** 1983. Formation of a novel phagosome by the Legionnaires disease bacterium (*Legionella pneumophila*) in human monocytes. *J. Exp. Med.* **158:**1319–1331.

77. **Horwitz, M. A., and F. R. Maxfield.** 1984. *Legionella pneumophila* inhibits acidification of its phagosome in human monocytes. *J. Cell Biol.* **99:**1936–1943.

78. **Horwitz, M. A.** 1983. The Legionnaires disease bacterium (*Legionella pneumophila*) inhibits phagosome-lysosome fusion in human monocytes. *J. Exp. Med.* **158:**2108–2126.

79. **Horwitz, M. A.** 1984. Phagocytosis of the Legionnaires disease bacterium (*Legionella pneumophila*) occurs by a novel mechanism: engulfment within a pseudopod coil. *Cell* **36:**27–33.

80. **Hsia, R.-C., Y. Pannekoek, E. Ingerowski, and P. Bavoil.** 1997. Type III secretion genes identify a putative virulence locus of *Chlamydia. Mol. Microbiol.* **25:**351–359.

81. **Hueck, C.** 1998. Type III protein secretion systems in bacterial pathogens of animals and plants. *Microbiol. Mol. Biol. Rev.* **62:**379–433.

82. **Ishibashi, Y., and T. Arai.** 1990. Specific inhibition of phagosome-lysosome fusion in murine macrophages mediated by *Salmonella typhimurium* infection. *FEMS Microbiol. Immunol.* **64:**35–55.

83. **Jacobs, W. R., and B. R. Bloom.** 1994. Molecular genetic strategies for identifying virulence determinants of *Mycobacterium tuberculosis. In* B. R. Bloom (ed.), *Tuberculosis: Pathogenesis, Prevention and Control.* ASM Press, Washington, D.C.

84. **Jahrus, A., B. Storrie, G. Griffith, and M. Desjardins.** 1994. Evidence for retrograde traffic between terminal lysosomes and the prelysosomal/late endosomal compartment. *J. Cell Sci.* **107:**145–157.

85. **Joiner, K.** 1997. Membrane-protein traffic in pathogen infected cells. *J. Clin. Investig.* **99:**1814–1816.

86. **Joiner, K. A.** 1994. Vacuolar membranes surrounding intracellular pathogens: where do they come from and what do they do? *Infect. Agents Dis.* **2:**215–219.

87. **Lawn, A. M., W. A. Blythe, and J. Taverne.** 1973. Interactions of TRIC agents with macrophages and BHK-21 cells observed by electron microscopy. *J. Hyg.* **71:**515–528.

88. **Leung, K., and B. Finlay.** 1991. Intracellular replication is essential for virulence of *Salmonella typhimurium. Proc. Natl. Acad. Sci. USA* **88:**11470–11474.

89. **Liou, W., H. Geuze, M. Geelen, and J. Slot.** 1997. The autophagic and endocytic pathways converge at the nascent autophagic vacuoles. *J. Cell Biol.* **136:**61–70.

90. **Lipsky, N. G., and R. E. Pagano.** 1985. Intracellular translocation of fluorescent sphingolipids in cultured fibroblasts: endogenously synthesized sphingomyelin and glucocerebroside analogues pass through the Golgi apparatus en route to the plasma membrane. *J. Cell. Biol.* **100:**27–34.

91. **Maara, A., S. Blander, M. A. Horwitz, and H. A. Shuman.** 1992. Identification of a *Legionella pneumophila* locus required for intracellular multiplication in human macrophages. *Proc. Natl. Acad. Sci. USA* **89:**9607–9611.

92. **Martin, W., and M. Muller.** 1998. The hydrogen hypothesis for the first eukaryote. *Nature* **392:**37–41.

93. **Matsumoto, A.** 1988. Structural characteristics of chlamydial bodies, p. 21–45. *In* A. L. Barron (ed.), *Microbiology of Chlamydia.* CRC Press, Boca Raton, Fla.

94. **Matsumoto, A., I. Bessho, K. Uehira, and T. Suda.** 1991. Morphological studies on the association of mitochondria with chlamydial inclusions. *J. Electron Microsc.* **40:**356–363.

95. **Matzanke, B., R. Bohnke, U. Mollmann, R. Reissbrodt, V. Schunemann, and A. Trautwein.** 1997. Iron uptake and intracellular metal transfer in mycobacteria mediated by xenosiderophores. *Biometals* **10:**193–203.

96. **McClarty, G.** 1994. Chlamydiae and the biochemistry of intracellular parasitism. *Trends Microbiol.* **2:**157–164.

97. **McDade, J. E., C. C. Shepherd, D. W. Frase, T. R. Tsai, M. A. Redus, W. R. Dowdle, and the Laboratory Investigation Team.** 1977. Legionnaires disease: isolation of a bacterium and demonstration of its role in other respiratory disease. *N. Engl. J. Med.* **297:**1197–1203.

98. **Meresse, S., S. Gorvel, and P. Chavrier.** 1995. The rab7 GTPase resides on a vesicular compartment connected to lysosomes. *J. Cell Sci.* **108:**3349–3358.

99. **Miller, S.** 1991. PhoP/PhoQ: macrophage-specific modulators of Salmonella virulence? *Mol. Microbiol.* **5:**2073–2078.

100. **Mor, N., and M. Goren.** 1987. Discrepancy in assessment of phagosome-lysosome fusion with two lysosomal markers in murine macrophages infected with *Candida albicans. Infect. Immun.* **55:**1663–1667.

101. **Moulder, J. W.** 1985. Comparative biology of intracellular parasitism. *Microbiol. Rev.* **49:**298–337.

102. **Moulder, J. W.** 1991. Interactions of chlamydiae with host cells in vitro. *Microbiol. Rev.* **55:**143–190.

103. **Muller, M.** 1993. The hydrogenosome. *J. Gen. Microbiol.* **139:**2879–2889.

104. **Oh, Y. K., C. Alpuche-Aranda, E. Berthiaume, T. Jinks, S. I. Miller, and J. R. Swanson.** 1996. Rapid and complete fusion of macrophage lysosomes with phagosomes containing *Salmonella typhimurium. Infect. Immun.* **64:**3877–3883.

105. **Oh, Y. K., and J. A. Swanson.** 1996. Different fates of phagocytosed particles after delivery into macrophage lysosomes. *J. Cell Biol.* **132:**585–593.

106. **Olkonnen, V., and H. Stenmark.** 1997. The role of Rab GTPases in membrane traffic. *Int. Rev. Cytol.* **176:**1–85.

107. **Paulnock, D.** 1994. The molecular biology of macrophage activation. *Immunol. Ser.* **60:**47–62.

108. **Pfeffer, S.** 1996. Transport vesicle docking: SNAREs and associates. *Annu. Rev. Cell Dev. Biol.* **12:**441–461.

109. **Pinder, J., R. Fowler, A. Dluezewski, L. Bannister, F. Lavin, G. Mitchell, R. Wilson, and W. Gratzer.** 1998. Actomyosin motor in the merozoite of the malaria parasite *Plasmodium falciparum*: implications for red cell invasion. *J. Cell Sci.* **111:**1831–1839.

110. **Pitt, A., L. Mayorga, P. Stahl, and A. Schwartz.** 1992. Alterations in the protein composition of maturing phagosomes. *J. Clin. Investig.* **90:**1978–1983.

111. **Pitt, A., L. S. Mayorga, A. L. Schwartz, and P. D. Stahl.** 1992. Transport of phagosomal components to an endosomal compartment. *J. Biol. Chem.* **267:**126–132.

112. **Pizarro-Cerdá, J., S. Méresse, R. G. Parton, G. van der Goot, A. Sola-Landa, I. Lopez-Goñi, E. Moreno, and J.-P. Gorvel.** 1998. *Brucella abortus* transits through the autophagic pathway and replicates in the endoplasmic reticulum of nonprofessional phagocytes. *Infect. Immun.* **66:**5711–5724.

113. **Pizarro-Cerdá, J., E. Moreno, V. San-** guedolce, J.-L. Mege, and J.-P. Gorvel. 1998. Virulent *Brucella abortus* prevents lysosome fusion and is distributed within autophagosome-like compartments. *Infect. Immun.* **66:**2387–2392.

114. **Prain, C. J., and J. H. Pearce.** 1989. Ultrastructural studies on the intracellular fate of *Chlamydia psittaci* (strain GPIC) and *Chlamydia trachomatis* (strain lymphogranuloma venereum 434): modulation of intracellular events and relationship with the endocytic mechanism. *J. Gen. Microbiol.* **135:**2107–2123.

115. **Purcell, M., and H. Shuman.** 1998. The *Legionella pneumophila icmGCDJBF* genes are required for killing human macrophages. *Infect. Immun.* **66:**2245–2255.

116. **Rabinovitch, M., and P. S. T. Veras.** 1996. Cohabitation of *Leishmania amazonensis* and *Coxiella burnetii. Trends Microbiol.* **4:**158–161.

117. **Ramakrishnan, L., and S. Falkow.** 1994. *Mycobacterium marinum* persists in cultured mammalian cells in a temperature-restricted fashion. *Infect. Immun.* **62:**3222–3229.

118. **Ramakrishnan, L., R. Valdivia, J. McKerrow, and S. Falkow.** 1997. *Mycobacterium marinum* causes both long-term subclinical infection and acute disease in the leopard frog (*Rana pipiens*). *Infect. Immun.* **65:**767–773.

119. **Rathman, M., L. Barker, and S. Falkow.** 1997. The unique trafficking pattern of *Salmonella typhimurium*-containing phagosomes in murine macrophages is independent of the mechanism of bacterial entry. *Infect. Immun.* **65:**1475–1485.

120. **Rathman, M., M. D. Sjaastad, and S. Falkow.** 1996. Acidification of phagosomes containing *Salmonella typhimurium* in murine macrophages. *Infect. Immun.* **64:**2765–2773.

121. **Rikihisa, Y.** 1991. The tribe Ehrlichieae and ehrlichial disease. *Clin. Microbiol. Rev.* **4:**286–308.

122. **Ristoph, J. D., K. W. Hedlund, and S. Gowda.** 1981. Chemically defined medium for *Legionella pneumophila* growth. *J. Clin. Microbiol.* **13:**115–119.

123. **Rittig, M. G., T. Haupl, and G. R. Burmester.** 1994. Coiling phagocytosis: a way for MHC class I presentation of bacterial antigens? *Int. Arch. Allergy Immunol.* **103:**4–10.

124. **Rockey, D. D., D. Grosenbach, D. E. Hruby, M. G. Peacock, R. A. Heizen, and T. Hackstadt.** 1996. *Chlamydia psittaci* IncA is phosphorylated by the host cell and is exposed on the cytoplasmic face of the developing inclusion. *Mol. Microbiol.* **24:**21–28.

125. **Rockey, D. D., R. A. Heizen, and T. Hackstadt.** 1995. Cloning and characterization

of a *Chlamydia psittaci* gene coding for a protein localized in the inclusion membrane of infected cells. *Mol. Microbiol.* **15**:617–626.

126. **Rothman, J., and F. Wieland.** 1996. Protein sorting by transport vesicles. *Science* **272**:227.

127. **Rothman, J. E.** 1994. Mechanisms of intracellular protein transport. *Nature* **372**:55–63.

128. **Roy, C., K. Berger, and R. Isberg.** 1998. *Legionella pneumophila* DotA protein is required for early phagosome trafficking decisions that occur within minutes of bacterial uptake. *Mol. Microbiol* **28**:663–674.

129. **Russell, D. G.** 1995. Mycobacterium and Leishmania: stowaways in the endosomal network. *Trends Cell Biol.* **5**:125–128.

130. **Russell, D. G.** 1998. What does "inhibition of phagosome-lysosome fusion" really mean? *Trends Microbiol.* **6**:212–214.

131. **Russell, D. G., J. Dant, and S. Sturgill-Koszycki.** 1996. *Mycobacterium avium-* and *Mycobacterium tuberculosis*-containing vacuoles are dynamic, fusion competent vesicles that are accessible to glycosphingolipids from the host cell plasmalemma. *J. Immunol.* **156**:4764–4773.

132. **Sadosky, A. B., L. A. Wiater, and H. A. Shuman.** 1993. Identification of *Legionella pneumophila* genes required for growth within and killing of human macrophages. *Infect. Immun.* **61**:5361–5373.

133. **Schachter, J.** 1988. The intracellular life of *Chlamydia. Curr. Top. Microbiol.* **138**:109–139.

134. **Schachter, J.** 1988. Overview of human disease, p. 153–165. *In* A. L. Barron (ed.), *Microbiology of Chlamydia*. CRC Press, Boca Raton, Fla.

135. **Schaible, U., S. Sturgill-Koszycki, P. Schlesinger, and D. Russell.** 1998. The mycobactericidal activity of activated macrophages is concomitant with distinct alterations in the *Mycobacterium avium* containing phagosome. *J. Immunol.* **160**:1290–1296.

136. **Schramm, N., C. R. Bagnell, and P. B. Wyrick.** 1996. Vesicles containing *Chlamydia trachomatis* serovar L2 remain above pH 6 within HEC-1B cells. *Infect. Immun.* **64**:1208–1214.

137. **Scidmore, M. A., E. R. Fischer, and T. Hackstadt.** 1996. Sphingolipids and glycoproteins are differentially trafficked to the *Chlamydia trachomatis* inclusion. *J. Cell Biol.* **134**:363–374.

138. **Scidmore, M. A., D. D. Rockey, E. R. Fischer, R. A. Heizen, and T. Hackstadt.** 1996. Vesicular interactions of the *Chlamydia trachomatis* inclusion are determined by early protein synthesis rather than route of entry. *Infect. Immun.* **64**:5366–5372.

139. **Segal, G., M. Purcell, and H. Shuman.** 1998. Host cell killing and bacterial conjugation require overlapping sets of genes within a 22 kb region

of the *Legionella pneumophila* genome. *Proc. Natl. Acad. Sci. USA* **95**:1669–1674.

140. **Segal, G., and H. Schuman.** 1997. Characterization of a new region required for macrophage killing by *Legionella pneumophila. Infect. Immun.* **65**:5057–5066.

141. **Simons, K., and E. Ikonen.** 1997. Functional rafts in cell membranes. *Nature* **387**:569–572.

142. **Sinai, A. P., and K. A. Joiner.** 1997. Safe haven: the cell biology of nonfusogenic pathogen vacuoles. *Annu. Rev. Microbiol.* **51**:415–462.

142a. **Sinai, A. P., S. Paul, M. Rabinovitch, G. Kaplan, and K. A. Joiner.** Co-infection of fibroblasts with *Coxiella burnetii* and *Toxoplasma gondii*: to each their own. *Microbes Infect.*, in press.

143. **Sinai, A. P., P. Webster, and K. A. Joiner.** 1997. Association of host cell endoplasmic reticulum and mitochondria with the *Toxoplasma gondii* parasitophorous vacuole membrane: a high affinity interaction. *J. Cell Sci.* **110**:2117–2128.

144. **Sola-Landa, A., J. Pizzaro-Cerda, M.-J. Grillo, E. Moreno, I. Moriyou, J.-M. Blasco, J.-P. Gorvel, and I. Lopez-Goni.** 1998. A two component regulatory system playing a critical role in plant pathogens and endosymbionts is present in *Brucella abortus* and controls cell invasion and virulence. *Mol. Microbiol.* **29**:125–138.

145. **Sollner, T., S. W. Whiteheart, M. Brunner, H. Erdjument-Bromage, S. Geromanos, P. Tempst, and J. E. Rothman.** 1993. SNAP receptors implicated in vesicle targeting and fusion. *Nature* **362**:318–324.

146. **Stephens, R., S. Kalman, C. Lammel, J. Fan, R. Marathe, L. Aravind, W. Mitchell, L. Olinger, R. Tatusov, Q. Zhao, E. Koonin, and R. Davis.** 1998. Genome sequence of an obligate intracellular pathogen of humans: *Chlamydia trachomatis. Science* **282**:754–759.

147. **Stephens, R. S.** 1993. Challenge of *Chlamydia* research. *Infect. Agents Dis.* **1**:279–293.

148. **Storrie, B., and M. Desjardin.** 1996. The biogenesis of lysosomes: is it a kiss and run, continuous fusion and fission process? *Bioessays* **18**:895–903.

149. **Sturgill-Koszycki, S., U. E. Schaible, and D. G. Russell.** 1996. *Mycobacterium*-containing phagosomes are accessible to early endosomes and reflect a transitional state in normal phagosome biogenesis. *EMBO J.* **15**:6960–6968.

150. **Sturgill-Koszycki, S., P. H. Schlesinger, P. Chakraborty, P. L. Haddix, H. L. Collins, A. K. Fok, R. D. Allen, S. L. Gluck, J. Heuser, and D. G. Russell.** 1994. Lack of acidification in *Mycobacterium* phagosomes produced by exclusion of the vesicular proton ATPase. *Science* **263**:678–681.

151. **Swanson, M. S., and R. R. Isberg.** 1995. Association of *Legionella pneumophila* with the macrophage endoplasmic reticulum. *Infect. Immun.* **63:**3609–3620.

152. **Swanson, M. S., and R. R. Isberg.** 1996. Identification of *Legionella pneumophila* mutants that have aberrant intracellular fates. *Infect. Immun.* **64:**2585–2594.

153. **Taraska, T., D. M. Ward, R. S. Ajioka, P. B. Wyrick, S. R. Davis-Kaplan, C. H. Davis, and J. Kaplan.** 1996. The late chlamydia inclusion membrane is not derived from the endocytic pathway and is relatively deficient in host proteins. *Infect. Immun.* **64:**3713–3727.

154. **Tardieux, I., P. Webster, J. Ravesloot, W. Boron, J. A. Lunn, J. E. Heuser, and N. W. Andrews.** 1992. Lysosome recruitment and fusion are early events required for trypanosome invasion of mammalian cells. *Cell* **71:**1117–1130.

155. **Tavare, J., W. A. Blythe, and R. C. Ballard.** 1974. Interactions of TRIC agents with macrophages: effects on lysosomal enzymes of the cell. *J. Hyg.* **72:**297–309.

156. **Tesh, M. J., S. A. Morse, and R. D. Miller.** 1983. Intermediary metabolism in *Legionella pneumophila*: utilization of amino acids and other compounds as energy sources. *J. Bacteriol.* **154:**1104–1109.

157. **Theriot, J. A.** 1995. The cell biology of infection by intracellular bacterial pathogens. *Annu. Rev. Cell Dev. Biol.* **11:**213–239.

158. **Tilney, L. G., and D. A. Portnoy.** 1989. Actin filaments and the growth, movement and spread of the intracellular bacterial parasite, *Listeria monocytogenes. J. Cell Biol.* **109:**1597–1608.

159. **Tribby, I. I. E., R. R. Friis, and J. W. Moulder.** 1973. Effect of chloramphenicol, rifampin, and nalidixic acid on *Chlamydia psittaci* grown in L cells. *J. Infect. Dis.* **127:**155–163.

160. **Valdavia, R., and S. Falkow.** 1997. Fluorescence-based isolation of bacterial genes expressed within host cells. *Science* **277:**2007–2011.

161. **Valdavia, R., A. Hromockyj, D. Monack, L. Ramakrishnan, and S. Falkow.** 1996. Application of green fluorescent protein (GFP) in the study of host-pathogen interaction. *Gene* **173:**47–52.

162. **Veras, P., C. de Chastellier, M. Moreau, V. Villiers, M. Thibon, D. Mattei, and M. Rabinovitch.** 1994. Fusion between large phagocytic vesicles: targeting of yeast and other particulates to phagolysosomes that shelter the bacterium *Coxiella burnetii* or the protozoan *Leishmania amazonensis* in Chinese hamster ovary cells. *J. Cell Sci.* **107:**3065–3076.

163. **Veras, P., C. Moulia, C. Dauguet, C. Tunis, M. Thibon, and M. Rabinovitch.** 1995. Entry and survival of *Leishmania amazonensis* amastigotes within phagolysosome-like vacuoles that shelter *Coxiella burnetii* in Chinese hamster ovary cells. *Infect. Immun.* **63:**3502–3506.

164. **Via, L., D. Deretic, R. Ulmer, N. Hibler, L. Huber, and V. Deretic.** 1997. Arrested mycobacteria phagosome maturation is caused by a block in vesicle fusion between stages controlled by Rab5 and Rab7. *J. Biol. Chem.* **272:**13326–13331.

165. **Vogel, J., H. Andrews, S. Wong, and R. Isberg.** 1998. Conjugative transfer by the virulence system of *Legionella pneumophila. Science* **279:**873–876.

166. **Warren, W. J., and R. D. Miller.** 1979. Growth of Legionnaires disease bacterium (*Legionella pneumophila*) in chemically defined medium. *J. Gen. Microbiol.* **10:**50–55.

167. **Webster, P., J. W. Ijdo, L. M. Chicoine, and E. Fikrig.** 1998. The agent of human granulocytic ehrlichiosis resides in an endosomal compartment. *J. Clin. Investig.* **101:**1932–1941.

168. **Wiater, L., K. Dunn, F. Maxfield, and H. Shuman.** 1998. Early events in phagosome establishment are required for intracellular survival of *Legionella pneumophila. Infect. Immun.* **66:**4450–4460.

169. **Winkler, H. H.** 1990. Rickettsia species (as organisms). *Annu. Rev. Cell. Biol.* **44:**131–153.

170. **Wyrick, P. B., and E. A. Brownridge.** 1978. Growth of *Chlamydia psittaci* in macrophages. *Infect. Immun.* **19:**1054–1060.

171. **Zeichner, S. L.** 1983. Isolation and characterization of macrophage phagosomes containing infectious and heat-inactivated *Chlamydia psittaci*: two phagosomes with different intracellular behaviors. *Infect. Immun.* **40:**956–966.

172. **Zeichner, S. L.** 1982. Isolation and characterization of phagosomes containing *Chlamydia psittaci* from L cells. *Infect. Immun.* **38:**325–342.

173. **Zhu, W., J. Arceneaux, M. Beggs, B. Byers, K. Eisenach, and M. Lundrigan.** 1998. Exochelin genes in *Mycobacterium smegmatis*: identification of an ABC transporter and two non-ribosomal peptide synthetase genes. *Mol. Microbiol.* **29:**629–639.

174. **Zychlinsky, A., M. C. Prevost, and P. Sansonetti.** 1992. *Shigella flexneri* induces apoptosis in infected macrophages. *Nature* **358:**167–169.

MECHANISMS FOR ESTABLISHING PERSISTENCE: IMMUNE MODULATION

Taraz Samandari, Myron M. Levine, and Marcelo B. Sztein

4

Bacteria have long been known to evade, subvert, or interfere with the proper functioning of the immune system. With the aid of powerful new techniques and the explosion of newly discovered molecules and mechanisms involved in the generation of effective immune responses, recent findings have demonstrated a remarkable diversity of such effects and have emphasized the complex nature of the interaction between the host's defense systems and the microorganisms' determination to gain and maintain a foothold. Several recognized mechanisms of immune avoidance, such as intracellular and extracellular sequestration, antigenic variation, and the presence of antiphagocytic capsules, are discussed elsewhere (94). In this chapter, we shall examine the increasingly common scenarios in which bacteria actively modulate the immune response to ensure their persistence.

THE IMMUNE SYSTEM IN PERSPECTIVE

In order to adequately appreciate the complex and diverse mechanisms by which bacteria affect the immune system, we provide a brief description of certain aspects of the human immune response. For a more detailed description of the mechanisms underlying the generation of immune responses the reader is referred to a number of recent reviews (47, 57, 111, 130, 133).

The mechanisms of protection against infectious agents may be divided into two complementary components: innate, or natural, immunity and specific, or acquired, immunity.

The components of native immunity include, among others, physical barriers (skin and mucosal surfaces), phagocytes (e.g., neutrophils and macrophages), natural killer (NK) cells, eosinophils, circulating molecules (e.g., complement), and such cytokines as alpha interferon (IFN-α), IFN-β, tumor necrosis factor alpha (TNF-α), and several interleukins (IL). Innate immune responses are triggered by foreign antigens and microorganisms and do not increase with successive exposures. For example, macrophages express CD14, a cell surface molecule that specifically binds lipopolysaccharide (LPS) complexed to LPS-binding protein (CD refers to "cluster of differentiation" for phenotypic markers on hematopoietic cells). Following exposure to LPS and other stimuli, macrophages secrete potent immunoregulatory cytokines, including IL-1β, IL-6, IL-12, and TNF-α. In turn, these

Taraz Samandari, Myron M. Levine, and Marcelo B. Sztein, Center for Vaccine Development, Departments of Medicine and Pediatrics, University of Maryland School of Medicine, Baltimore, MD 21201.

Persistent Bacterial Infections, Edited by J. P. Nataro, M. J. Blaser, and S. Cunningham-Rundles, © 2000 ASM Press, Washington, D.C.

proinflammatory cytokines induce fever, enhance the ability of macrophages to kill phagocytosed bacteria, trigger production of other cytokines in other cells, induce the acute-phase response, and modulate the specific arm of the immune response. When bacteria are phagocytosed by macrophages and neutrophils, a number of bacterial killing mechanisms are activated, including oxygen-dependent mechanisms (superoxide [O_2^-], hydroxyl radicals [$^{\cdot}OH$], H_2O_2, and singlet oxygen [$O^{\cdot}$]; i.e., "the oxidative, or respiratory, burst") and the fusion of lysosomes bearing digestive enzymes with the phagosome. Macrophages and neutrophils express nitric oxide synthase, producing nitric oxide (NO), which is toxic for some bacteria and fungi.

In contrast to innate immunity, the effector mechanisms of acquired immunity—which include antibodies, cytotoxic T lymphocytes, and T-lymphocyte-derived cytokines (such as IFN-γ and IL-4)—are induced following exposure to antigens and increase in magnitude with successive exposure to the inciting antigens. The chief cell types involved in the specific immune response are the T and B lymphocytes.

B cells, derived from the bone marrow, are the precursors of antibody-secreting cells (plasma cells). B cells recognize antigens through immunoglobulin (Ig) receptors on their surfaces. The binding of B cells to a specific antigen leads to their clonal expansion and switching to the expression of a specific antibody isotype (e.g., IgM to IgG, -E, or -A) under the influence of cytokines derived from helper T cells, macrophages, and other cell types. Somatically mutated, high-affinity B cells form the basis for B-cell memory. Antibodies are particularly effective against extracellular microbes and neutralize microbial toxins through several mechanisms. For example, IgG binding to specific epitopes present on an infecting organism leads to opsonization and therefore increased phagocytosis. Neutrophils, macrophages, and eosinophils, but particularly NK cells, can lyse bacteria or infected cells by binding the antibody attached to a microbial antigen via an Fc receptor, a mechanism known as antibody-dependent cell-mediated cytotoxicity. The binding of human IgG1, IgG3, and IgM to microbes also activates the complement pathway, which leads to lysis, opsonization, and phagocytosis of the microorganism. Toxins are neutralized by the formation of antigen-antibody complexes. "T-dependent" antigens require antigen-induced activation of helper T cells to elicit an antibody response, while "T-independent" antigens can stimulate B cells to produce antibody without T-cell help. Most T-independent antigens are large polymeric molecules with repeated epitopes (such as polysaccharides), capable of cross-linking surface Ig.

T cells (lymphocytes which develop in the thymus), in contrast to B cells, recognize peptides derived from protein antigens that are presented on the surfaces of antigen-presenting cells (APC) in conjunction with either class I (HLA-A, -B, and -C in humans) or class II (HLA-DP, -DQ, and -DR in humans) major histocompatibility complex (MHC) molecules. T cells recognize the peptide through a T-cell receptor (TCR) specific for that antigen. The two main populations of T cells bear either CD8 or CD4 surface glycoproteins, which act as coreceptors (accessory molecules) by binding MHC class I (found in all cells) and class II molecules (found in professional APC, such as dendritic cells, macrophages, B cells, and Langerhans cells), respectively. CD4$^+$ cells (T helper [Th] cells) are mainly involved in the inflammatory response and in providing help for antibody production by B cells, and CD8$^+$ cells (T-cytotoxic [Tc] cells) comprise the majority of cytotoxic-T-lymphocyte (CTL) activity in class I MHC-restricted killing of pathogenic organisms. There are two main mechanisms of immune-mediated killing of target cells (e.g., infected cells or tumor cells): (i) secretion of the pore-forming protein perforin (used by both CD8$^+$ CTLs and NK cells) and (ii) interaction of Fas ligand (FasL) on activated CTLs with the apoptosis-inducing Fas molecule (CD95) on the target cells. When FasL on CD8$^+$ CTLs binds Fas on a target cell, a key molecule that is activated is IL-1β-converting enzyme (ICE, or caspase-1), a cysteine protease which, along with other enzymes, ultimately induces DNA fragmentation of the target cell.

Successful antigen-specific activation of T cells resulting in T-cell expansion and differentiation requires first a signal provided by the interaction of TCRs on the surfaces of T cells with MHC-antigen complexes on APC and a second, complementary signal provided by soluble factors, such as IL-2, or by the binding of CD28 to members of the B7 family on the APC that helps to stabilize the T cell-APC interactions. The activation of T cells results in the expression of new surface molecules, such as CD45RO (the activated form of CD45RA found on naïve T cells) and CD69, which is also seen in activated early B cells and monocytes.

It is important to mention that nonprotein antigens, such as microbial (particularly mycobacterial) lipid and glycolipid antigens, can be presented to T cells in a restricted fashion by nonclassical MHC molecules, such as CD1, that are differentially expressed on APC and cells of the gastrointestinal epithelium.

T-cell activation triggered by cross-linking of TCRs by antigen-MHC complexes, aided by costimulatory molecules, results in the production of a multitude of molecules with strong immunoregulatory properties, collectively known as cytokines. Cytokines are proteins produced by leukocytes (e.g., lymphocytes, APC, and NK cells), as well as by cells not typically considered part of the immune system (e.g., keratinocytes, fibroblasts, and endothelial cells). Most cytokines share a number of characteristics: (i) they may act on many cell types (pleiotropism), sometimes exerting more than one effect on a single target cell; (ii) their production following cell activation requires de novo RNA and protein synthesis and is transient; (iii) they are redundant in that similar activities are typically performed by more than one cytokine; (iv) often, production of one cytokine is followed by the release of other cytokines, producing a "cascading effect"; (v) they

regulate each other either negatively or positively; (vi) they exert their effects by interacting with high-affinity specific receptors on the target cell(s); and (vii) in most cases their effect is autocrine and/or paracrine.

Acting in concert, cytokines not only modulate the growth, maturation, and differentiation of all cells involved in the generation of the specific immune response, they also strongly regulate the innate immune responses. Cytokines that play key roles in the modulation of immune responses include IL-1, IL-2, IL-4, IL-6, IL-8, IL-10, IL-12, TNF-α, TNF-β, IFN-γ, and transforming growth factor β (TGF-β). IL-1 is principally made by macrophages and fibroblasts and induces fever, acute-phase proteins, and prostaglandin synthesis, among other effects. IL-2, produced by T cells, activates other T cells and NK cells and stimulates T- and B-cell division. IL-4 is made by Th2 cells (see below) and bone marrow stroma; it activates B cells and promotes class switching to IgG1 and IgE. IL-6 is made by macrophages, Th2 cells, and endothelial cells; it induces fever, secretion of acute-phase proteins, and the growth and differentiation of B and T cells. IL-8, produced by monocytes and other cell types, is important in chemotaxis and activation of neutrophils. IL-10 is made by Th2 cells and plays an important inhibitory role in cytokine synthesis by Th1 cells (see below). IL-12, which is made by monocytes/macrophages, induces Th1-cell development. IFN-γ, principally made by type 1 T cells, exhibits a wide variety of effects, including macrophage activation, stimulation of the differentiation of CTLs, enhancement of class I and II expression on APC, and inhibition of the generation of type 2 T cells (see below). TNF-α is secreted principally by macrophages and T cells, and TNF-β is produced by T cells. In addition to its cytotoxic effect on tumor cells, TNF-α causes the cachexia seen in some chronic diseases, induces acute-phase proteins, enhances the adhesiveness of the endothelium for leukocytes, and induces IFN-γ, IL-6, IL-1, and other cytokines. TGF-β, which is made by B and T cells among many others, is strongly inhibitory of immune responses, since it prevents proliferation of both B and T cells, induces isotype switching to IgA, and promotes wound repair and angiogenesis.

One of the single most important findings concerning protection against infectious diseases was the realization of the existence of distinct T-cell (either Th or Tc) subpopulations that exhibit discrete or overlapping patterns of cytokine production. These subsets are designated type 1 (Th1 or Tc1) and type 2 (Th2 or Tc2). Th1 cells produce IFN-γ, IL-2, and TNF-β, while Th2 cells produce IL-4, IL-5, IL-6, IL-9, IL-10, and IL-13. The majority of CD8$^+$ T cells secrete a Th1-like pattern; however, both Tc1 and Tc2 subsets mediate CTL activity.

Typically, type 1 responses are involved in cell-mediated immune responses, such as CTL activity, delayed-type hypersensitivity (DTH), antibody-dependent cell-mediated cytotoxicity, and macrophage activation, and in providing help for the production of certain Ig isotypes (IgG2a in mice and IgG1 in humans). Consequently, type 1 responses have been associated with beneficial responses in infections caused by protozoa (e.g., *Trypanosoma cruzi*), viruses (e.g., influenza virus), bacteria (e.g., *Salmonella enterica* serovar Typhi)—particularly those that are intracellular—and fungi (e.g., *Candida*). In contrast, Th1 responses have been associated with detrimental responses in helminthic infections and pathological conditions, such as autoimmune disorders and transplant rejection. Type 2 responses, on the other hand, provide help for Ig production by B cells, including IgE and IgG (IgG1 in mice and IgG4 in humans). Accordingly, type 2 responses are found to be beneficial in infections caused by helminths (e.g., *Brugia malayi*) and some bacteria (e.g., *Borrelia burgdorferi*) and detrimental in infections caused by protozoans (e.g., *Leishmania major*) and certain viruses (e.g., herpes simplex virus) and in pathological conditions, such as allergies and atopic asthma. Type 1 and type 2 responses are, to a considerable extent, mutually inhibitory phenotypes, leading to the predominance of either type 1 or type 2 responses. This is largely based on the inhibitory effects of type 1 cytokines on type 2 responses and vice versa. It should be noted that the distinction between type 1 and type 2 phenotypes is more marked in laboratory mice than in humans.

It has long been known that certain T cells are suppressive of the immune response. Whereas a distinct population of suppressor cells was once thought to exist, it is now believed that these "suppressor" T cells are sets of T cells with distinct cytokine-producing patterns that oppose or redirect the actions of other immune cells. Some T cells that are capable of producing TGF-β, which has broad antiinflammatory and immunosuppressive effects, may indeed act as suppressor T cells.

The presentation of antigens to T cells involves a series of intracellular events within APC, including generation of antigenic peptide fragments, binding of these peptides to MHC molecules to form stable peptide-MHC complexes, and transport of the complexes to the cell surface, where they can be recognized by TCRs on the surfaces of T cells. There are two main "classical" pathways of antigen processing and presentation. One of these pathways, the cytosolic pathway, associated with class I MHC molecules, is predominantly used for presentation of peptides produced endogenously in the APC, such as viral proteins, proteins secreted by intracellular bacteria (e.g., *Salmonella* serovar Typhi), tumor antigens, and self-peptides. Peptides synthesized intracellularly are sampled and degraded by a proteasome complex after being targeted for proteolysis by becoming covalently linked to ubiquitin. Small peptide fragments are then transferred into the endoplasmic reticulum by *TAP1* and *TAP2* gene products, subsequently become associated with a newly synthesized class I MHC, and are transported to the cell surface. The second classical pathway of antigen processing and presentation, the endosomal pathway, which is predominantly used for presentation of soluble exogenous antigens such as extracellular bacterial products, involves (i) the capture of the antigen by an APC, either through binding to a specific receptor or by uptake in the fluid phase by macropinocytosis; (ii) proteolytic digestion in both endosomal and lysosomal compartments; and finally, (iii) association with class II MHC molecules before expression on the cell surface. It is important to note that there are poorly understood alternative pathways in antigen processing and presentation for both class I and class II MHC molecules. For example, although live *S. enterica* serovar Typhi cannot escape the vacuole, the APC manages to present *S. enterica* serovar Typhi peptides in the context of class I MHC.

The TCR of the vast majority of T cells is a heterodimer composed of an α- and a β-chain covalently linked. Whereas the TCR is responsible for recognition and binding to the MHC-peptide antigen complex, its ability to trigger cell activation depends on noncovalent association with several CD3 proteins that reside on the T-cell surface. Most CD3 proteins have tyrosine phosphorylation motifs in their cytoplasmic tails that are phosphorylated upon TCR-MHC-peptide binding (or mitogenic stimulation) and initiate a cascade of phosphorylation events that activate such protein kinases as the MAP kinases ERK1 and ERK2. The phosphorylation activity—among other events—induces the release from intracellular stores of Ca^{2+}, which plays an essential role in the stimulation of NFAT and NF-κB transcription factors, which in turn are critical for the activation of the IL-2, IL-4, TNF-α, and IL-2 receptor α-chain (IL-2Rα) genes. Following activation of the transcription factors, a number of cell surface molecules—such as CD69, CD25 (IL-2Rα), and CD45RO—are expressed on the surface and play critical roles in the activation, differentiation, and proliferation of T cells.

If the second signal provided by accessory molecules (the first being TCR-CD3 binding) is absent, it leads to T-cell anergy. It has been discovered that CD28, which binds members of the B7 family of surface molecules on APC, is a key molecule for T-cell activation. Other such costimulatory molecules include CD5, CTLA-4, CD2, CD40L, and intercellular adhesion molecule 1 (ICAM-1, or CD54).

ICAM-1 on the Th lymphocyte binds leukocyte function-associated antigen 1 (LFA-1, or $\alpha_L\beta_2$ integrin) on APC. In addition to CD4, CD8, CD28, CTLA-4, and CD2, a growing number of other accessory (adhesion) molecules on the T-cell membrane also contribute to optimal T-cell activation by fostering closer T-cell–APC cell-cell interactions through the binding of specific ligands on APC and other cells, as well as extracellular matrices, and, in some cases, by providing additional activation signals. Because of the key role that these molecules play in regulating the trafficking of lymphocytes to peripheral tissues, they are also commonly called homing receptors. Chief among these accessory and adhesion molecules are CD40-CD40 ligand, those belonging to the integrin superfamily (e.g., CD11b [also called Mac-1], which functions to promote adhesion of monocytes and neutrophils to vascular endothelium), and selectins.

A second type of TCR, consisting of γ-δ heterodimers, is found in significant numbers in the mucosal surfaces of the gastrointestinal tract, and most do not express CD4 or CD8 molecules. The vast majority of γδ T cells do not recognize antigen peptides in the context of classical MHC I or II molecules, may directly recognize antigens without requiring antigen processing, and appear to play a significant role in protection against such organisms as *Leishmania*, *Mycobacterium*, *Plasmodium*, and *Salmonella*.

It should also be noted that superantigens are a group of bacterial and viral proteins that, without processing, trigger activation of up to 20% of T cells, including CD4$^+$ and CD8$^+$ αβ TCR, as well as γδ T cells. This activation is triggered by high-affinity binding of these superantigens to the lateral sides of class II MHC molecules on APC and to the β-chain (Vβ) of αβ T cells. Superantigens have been identified in bacteria and viruses and include staphylococcal enterotoxin A (SEA), SEB, SEC, SED, and SEE; toxic shock syndrome toxin 1 (TSST-1); toxins produced by streptococci, *Yersinia*, and *Mycoplasma*; and certain retroviral glycoproteins.

TABLE 1 Bacterial disruption of selected immune mechanisms

Immune defense mechanism	Bacteria or purified bacterial molecule
Antibody; inhibition of binding	*H. pylori, N. gonorrhoeae, N. meningitidis, H. influenzae,* protein A of *Staphylococcus, S. pneumoniae, Streptococcus sanguis, S. pyogenes, V. cholerae*
Antibody; inhibition of production	*A. actinomycetemcomitans, L. monocytogenes, N. meningitidis, P. aeruginosa, S. enterica* serovar Typhimurium, *Streptococcus mutans, S. aureus, C. trachomatis*
Antibody; polyclonal production	Endotoxin of *S. enterica* serovar Typhi, *M. leprae, Mycoplasma pneumoniae, T. pallidum*
APC; interference with antigen uptake	*H. pylori, S. enterica* serovar Typhi
APC; interference with antigen processing	*L. monocytogenes, S. flexneri, S. enterica* serovar Typhimurium
APC; interference with antigen presentation (including MHC expression)	*E. coli, L. pneumophila, L. monocytogenes, M. tuberculosis, Mycoplasma fermentans, Pasteurella haemolytica, P. aeruginosa, S. enterica* serovar Enteritidis, *S. aureus, T. pallidum*
APC; interference with costimulatory molecule presentation	*M. tuberculosis, M. avium*
APC; interference by unknown mechanism	SEA
B cell; induction of apoptosis	*A. actinomycetemcomitans,* verotoxin-producing *E. coli, Porphyromonas gingivalis, S. flexneri,* staphylococcal toxic shock syndrome toxin 1
Cell-mediated immunity; suppression of activity	*P. aeruginosa, M. leprae, V. cholerae*
Complement; interference with binding	*E. coli, N. meningitidis, N. gonorrhoeae, P. aeruginosa, S. pyogenes, S. aureus, Citrobacter freundii*
Cytokine; cleavage	*L. pneumophila, P. aeruginosa, Serratia marcescens, S. aureus, L. monocytogenes*
Cytokine; interference with binding	*Y. pestis*
Cytokine; interference by unknown mechanism	*B. burgdorferi, E. chaffeensis,* EPEC, EHEC, lactobacilli, *L. pneumophila, M. bovis, P. aeruginosa, S. enterica* serovar Typhimurium, *V. cholerae, Y. pseudotuberculosis, Y. enterocolitica, Y. pestis*
Cytokine receptor; interference	*L. monocytogenes, M. avium, Prevotella intermedia, S. enterica* serovar Typhimurium, *S. flexneri, V. cholerae*
Dendritic cell; induction of apoptosis	*L. monocytogenes*
Lymphocyte; induction of apoptosis	Gram-negative bacterial LPS, *Rickettsia tsutsugamushi*
Lymphocyte; inhibition of proliferation	*A. actinomycetemcomitans, B. fragilis, B. pertussis, B. burgdorferi, Coxiella burnetii,* EPEC, EHEC, *Fusobacterium nucleatum, H. pylori,* lactobacilli, *L. pneumophila, L. monocytogenes, M. avium, M. intracellulare-M. avium, M. leprae, M. arthritidis, P. intermedia, P. aeruginosa, S. enterica* serovar Enteritidis, *S. enterica* serovar Typhi, *S. enterica* serovar Typhimurium, *S. aureus,* SEA, SEB, SEE, *V. cholerae* exotoxin

(continued)

TABLE 1 *(continued)*

Immune defense mechanism	Bacteria or purified bacterial molecule
Macrophage; induction of apoptosis	*A. actinomycetemcomitans, B. pertussis, Burkholderia cepacia, Chlamydia psittaci, C. difficile, E. coli, L. pneumophila, Leptospira interrogans, M. avium, M. tuberculosis* (H37Ra and H37Rv), *P. aeruginosa, S. enterica* serovar Enteritidis, *S. enterica* serovar Typhimurium, *S. flexneri, S. sonnei, S. aureus, S. pyogenes, Y. enterocolitica, Y. pseudotuberculosis*
Macrophage; inhibition of induction of apoptosis	*M. bovis* BCG, *M. tuberculosis*, endotoxin-associated protein of *S. enterica* serovar Typhimurium
NK cell; inhibition of function	*S. enterica* serovar Typhimurium
Phagosome-lysosome fusion; inhibition	*Afipia felis, B. pertussis, Chlamydia, Ehrlichia, L. pneumophila, Mycobacterium kansasii, M. avium, Mycobacterium smegmatis, Mycobacterium phlei, Rickettsia, S. enterica* serovar Typhimurium, *Y. enterocolitica*
PMN; induction of apoptosis	*B. pertussis, Bartonella cepacia, E. coli, P. haemolytica*
PMN; inhibition of function	*A. actinomycetemcomitans; Bartonella henselae;* LPS of *E. coli, K. pneumoniae, V. cholerae, S. flexneri, S. enterica* serovar Typhosa and *P. aeruginosa; Neisseria; Y. enterocolitica; Y. pestis*
T cell; induction of apoptosis	Toxin A of *C. difficile, M. tuberculosis, P. gingivalis*, enterotoxins of *Staphylococcus, S. flexneri*
T cell; suppression of function	*C. trachomatis, L. monocytogenes, P. aeruginosa, L. pneumophila, P. intermedia*, LPS of *E. coli, K. pneumoniae, P. aeruginosa, S. pneumoniae, T. pallidum*

MECHANISMS OF BACTERIAL INTERFERENCE WITH THE IMMUNE SYSTEM

As complicated as the above scheme is, microbial pathogens can suppress or subvert nearly every component of the human immune system (Table 1).

Eluding Antibody Responses

Infection of mice with certain microbial pathogens results in a general reduction in the production of antibodies against nonmicrobial heterologous antigens. In *Chlamydia trachomatis* infections, this effect may be mediated by T suppressor activity (80). *Salmonella, Pseudomonas aeruginosa*, and hemolysin-bearing *Listeria monocytogenes* have also been described as producing such an effect (see below).

Specific microbial molecules may actually bind antibodies or inhibit the production of antibodies at the B-cell level. In vitro studies have shown that two M proteins of *Streptococcus pyogenes*, Arp and Sir, have high-affinity binding sites for Ig as well as the complement binding protein C4BP (132). The immunosuppressive factor of *Actinobacillus actinomycetemcomitans*, an agent of periodontal disease, inhibits B-cell proliferation, possibly through the activation of a regulatory subpopulation of B lymphocytes (126). In addition, a purified 80- to 85-kDa toxin of *A. actinomycetemcomitans* induces apoptosis of the HS-72 B-cell hybridoma by a pathway inhibitable by overexpression of Bcl-2 (107). Endo-β-N-acetylglucosamine of *Staphylococcus aureus* (138) and the pigment, pyocyanine, of *P. aeruginosa* (137) inhibit Ig secretion by B cells. The verotoxin (or Shiga-like toxin) of *Escherichia coli* may induce apoptosis of IgG and IgA B cells (82).

Outwitting the APC

Microorganisms have been shown to inhibit APC function at several points during antigen uptake, processing, and presentation. Opsonized *Treponema pallidum* is notorious for slowing macrophage phagocytosis to a greater extent than other bacteria (1). The 36- to 38-kDa porins of *Yersinia enterocolitica* have also been shown to inhibit phagocytosis (136). Indeed, *Yersinia* species possess a sophisticated array of secreted antiphagocytic factors (see below). Enteropathogenic *E. coli* (EPEC) secretes the Tir protein, which is inserted into the host cell membrane and is tyrosine phosphorylated. The Tir protein binds an EPEC outer membrane protein, intimin. Both the intimin and Tir proteins appear to be important for the inhibition of phagocytosis (36).

Since MHC molecules are critical to the presentation of antigens to T cells, another important mechanism used by certain microorganisms to inhibit the immune response is the reduction of expression of MHC in APC. Downregulation of class I and/or class II MHC molecules in APC has been described during infection with *Legionella pneumophila* (22), *L. monocytogenes* (49, 140), *Mycoplasma fermentans* (34), and *Pasteurella haemolytica* (53a). Moreover, both living and opsonized *S. enterica* serovar Enteritidis, *S. aureus*, *E. coli*, and *P. aeruginosa* reduce HLA-DQ, CD54, and CD14, leading to altered antigen presentation by macrophages in vitro (113).

Some bacteria downregulate important costimulatory, adhesion, or accessory molecules. These include mycobacteria (120, 128, 135), *Helicobacter pylori* (66, 67), *S. enterica* serovar Typhi (148), and *S. enterica* serovar Typhimurium (145). In vitro infections with *S. enterica* serovar Typhimurium, *L. monocytogenes*, and *Shigella flexneri* specifically downregulate transcription of the *mss1* gene, which is involved in the ubiquitination of class I presented antigens (123). Finally, SEB has also been shown to render APC functions defective (101).

Primarily utilizing macrophage model systems, many investigators have demonstrated the inhibition of phagolysosomal fusion by intracellular microorganisms (see chapter 3).

Alteration of Cytokine Production Patterns

One of the most important mechanisms employed by bacteria to subvert the immune system is affecting the production of, or otherwise interfering with, critical immunoregulatory cytokines and/or the expression of their receptors. An excellent recent review by Wilson et al. focused upon the disruption of cytokine patterns by bacteria (147).

It has been shown that the alkaline protease and elastase of *P. aeruginosa* specifically digest and thus inactivate recombinant human IFN-γ and TNF-α (110). *L. pneumophila* protease cleaves recombinant IL-2 (95). *Yersinia pestis* possesses an outer membrane usher protein, Caf1 A, that has specific high-affinity binding to human IL-1β (149). *S. flexneri* possesses a high-affinity TNF-α receptor. TNF-α pretreatment of *S. flexneri* increases macrophage uptake of the bacterium and invasion of HeLa cells (83). Several bacteria interfere with cytokine receptors on immune cells; examples include *Mycobacterium avium* (32), *L. monocytogenes* (27), and *Prevotella intermedia* (125). The metalloproteinase of *Serratia marcescens* cleaves IL-6 receptors from the surfaces of monocytes, as do the supernatants of *S. aureus*, *P. aeruginosa*, and *L. monocytogenes* (141). An 87-kDa protein, STI, of *S. enterica* serovar Typhimurium suppresses expression of the β and γ chains of IL-2R on T cells (89, 90), and the A subunit of cholera toxin was shown to downregulate IL-12 receptor expression on T cells (15).

Many bacteria and their toxins have been shown to inhibit the production of inflammatory cytokines, particularly IL-1, TNF-α, and IL-6. These offenders include *Ehrlichia chaffeensis* (78), *E. coli* (37, 68), *Yersinia* species (8, 13, 103, 109, 118, 119, 121), exotoxin A of *P. aeruginosa* (127), and the A subunit of cholera toxin (15). Henderson and colleagues hypothesized that since exotoxins are such potent modulators of the cytokine response, treatment may be directed against specific cytokines in bacterial infections where exotoxins play an important role or exotoxins themselves may be used therapeutically as immunomodulatory agents

(45). Production of IL-2, a key molecule involved in T-cell proliferation, has been shown to be suppressed by EPEC, *Lactobacillus* (64, 65), and *Legionella* (95).

Excessive production of certain cytokines may create a permissive environment for mycobacterial survival. Mice transgenically expressing IL-10 from the T-cell compartment are unable to clear *Mycobacterium bovis* BCG infection in spite of abundant amounts of T-cell-derived IFN-γ, suggesting that IL-10 probably mediates an inhibitory effect upon the macrophage (102). In an in vitro study, an excessive production of IL-6 secondary to BCG infection was shown to suppress T-cell responses (139).

Live *T. pallidum* reduces mitogen-stimulated IFN-γ production from rabbit splenocytes and, by an indomethacin-reversible mechanism, stimulates IL-1 production by adherent splenocytes (134). The *yop-1* gene product of *Yersinia* enables the bacterium to overcome the inhibition of invasion caused by IFN-α (17).

It is well known that parasites such as *Leishmania* cause shifts in the production of Th1 and Th2 cytokines in order to improve their survival. This might also be a mechanism used by bacteria to evade the host's immune responses. In a mouse model of *B. burgdorferi*, it was shown that CD4[+] cells and B cells in a Lyme disease-susceptible strain of mice (C3H/HeJ) produce Th2 cytokines whereas inherently disease-resistant BALB/c mice do not (150).

Inhibition of Lymphocyte Proliferation

Inhibition of mitogen-induced lymphocyte proliferation by whole live bacteria, soluble or particulate preparations of the bacteria, and sometimes purified molecules is arguably the most common observation in the literature concerning inhibition of the host's immune response. When lymphocytes—whether B or T cells—recognize a foreign antigen, they proliferate. Expansion of the pool of specific lymphocytes through proliferation is a critical event in mounting a substantive response following exposure to specific antigens. The inhibition of lymphocyte proliferation is discussed below in detail for mycobacteria, *H. pylori*, *Listeria*, *Pseudomonas*, and *Salmonella*. Inhibition of lymphocyte proliferation by many products derived from bacteria has also been reported, including the leukotoxin of periodontopathogenic *A. actinomycetemcomitans* (114); the immunosuppressive factor of this same organism, which was shown to inhibit IgG and IgM production by reducing B-cell proliferation (126); butyric, propionic, and isobutyric acids of anaerobic bacteria of subgingival plaques (30), with butyric acid exerting a selective effect on B cells (31); *Bacteroides fragilis* (116); sonicated extracts of *B. burgdorferi* (19) and *Fusobacterium nucleatum*, a cause of peritonsillar abscesses (124); a soluble T-cell mitogen, MAM, derived from *Mycoplasma arthritidis* (23); a heat-labile 50-kDa molecule of the periodontopathogenic *P. intermedia* (125); living or opsonized *S. aureus* (113); SEB (101); and *S. aureus* endo-β-*N*-acetylglucosamine (138). Finally, we have recently shown that killed whole-cell *S. flexneri* inhibits human lymphocyte proliferation in response to stimulation with heterologous antigen (148). Despite strong, specific memory cytokine responses to *Shigella* antigens, we have also observed a lack of proliferation in response to *Shigella* antigens by peripheral blood mononuclear cells (PBMC) of individuals exposed to *Shigella dysenteriae* (120a). The mechanism of this suppression of proliferation remains to be elucidated.

Apoptosis of Immune Cells

In addition to the well-known ability of many bacteria to induce cell necrosis, numerous pathogens have also been found to trigger programmed cell death in both immune and non-immune cells. By inducing apoptosis in immune cells, bacteria may gain a foothold in the host, multiply, and spread within the body.

Many investigators have examined the effects of live whole bacteria or purified molecules from bacteria on macrophage cell lines. For example, infection of the murine macrophage cell line J774.1 with the gram-negative anaerobe *A. actinomycetemcomitans* results in apoptosis by a mechanism that is dependent on cellular entry and protein phosphorylation (60). A similar effect is observed in *Leptospira interrogans* (92). Live whole *L. pneumophila* (100) was shown to induce apoptosis in a macrophage cell line, HL-60. *Y. enterocolitica* appears to impair the activation of the transcription factor NF-κB, thereby inhibiting TNF-α production and triggering apoptosis in J774A.1 macrophages (118). Purified molecules that induce apoptosis in macrophage cell lines include the leukotoxin of *A. actinomycetemcomitans* (69) and IpaB of *S. flexneri* (151). IpaB is thought to bind specifically to caspase 1, thus providing the apoptotic trigger.

The induction of apoptosis in monocytes/macrophages has been shown to be triggered by a number of bacteria or purified bacterial products in vivo, as well as in vitro in primary and short-term cultures. Bacteria able to mediate this phenomenon include live whole hemolysin⁺ and adenylate cyclase⁺ *Bordetella pertussis* (62), *Chlamydia psittaci* (by a caspase-independent mechanism) (108), *Mycobacterium tuberculosis* (61), clinical isolates of *S. flexneri* and *Shigella sonnei* (40), *S. enterica* serovar Typhimurium (99), *Y. enterocolitica* bearing a functional type III secretion pathway and the *yopP* gene (93), and *S. aureus*, *E. coli*, *P. aeruginosa*, and *S. enterica* serovar Enteritidis (7). Certain molecules may elicit activation-induced cell death in monocytes/macrophages. These include the hemolysin of *Burkholderia cepacia* (54), a 68-kDa protein of *M. avium* (44), IpaB of *Shigella* (48), and exotoxin B of *S. pyogenes* (73). APC other than macrophages have also been shown to be susceptible to apoptosis. For example, purified lysteriolysin and lysteriolysin-expressing *L. monocytogenes* isolates were shown to cause dendritic cells to undergo apoptosis (41).

Macrophage apoptosis has also been demonstrated in vivo in bronchoalveolar lavage fluids of mice intranasally infected with adenyl-ate cyclase-hemolysin⁺ *B. pertussis* (39) and by *S. flexneri* in rabbit Peyer's patches (152). *Yersinia pseudotuberculosis* YopJ mediates apoptosis in murine macrophages; when the gene is mutated, the 50% lethal dose in mice infected with the bacteria increases 64-fold (98).

Apoptosis of polymorphonuclear neutrophils (PMN) has also been observed. Bacteria and bacterial products shown to induce apoptosis of PMN include adenylate cyclase-hemolysin⁺ *B. pertussis* (39), the hemolysin of *B. cepacia* (54), the leukotoxin of *P. haemolytica* (129), and *E. coli* (143).

The induction of apoptosis in lymphocytes has also been shown in in vivo experiments. For example, LPS administered to pigs induced apoptosis in lymphocytes of the thymus and mesenteric lymph nodes and correlated with increased serum TNF-α and cortisol levels (105). Histology of lymphocytes of the lymph node and spleen demonstrated evidence of apoptosis when *Rickettsia tsutsugamushi* was administered to mice (59). When virulent *S. flexneri* was administered to rabbits, apoptosis of macrophages, B cells, and T cells was seen in the Peyer's patches (152). LPS of *Porphyromonas gingivalis*, possibly via TNF-α, induces apoptosis of Ig- and Ia-expressing B cells in mice (55). TSST-1 of *Staphylococcus* has been observed to stimulate Ig secretion of B cells at low doses but also to increase Fas expression and induce IFN-γ-dependent apoptosis of B cells at high doses (50).

In vivo, T-cell apoptosis has been described as an effect of the LPSs of gram-negative bacteria (18) and the LPS of the anaerobe *P. gingivalis* (55). When Wang et al. infected mice with *E. coli*, *Klebsiella pneumoniae*, *P. aeruginosa*, or *Streptococcus pneumoniae*, thymic atrophy was induced by all of the bacteria. There was a concomitant decrease in CD4⁺ CD8⁺ thymocytes. The onset of atrophy was slowest in *S. pneumoniae* infections. LPS by itself caused apoptosis in LPS responder mice (C3H/HeN) but not LPS nonresponder mice (C3H/HeJ). Upon further examination, these investigators showed that monoclonal antibodies directed against TNF-α completely inhibited *E. coli*-induced atrophy (142). T-cell apoptosis in the whole animal may also be induced by SEB (115).

In vitro, T-cell apoptosis has been shown to be caused by several purified bacterial molecules, including toxin A of *C. difficile*, by a TNF-α-independent mechanism (85); enterotoxin of *Staphylococcus*, by a CD11a-CD18-dependent pathway (24); and by the volatile fatty acid metabolite, butyric acid, of periodontopathogenic bacteria (74). SEA activates CD8$^+$ cells to suppress CD4$^+$-T-cell proliferation by Fas-FasL-mediated apoptosis (104). Finally, *M. tuberculosis*-reactive γδ T cells (Vγ9$^+$ Vδ2$^+$) were shown to undergo apoptosis when exposed to the live microorganism by a Fas-FasL mechanism (81, 86).

It is not always clear whether apoptosis is of benefit to the host or to the invading microorganism. Indeed, inhibition of apoptosis has been described as a mechanism of survival by mycobacteria (6, 29, 71), and the endotoxin-associated protein of *S. enterica* serovar Typhimurium appears to block monocyte apoptosis, resulting in immunostimulation (87). In certain situations the timing of programmed cell death may benefit either host or pathogen. Based upon experiments with *Salmonella* and enteroinvasive *E. coli*, Kim and colleagues suggested that a 12- to 18-h delay (compared to apoptosis of monocytes) observed in the apoptosis of human intestinal epithelial cells may serve either to allow epithelial cells to generate signals important for an inflammatory response or to permit the bacteria enough time to adapt to the intracellular environment before further invasion (63).

Disruption of Neutrophil Activity

Neutrophils (or PMN) play a crucial role in the response to bacterial infections. First, through chemotaxis, they migrate to the site of tissue injury by "sensing" soluble factors. They then ingest invading microorganisms by phagocytosis, which is optimized by bound antibody or complement. Finally, neutrophils destroy the pathogen in the phagosome by the fusion of granules containing a variety of effector proteins. A special neutrophil enzyme complex,

NADPH oxidase, generates toxic oxygen metabolites that kill phagocytosed microorganisms.

Leukotoxins, such as that produced by *A. actinomycetemcomitans*, are toxic to PMN (114). *Bartonella henselae* inhibits PMN chemotaxis, degranulation, and oxidative metabolism (35). After intravenous injection with *E. coli* LPS, rabbit PMN chemotaxis to complement (C5) is inhibited (117). In another study, endotoxins of *E. coli*, *K. pneumoniae*, *Vibrio cholerae*, *S. flexneri*, *S. enterica* serovar Typhosa, and *P. aeruginosa* were demonstrated to inhibit neutrophil chemotaxis in response to IL-8 (9). The purified porins of *Neisseria* were shown to inhibit actin polymerization, degranulation, opsonin receptor expression, and phagocytosis in human neutrophils (10). Finally, a *Yersinia* 36- to 38-kDa porin (136) and the 70-kDa secreted V antigen (144) have been shown to inhibit PMN chemotaxis.

Interference with T-Cell Function

Given the central role of T cells in the generation and maintenance of immunity, the suppression of the T-cell response is probably a key mechanism permitting persistent bacterial infection. As described above, this may be effected by stopping the APC from presenting antigen to the T cell, by inhibiting lymphocyte proliferation, by altering cytokine patterns, or by inducing apoptosis in T cells. There are also instances where bacteria exert a more specific effect upon T cells. For example, when APC are treated with listeriolysin O, a hemolysin of *Listeria*, they irreversibly inhibit antigen-specific T cells (25). *Pseudomonas* exotoxin A suppresses antigen stimulation of T cells in vitro (52). A *Legionella* protease specifically cleaves the CD4 molecule but no other T-cell surface protein (95). IL-2R and CD69, a molecule that is involved in T-cell activation, are downregulated in T cells by sonic extracts of *P. intermedia* (125). The stimulation of T suppressor activity has been noted in *C. trachomatis* (80) and the lipid A proximal inner core region of the oligosaccharide of some gram-negative bacterial LPSs (5).

In addition, memory T cells of mice that received SEB were anergized by it (79), and *B. pertussis* appears to inhibit T-cell proliferation to exogenous antigens through either its filamentous hemagglutinin or its adenylate cyclase toxin (14). Finally, the unresponsiveness of lymphocytes from patients with Q fever endocarditis (*Coxiella burnetii*) appears to be mediated by T suppressor cells that secrete a lymphokine which stimulates PGE_2 production by monocytes (70).

IMMUNE EVASION MECHANISMS OF SELECTED BACTERIA

E. coli

Several pathotypes of *E. coli* have been described, and some have been implicated in persistent diarrheal syndromes. Klapproth and coworkers have shown that lysates from EPEC and enterohemorrhagic *E. coli* (EHEC), but not from other *E. coli*, inhibit mitogen-stimulated expression of IL-2, IL-4, IL-5, and IFN-γ by human PBMC. More specifically, supernatants of EPEC were able to inhibit IL-2 and IL-5 secretion but did not affect IL-8 production or CD25 expression (64, 65). Recent observations by these investigators implicate lymphostatin, a predicted 366-kDa EPEC and EHEC gene product, as the factor that exerts this inhibitory effect upon cytokines, leading to inhibition of mitogen-induced lymphocyte proliferation (J. M. Klapproth, I. C. A. Scaletsky, B. P. McNamara, L. C. Lai, C. Malstrom, S. P. James, and M. S. Donnenberg, submitted for publication). Konig and Konig determined that at nontoxic concentrations, *E. coli* α-hemolysin depressed the spontaneous and *E. coli*-induced production of several proinflammatory cytokines: TNF-α, IL-6, and IL-1β (68). Granowitz and colleagues determined that within 6 h after human volunteers were injected intravenously with *E. coli* LPS, there was a suppression of stimulus-induced production of IL-1, TNF-α, and IL-6 in circulating CD14+ cells (monocytes) (37).

E. coli also appears to exert several effects upon neutrophils and macrophages. Goosney et al. utilized several mutant EPEC strains to describe an inhibition of phagocytosis in macrophages. This antiphagocytotic activity was dependent upon a type III secretion pathway, involved tyrosine dephosphorylation, and required intimin-Tir binding (36). Others have observed an inhibition of neutrophil chemotaxis to complement (C5) after injection of rabbits with the LPS of *E. coli* (117). Interestingly, Watson and colleagues showed that *E. coli* induces apoptosis of neutrophils via an oxygen-dependent mechanism but felt that this may be of greatest benefit to the host during gram-negative septicemia (143).

Induction of apoptosis by *E. coli* has been demonstrated not only in neutrophils but also in B cells by the Shiga-like toxin of verotoxin-elaborating *E. coli*. Verotoxin type 1 (VT1) specifically binds CD77, a human B-cell differentiation antigen which is a glycosphingolipid, globotriaosyl ceramide (Gb_3). VT1 abrogates IgG B-cell responses but not IgM B-cell or T-cell responses in vitro. Furthermore, VT1-treated pigs are immunocompromised. Thus, VT1 may target antibody-producing cells to prevent an effective immune response (82).

In summary, various investigators have demonstrated that *E. coli* exhibits an ability to inhibit production of inflammatory cytokines, suppress lymphocyte proliferation, inhibit phagocytosis, and induce apoptosis in neutrophils and B cells.

H. pylori

Several laboratories have described the inhibition of lymphocyte proliferation in response to antigens and mitogens by *H. pylori*. Chmiela and coworkers determined that cytoplasmic but not bacterial cell surface antigens completely inhibit phytohemagglutinin proliferation by human lymphocytes (20, 21). Knipp et al. determined that this effect was induced at least in part by reduction of CD25 (IL-2R) expression on CD14+ cells (monocytes). They also narrowed the cause of the antiproliferation activity to an approximately 100-kDa *H. pylori* protein, PIP (for proliferation-inhibiting protein) (66, 67). As for cytokine production, when supernatants from antral biopsies from patients infected with *H. pylori* were compared with those of healthy control subjects, it was found that both IL-10 and TNF-α were significantly elevated in the patients. The investigators speculated that IL-10 may contribute to immune suppression (12).

It is known that *H. pylori* elicits both serum and mucosal antibody responses in infected patients. However, *H. pylori* directly stained from gastric biopsy specimens demonstrated poor IgG and IgA binding, whereas cultured bacteria stained readily (26). The authors concluded that, although the reasons for the lack of antibody deposition on gastric *H. pylori* are uncertain, it might be an important mechanism used by *H. pylori* to evade the host's humoral immune response.

Using an in vitro model with a murine macrophage cell line, Wilson and colleagues determined that *H. pylori* stimulates inducible nitric oxide synthase expression and activity (146). This activity was enhanced by IFN-γ, and both LPS-dependent and -independent mechanisms contributed to this effect. Since high-output nitric oxide production is associated with immune activation and tissue injury, this manipulation of macrophages may play an important role in the pathology of *H. pylori*. This is significant, since NO overexpression has been implicated as a cause of chronic disease due to *Salmonella* and *Listeria*, as described below.

In summary, some of the major mechanisms employed by *H. pylori* to thwart the immune response are evasion of the antibody response in vivo, inhibition of lymphocyte proliferation, manipulation of cytokine responses, and increase of inducible NO synthase activity in macrophages.

Listeria

Although many gram-positive organisms have immunosuppressive effects similar to those described above for gram-negative bacteria, the best studied is the facultative anaerobe *L. monocytogenes*. *L. monocytogenes* enters the human host via the gastrointestinal tract, from which it invades the reticuloendothelial system. In immunocompromised hosts, *L. monocytogenes* can establish a chronic and often lethal disseminated infection. Although the modulation of host cell signal transduction pathways by *L. monocytogenes* is not specifically discussed in this text, a recent review is available (72).

Listeriolysin O, a secreted hemolysin, appears to give the organism several advantages with respect to the immune system. Hemolysin⁺ strains, but not hemolysin⁻ mutants, are capable of inducing a transient inhibition of antibody responses to *Listeria* in vivo, as well as to heterologous T-cell-dependent and T-cell-independent antigens (42). Another group of investigators observed that stimulation of MHC class II-dependent T cells by native antigens, but not by peptides, is inhibited upon pretreatment of APC with listeriolysin O. This inhibition was not due to a lack of processing of the antigen by APC but was the result of an irreversible inactivation of epitope-specific T cells (25). These same investigators demonstrated that both purified listeriolysin O and *L. monocytogenes* expressing listeriolysin, but not strains incapable of producing listeriolysin, induced apoptosis of dendritic cells (41).

Infection of bone marrow-derived macrophages by *L. monocytogenes* resulted in the downregulation of TNF-α receptor I (TNF-RI) and IFN-γ receptor mRNA but an upregulation of TNF-RII mRNA in a time- and dose-dependent fashion. Induction of proinflammatory cytokines, including TNF-α, took place independently of autocrine TNF-α signaling via TNF-RI. No alteration in cytokine receptor mRNA was noted with the nonpathogenic species *Listeria innocua* (27). Schwan et al. demonstrated that *L. monocytogenes* (among other bacteria) is capable of downregulating the macrophage *mss1* gene, which is involved in the ubiquitination pathway for antigen processing (123).

L. monocytogenes interferes with signal transduction pathways in macrophages. Whereas there is a transient activation of NF-κB during the adhesion of virulent as well as avirulent listeriae to the cell surface, a long-lasting NF-κB activation is effected only by virulent strains expressing the virulence genes *plcA* and *plcB*, which encode phospholipases and are associated with proteolytic degradation of IκBβ (43). NF-κB plays a central role in the transcription of cytokines that are proinflammatory and that stimulate lymphocyte activation.

The NO pathway has also been implicated as one of the mechanisms targeted by *Listeria* to subvert the host's immune system. Reactive nitrogen intermediates (RNI) such as NO are synthesized not only by neutrophils and macrophages but also by endothelial cells, mast cells, and hepatocytes. RNI exert potent antimicrobial activity against a variety of pathogens, including mycobacteria, helminths, protozoans, and fungi. When nonimmune mice were infected by intravenous injection with a sublethal dose of *L. monocytogenes*, Gregory et al. discovered that in primary infections, a marked increase in RNI occurs in parenchymal and nonparenchymal hepatocytes that actually promotes replication of the bacteria. Mice administered an inhibitor of RNI production, N^G-monomethyl-L-arginine (NMMA), exhibited 10- to 100-fold reduction in the number of *Listeria* in their livers. They observed that in vitro NMMA stimulated antigen-specific proliferation of T lymphocytes derived from *Listeria*-infected mice at concentrations that inhibited RNI production. This suggests that during primary infections *Listeria* induces such large quantities of RNI that lymphocyte proliferation is inhibited and the bacteria prolong their survival (38). MacFarlane and coworkers found that *Listeria* infection of mice resulted in a suppression of their antibody response to sheep erythrocytes that correlated with an increase in nitrite production. Treatment of splenocytes in vitro with NMMA completely reversed this inhibition of antibody production. Lymphocyte proliferation in response to mitogen was also inhibited in *Listeria*-infected mice. This response was only partially reversed by NMMA (84).

In summary, *L. monocytogenes* may induce immunosuppression in the host by targeting a wide spectrum of mechanisms, including suppression of the antibody response, interference in signal transduction pathways, inhibition of MHC class II antigen presentation, disruption of the mechanisms of antigen processing in the APC and apoptosis of APC, modulation of cytokine receptors, and upregulation of RNI.

Mycobacteria

Investigators at several laboratories have described the inhibition of lymphocyte proliferation by mycobacteria. When mice were heavily infected with *M. avium* and *Mycobacterium simiae*, their T-cell proliferation in response to mitogen and alloantigens was inhibited. Immunosuppression was also suggested in vivo by depressed DTH; however, since the mice were able to undergo regression of tumors, it was concluded that the observed immunosuppression was not a generalized phenomenon (108a). Tsuyuguchi et al. demonstrated inhibition of lymphocyte proliferation in vitro by *M. avium-Mycobacterium intracellulare* complex. These authors observed a reduced expression of accessory molecules CD11b and CD14 in monocytes (135). By examining T-cell proliferation in response to mitogens and antigens in patients with both lepromatous and tuberculoid leprosy, Kaplan and coworkers discovered that soluble or particulate preparations of *Mycobacterium leprae* inhibited lymphoproliferation in both types of patients. They further determined that lipoarabinomannan B (LAM-B) of both *M. leprae* and *M. tuberculosis* suppressed lymphoproliferation in patients with tuberculoid leprosy and suggested that this phenomenon was mediated to a certain extent by CD8$^+$ T cells (58). Others found that the phenolic glycolipid (gly-I) of *M. leprae* inhibited proliferation of lymphocytes from patients with lepromatous leprosy and also suggested that T suppressors were involved (91). Vanheyningen and colleagues found that macrophages infected with *M. bovis* BCG as well as *M. avium* 101, but not *L. monocytogenes* or *Leishmania mexicana*, were inhibited in their ability to stimulate T cells. The inhibition was not due to decreases in macrophage viability, antigen uptake, or cell surface expression of MHC class II or other accessory molecules necessary for antigen presentation. They concluded that the approximately 10,000-fold more IL-6 made by mycobacterium-infected macrophages induced this effect (139).

Mycobacterial infections have profound effects upon the regulation of cytokines. It is still controversial whether the secretion of inhibitory cytokines by macrophages or an imbalance between the inflammatory cytokine response and the protective type 1 response is the predominant mechanism that allows mycobacteria to persist in the host for extended periods of time.

Mycobacteria have also been shown to have potent effects on APC. Some mouse strains are inherently susceptible to *M. tuberculosis*, whereas other strains are inherently resistant. Saha et al. observed that after infection with *M. tuberculosis*, suppression of mitogen-induced lymphoproliferation occurred in an inherently susceptible strain of mice (BALB/c) but not in a resistant strain (C3H/HeJ). They attributed this phenomenon and the inhibition of DTH in vivo to the inability of macrophages to deliver costimulatory signals to Th cells, as demonstrated by the downregulation of B7 in BALB/c mice and not in C3H/HeJ mice (120). Other investigators have found that live, but not heat-killed, *M. tuberculosis* specifically downregulates CD1 mRNA, but not MHC class I or class II. Given that CD1 is an important molecule in the presentation of mycobacterial lipids and glycolipids, this may be an important mechanism for immune evasion by *M. tuberculosis* (128). LAM from a virulent strain of *M. tuberculosis*, but not that from a nonvirulent strain, is a much less potent activator of NF-κB in macrophages (16). Since NF-κB is a critical component in the regulation of many genes central to immune function, the ability of LAM from a virulent strain to avoid activation of the macrophage provides yet another insight into its ability to subvert APC function.

The induction or inhibition of apoptosis of macrophages by mycobacteria is controversial. Generally speaking, it was suggested that macrophage apoptosis limits growth of the microorganism (33, 97). When human alveolar macrophages are infected with either the nonvirulent H37Ra or the virulent H37Rv strain of *M. tuberculosis*, increased macrophage mortality is observed. The cytolytic mechanism was determined to be apoptosis and may be mediated at least in part by TNF-α (61). When Hayashi and colleagues treated the human monocyte cell line THP-1 with either a sonicated preparation of *M. avium* or a purified 68-kDa protein, dose-dependent apoptosis was observed. They determined that the apoptotic mechanism was dependent on the generation of free oxygen radicals (44). On the other hand, Durrbaum-Landmann and coworkers observed that infection of human monocytes from healthy donors in vitro with low numbers of viable *M. tuberculosis* H37Rv cells prevented spontaneously occurring apoptosis in monocytes (29). Investigators at the Pasteur Institute reported that both live and heat-killed *M. bovis* BCG prevented apoptosis of resting human monocytes. BCG infections were also accompanied by an impairment of the capacity of monocytes to secrete IL-10 (which induces human monocyte apoptosis) and by an induction of the capacity to secrete TNF-α (71). Infection of human alveolar macrophages with the virulent H37Rv strain of *M. tuberculosis* induces substantially less apoptosis than infection with the nonvirulent H37Ra strain. They determined that H37Rv induced an IL-10-dependent release of soluble TNF-RII, resulting in reduced TNF-α bioactivity (6).

γδ T cells are thought to play an important role in defense against mycobacterial infections (28, 75, 96). Both American and European investigators have found *M. tuberculosis* to induce apoptosis of γδ T cells. Li and coworkers found that *M. tuberculosis* antigens induced apoptosis in a large proportion of peripherally isolated $V\gamma^{9+} V\delta^{2+}$ T cells of both healthy individuals and patients with tuberculosis. They determined that the apoptosis was mediated through the Fas-FasL pathway (81). Manfredi and colleagues determined that mycobacterial antigens induce expression of FasL (CD95L) in γδ T cells which undergo apoptosis triggered by Fas[+] leukocytes (86).

In summary, the many mechanisms used by mycobacteria to evade or interfere with the host's immune response include stimulating the secretion of inhibitory cytokines, inhibiting lymphocyte proliferation, altering costimulatory and antigen-presenting molecules on the surfaces of APC, inducing apoptosis of $\gamma\delta$ T cells, and either stimulating or preventing the apoptosis of APC.

P. aeruginosa

P. aeruginosa commonly causes persistent infections in patients with cystic fibrosis (see chapter 15). Several investigators have found that P. aeruginosa or its products inhibit lymphocyte proliferation. For example, in vitro proliferation of human peripheral blood lymphocytes in response to tetanus toxoid and other antigens was shown to be inhibited by the whole live microbe. Issekutz et al. found this to be mediated by suppressor monocytes (56). When testing the effect of Pseudomonas slime extract in vivo by measuring the proliferation of murine splenocytes in response to serovar Typhimurium, Polish scientists found that the mediator of proliferation inhibition is passively transferrable to normal mice (77). Pyocyanine, a pseudomonal phenazine pigment, was shown to inhibit lymphocyte proliferation in vitro in a dose-dependent manner, reducing IL-2 production and IL-2R expression (106). Ulmer and colleagues found that the inhibition of proliferation induced by pyocyanine inhibited immune globulin secretion by B cells and found an associated increase in TNF-α and IL-1 secretion from monocytes with both LPS and pyocyanine (137). Other workers have found that exotoxin A of P. aeruginosa suppresses lymphoproliferation in vitro at nontoxic doses (127). When mice are coimmunized with exotoxin A and either T-dependent or T-independent antigens, the antibody response is suppressed in a dose-dependent fashion (51).

Investigators at several laboratories have discovered that whole Pseudomonas inhibits cell-mediated immunity in vivo. Petit and Daguet have summarized their findings, listing P. aeruginosa's ability to interfere with the nonspecific immune system—complement, neutrophils, and macrophages—as well as cell-mediated immunity, such as delayed survival of skin homografts and suppression of DTH and acquired cellular resistance to L. monocytogenes (112). Blackwood et al. injected mice with P. aeruginosa and assessed their ability to respond to L. monocytogenes. The clearance of L. monocytogenes from mouse spleens was decreased by prior Pseudomonas infection, as was DTH to a sublethal Listeria dose. P. aeruginosa administered to L. monocytogenes-sensitized mice at the time of footpad challenge was suppressive, although these mice responded normally upon reinfection. Thus, P. aeruginosa induced two types of suppression of L. monocytogenes infection: a transient suppression, affecting the DTH response to challenge but not resensitization, and a longer-lasting suppression that did not permit mice exposed to P. aeruginosa at the time of Listeria sensitization to respond to subsequent Listeria exposure (11). In attempting to model the condition of critically ill patients, Marshall and colleagues gavaged rats daily for 3 weeks with killed P. aeruginosa, Staphylococcus epidermidis, or Candida. Only animals given Pseudomonas demonstrated an impaired ability to localize a subcutaneous S. aureus challenge, suggesting an impairment of cell-mediated immunity (88).

Endotoxin from P. aeruginosa was also shown to inhibit chemotaxis to IL-8, perhaps explaining why neutrophil accumulation is suppressed in inflammatory lesions (9). An alkaline protease and an elastase elaborated by P. aeruginosa specifically inactivate human IFN-γ and TNF-α in vitro; the former cytokine is secreted by T lymphocytes and NK cells and the latter is secreted primarily by macrophages/monocytes (110). Other investigators have determined that exotoxin A of P. aeruginosa decreases TNF-α, lymphotoxin (TNF-β), and IFN-γ secretion from both macrophages and lymphocytes (127).

Apoptosis of APC and T cells is a feature of Pseudomonas infections as well. Wang and colleagues injected mice intraperitoneally with P. aeruginosa and observed thymic atrophy. The predominant cell type lost was CD4$^+$ CD8$^+$

cells (142). LPS, when given at subimmunogenic doses to animals, resulted in a negative modulation of the antibody response to polysaccharide or LPS via putative suppressor T cells (131). When monocytes were exposed to whole live *P. aeruginosa*, they underwent apoptosis 2 to 4 h after phagocytosis, whereas spontaneous apoptosis takes place at 48 h (7). Finally, Pryjma and coworkers determined that either living or opsonized *P. aeruginosa* inhibited lymphocyte proliferation to tetanus toxoid and mitogens and further observed a decrease in the expression of CD54, CD14, and HLA-DQ on the surfaces of macrophages (113).

In summary, as described above in the case of other organisms, *P. aeruginosa* demonstrates an ability to evade or suppress the immune system by a variety of mechanisms, i.e., inhibiting lymphocyte proliferation, modulating important costimulatory molecules on the APC surface, inducing apoptosis of T cells and macrophages, suppressing cytokine production, and inhibiting the efficacy of complement and neutrophils.

Salmonella

S. enterica, and especially serovar Typhi, disseminates from the gastrointestinal tract and can establish a persistent infection of the reticuloendothelial system. In both animal and human models, *Salmonella* has been described as subverting the host's immune response by a number of mechanisms.

It is well established that mice infected with serovar Typhimurium develop an immunosuppressive state manifested by poor proliferation in response to heterologous antigens and the impaired ability to mount an antibody response to sheep erythrocyte antigens (2). Huang and colleagues found this immunosuppression to be induced by a soluble factor and reversed by IL-4, but not by an excess of IL-2. Further studies showed this phenomenon to be completely reversed by NMMA, an inhibitor of nitric oxide synthase, implicating NO as the mediator of immunosuppression (53). In addition to IL-4, anti-IFN-γ monoclonal antibody was also found to reverse the observed

immunosuppression (3). Reports from the same laboratory indicated that NK cells regulate the induction of NO-mediated immunosuppression through the production of IFN-γ (122). Working with an in vitro murine splenocyte proliferation model, Matsui and coworkers isolated an 87-kDa protein, STI (for *Salmonella typhimurium*-derived inhibitor), that inhibited mitogen-induced proliferation of T lymphocytes and was associated with a defect in the IL-2R function (89, 90). Using serovar Typhimurium PhoP mutants, Wick et al. demonstrated that the PhoP-regulated gene products have the ability to decrease the processing and presentation of serovar Typhimurium antigen by macrophages (145). Schwan and Kopecko detected transcriptional downregulation of the *mss1* gene in murine J774A.1 macrophages following uptake of serovar Typhimurium. MSS1 composes the ATPase part of the 26S protease that degrades ubiquitinated proteins and thus may further contribute to the inhibition of antigen presentation by macrophages (123).

Evidence for *Salmonella*-mediated immunosuppression has also been demonstrated in humans. Using human PBMC, we have recently demonstrated that purified serovar Typhi flagellin (55 kDa) inhibit proliferation to tetanus toxoid in a dose-dependent manner. This suppression of proliferation was not dependent on NO, prostaglandins, or oxygen radicals and was not reversed by monoclonal antibodies to the inflammatory cytokines TNF-α, IL-1β, IL-6, and IL-10. We observed that the immunosuppressive effects of serovar Typhi flagellin were most likely mediated by altering macrophage presentation of antigen (tetanus toxoid) through inhibition of the uptake of soluble antigen and downregulation of the expression of CD54 (ICAM-1), a critical costimulatory molecule in APC (148). Similar mechanisms of suppression have also been reported by Pryjma and coworkers, who found a correlation between the suppression of PBMC proliferation by serovar Enteritidis and reduced expression of ICAM-1, CD14 (LPS receptor), and HLA-DQ on macrophages (113).

Salmonella has also been shown to induce apoptosis in monocytes/macrophages. Monack and colleagues showed that serovar Typhimurium stimulates activation-induced cell death in RAW264.7 macrophages and, to a greater degree, in murine bone marrow-derived macrophages, while bacterial mutants incapable of causing host cell membrane ruffling (and thus invasion) did not (99). Baran et al. demonstrated that whereas monocytes spontaneously undergo apoptosis in 48 h, serovar Enteritidis reduces this process to 2 to 4 h after phagocytosis (7). Hersh et al. have demonstrated that the secreted *Salmonella* invasin, SipB, induces apoptosis when microinjected into macrophages. Similar to its *Shigella* analog, IpaB, SipB binds caspase-1 and by this route initiates the apoptotic cascade (46). Interestingly, Mangan and coworkers showed that purified *Salmonella* endotoxin-associated protein promotes the survival of monocytes by blocking apoptosis and increasing IL-1, HLA-DR, and IL-2R expression (87). There is heated debate regarding the evasion of the immune system in *Salmonella* via inhibition of phagolysosomal fusion. A thorough discussion of this subject has been included in chapter 3.

In summary, a considerable body of evidence indicates that *Salmonella* inhibits lymphocyte proliferation (and thus potentially both cellular and humoral immunity) by acting primarily on antigen-presenting cells (monocytes/macrophages). Antigen uptake, antigen processing (via ubiquitination), and antigen presentation, including MHC class II, LPS receptor expression, and expression of costimulatory molecules, can all be affected by the bacterium. A high level of NO production by macrophages stimulated by IFN-γ from NK cells may also contribute to *Salmonella*-induced immunosuppression.

Yersinia

Y. pseudotuberculosis and, to a lesser extent, *Y. enterocolitica* can induce persistent infections and have become prototypical bacterial immune modulators. Most of the previously described mechanisms of immune subversion by *Yersinia* have depended on its ability to overcome inflammatory cytokines, particularly TNF-α. Importantly, this has been demonstrated in several laboratories to be advantageous to the microbe in vivo, as described below.

The *Yersinia* plasmid-encoded Yop virulon enables extracellularly adhering bacteria to inject toxic effector proteins, which are encoded by the so-called Lcr (for low-calcium response) plasmid. The Yop virulon includes a type III secretion system (Ysc), at least two translocator proteins (YopB and YopD), and a set of intracellular Yop effectors (YopE, YopH, YopO, YopM, YopP, and probably others). YopB, a secreted 41-kDa protein of *Y. enterocolitica*, suppresses TNF-α transcription and secretion in macrophages but not IL-1 or IL-6 production. Administration of anti-YopB antiserum to mice prior to infection with *Y. enterocolitica* increased TNF activity levels in Peyer's patches and coincided with a reduction in bacterial growth (8). In the J774A.1 murine macrophage cell line, Ruckdeschel and coworkers have shown that *Y. enterocolitica* deactivates MAP kinase, causing a decrease in TNF-α transcription and release (119). They demonstrated further that the activation of the transcription activator NF-κB was impaired by the virulent organism, leading to inhibition of TNF-α release (118). Using *yopP* (called *yopJ* in *Y. pseudotuberculosis*) knockout mutants in the same model system, Boland et al. showed that YopP was responsible for inhibition of the MAP kinase ERK-2 and of TNF-α release (13). Two other groups have demonstrated the importance of the *yopJ-yopP* locus in the inhibition of inflammatory cytokines. In *Y. pseudotuberculosis*, the *yopJ* locus mediates inhibition of NF-κB activation and cytokine expression, leading to greatly reduced inflammatory responses (121). In a murine macrophage cell line, the *yopJ* locus downregulates MAP kinases and inhibits TNF-α (109). Although its significance remains unknown, *Y. pestis* elaborates an outer membrane usher protein, Caf1A, that demonstrates specific high-affinity binding of human IL-1β (149).

Several investigators have noted that the

Yersinia immune assault is not limited to the inhibition of inflammatory cytokine transcription and release but may also trigger apoptosis of macrophages. Apoptosis has been demonstrated in the infection of a murine macrophage cell line by *Y. enterocolitica* (118). Additionally, it has been discovered that this process requires functional type III secretion and translocation and involves YopP, presumably acting as the effector protein (93). YopP bears a high sequence similarity to AvrRxv, a virulence protein from a plant-pathogenic bacterium. Apoptosis of macrophages was observed in the lymph nodes and spleens of mice infected with *Y. pseudotuberculosis*. The oral 50% lethal dose for a YopJ mutant *Y. pseudotuberculosis* increased 64-fold compared with that of the wild type, and it was unable to induce apoptosis above background levels (98).

Yersinia has a sophisticated antiphagocytic defense mediated by the Ysc secretion system. YopH is directly antiphagocytic via dephosphorylation of cytoskeletal proteins (4). The suppressor effect on TNF-α production, accompanied by a lack of TNF-α mRNA, is distinct from the ability of *Y. enterocolitica* to resist phagocytosis (119). Preincubation of human neutrophils and monocytes with 36- to 38-kDa porins led to an inhibition of phagocytosis and phagosome-lysosome fusion and enhanced nitrite production. Furthermore, these *Yersinia* porins inhibited chemotaxis and adherence (136). V antigen, a secreted protein encoded by the Lcr plasmid of *Yersinia* species, was shown to inhibit PMN chemotaxis and migration both in vivo and in vitro (144).

In summary, *Yersinia* has been demonstrated to inhibit the functions of PMN, to overcome the effects of cytokines that prevent host cell invasion, and to downregulate inflammatory-cytokine transcription and release by macrophages, as well as to induce apoptosis of APC.

CONCLUSIONS

Virtually all the major components of the immune system may be affected by pathogenic microorganisms. These diverse mechanisms of immune subversion are not limited to intracellular or extracellular, gram-negative or gram-positive, aerobic or anaerobic bacteria. In fact, for each bacterial species examined here, multiple and diverse components required for an effective immune response have been shown to be disrupted.

The vast majority of mechanisms described above have been demonstrated in vitro. It remains to be proven whether one or more of these mechanisms of immune interference are clinically important. Indeed, in only a handful of cases have these mechanisms been demonstrated to promote bacterial survival in vivo. Future studies, perhaps with volunteers, will help establish the validity of these observations.

Through an in-depth examination of the mechanisms used by our microbial adversaries to evade or otherwise subvert the host's immune response, we may be able to devise more effective live vaccines and develop novel therapeutic strategies for the treatment of persistent infections, as well as to discover valuable immunomodulatory agents.

REFERENCES

1. **Alder, J. D., L. Friess, M. Tengowski, and R. F. Schell.** 1990. Phagocytosis of opsonized *Treponema pallidum* subsp. *pallidum* proceeds slowly. *Infect. Immun.* **58:**1167–1173.
2. **al-Ramadi, B. K., Y. W. Chen, J. J. J. Meissler, and T. K. Eisenstein.** 1991. Immunosuppression induced by attenuated *Salmonella.* Reversal by IL-4. *J. Immunol.* **147:**1954–1961.
3. **al-Ramadi, B. K., J. J. J. Meissler, D. Huang, and T. K. Eisenstein.** 1992. Immunosuppression induced by nitric oxide and its inhibition by interleukin-4. *Eur. J. Immunol.* **22:**2249–2254.
4. **Andersson, K., N. Carballeira, K. E. Magnusson, C. Persson, O. Stendahl, H. Wolf-Watz, and M. Fallman.** 1996. YopH of *Yersinia pseudotuberculosis* interrupts early phosphotyrosine signalling associated with phagocytosis. *Mol. Microbiol.* **20:**1057–1069.
5. **Baker, P. J., T. Hraba, C. E. Taylor, P. W. Stashak, M. B. Fauntleroy, U. Zahringer, K. Takayama, T. R. Sievert, X. Hronowski, and R. J. Cotter.** 1994. Molecular structures that influence the immunomodulatory properties of the lipid A and inner core region oligosaccharides of bacterial lipopolysaccharides. *Infect. Immun.* **62:**2257–2269.
6. **Balcewicz-Sablinska, M. K., J. Keane, H. Kornfeld, and H. G. Remold.** 1998. Patho-

genic *Mycobacterium tuberculosis* evades apoptosis of host macrophages by release of TNF-R2, resulting in inactivation of TNF-alpha. *J. Immunol.* **161:** 2636–2641.

7. **Baran, J., K. Guzik, W. Hryniewicz, M. Ernst, H. D. Flad, and J. Pryjma.** 1996. Apoptosis of monocytes and prolonged survival of granulocytes as a result of phagocytosis of bacteria. *Infect. Immun.* **64:**4242–4248.

8. **Beuscher, H. U., F. Rodel, A. Forsberg, and M. Rollinghoff.** 1995. Bacterial evasion of host immune defense: *Yersinia enterocolitica* encodes a suppressor for tumor necrosis factor alpha expression. *Infect. Immun.* **63:**1270–1277.

9. **Bignold, L. P., S. D. Rogers, T. M. Siaw, and J. Bahnisch.** 1991. Inhibition of chemotaxis of neutrophil leukocytes to interleukin-8 by endotoxins of various bacteria. *Infect. Immun.* **59:** 4255–4258.

10. **Bjerknes, R., H. K. Guttormsen, C. O. Solberg, and L. M. Wetzler.** 1995. Neisserial porins inhibit human neutrophil actin polymerization, degranulation, opsonin receptor expression, and phagocytosis but prime the neutrophils to increase their oxidative burst. *Infect. Immun.* **63:** 160–167.

11. **Blackwood, L. L., T. Lin, and J. I. Rowe.** 1987. Suppression of the delayed-type hypersensitivity and cell-mediated immune responses to *Listeria monocytogenes* induced by *Pseudomonas aeruginosa*. *Infect. Immun.* **55:**639–644.

12. **Bodger, K., J. I. Wyatt, and R. V. Heatley.** 1997. Gastric mucosal secretion of interleukin-10: relations to histopathology, *Helicobacter pylori* status, and tumour necrosis factor-alpha secretion. *Gut* **40:**739–744.

13. **Boland, A., and G. R. Cornelis.** 1998. Role of YopP in suppression of tumor necrosis factor alpha release by macrophages during *Yersinia* infection. *Infect. Immun.* **66:**1878–1884.

14. **Boschwitz, J. S., J. W. Batanghari, H. Kedem, and D. A. Relman.** 1997. *Bordetella pertussis* infection of human monocytes inhibits antigen-dependent CD4 T cell proliferation. *J. Infect. Dis.* **176:**678–686.

15. **Braun, M. C., J. He, C. Y. Wu, and B. L. Kelsall.** 1999. Cholera toxin suppresses interleukin (IL)-12 production and IL-12 receptor beta1 and beta2 chain expression. *J. Exp. Med.* **189:** 541–552.

16. **Brown, M. C., and S. M. Taffet.** 1995. Lipoarabinomannans derived from different strains of *Mycobacterium tuberculosis* differentially stimulate the activation of NF-κB and KBF1 in murine macrophages. *Infect. Immun.* **63:**1960–1968.

17. **Bukholm, G., G. Kapperud, and M. Skurnik.** 1990. Genetic evidence that the *yopA* gene-en-

coded *Yersinia* outer membrane protein Yop1 mediates inhibition of the anti-invasive effect of interferon. *Infect. Immun.* **58:**2245–2251.

18. **Castro, A., V. Bemer, A. Nobrega, A. Coutinho, and P. Truffa-Bachi.** 1998. Administration to mouse of endotoxin from gram-negative bacteria leads to activation and apoptosis of T lymphocytes. *Eur. J. Immunol.* **28:**488–495.

19. **Chiao, J. W., C. Pavia, M. Riley, W. Altmann-Lasekan, M. Abolhassani, K. Liegner, and A. Mittelman.** 1994. Antigens of Lyme disease of spirochaete *Borrelia burgdorferi* inhibits antigen or mitogen-induced lymphocyte proliferation. *FEMS Immunol. Med. Microbiol.* **8:**151–155.

20. **Chmiela, M., J. A. Lelwala-Guruge, T. Wadstrom, and W. Rudnicka.** 1996. The stimulation and inhibition of T cell proliferation by *Helicobacter pylori* components. *J. Physiol. Pharmacol.* **47:**195–202.

21. **Chmiela, M., B. Paziak-Domanska, A. Ljungh, T. Wadstrom, and W. Rudnicka.** 1996. The proliferation of human T lymphocytes stimulated by *Helicobacter pylori* antigens. *Immunobiology* **195:**199–208.

22. **Clemens, D. L., and M. A. Horwitz.** 1993. Hypoexpression of major histocompatibility complex molecules on *Legionella pneumophila* phagosomes and phagolysosomes. *Infect. Immun.* **61:** 2803–2812.

23. **Cole, B. C., and D. J. Wells.** 1990. Immunosuppressive properties of the *Mycoplasma arthritidis* T-cell mitogen in vivo: inhibition of proliferative responses to T-cell mitogens. *Infect. Immun.* **58:** 228–236.

24. **Damle, N. K., G. Leytze, K. Klussman, and J. A. Ledbetter.** 1993. Activation with superantigens induces programmed death in antigen-primed CD4+ class II+ major histocompatibility complex T lymphocytes via a CD11a/CD18-dependent mechanism. *Eur. J. Immunol.* **23:** 1513–1522.

25. **Darji, A., B. Stockinger, J. Wehland, T. Chakraborty, and S. Weiss.** 1997. Antigen-specific T cell receptor antagonism by antigen-presenting cells treated with the hemolysin of *Listeria monocytogenes*: a novel type of immune escape. *Eur. J. Immunol.* **27:**1696–1703.

26. **Darwin, P. E., M. B. Sztein, Q. X. Zheng, S. P. James, and G. T. Fantry.** 1996. Immune evasion by *Helicobacter pylori*: gastric spiral bacteria lack surface immunoglobulin deposition and reactivity with homologous antibodies. *Helicobacter* **1:** 20–27.

27. **Demuth, A., W. Goebel, H. U. Beuscher, and M. Kuhn.** 1996. Differential regulation of cytokine and cytokine receptor mRNA expression upon infection of bone marrow-derived

macrophages with *Listeria monocytogenes*. *Infect. Immun.* **64**:3475–3483.

28. **D'Souza, C. D., A. M. Cooper, A. A. Frank, R. J. Mazzaccaro, B. R. Bloom, and I. M. Orme.** 1997. An anti-inflammatory role for gamma delta T lymphocytes in acquired immunity to *Mycobacterium tuberculosis*. *J. Immunol.* **158**: 1217–1221.

29. **Durrbaum-Landmann, I., J. Gercken, H. D. Flad, and M. Ernst.** 1996. Effect of in vitro infection of human monocytes with low numbers of *Mycobacterium tuberculosis* bacteria on monocyte apoptosis. *Infect. Immun.* **64**:5384–5389.

30. **Eftimiadi, C., P. Stashenko, M. Tonetti, P. E. Mangiante, R. Massara, S. Zupo, and M. Ferrarini.** 1991. Divergent effect of the anaerobic bacteria by-product butyric acid on the immune response: suppression of T-lymphocyte proliferation and stimulation of interleukin-1 beta production. *Oral Microbiol. Immunol.* **6**:17–23.

31. **Eftimiadi, C., S. Valente, S. Mangiante, and M. Ferrarini.** 1995. Butyric acid, a metabolic end product of anaerobic bacteria, inhibits B-lymphocyte function. *Minerva Stomatol.* **44**:445–447.

32. **Eriks, I. S., and C. L. Emerson.** 1997. Temporal effect of tumor necrosis factor alpha on murine macrophages infected with *Mycobacterium avium*. *Infect. Immun.* **65**:2100–2106.

33. **Fratazzi, C., R. D. Arbeit, C. Carini, and H. G. Remold.** 1997. Programmed cell death of *Mycobacterium avium* serovar 4-infected human macrophages prevents the mycobacteria from spreading and induces mycobacterial growth inhibition by freshly added, uninfected macrophages. *J. Immunol.* **158**:4320–4327.

34. **Frisch, M., G. Gradehandt, and P. F. Muhlradt.** 1996. *Mycoplasma fermentans*-derived lipid inhibits class II major histocompatibility complex expression without mediation by interleukin-6, interleukin-10, tumor necrosis factor, transforming growth factor-beta, type I interferon, prostaglandins or nitric oxide. *Eur. J. Immunol.* **26**: 1050–1057.

35. **Fumarola, D., S. Pece, R. Fumarulo, R. Petruzzelli, B. Greco, G. Giuliani, A. B. Maffione, and E. Jirillo.** 1994. Downregulation of human polymorphonuclear cell activities exerted by microorganisms belonging to the alpha-2 subgroup of *Proteobacteria* (*Afipia felis* and *Rochalimaea henselae*). *Immunopharmacol. Immunotoxicol.* **16**:449–461.

36. **Goosney, D. L., J. Celli, B. Kenny, and B. B. Finlay.** 1999. Enteropathogenic *Escherichia coli* inhibits phagocytosis. *Infect. Immun.* **67**:490–495.

37. **Granowitz, E. V., R. Porat, J. W. Mier, S. F. Orencole, G. Kaplanski, E. A. Lynch, K. Ye, E. Vannier, S. M. Wolff, and C. A. Dinarello.** 1993. Intravenous endotoxin suppresses the cytokine response of peripheral blood mononuclear cells of healthy humans. *J. Immunol.* **151**: 1637–1645.

38. **Gregory, S. H., E. J. Wing, R. A. Hoffman, and R. L. Simmons.** 1993. Reactive nitrogen intermediates suppress the primary immunologic response to *Listeria*. *J. Immunol.* **150**:2901–2909.

39. **Gueirard, P., A. Druilhe, M. Pretolani, and N. Guiso.** 1998. Role of adenylate cyclase-hemolysin in alveolar macrophage apoptosis during *Bordetella pertussis* infection in vivo. *Infect. Immun.* **66**:1718–1725.

40. **Guichon, A., and A. Zychlinsky.** 1997. Clinical isolates of *Shigella* species induce apoptosis in macrophages. *J. Infect. Dis.* **175**:470–473.

41. **Guzman, C. A., E. Domann, M. Rohde, D. Bruder, A. Darji, S. Weiss, J. Wehland, T. Chakraborty, and K. N. Timmis.** 1996. Apoptosis of mouse dendritic cells is triggered by listeriolysin, the major virulence determinant of *Listeria monocytogenes*. *Mol. Microbiol.* **20**:119–126.

42. **Hage-Chahine, C. M., G. Del Giudice, P. H. Lambert, and J. C. Pechere.** 1992. Hemolysin-producing *Listeria monocytogenes* affects the immune response to T-cell-dependent and T-cell-independent antigens. *Infect. Immun.* **60**: 1415–1421.

43. **Hauf, N., W. Goebel, F. Fiedler, Z. Sokolovic, and M. Kuhn.** 1997. *Listeria monocytogenes* infection of P388D1 macrophages results in a biphasic NF-kappaB (RelA/p50) activation induced by lipoteichoic acid and bacterial phospholipases and mediated by IkappaBalpha and IkappaBbeta degradation. *Proc. Natl. Acad. Sci. USA* **94**: 9394–9399.

44. **Hayashi, T., A. Catanzaro, and S. P. Rao.** 1997. Apoptosis of human monocytes and macrophages by *Mycobacterium avium* sonicate. *Infect. Immun.* **65**:5262–5271.

45. **Henderson, B., M. Wilson, and B. Wren.** 1997. Are bacterial exotoxins cytokine network regulators? *Trends. Microbiol.* **5**:454–458.

46. **Hersh, D., D. M. Monack, M. R. Smith, N. Ghori, S. Falkow, and A. Zychlinsky.** 1999. The *Salmonella* invasin SipB induces macrophage apoptosis by binding to caspase-1. *Proc. Natl. Acad. Sci. USA* **96**:2396–2401.

47. **Herzenberg, L. A., D. M. Weir, and C. Blackwell.** 1996. *Weir's Handbook of Experimental Immunology*. Blackwell Science, Inc., Cambridge, Mass.

48. **Hilbi, H., Y. Chen, K. Thirumalai, and A. Zychlinsky.** 1997. The interleukin 1β-converting enzyme, caspase 1, is activated during *Shigella flexneri*-induced apoptosis in human monocyte-

derived macrophages. *Infect. Immun.* **65:** 5165–5170.

49. **Hiltbold, E. M., and H. K. Ziegler.** 1996. Interferon-gamma and interleukin-10 have cross-regulatory roles in modulating the class I and class II MHC-mediated presentation of epitopes of *Listeria monocytogenes* by infected macrophages. *J. Interferon Cytokine Res.* **16:**547–554.

50. **Hofer, M. F., K. Newell, R. C. Duke, P. M. Schlievert, J. H. Freed, and D. Y. Leung.** 1996. Differential effects of staphylococcal toxic shock syndrome toxin-1 on B cell apoptosis. *Proc. Natl. Acad. Sci. USA* **93:**5425–5430.

51. **Holt, P. S., and M. L. Misfeldt.** 1984. Alteration of murine immune response by *Pseudomonas aeruginosa* exotoxin A. *Infect. Immun.* **45:**227–233.

52. **Holt, P. S., and M. L. Misfeldt.** 1986. Variables which affect suppression of the immune response induced by *Pseudomonas aeruginosa* exotoxin A. *Infect. Immun.* **52:**96–100.

53. **Huang, D., M. G. Schwacha, and T. K. Eisenstein.** 1996. Attenuated *Salmonella* vaccine-induced suppression of murine spleen cell responses to mitogen is mediated by macrophage nitric oxide: quantitative aspects. *Infect. Immun.* **64:**3786–3792.

53a.**Hughes, H. P., M. Campos, L. McDougall, T. K. Beskorwayne, A. A. Potter, and L. A. Babiuk.** 1994. Regulation of major histocompatibility complex class II expression by *Pasteurella haemolytica* leukotoxin. *Infect. Immun.* **62:** 1609–1615.

54. **Hutchison, M. L., I. R. Poxton, and J. R. Govan.** 1998. *Burkholderia cepacia* produces a hemolysin that is capable of inducing apoptosis and degranulation of mammalian phagocytes. *Infect. Immun.* **66:**2033–2039.

55. **Isogai, E., H. Isogal, K. Kimura, N. Fujii, S. Takagi, K. Hirose, and M. Hayashi.** 1996. In vivo induction of apoptosis and immune responses in mice by administration of lipopolysaccharide from *Porphyromonas gingivalis*. *Infect. Immun.* **64:** 1461–1466.

56. **Issekutz, T. B., and J. M. Stoltz.** 1985. Suppression of lymphocyte proliferation by *Pseudomonas aeruginosa*: mediation by *Pseudomonas*-activated suppressor monocytes. *Infect. Immun.* **48:** 832–838.

57. **Janeway, C. A., P. Travers, M. Walport, and J. D. Capra.** 1999. *Immunobiology: the Immune System in Health and Disease.* Elsevier Science, Ltd., London, United Kingdom.

58. **Kaplan, G., R. R. Gandhi, D. E. Weinstein, W. R. Levis, M. E. Patarroyo, P. J. Brennan, and Z. A. Cohn.** 1987. *Mycobacterium leprae* antigen-induced suppression of T cell proliferation in vitro. *J. Immunol.* **138:**3028–3034.

59. **Kasuya, S., I. Nagano, T. Ikeda, C. Goto, K. Shimokawa, and Y. Takahashi.** 1996. Apoptosis of lymphocytes in mice induced by infection with *Rickettsia tsutsugamushi*. *Infect. Immun.* **64:**3937–3941.

60. **Kato, S., M. Muro, S. Akifusa, N. Hanada, I. Semba, T. Fujii, Y. Kowashi, and T. Nishihara.** 1995. Evidence for apoptosis of murine macrophages by *Actinobacillus actinomycetemcomitans* infection. *Infect. Immun.* **63:**3914–3919.

61. **Keane, J., M. K. Balcewicz-Sablinska, H. G. Remold, G. L. Chupp, B. B. Meek, M. J. Fenton, and H. Kornfeld.** 1997. Infection by *Mycobacterium tuberculosis* promotes human alveolar macrophage apoptosis. *Infect. Immun.* **65:** 298–304.

62. **Khelef, N., A. Zychlinsky, and N. Guiso.** 1993. *Bordetella pertussis* induces apoptosis in macrophages: role of adenylate cyclase-hemolysin. *Infect. Immun.* **61:**4064–4071.

63. **Kim, J. M., L. Eckmann, T. C. Savidge, D. C. Lowe, T. Witthoft, and M. F. Kagnoff.** 1998. Apoptosis of human intestinal epithelial cells after bacterial invasion. *J. Clin. Investig.* **102:** 1815–1823.

64. **Klapproth, J. M., M. S. Donnenberg, J. M. Abraham, and S. P. James.** 1996. Products of enteropathogenic *E. coli* inhibit lymphokine production by gastrointestinal lymphocytes. *Am. J. Physiol.* **271:**G841–G848.

65. **Klapproth, J. M., M. S. Donnenberg, J. M. Abraham, H. L. Mobley, and S. P. James.** 1995. Products of enteropathogenic *Escherichia coli* inhibit lymphocyte activation and lymphokine production. *Infect. Immun.* **63:**2248–2254.

66. **Knipp, U., S. Birkholz, W. Kaup, K. Mahnke, and W. Opferkuch.** 1994. Suppression of human mononuclear cell response by *Helicobacter pylori*: effects on isolated monocytes and lymphocytes. *FEMS Immunol. Med. Microbiol.* **8:**157–166.

67. **Knipp, U., S. Birkholz, W. Kaup, and W. Opferkuch.** 1996. Partial characterization of a cell proliferation-inhibiting protein produced by *Helicobacter pylori*. *Infect. Immun.* **64:**3491–3496.

68. **Konig, B., and W. Konig.** 1993. Induction and suppression of cytokine release (tumour necrosis factor-alpha; interleukin-6, interleukin-1 beta) by *Escherichia coli* pathogenicity factors (adhesins, alpha-haemolysin). *Immunology* **78:**526–533.

69. **Korostoff, J., J. F. Wang, I. Kieba, M. Miller, B. J. Shenker, and E. T. Lally.** 1998. *Actinobacillus actinomycetemcomitans* leukotoxin induces apoptosis in HL-60 cells. *Infect. Immun.* **66:** 4474–4483.

70. **Koster, F. T., J. C. Williams, and J. S. Goodwin.** 1985. Cellular immunity in Q fever: modu-

lation of responsiveness by a suppressor T cell-monocyte circuit. *J. Immunol.* **135**:1067–1072.

71. **Kremer, L., J. Estaquier, E. Brandt, J. C. Ameisen, and C. Locht.** 1997. *Mycobacterium bovis* Bacillus Calmette Guerin infection prevents apoptosis of resting human monocytes. *Eur. J. Immunol.* **27**:2450–2456.

72. **Kuhn, M., and W. Goebel.** 1998. Host cell signalling during *Listeria monocytogenes* infection. *Trends Microbiol.* **6**:11–15.

73. **Kuo, C. F., J. J. Wu, P. J. Tsai, F. J. Kao, H. Y. Lei, M. T. Lin, and Y. S. Lin.** 1999. Streptococcal pyrogenic exotoxin B induces apoptosis and reduces phagocytic activity in U937 cells. *Infect. Immun.* **67**:126–130.

74. **Kurita-Ochiai, T., K. Fukushima, and K. Ochiai.** 1997. Butyric acid-induced apoptosis of murine thymocytes, splenic T cells, and human Jurkat T cells. *Infect. Immun.* **65**:35–41.

75. **Ladel, C. H., C. Blum, A. Dreher, K. Reifenberg, and S. H. Kaufmann.** 1995. Protective role of gamma/delta T cells and alpha/beta T cells in tuberculosis *Eur. J. Immunol.* **25**: 2877–2881. (Erratum, **25**:3525.)

76. **Laffineur, E., N. Genetet, and J. Leonil.** 1996. Immunomodulatory activity of beta-casein permeate medium fermented by lactic acid bacteria. *J. Dairy. Sci.* **79**:2112–2120.

77. **Lagowska-Zlotorzycka, M., A. Czarny, and M. Mulczyk.** 1987. Effect of slime extract from *Pseudomonas aeruginosa* on cell mediated immunity induced in mice by Salmonella typhimurium. *Arch. Immunol. Ther. Exp.* **35**:277–281.

78. **Lee, E. H., and Y. Rikihisa.** 1996. Absence of tumor necrosis factor alpha, interleukin-6 (IL-6), and granulocyte-macrophage colony-stimulating factor expression but presence of IL-1β, IL-8, and IL-10 expression in human monocytes exposed to viable or killed *Ehrlichia chaffeensis. Infect. Immun.* **64**:4211–4219.

79. **Lee, W. T., and E. S. Vitetta.** 1992. Memory T cells are anergic to the superantigen staphylococcal enterotoxin B. *J. Exp. Med.* **176**:575–579.

80. **Levitt, D., and R. Corlett.** 1988. Patterns of immunoenhancement and suppression induced by *Chlamydia trachomatis* in vivo and in vitro. *J. Immunol.* **140**:273–276.

81. **Li, B., H. Bassiri, M. D. Rossman, P. Kramer, A. F. Eyuboglu, M. Torres, E. Sada, T. Imir, and S. R. Carding.** 1998. Involvement of the Fas/Fas ligand pathway in activation-induced cell death of mycobacteria-reactive human gamma delta T cells: a mechanism for the loss of gamma delta T cells in patients with pulmonary tuberculosis. *J. Immunol.* **161**:1558–1567.

82. **Lingwood, C. A.** 1996. Role of verotoxin re-

ceptors in pathogenesis. *Trends Microbiol.* **4:** 147–153.

83. **Luo, G., D. W. Niesel, R. A. Shaban, E. A. Grimm, and G. R. Klimpel.** 1993. Tumor necrosis factor alpha binding to bacteria: evidence for a high-affinity receptor and alteration of bacterial virulence properties. *Infect. Immun.* **61**:830–835.

84. **MacFarlane, A. S., D. Huang, M. G. Schwacha, J. J. J. Meissler, J. P. Gaughan, and T. K. Eisenstein.** 1998. Nitric oxide mediates immunosuppression induced by *Listeria monocytogenes* infection: quantitative studies. *Microb. Pathog.* **25**:267–277.

85. **Mahida, Y. R., A. Galvin, S. Makh, S. Hyde, L. Sanfilippo, S. P. Borriello, and H. F. Sewell.** 1998. Effect of *Clostridium difficile* toxin A on human colonic lamina propria cells: early loss of macrophages followed by T-cell apoptosis. *Infect. Immun.* **66**:5462–5469.

86. **Manfredi, A. A., S. Heltai, P. Rovere, C. Sciorati, C. Paolucci, G. Galati, C. Rugarli, R. Vaiani, E. Clementi, and M. Ferrarini.** 1998. *Mycobacterium tuberculosis* exploits the CD95/CD95 ligand system of gammadelta T cells to cause apoptosis. *Eur. J. Immunol.* **28**:1798–1806.

87. **Mangan, D. F., S. M. Wahl, B. M. Sultzer, and S. E. Mergenhagen.** 1992. Stimulation of human monocytes by endotoxin-associated protein: inhibition of programmed cell death (apoptosis) and potential significance in adjuvanticity. *Infect. Immun.* **60**:1684–1686.

88. **Marshall, J. C., N. V. Christou, and J. L. Meakins.** 1988. Immunomodulation by altered gastrointestinal tract flora. The effects of orally administered, killed *Staphylococcus epidermidis, Candida,* and *Pseudomonas* on systemic immune responses. *Arch. Surg.* **123**:1465–1469.

89. **Matsui, K.** 1996. Purification of a product from *Salmonella typhimurium* with the ability to inhibit mitogen-induced proliferation of murine splenic T-lymphocytes. *FEMS Immunol. Med. Microbiol.* **13**:155–160.

90. **Matsui, K.** 1996. Purified protein from *Salmonella typhimurium* inhibits the interleukin-2 response of murine splenic T-lymphocytes activated with anti-CD3 antibody. *Microbiol. Immunol.* **40:** 681–684.

91. **Mehra, V., P. J. Brennan, E. Rada, J. Convit, and B. R. Bloom.** 1984. Lymphocyte suppression in leprosy induced by unique *M. leprae* glycolipid. *Nature* **308**:194–196.

92. **Merien, F., G. Baranton, and P. Perolat.** 1997. Invasion of Vero cells and induction of apoptosis in macrophages by pathogenic *Leptospira interrogans* are correlated with virulence. *Infect. Immun.* **65**:729–738.

93. **Mills, S. D., A. Boland, M. P. Sory, P. van**

. der Smissen, C. Kerbourch, B. B. Finlay, and G. R. Cornelis. 1997. *Yersinia enterocolitica* induces apoptosis in macrophages by a process requiring functional type III secretion and translocation mechanisms and involving YopP, presumably acting as an effector protein. *Proc. Natl. Acad. Sci. USA* **94**:12638–12643.

94. **Mims, C. A., N. J. Dimmock, A. Nash, and J. Stephen.** 1995. *Mims' Pathogenesis of Infectious Disease.* Academic Press, Ltd., London, United Kingdom.

95. **Mintz, C. S., R. D. Miller, N. S. Gutgsell, and T. Malek.** 1993. *Legionella pneumophila* protease inactivates interleukin-2 and cleaves CD4 on human T cells. *Infect. Immun.* **61**:3416–3421.

96. **Modlin, R. L., C. Pirmez, F. M. Hofman, V. Torigian, K. Uyemura, T. H. Rea, B. R. Bloom, and M. B. Brenner.** 1989. Lymphocytes bearing antigen-specific gamma delta T-cell receptors accumulate in human infectious disease lesions. *Nature* **339**:544–548.

97. **Molloy, A., P. Laochumroonvorapong, and G. Kaplan.** 1994. Apoptosis, but not necrosis, of infected monocytes is coupled with killing of intracellular bacillus Calmette-Guerin. *J. Exp. Med.* **180**:1499–1509.

98. **Monack, D. M., J. Mecsas, D. Bouley, and S. Falkow.** 1998. *Yersinia*-induced apoptosis in vivo aids in the establishment of a systemic infection of mice. *J. Exp. Med.* **188**:2127–2137.

99. **Monack, D. M., B. Raupach, A. E. Hromockyj, and S. Falkow.** 1996. *Salmonella typhimurium* invasion induces apoptosis in infected macrophages. *Proc. Natl. Acad. Sci. USA* **93**: 9833–9838.

100. **Muller, A., J. Hacker, and B. C. Brand.** 1996. Evidence for apoptosis of human macrophage-like HL-60 cells by *Legionella pneumophila* infection. *Infect. Immun.* **64**:4900–4906.

101. **Muraille, E., T. De Smedt, F. Andris, B. Pajak, M. Armant, J. Urbain, M. Moser, and O. Leo.** 1997. Staphylococcal enterotoxin B induces an early and transient state of immunosuppression characterized by V beta-unrestricted T cell unresponsiveness and defective antigen-presenting cell functions. *J. Immunol.* **158**: 2638–2647.

102. **Murray, P. J., L. Wang, C. Onufryk, R. I. Tepper, and R. A. Young.** 1997. T cell-derived IL-10 antagonizes macrophage function in mycobacterial infection. *J. Immunol.* **158**: 315–321.

103. **Nakajima, R., and R. R. Brubaker.** 1993. Association between virulence of *Yersinia pestis* and suppression of gamma interferon and tumor necrosis factor alpha. *Infect. Immun.* **61**:23–31.

104. **Noble, A., G. A. Pestano, and H. Cantor.** 1998. Suppression of immune responses by CD8 cells. I. Superantigen-activated CD8 cells induce unidirectional Fas-mediated apoptosis of antigen-activated CD4 cells. *J. Immunol.* **160**: 559–565.

105. **Norimatsu, M., T. Ono, A. Aoki, K. Ohishi, T. Takahashi, G. Watanabe, K. Taya, S. Sasamoto, and Y. Tamura.** 1995. Lipopolysaccharide-induced apoptosis in swine lymphocytes in vivo. *Infect. Immun.* **63**: 1122–1126.

106. **Nutman, J., M. Berger, P. A. Chase, D. G. Dearborn, K. M. Miller, R. L. Waller, and R. U. Sorensen.** 1987. Studies on the mechanism of T cell inhibition by the *Pseudomonas aeruginosa* phenazine pigment pyocyanine. *J. Immunol.* **138**:3481–3487.

107. **Ohguchi, M., A. Ishisaki, N. Okahashi, M. Koide, T. Koseki, K. Yamato, T. Noguchi, and T. Nishihara.** 1998. *Actinobacillus actinomycetmcomitans* toxin induces both cell cycle arrest in the G2/M phase and apoptosis. *Infect. Immun.* **66**:5980–5987.

108. **Ojcius, D. M., P. Souque, J. L. Perfettini, and A. Dautry-Varsat.** 1998. Apoptosis of epithelial cells and macrophages due to infection with the obligate intracellular pathogen *Chlamydia psittaci. J. Immunol.* **161**:4220–4226.

108a. **Orme, I. M., and F. M. Collins.** 1984. Immune response to atypical mycobacteria: immunocompetence of heavily infected mice measured in vivo fails to substantiate immunosuppression data obtained in vitro. *Infect. Immun.* **43**: 32–37.

109. **Palmer, L. E., S. Hobbie, J. E. Galan, and J. B. Bliska.** 1998. YopJ of *Yersinia pseudotuberculosis* is required for the inhibition of macrophage TNF-alpha production and downregulation of the MAP kinases p38 and JNK. *Mol. Microbiol.* **27**:953–965.

110. **Parmely, M., A. Gale, M. Clabaugh, R. Horvat, and W. W. Zhou.** 1990. Proteolytic inactivation of cytokines by *Pseudomonas aeruginosa. Infect. Immun.* **58**:3009–3014.

111. **Paul, W. E.** 1998. *Fundamental Immunology.* Lippincott-Raven, Philadelphia, Pa.

112. **Petit, J. C., and G. L. Daguet.** 1983. Interference of *Pseudomonas aeruginosa* with immunospecific host defenses. *Biomed. Pharmacother.* **37**: 422–428.

113. **Pryjma, J., J. Baran, M. Ernst, M. Woloszyn, and H. D. Flad.** 1994. Altered antigen-presenting capacity of human monocytes after phagocytosis of bacteria. *Infect. Immun.* **62**: 1961–1967.

114. **Rabie, G., E. T. Lally, and B. J. Shenker.** 1988. Immunosuppressive properties of *Actino-*

bacillus actinomycetemcomitans leukotoxin. *Infect. Immun.* **56:**122–127.

115. **Renno, T., M. Hahne, and H. R. MacDonald.** 1995. Proliferation is a prerequisite for bacterial superantigen-induced T cell apoptosis in vivo. *J. Exp. Med.* **181:**2283–2287.

116. **Rodloff, A. C., P. Widera, S. Ehlers, T. Montag, M. Lucas, G. Schmidt, and H. Hahn.** 1990. Suppression of blastogenic transformation of lymphocytes by *Bacteroides fragilis* in vitro and in vivo. *Zentbl. Bakteriol.* **274:**406–416.

117. **Rosenbaum, J. T., K. T. Hartiala, R. O. Webster, E. L. J. Howes, and I. M. Goldstein.** 1983. Antiinflammatory effects of endotoxin. Inhibition of rabbit polymorphonuclear leukocyte responses to complement (C5)-derived peptides in vivo and in vitro. *Am. J. Pathol.* **113:**291–299.

118. **Ruckdeschel, K., S. Harb, A. Roggenkamp, M. Hornef, R. Zumbihl, S. Kohler, J. Heesemann, and B. Rouot.** 1998. *Yersinia enterocolitica* impairs activation of transcription factor NF-kappaB: involvement in the induction of programmed cell death and in the suppression of the macrophage tumor necrosis factor alpha production. *J. Exp. Med.* **187:**1069–1079.

119. **Ruckdeschel, K., J. Machold, A. Roggenkamp, S. Schubert, J. Pierre, R. Zumbihl, J. P. Liautard, J. Heesemann, and B. Rouot.** 1997. *Yersinia enterocolitica* promotes deactivation of macrophage mitogen-activated protein kinases extracellular signal-regulated kinase-1/2, p38, and c-Jun NH2-terminal kinase. Correlation with its inhibitory effect on tumor necrosis factor-alpha production. *J. Biol. Chem.* **272:**15920–15927.

120. **Saha, B., G. Das, H. Vohra, N. K. Ganguly, and G. C. Mishra.** 1994. Macrophage-T cell interaction in experimental mycobacterial infection. Selective regulation of co-stimulatory molecules on *Mycobacterium*-infected macrophages and its implication in the suppression of cell-mediated immune response. *Eur. J. Immunol.* **24:**2618–2624.

120a. **Samandari, T., K. L. Kotloff, G. A. Losonsky, W. D. Picking, M. M. Levine, and M. B. Sztein.** Production of interferon-gamma and IL-10 to Shigella invasins by mononuclear cells from volunteers orally inoculated with a Shiga toxin-deleted Shigella dysenteriae strain. *J. Immun.*, in press.

121. **Schesser, K., A. K. Spiik, J. M. Dukuzumuremyi, M. F. Neurath, S. Pettersson, and H. Wolf-Watz.** 1998. The *yopJ* locus is required for *Yersinia*-mediated inhibition of NF-kappaB activation and cytokine expression: YopJ contains a eukaryotic SH2-like domain that is essen-

tial for its repressive activity. *Mol. Microbiol.* **28:**1067–1079.

122. **Schwacha, M. G., J. J. J. Meissler, and T. K. Eisenstein.** 1998. *Salmonella typhimurium* infection in mice induces nitric oxide-mediated immunosuppression through a natural killer cell-dependent pathway. *Infect. Immun.* **66:**5862–5866.

123. **Schwan, W. R., and D. J. Kopecko.** 1997. Uptake of pathogenic intracellular bacteria into human and murine macrophages downregulates the eukaryotic 26S protease complex ATPase gene. *Infect. Immun.* **65:**4754–4760.

124. **Shenker, B. J., and J. M. DiRienzo.** 1984. Suppression of human peripheral blood lymphocytes by *Fusobacterium nucleatum. J. Immun.* **132:**2357–2362.

125. **Shenker, B. J., L. Vitale, and J. Slots.** 1991. Immunosuppressive effects of *Prevotella intermedia* on in vitro human lymphocyte activation. *Infect. Immun.* **59:**4583–4589.

126. **Shenker, B. J., L. A. Vitale, and D. A. Welham.** 1990. Immune suppression induced by *Actinobacillus actinomycetemcomitans*: effects on immunoglobulin production by human B cells. *Infect. Immun.* **58:**3856–3862.

127. **Staugas, R. E., D. P. Harvey, A. Ferrante, M. Nandoskar, and A. C. Allison.** 1992. Induction of tumor necrosis factor (TNF) and interleukin-1 (IL-1) by *Pseudomonas aeruginosa* and exotoxin A-induced suppression of lymphoproliferation and TNF, lymphotoxin, gamma interferon, and IL-1 production in human leukocytes. *Infect. Immun.* **60:**3162–3168.

128. **Stenger, S., K. R. Niazi, and R. L. Modlin.** 1998. Down-regulation of CD1 on antigen-presenting cells by infection with *Mycobacterium tuberculosis. J. Immun.* **161:**3582–3588.

129. **Stevens, P. K., and C. J. Czuprynski.** 1996. *Pasteurella haemolytica* leukotoxin induces bovine leukocytes to undergo morphologic changes consistent with apoptosis in vitro. *Infect. Immun.* **64:**2687–2694.

130. **Sztein, M. B., and G. F. Mitchell.** 1997. Recent advances in immunology: impact on vaccine development, p. 99–126. *In* M. M. Levine, G. C. Woodrow, J. B. Kaper, and G. S. Cobon (ed.), *New Generation Vaccines.* Marcel Dekker, Inc., New York, N.Y.

131. **Taylor, C. E., and R. Bright.** 1989. T-cell modulation of the antibody response to bacterial polysaccharide antigens. *Infect. Immun.* **57:**180–185.

132. **Thern, A., L. Stenberg, B. Dahlback, and G. Lindahl.** 1995. Ig-binding surface proteins of *Streptococcus pyogenes* also bind human C4b-binding protein (C4BP), a regulatory component

of the complement system. *J. Immunol.* **154:** 375–386.

133. **Thomson, A.** 1998. *The Cytokine Handbook.* Academic Press, Ltd., London, United Kingdom.

134. **Tomai, M. A., and T. J. Fitzgerald.** 1991. Splenic macrophage function in early syphilitic infection is complex. Stimulation versus downregulation. *J. Immunol.* **146:**3171–3176.

135. **Tsuyuguchi, I., H. Kawasumi, T. Takashima, T. Tsuyuguchi, and S. Kishimoto.** 1990. *Mycobacterium avium-Mycobacterium intracellulare* complex-induced suppression of T-cell proliferation in vitro by regulation of monocyte accessory cell activity. *Infect. Immun.* **58:** 1369–1378.

136. **Tufano, M. A., F. Rossano, P. Catalanotti, G. Liguori, A. Marinelli, A. Baroni, and P. Marinelli.** 1994. Properties of *Yersinia enterocolitica* porins: interference with biological functions of phagocytes, nitric oxide production and selective cytokine release. *Res. Microbiol.* **145:** 297–307.

137. **Ulmer, A. J., J. Pryjma, Z. Tarnok, M. Ernst, and H. D. Flad.** 1990. Inhibitory and stimulatory effects of *Pseudomonas aeruginosa* pyocyanine on human T and B lymphocytes and human monocytes. *Infect. Immun.* **58:**808–815.

138. **Valisena, S., P. E. Varaldo, and G. Satta.** 1991. Staphylococcal endo-beta-N-acetylglucosaminidase inhibits response of human lymphocytes to mitogens and interferes with production of antibodies in mice. *J. Clin. Investig.* **87:** 1969–1976.

139. **VanHeyningen, T. K., H. L. Collins, and D. G. Russell.** 1997. IL-6 produced by macrophages infected with *Mycobacterium* species suppresses T cell responses. *J. Immunol.* **158:** 330–337.

140. **Virgin, H. W., G. F. Wittenberg, G. J. Bancroft, and E. R. Unanue.** 1985. Suppression of immune response to *Listeria monocytogenes*: mechanism(s) of immune complex suppression. *Infect. Immun.* **50:**343–353.

141. **Vollmer, P., I. Walev, S. Rose-John, and S. Bhakdi.** 1996. Novel pathogenic mechanism of microbial metalloproteinases: liberation of membrane-anchored molecules in biologically active form exemplified by studies with the human interleukin-6 receptor. *Infect. Immun.* **64:**3646–3651.

142. **Wang, S. D., K. J. Huang, Y. S. Lin, and**

H. Y. Lei. 1994. Sepsis-induced apoptosis of the thymocytes in mice. *J. Immunol.* **152:**5014–5021.

143. **Watson, R. W., H. P. Redmond, J. H. Wang, C. Condron, and D. Bouchier-Hayes.** 1996. Neutrophils undergo apoptosis following ingestion of *Escherichia coli. J. Immunol.* **156:**3986–3992.

144. **Welkos, S., A. Friedlander, D. McDowell, J. Weeks, and S. Tobery.** 1998. V antigen of *Yersinia pestis* inhibits neutrophil chemotaxis. *Microb. Pathog.* **24:**185–196.

145. **Wick, M. J., C. V. Harding, N. J. Twesten, S. J. Normark, and J. D. Pfeifer.** 1995. The phoP locus influences processing and presentation of *Salmonella typhimurium* antigens by activated macrophages. *Mol. Microbiol.* **16:**465–476.

146. **Wilson, K. T., K. S. Ramanujam, H. L. Mobley, R. F. Musselman, S. P. James, and S. J. Meltzer.** 1996. *Helicobacter pylori* stimulates inducible nitric oxide synthase expression and activity in a murine macrophage cell line. *Gastroenterology* **111:**1524–1533.

147. **Wilson, M., R. Seymour, and B. Henderson.** 1998. Bacterial perturbation of cytokine networks. *Infect. Immun.* **66:**2401–2409.

148. **Wyant, T. L., M. K. Tanner, and M. B. Sztein.** 1999. Potent immunoregulatory effects of *Salmonella typhi* flagella on antigenic stimulation of human peripheral blood mononuclear cells. *Infect. Immun.* **67:**1338–1346.

149. **Zav'yalov, V. P., T. V. Chernovskaya, E. V. Navolotskaya, A. V. Karlyshev, S. MacIntyre, A. M. Vasiliev, and V. M. Abramov.** 1995. Specific high affinity binding of human interleukin 1 beta by CaflA usher protein of *Yersinia pestis. FEBS Lett.* **371:**65–68.

150. **Zeidner, N., M. L. Mbow, M. Dolan, R. Massung, E. Baca, and J. Piesman.** 1997. Effects of *Ixodes scapularis* and *Borrelia burgdorferi* on modulation of the host immune response: induction of a TH2 cytokine response in Lyme disease-susceptible (C3H/HeJ) mice but not in disease-resistant (BALB/c) mice. *Infect. Immun.* **65:** 3100–3106.

151. **Zychlinsky, A., M. C. Prevost, and P. J. Sansonetti.** 1992. *Shigella flexneri* induces apoptosis in infected macrophages. *Nature* **358:** 167–169.

152. **Zychlinsky, A., K. Thirumalai, J. Arondel, J. R. Cantey, A. O. Aliprantis, and P. J. Sansonetti.** 1996. In vivo apoptosis in *Shigella flexneri* infections. *Infect. Immun.* **64:**5357–5365.

MATHEMATICAL MODELS OF COLONIZATION AND PERSISTENCE IN BACTERIAL INFECTIONS

Denise E. Kirschner and Rolf Freter

5

After decades of research focusing on infected patients and experimental animals, most modern research on microbial pathogenesis takes place at the level of cellular and biochemical mechanisms governing host-parasite interaction; however, studies at many scales will undoubtedly be needed for a deeper understanding of infectious diseases. For example, linking pathogen-specific information to that on the immune system will be critical for understanding the dynamics of most bacterial infections. Components of host-pathogen systems are sufficiently numerous and their interactions sufficiently complex that intuition alone is insufficient to fully understand the dynamics of the interactions. Here, mathematical modeling becomes an important experimental tool. In this chapter, we will focus on mathematical models of colonization and persistent bacterial infections. We will review the modeling method and the state of the field and then focus on three key areas where modeling has, and will continue to have, an impact: the ecology of the indigenous microflora and its plasmids, *Helicobacter pylori* colonization, and host-pathogen interactions with *Mycobacterium tuberculosis*.

This is by no means a complete list of bacterial pathogens that have been explored with modeling; models of other bacterial infections will certainly emerge over the next decade and beyond.

MODELING PRINCIPLES

In many infectious diseases, particularly those arising from persistent infections with pathogens such as *M. tuberculosis* and *H. pylori,* we are far from understanding the mechanisms of disease progression. The strength of the modeling process is that it can lend insight and clarification to existing data and theories. Mathematical models thus provide a unique approach to representing and studying the integrated behavior of complex biological systems. The use of mathematical models also enables us to compare and contrast existing theories of the dynamic interactions in a complex system.

Mathematical models of host-pathogen dynamics are formulated on the basis of specific assumptions regarding the system's components and their interactions. In the same way that an experimental animal model can play a key role in our understanding of a human biological system (allowing for comparative biology), a mathematical model can lend valuable insights into complex interactions and reveal key governing parameters. An important dis-

Denise E. Kirschner and Rolf Freter, Department of Microbiology and Immunology, The University of Michigan Medical School, Ann Arbor, MI 48109-0620.

Persistent Bacterial Infections, Edited by J. P. Nataro, M. J. Blaser, and S. Cunningham-Rundles, © 2000 ASM Press, Washington, D.C.

tinction to make is that unlike statistical methods that rely solely on the analysis of empirical data, mathematical models of host-pathogen interactions are based on assumptions about the host-bacterial dynamics and use data to estimate the rate constants that govern the interactions. Host-pathogen models are based on mechanistic assumptions and can therefore be used effectively to compare and contrast alternative hypotheses concerning mechanisms of pathogenesis. Thus, it should be understood that the main purpose of mathematical modeling is to determine the interplay among specific interacting factors in infection and not merely to achieve correlations within empirical data. A good model, therefore, uses parameters that represent defined biological entities (e.g., growth rates, nutrient uptake, etc.) rather than numerically derived values that merely serve to align the model solutions with experimental data. Also, a key strength of modeling is that it reveals various sensitivities to the parameters and initial conditions involved in the model, indicating which processes and interactions are dominant in the dynamics. For example, the outcome of an infection initiated with an inoculum of 10 bacteria might be shown to be qualitatively different from that of one initiated with 10^4 bacteria, thus illustrating a sensitivity to this parameter. The choice of mathematical method is based on several considerations about the system being studied. For example, whether the time frame of a study is short or long, whether the population sizes are large or small, whether the system has randomness present or is strictly determinable, and/or the types of questions being posed about the system all determine the modeling technique that is most appropriate.

As in experimentation, modeling research develops by iterative refinement; thus, the models can progressively incorporate greater detail as it becomes available. A criticism of modeling is that the models are only as good as the knowledge, data, and assumptions which they are based on. This point actually highlights their strength in that specific hypotheses can be tested and compared. A successful mathe-

matical model will not necessarily answer a question but instead will pose questions about the system. It also should suggest experiments that can be conducted to clarify understanding of the system. Once a host-pathogen system can be reliably described with a mathematical model, it becomes possible to explore the effects of perturbing elements of the system that may be problematic, or even impossible, to address experimentally. If the predictions of a mathematical model are incompatible with experimental data and the underlying theory, it proves conclusively that the theory is incomplete or faulty. However, if the predictions of a mathematical model agree with the data, this represents strong evidence for the correctness of the theory but does not itself constitute conclusive proof of its validity.

Some of the earliest mathematical modeling, of population growth, was done in 1798 by Malthus. The simple idea he used was that of exponential growth. Exponential-growth models assume that the rate of change of a population at time t, namely, $P(t)$, is proportional to itself, and this can be represented mathematically as

$$\frac{dP(t)}{dt} = kP(t) \tag{1}$$

where k is the growth rate constant of that change. The mathematical solution to this differential equation, where P_0 represents the initial population size, is $P(t) = P_0 e^{kt}$. The graph of this function is shown on a log scale in Fig. 1B.

Although Malthus was attempting at the time to predict how the human population was growing, this proportionality assumption could be applied to other populations, such as those of bacteria. Of course for any population, this model of exponential growth cannot hold true over a long time frame. For example, the actual growth curve of bacteria is given in Fig. 1A. Thus, the model should be modified to include greater complexity about the system to better capture known dynamics. This modification elaborates a key step in the modeling processes—that of iteration. Finer as well as

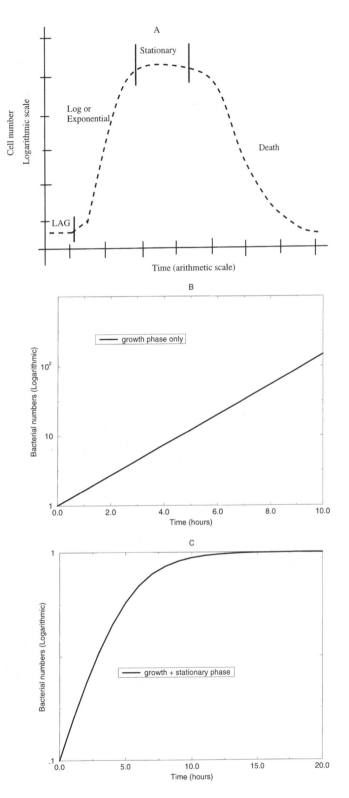

FIGURE 1 (A) Classical complete growth curve for bacteria. (B) Model of exponential growth phase only. (C) Model of exponential and stationary phases of growth.

broader details can be included in the system to better capture its behavior. To that end, in our example of population growth, we consider the concept of a population carrying capacity, defined as K. This is a general term that can encompass various elements affecting the growth of the population. For example, consider the situation of bacteria growing in culture. These bacteria are limited by, among other things, the volume of the culture (which could moderate toxic effects) as well as the availability of oxygen and nutrients in the medium (which could account for competition between bacteria). The parameter K would then be a measure of these elements in the particular experimental system. To introduce these ideas mathematically, we multiply the existing model, equation 1, by a term, $1 - (P/K)$, as follows:

$$\frac{dP(t)}{dt} = kP(t) \left(1 - \frac{P(t)}{K}\right) \quad (2)$$
$$= kP(t) - \frac{k(P(t))^2}{K}$$

Notice that the growth term remains the same as before (i.e., kP), but now the carrying capacity, K, and interaction between bacteria, P^2, both inhibit that growth (via the minus sign). The mathematical solution of the differential equation in equation 2 is not as tractable as our first model (equation 1); this is due to the now nonlinear nature of the equation (i.e., the P^2 term). The graph of the solution function can, however, be obtained through computer simulation and is given in Fig. 1C. Notice that through this simple modification to the system we are able to predict both the growth and stationary phases of the well-known bacterial growth curve. To fully capture all the stages (including lag and death) shown in Fig. 1A, we would again have to modify the model. While the equations can accurately trace the bacterial growth curve, they are not yet useful as models to understand growth, because the parameters k and K were not chosen as functions of basic biological mechanisms. This could be improved, however, by expressing k as a function of nutrient

concentration, temperature, rates of nutrient uptake, etc., and K as a function of the accumulation of toxic metabolites, oxygen concentration, etc.

Testing and validation are other elements of the modeling process. A key method for addressing these lies in the comparison of the model output with experimental and/or clinical data. The typical goal of the modeling method is to determine if the assumptions about the interactions of the elements of the system lead to the dynamics seen either clinically or experimentally. This would then indicate that the interactions included in the model sufficiently capture some of the key biological dynamics. It should be noted that many times if data are not available with which to test the model, the model itself can suggest which experiments are needed.

No other modeling of population growth was done until the mid- to late 20th century. Recently, models of host interactions with microbes have begun to appear, including relatively few models that explore bacterium-host-level interactions (9, 11, 26, 27, 38, 39, 50, 51). We will discuss in detail below the key findings of some of these models. The models by Lipsitch and Levin (50, 51) focus on antimicrobial chemotherapy, while the one by Gordon and Riley (27) is a first work on urinary tract bacterial infections. Two other models by Antia et al. (7, 8) explored mycoparasite immune dynamics. The first of these (8) considered the dynamics of parasites during acute infections. The model incorporates a generic population of parasites together with an immune response. The investigators assumed that the virulence of the organism is proportional to its growth rate in the host. Their results indicated that optimal transmission of parasites would result if the parasite had an intermediate rate of growth (not high as in *Escherichia coli* or low as in *M. tuberculosis*), and they argue that this would result in the evolution and maintenance of an intermediate level of parasite virulence. Their second model (7) considered a different set of hypotheses for the dynamics of persistent mycobacterial infections. This model predicted that the initial persistence of the parasite may be achieved by very-slow-growing parasites or by parasites having a refuge that is inaccessible to the immune response. They also suggested that escape from immune control at a later time might be a consequence of two processes: antigen deletion of T cells in the thymus and the presence of a limit to the maximal number of divisions a T cell can undergo (i.e., a "Hayflick limit"). In their scenario, the persistent parasite antigens prevent the generation of new parasite-specific cells from the thymus and the existing parasite-specific cells are eventually eliminated as they reach the Hayflick limit.

Epidemic models of infectious diseases have been developed since the middle of the 1900s. Hundreds of mathematical models have been published exploring the effects of both bacterial and viral pathogens on different subgroups of human populations. Many of the results have defined paradigms in epidemiology, such as the notion of a core population in sexually transmitted diseases (31) as well as ways to determine herd immunity levels for vaccination policies (3). Relating to persistent bacterial infections, key pathogens that have been studied are *Neisseria gonorrhoeae* (31), *M. tuberculosis* (13, 14, 16, 17, 58), and *Treponema pallidum* (10). Such important issues as drug resistance, rate of spread of infection, trends of the epidemics, and the effects of treatment and vaccination all have been insightfully addressed through these modeling approaches.

Models of persistent viral infections, namely, human immunodeficiency virus (HIV)-host models, also have a successful recent history. Many of the key results that have shaped our understanding of the T-cell and viral dynamics in HIV disease have come from mathematical modeling approaches (32, 68, 75). Many others have provided insight into HIV-immune system dynamics as well as disease progression (1, 4–6, 40–46, 54, 55, 63, 64, 67). For example, a recent model developed by one of us (D.E.K.) examined the role of the thymus in pediatric HIV type 1 infection (41).

Until this work, there was no clear explanation for the different disease progressions in pediatric versus adult HIV infections. The model was able to show that infection in the thymus not only can supplement peripheral infection but can help explain the faster progression in pediatric cases, as well as the early and high viral burden. This is based on the fact that the thymus is most active in children and involutes in adulthood. Subsequent clinical data have confirmed that the thymus does play a key role (60).

COLONIZATION BY BACTERIA IN THE LARGE INTESTINE

Two studies by one of us (R.F.) lend themselves to illustrating that some problems in persistent infections (or, for that matter, in any area of microbiology) can be studied most effectively by integrating experimental or clinical observations with mathematical modeling. In the following discussion, we demonstrate some of the unique contributions mathematical modeling can make to the study of complex problems in host-microbe interactions. Space does not permit a detailed recounting of the experimental details of each investigation; these are available, however, in the original publications (23, 25, 26).

The indigenous microflora of the mammalian large intestine is a stable ecosystem, comprising more than 400 different kinds of bacteria, most of them strict anaerobes. The study of the indigenous microflora represents a subspecialty of ecology—the science that considers the relations and interactions of organisms with their environment and with each other. The microflora is usually in the climax stage of ecological succession, meaning that it will prevent colonization by exogenous bacteria, including potential pathogens, entering from the environment. Because of this colonization resistance, the microflora forms a host defense mechanism in the intestine that is even more effective than the much better understood immunological mechanisms. Colonization is the first step in the pathogenesis of persistent (as well as most other) infections, and for this reason, insight into the principles underlying colonization by the indigenous flora is a necessary step toward an eventual understanding of the main topic of this volume. In the absence of a generally accepted definition, we define colonization here as the state in which the population size of the colonizing microorganism in (or on) the host remains constant, i.e., when the number of microorganisms that are killed or otherwise removed from a given site is precisely compensated for by multiplication of the remaining microorganisms.

Colonization of the large intestine by several hundred different kinds of bacteria is obviously a complex process involving many parameters, such as microbial multiplication rates, nutrient concentration, rates of adhesion to the gut wall, rate of removal by intestinal peristalsis, etc. Critical to the performance of natural ecosystems is the manner in which these various elements interact. Such interactions are usually difficult to appreciate when the individual microbial populations, and the ecological mechanisms controlling them, are studied in isolation rather than under the physiological and ecological conditions existing in a complex environment harboring these diverse populations. For example, under the different conditions prevailing in various natural environments, such as the lumen or the wall of the large intestine, a parameter that is potentially able to control the population size of an indigenous bacterium may be quantitatively most important or it may be partially or totally eclipsed in effectiveness by other mechanisms. For this reason, colonization is still imperfectly understood, with most investigators studying individual mechanisms.

In the first study to be discussed, we used an in vitro model as well as a mathematical model. The in vitro model was an anaerobic continuous-flow (CF) culture of the entire flora of a mouse cecum. Such a culture had been shown to duplicate bacterial interactions as they occur in the mouse large intestine (23). The mathematical model of this system made the following assumptions.

1. A resident strain of *E. coli* colonizes the large intestine (or CF culture). An invader strain is ingested once, and in large numbers.

2. Resident and invaders have exactly the same properties.

3. Both strains compete for the same adhesion sites on the wall of the intestine or CF culture.

4. Offspring of adherent strains occupy additional sites or, when most sites are filled, are shed into the lumen.

5. Adhesion is reversible, and adherent bacteria are slowly shed into the lumen.

6. Both resident and invader strains compete for the same limiting nutrient. (Thus, the relations between growth rates and limiting-nutrient concentrations were modeled by classical Monod kinetics.)

In a typical experiment, such as that shown in Fig. 2, normal mice were inoculated with a culture of the *E. coli* invader strain (marked with streptomycin resistance). Inoculation was directly into the stomach by means of a blunt feeding needle. At intervals thereafter, the ani-

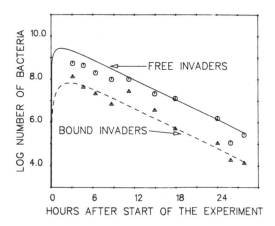

FIGURE 2 Passage of *E. coli* invaders through mouse cecum. The symbols represent experimental data: the circles are the bacteria suspended in the lumen, and the triangles are the adherent population. The curves represent the best-fit estimates generated by the mathematical model for each of the two experimental populations. (Reprinted from *Microecology and Therapy* [25] with permission from publisher.)

mals were euthanized and the number of invaders in the lumen or adherent to the wall of the large intestine was determined by culture of the homogenized specimens. In Fig. 2, these experimental data are represented by symbols. The mathematical model of this system was also employed. The model system was solved, and its output was run through a computer program that incrementally varied the parameters of interest (e.g., the rate constants of adhesion and elution) until an optimal fit to the data was obtained (shown by the curves in Fig. 2).

The parameter estimates thus obtained (e.g., the rate constants of adhesion and elution, flow through the system, multiplication, etc.) were then incorporated into the mathematical model. The output of the model was then studied to answer some of the original questions we posed. For example, the major feature of the indigenous flora is that it confers colonization resistance. This is seen in Fig. 2, where the population size of the invaders decreases without their ever being able to colonize (i.e., to achieve a stable population size). This is in spite of the fact that the resident *E. coli* bacteria in these experiments (not shown) formed stable populations (which is part of the definition of a normal mouse). In light of the importance of this feature for human and animal health, numerous hypotheses have been proposed over the past decades to explain the elimination of invaders by the indigenous flora, e.g., the production of toxic substances or competition for nutrients or for adhesion sites. Unfortunately, none of these hypotheses were able to account for the observation that whatever mechanism caused the invaders to be eliminated had no effect on a physiologically identical resident. The explanations furnished by the mathematical model are shown in Fig. 3 (top).

As may be seen in Fig. 3, when an invader strain is introduced at the 50-h mark, it is eliminated rapidly from the mouse intestine. This is in spite of the fact that the rate of elimination of bacteria from the large intestine is lower than the optimal growth rate of the bacteria. In other words, in the absence of an indigenous

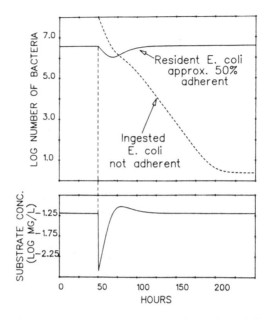

FIGURE 3 (Top) Prediction by the mathematical model of the fate of an *E. coli* strain that invades the large intestine of an animal that already harbors an adherent *E. coli* resident strain. (Bottom) Concentration of limiting nutrient in the system. (Reprinted from reference 24 with permission.)

flora, the invader strain can form large stable populations in the lumen, even without adherence to the gut wall. Moreover, as mentioned above, resident and invader strains have the same properties (in paired experiments in mice one can exchange the strains used as residents and invaders without changing the finding that it is the invader that is always eliminated). Why then is the invader strain at such a striking disadvantage? The mathematical model shows that the large number of invaders causes a temporary decrease in the concentration of the limiting nutrient (Fig. 3, bottom), but when the nutrient concentration quickly returns to normal, the invader population is still decreasing. The mathematical model furnishes an explanation for this phenomenon. In a CF culture, or the large intestine, a large portion of the resident strain adheres to the wall. In the adherent state, its rate of elimination by the flow of nutrient through the gut or through the CF culture is lower than that of bacteria suspended in the lumen. Consequently, the growth rate that an adherent strain must achieve in order to maintain a constant population (i.e., to have a growth rate equal to its rate of elimination) must be lower than that required for a suspended, nonadherent population. According to classical CF culture theory, the concentration of limiting nutrient that will establish itself in the culture will be exactly that which will allow the resident strain to maintain a growth rate equal to its rate of elimination. However, when an invader strain having the same properties as the resident invades, it will initially be suspended in the lumen and, consequently, have a higher rate of elimination. For this reason it would require a higher concentration of nutrient to maintain its population at a constant level. Not finding an adequately high nutrient concentration, the invader strain will grow too slowly and will be eliminated. Elimination will continue until the small remaining invader population has found adhesion sites and has subsequently achieved the lower rate of elimination typical of adherent bacteria (at about 200 h [Fig. 3]). Consequently, it will then be able to maintain a constant population at the prevailing nutrient concentration. The mathematical model indicated that this slow adhesion was not due to a lack of free adhesion sites but rather was a function of the relatively low rate constant of adhesion of the invader strain. In other words, the rate of adhesion of the invader was so low that most of its population had already been eliminated by the time it could form significantly large adherent populations.

The mathematical model further indicated that in the absence of adhesion on the part of the indigenous microflora, there would be no resistance to colonization by invading bacteria. Thus, adhesion of bacteria in the large intestine is not required for colonization because of the low rate of elimination of contents from this organ (in contrast to colonization of the small intestine), but adhesion in the large intestine is required for the protective function of the indigenous flora against colonization by invading bacteria.

This theory was developed with the aid of mathematical modeling. Was the mathematical model essential? In retrospect, it is not entirely impossible that the relationship among adhesion, nutrient concentration, and resistance to colonization could have been derived through experimentation alone. However, the constant guidance obtained through mathematical modeling made the study much more efficient.

PLASMID TRANSFER AMONG BACTERIA IN THE LARGE INTESTINE

The second example to illustrate the role of a mathematical model is a study of plasmid transfer among bacteria in the large intestine. As in the first study, it involves CF cultures as in vitro models, in vivo animal experiments (which gave essentially similar results), and published data from human experiments. Genes for drug resistance and virulence factors of bacteria are often located on plasmids, as are sequences inserted by recombinant DNA techniques. Plasmids may then transfer to other bacteria, thereby increasing the genetic complements of their new host microorganisms. When plasmids specify resistance to antibiotics or virulence factors, there is a strong possibility that plasmid-bearing bacteria may transfer such genetic components in vivo to normally saprophytic members of the indigenous flora of the large intestine, with potentially disastrous results. Because of this, a constant stream of studies concerning plasmid transfers in vitro and in vivo were published until about the mid-1980s. The resulting conclusions were consistent but rather confusing. Nevertheless, interpretation of that literature clearly permits the following generalizations to be made. Even among pairs of bacteria that readily permit plasmid transfers in vitro, very little or no plasmid transfer occurs in the normal gut, i.e., one that is colonized by an undisturbed microflora. In contrast, when the microflora is absent, as in germfree or newborn animals, or when it is incomplete or disturbed, as in the very young or in antibiotic-treated animals, then plasmid transfer can be observed as readily as during in vitro matings.

The fact that a normal intestine does not readily permit plasmid transfer has given rise to numerous speculations about the reason, such as that inhibitors of plasmid transfer are produced by organisms of the indigenous microflora, especially short-chain fatty acids; that the anaerobic conditions prevailing in the large intestine may be nonconducive; that the growth phases of donor and recipient bacteria may be different; and that the inherent efficiency with which potential recipients can accept a plasmid, the demonstrable negative effect of some plasmids on the growth rate of their host bacteria, and fragmentation or segregation of the plasmid in vivo are all relevant (see reference 26 for a review and further references). Contradictory experimental results made it impossible to make definitive choices among these various hypotheses. The major obstacle to progress was the lack of a rational method of describing the fertility of a given pair of donor and recipient strains for a given plasmid. A major step forward was made by Levin and Rice (47), who developed a mathematical model based on mass-action kinetics and determined the transfer rate constants for various plasmids in mixed static and CF cultures containing only the recipient and donor strains. The transfer rate constant (γ) was then taken by these authors as a measure of the fertility of a given mating. Thus, the transfer rate constant, γ_1, was determined as $dN_\star(t)/dt = \gamma_1 N_+(t)N(t)$, with $N_\star(t)$ denoting the concentration of transconjugants, $N_+(t)$ representing the concentration of the original donors, and $N(t)$ being the concentration of recipient bacteria. In the pure-culture experiments by Levin et al. (48), plasmid transfer occurred quite rapidly, so that these authors could neglect the contribution from recent transconjugants. In contrast, transfers in the presence of the indigenous microflora were slow, and the contribution of recent transconjugants became significant. That was particularly true with those plasmids whose fertility is increased for a few generations after transfer. Accordingly, a second transfer rate constant was defined by us (24) as $dN_\star(t)/dt = \gamma_2 N_\star(t)N(t)$. The concentration of transconjugants in a CF culture of

mouse intestinal flora or in the mouse gut itself was then described as a combination of the two models, namely, $dN_\star(t)/dt = \gamma_1 N_+(t)N(t) + \gamma_2 N_\star(t)N(t) + (\psi_\star - \rho)N_\star(t)$, with $\psi_\star$ representing the rate constant of multiplication of the transconjugants and ρ representing the flow rate of contents through the CF culture or the gut.

The mathematical-modeling experiments were conducted in a manner analogous to the one described above, and the best-fit transfer rate constants were determined. This model was not very efficient in matching the experimental data points to those calculated. Much better results were obtained when additional terms were introduced to account for the depression of fertility of transconjugants for a few generations after transfer of the plasmid, the loss of donor population to transconjugants, and the segregation of the plasmids. In a total of 68 experiments in CF cultures and 5 in vivo experiments in the mouse gut, the most surprising result was that fertility, defined above as the transfer rate constants for a given mating, was not appreciably different in CF cultures free of indigenous flora, in CF cultures of normal mouse flora, and in normal mice. These results imply that the environment of the gut, contrary to common intuitive assumptions, did not impair plasmid transfer at all. The low plasmid transfer rates in the gut were entirely due to the kinetics of the gut environment, i.e., low concentrations of donors and/or recipients. As a final test, data published by E. S. Anderson (2) on human volunteers were inserted into the mathematical model (Fig. 4). Anderson had fed plasmid-bearing *E. coli* bacteria to volunteers and was able to recover transconjugants only on the first day after ingestion of the donor strain by the volunteers. Our model shows that this would be expected if transfer in the human gut were analogous to that in the mouse or in CF cultures of mouse flora.

The sensitivity of the culture method employed by Anderson was 10 bacteria per ml (or g) of feces, a concentration which was found only once, on day 1. For subsequent days, the mathematical model postulated lower numbers

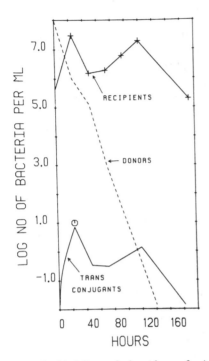

FIGURE 4 Modeling of plasmid transfer in the human gut, based on data published by Anderson (2). The symbols represent Anderson's data; the lines were calculated by the mathematical models based on parameters derived from computer-generated best-fit estimates for mice and from CF cultures of mouse intestinal floras. (Reprinted from reference 26 with permission.)

of transconjugants in the stool. These were not detected by the culture methods used, prompting the earlier authors to assume that all transconjugants had disappeared. This and other reconstructions of human experiments reported in the literature are consistent with the conclusion that the quantitative aspects of fertility and plasmid transfer in the human gut are similar to those in our mice and CF cultures. It appears that plasmid transfer occurs consistently in the human gut but that the resulting transconjugant populations are too small to be detected with the culture methods available to earlier investigators.

The latter study is an example where the availability of a mathematical model was a necessary condition for success. There was no other way to have arrived at the meaningful parameters and the transfer rate constants without the mathematical model or the computer to perform the tedious calculations.

DYNAMICS OF *H. PYLORI* COLONIZATION

H. pylori is a bacterial pathogen of the gastrointestinal tract that persists for decades. *H. pylori* induces chronic gastric inflammation that results in peptic ulcer disease or gastric cancer in a small set of infected persons (29). *H. pylori* is tropic for the acid-rich stomach, which is essentially sterile, and the immune response, although present (22), appears to be ineffective (19). A key question, then, is how can *H. pylori* colonize this environment in the face of peristalsis and very low pH?

To address this issue, we posed a regulatory feedback system based on both bacterial and host characteristics as a mechanism enabling *H. pylori* to colonize. We then created a mathematical model to explore this theoretical construct. It indicates that the proposed feedback network produces the observed colonization as well as ruling out other conceptual models of persistence (39). A summary of the modeling results is presented below.

Model of Colonization and Persistence

Adherence is a virulence attribute for many pathogenic bacteria, and in particular, for gastrointestinal pathogens that must evade peristalsis or sloughing. For *H. pylori*, adherence plays a key role in survival, since the mucus layer in which most *H. pylori* organisms reside is washed away multiple times per day (62). *H. pylori* adheres to the gastric epithelium lining the lower stomach and forms adherence pedestals (30, 73). These epithelial cells are also sloughed, although at a lower rate than mucus is shed (49). We assume that the adherent phenotype is more advantageous than the free-swimming phenotype because of proximity of the adherent bacteria to nutrients, a lower washout rate, and the fact that the pH at the epithelial cells is in the range for bacterial growth. Thus, the model incorporates migration of *H. pylori* from the mucus compartment to adhere to the cell surface. Since the adherent *H. pylori* cells divide, and the carrying capacity of the tissue is most likely near saturation, most of the new daughter cells must migrate back into the mucus layer. Thus, in our model of *H. pylori* colonization, the small portion of the bacterial population that adheres to the epithelial cells is crucial to persistence. In comparing these ideas with the situation in the colon, it has been assumed that the indigenous colonic bacteria associate with the mucus gel and epithelium; however, they do not serve as a reservoir for the mucus-living bacteria, as is specified in the *H. pylori* model. Further, microbial colonization of the colon and stomach is dissimilar in environmental pH, nutrient sources, and interspecies competition, among other factors. Thus, this model of colonization is unique to *H. pylori*.

Recent estimates of the population size of colonizing *H. pylori* in the mucus gel range from 10^4 to 10^5 per mm^3 (62). In the same study, histological assays indicated that the *H. pylori* population on the epithelial layer ranges from 10^1 to 10^3 per mm^3. Thus, we assume that free-living and adherent *H. pylori* cells represent 99 and 1% of the *H. pylori* populations, respectively. This high ratio of mucus-living to adherent bacteria, although characteristic, is not necessary for colonization, as low concentrations of *H. pylori* may be present in the mucus during persistence. We show with our model that it is the adherent population that serves to sustain colonization by acting as a core population (where a small proportion of the population serves to sustain an epidemic, as in sexually transmitted diseases) and that the mucus population acts both to replenish the adherent population and for transmission to new hosts.

The Theoretical Construct

To describe the complex interactions between *H. pylori* and the host, we propose a model in which these colonizing organisms together with the host regulate their responses in both a positive and a negative autoregulatory fashion (Fig. 5).

In this model, bacteria release proinflammatory effectors (such as urease), increasing the pH of the local environment and provoking a host response that leads to tissue damage (via inflammation) with subsequent nutrient release; the bacteria then grow in response to this growth-limiting nutrient. However, in the long term, uncontrolled inflammation may be deleterious for *H. pylori*, since its niche would be lost (33, 36). Experimental observation indicates that *H. pylori* surface molecules, such as lipopolysaccharide, have low proinflammatory activities (57). Thus, we assume that *H. pylori* can down-regulate effector production. Released host nutrients may also activate *H. pylori* signal transduction pathways that repress synthesis of bacterial proinflammatory effectors (12) and nitrogen repression (20) of cloned *H. pylori* urease; this is consistent with our hypothesis, since urease and its products have proinflammatory activities (52, 72). Inflammation may be damaging when infection cannot be eradicated, leading to impairment of tissue structure and function. Experimental data show that the cellular response to *H. pylori* infection appears to be suppressed even in the early stages of colonization (37, 70). The elements of this highly regulated feedback model are summarized in a schematic diagram in Fig. 5.

Using this proposed feedback model for *H. pylori* colonization, we created a mathematical model that examined these interactions and described the sensitivity of the system to changes of the interaction rates.

THE MATHEMATICAL MODEL

We define four populations and describe their interactions by using differential equations that monitor their rates of change, where $M(t)$ is the concentration of *H. pylori* cells in the mucus gel per cubic millimeter at any time and $A(t)$ is the concentration of *H. pylori* cells adherent to the epithelial cells per cubic millimeter. We also define $N(t)$, representing the nutrient concentration (assumed proportional to inflamma-

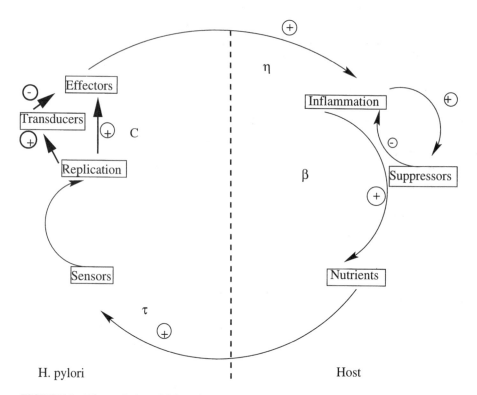

FIGURE 5 Theoretical model describing interactions of *H. pylori* with the host, incorporating positive and negative feedback regulation. Effectors released by *H. pylori* interact with the mucosa and induce inflammation. Inflammation leads to the release of nutrients that are taken up by *H. pylori,* allowing replication and further release of effectors. The bacteria sense inflammation indicators and down-regulate effector production, while the host also down-regulates the inflammatory response. The interactions within this system are governed by the four parameters τ, C, β, and η, which are not presently measurable. Therefore, mathematical modeling can play the unique role of elaborating these host-pathogen interactions. (Adapted from reference 1.)

tion), and $E(t)$, the total effector concentration released by *H. pylori* that leads to inflammation and nutrient release. A schematic representation of the mathematical model is given in Fig. 6.

PARAMETER ESTIMATION

To complete the development of a mathematical model, we must define values for the parameters and initial conditions for the rate constants in the model. This is a key place where experimental results are incorporated into the models. We chose millimeters^{-3} as the units marking the volume of population concentrations and measured time in days. Note that the model is robust with small changes in the

choices of these parameter values. We illustrate the process of estimation for some of the key parameters in the model. As mentioned above, during colonization *H. pylori* density ranges from 10^4 to 10^5 per mm^3 in the mucus gel and from 10^1 to 10^3 per mm^3 on the epithelial layer (62); thus, we select the initial population size of mucus-living *H. pylori* to be 10^5/ml and that of the adherent bacteria to be 500/ml. Epithelial cells slough every 2 to 3 days (37); thus, the rate (μ_A) is 0.3/day. Estimating that the mucus sheds at a rate at least two to three times higher than that of the epithelial cells, μ_M is 0.85/day. The growth of *H. pylori* can be determined from the doubling time based on logistic growth (see equation 2). If we assume the in

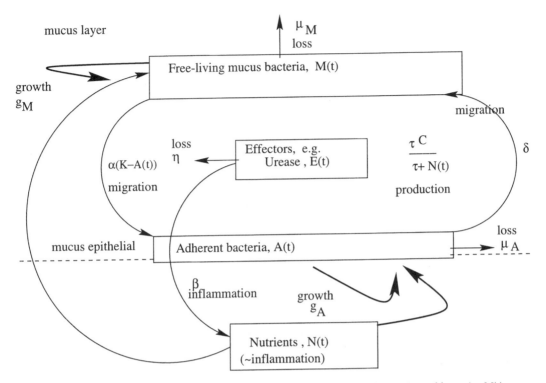

FIGURE 6 Mathematical model describing the interaction of *H. pylori* and host. Mucosal bacteria, $M(t)$, grow proportionally to nutrient at rate rg_M and are cleared continuously by peristalsis at the rate μ_M. They also migrate to the adherent sites [at rate $\alpha(K - A(t))$] and gain in numbers due to migration from the adherent sites (at rate δ). Adherent bacteria, $A(t)$, follow a similar dynamic, with opposite migration. Nutrients, $N(t)$, are produced proportionally to effector amounts (at rate β) and are taken up by the adherent and mucosal populations (at rates g_M and g_A, respectively). Effectors are produced by both mucosal and adherent bacteria [at rate $\tau C/\tau + N(t)$] and degrade nonspecifically at rate η.

vivo doubling time of *H. pylori* is 1 h ($D = 0.0416$ day), then using the formula $r = \ln 2/D$, the growth rate (r) is 16.66/day.

The four parameters, C, β, η, and τ, defined in the feedback system (Fig. 5) play a key role in the dynamics of the system; values for these parameters are not presently known and cannot be experimentally measured. Except for the parameter τ, they are each bifurcation parameters, i.e., changes in their values can cause significant change in the resulting dynamics. This is not surprising, since a fine–tuned feedback system may be crucial for the unprecedented survival of *H. pylori* in the human stomach.

To study the model, we numerically solve the complex mathematical system that describes the scheme in Fig. 6; the time-series

solution, showing the system immediately going into steady state, is shown in Fig. 7. Thus, the bacteria have completely colonized the system and are in equilibrium (c.f. reference 39).

This model can now be tested for a variety of different influences, such as competition between strains, host perturbations, and other biological variations. For example, we study the question of competition between different *H. pylori* strains. Clinical studies indicate that humans may be simultaneously colonized with (at least) two different strains of *H. pylori*. For example, *cagA*[+] and mutant *cagA* (34, 74) have been shown to be associated with different outcomes of infection (34, 74). We found with the mathematical model of these interactions

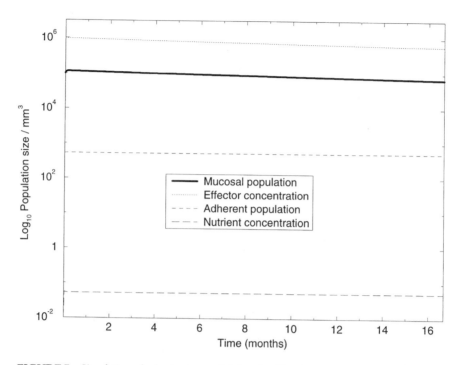

FIGURE 7 Simulation of colonization model showing *H. pylori* persistence. The four populations shown are the mucosal bacteria, the adherent bacteria, and the effector and nutrient concentrations. Notice that within a year the populations enter a steady-state in which they will remain indefinitely unless there is some perturbation in the system.

that only where genotypic differences did not alter the apparent phenotype of the strains with respect to growth, acquisition of nutrients, etc. (i.e., differences in one or more of the parameters), could there be persistent coexistence. If the phenotypes varied to any measurable degree based on known characteristics, then coexistence was only temporary and eventually the strain with the advantage competitively excluded the other over a time frame that was inversely correlated with the magnitude of the phenotypic difference (11, 39). Therefore, a clinical biopsy may reveal the presence of multiple strains within a given host; however, their concentration levels and long-term existence patterns may be very different.

The Effect of a Developing Host Response on Colonization

The system discussed above was designed to model the steady-state condition that exists for

the majority of *H. pylori* cells resident in the human stomach, where we assumed that any host response was already in a down-regulated steady state. During infection, however, there are a variety of host responses to *H. pylori*. For example, there are both humoral and cellular immune responses (19, 22), although both appear to be ineffective in clearing the bacteria and preventing colonization in most individuals. Our present model of colonization does not account for the initial events in infection, just after an inoculum is introduced into a naive host. In a second study (11), we examined the initial events by including a generalized host response.

To elaborate the early dynamics of *H. pylori* colonization, we developed a new model that incorporates the role of the developing host response. The model allows us to examine both the initial events following *H. pylori* introduction into a naive host and the development of colonization. This model also allows us to predict the effects of host perturbations on the *H. pylori* populations and the resulting consequences. Incorporation of the dynamic host response into a model of *H. pylori* colonization is critical if we are to understand the initial features of the interactions between microbe and host, as well as the phenomena that permit persistence to develop. Thus, we extended our earlier model to incorporate characteristics of the host-microbial interaction that had not been addressed previously. In the new model, the major role of the host response is to down-regulate tissue inflammation and its exudate into the gastric lumen, which we have assumed to be the major nutrient source for *H. pylori*. We were able to show that the strength of the host response plays a key role in deciding whether persistent infection can be established.

We describe a new population reflecting the intensity of the host response to *H. pylori* (H_R) (11). The growth rate of the host response is reflected by k_1. The host response initially grows as a function of the bacterial population, but this growth has a limited capacity, which is represented by k_2 (69). In this model, we assume that adherent *H. pylori*, (A), will have a greater impact on the host response than will the mucus-living *H. pylori*, (M), due to its proximity to host epithelial cells. The new equation is

$$\frac{dH_R(t)}{dt} = k_1(M(t) + k_3A(t))(k_2 - H_R(t)). \quad (3)$$

The equation marking the change in nutrients (proportional to inflammation) in the earlier model is now altered to reflect the host's developing response to introduction of *H. pylori*. The source of nutrients now represents the proportional relationship between effectors, E, and the limiting effects of the host response, H_R: if H_R is small, the term acts as it did in the previous model, but if it is large, then the production rate of the nutrients is limited.

Exploring the Host Response Model

If we solve the new system of equations together with the new initial starting values that

reflect beginning at conditions reflecting the inoculum, we see that the model yields two qualitatively different outcomes (Fig. 8). For small values of k_2, the host response capacity, the model predicts that the system will develop into persistent colonization (Fig. 8A). For large values of k_2, the model predicts the system will undergo transient colonization and the bacterial population will eventually be cleared (Fig. 8B). Notice in Fig. 8A and B how different values for the parameter k_2 alter the host response curves. This indicates that under certain host responses, the bacteria either can be cleared or will establish persistence. This model can also be used to test how other variations in the host response will affect the predicted model outcomes.

DYNAMICS OF THE HOST IMMUNE RESPONSE AND *M. TUBERCULOSIS*

Tuberculosis (TB) has been a leading cause of death in the world for centuries. Today it remains the number one cause of death by infectious disease worldwide—3.1 million deaths per year. TB is not only one of our oldest microbial disease enemies, it remains one of the most formidable: an estimated one-third of the world population has latent TB. Thus, there is a great need to elucidate the mechanisms of TB progression. Key issues are to understand the immunologic mechanisms that are involved in establishing and maintaining latent infection (resolution) and those that lead to reactivation of *M. tuberculosis* and development of active disease. There exists an enormous body of literature regarding the individual elements of both pathogenic mechanisms and the immune response to *M. tuberculosis*; however, little is known about combined interactions or the balance among these processes. This lack of knowledge is reflected in the limited number of antibiotic therapies that are currently effective against multidrug-resistant strains. The therapy limitations, coupled with the emergence of multidrug resistance, make the development of alternative therapeutic approaches even more pressing. Preliminary efforts in one

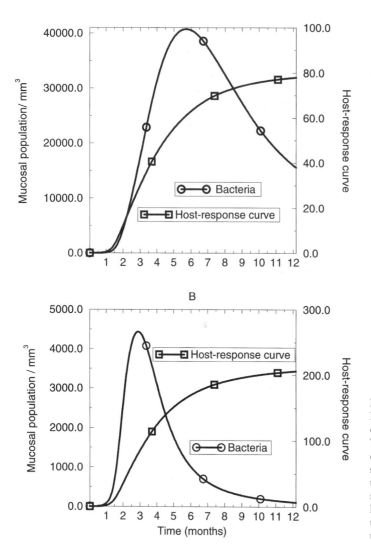

FIGURE 8 Model dynamics. (A) Initial transient dynamics and development of persistent colonization. The results are obtained by numerically solving the modified model system. (B) Transient colonization that results from a much larger host response (due to an increase in the host carrying capacity). Note how this larger host response causes a timely elimination of the bacteria.

of our laboratories (D.E.K.) focus on elucidating the mechanisms of disease progression through investigation of the regulation of the immune response to *M. tuberculosis* infection. Our long-term goal is to explain the establishment and maintenance of latency in *M. tuberculosis* infection. TB is a unique disease in that 90% of persons establish a latent infection; however, 5% progress rapidly and 5% progress slowly to active disease over their lifetimes (18, 71). Our particular focus is to predict why some individuals clear *M. tuberculosis* infection while others develop latent infection essentially

for life, and why still others develop active disease, via either a fast or slow disease course. The immune mechanisms that are involved in these alternative disease trajectories are crucial, and these mechanisms are the focus of our present and continuing work.

We have shown above the detailed elements involved in various approaches to modeling. Therefore, in the interest of brevity and because this work is still very much in progress, we will only outline our preliminary results in this section.

During infection, immune cells secrete cytokines that modulate the immune response in both a positive and a negative fashion. Cytokines have been shown to be involved in the dynamics of *M. tuberculosis* infection, specifically by influencing the differentiation of CD4[+] T cells into either TH1 or TH2 cells. Mosmann and colleagues (56) discovered that, upon stimulation, CD4[+] T cells further differentiate into TH1 and TH2 subsets that are distinguished on the basis of the cytokine profiles they produce. TH1 cells are not only responsible for stimulating macrophages to engulf and kill foreign particles but also for activating CD8[+] T cells, which then differentiate into cytotoxic T lymphocytes that can kill infected cells directly. TH2 cells down-regulate the cell-mediated response while up-regulating the humoral (antibody) response.

Models that qualitatively and quantitatively characterize the balance of the TH1- and TH2-type response can be useful in delineating the mechanisms of disease progression in *M. tuberculosis* infection. During infection, there are two types of cellular immune responses: an activated macrophage response (governed by a TH1 response), leading to a delayed-type hypersensitivity (DTH) reaction that on its own is not able to effect resolution, and a T-cell-regulated, macrophage-suppressing response resulting in the down-regulation of the DTH reaction (governed by a TH2 response) that can effect resolution.

Although the events in the immunology and pathology of *M. tuberculosis* infection are not well characterized, numerous factors that regulate immune processes have been implicated in the development of TB. These processes include cell-pathogen and cell-cell interactions as well as the production and action of cytokines that facilitate these interactions. In particular, the progression of disease may depend upon the dominant cytokine phenotype. The initiation of a TH1 cytokine response by an inciting agent may result in a vigorous DTH response with the expression of gamma interferon (IFN-γ) and interleukin 12. An effective response spearheaded by elevated levels of IFN-γ usually will clear the inciting agent and

ensure that granuloma formation takes place. On the other hand, TH2 cytokines result in a cessation of the TH1 response, which may ultimately prevent the lung environment from being destroyed by an overly active DTH response. We devised a hypothesis that the stages of TB depend on the balance of TH1 and TH2 cytokines that are generated during the expression of disease. We are testing this hypothesis through mathematical modeling.

Primary TB, the response following the first exposure to *M. tuberculosis*, usually develops in the alveoli of the lung at the peripheral midzone after droplets containing the bacteria are inhaled. The bacteria are then ingested by resident alveolar macrophages and begin to multiply (15). These cells are poor at destroying their occupants because *M. tuberculosis* has the ability to prevent the phagosome-lysosome fusion in insufficiently activated macrophages (53, 59). Eventually, an infected macrophage either bursts due to the large number of bacteria multiplying within or it circulates out through the lymphatic ducts to the lymph nodes (transporting bacteria and antigen), where the specific immune response is initiated. Here, CD4[+] T cells are activated to become TH1 and TH2 cells. TH1 cells, which are thought to be the dominant type in the immune response to TB infection (28), must migrate to the site of infection, activate macrophages to facilitate killing the ingested bacteria, orchestrate the DTH response, kill (or stimulate cytotoxic T lymphocytes to kill) macrophages that are unable to destroy their ingested bacteria.

Many recent studies explore the role of cytokine profiles in infection with *M. tuberculosis* (e.g., references 21, 35, 61, 65, and 66). The relevant immune responses involve a complex interplay of cellular immune processes and cytokine mediators. To distinguish among the cellular immune processes for modeling, we first define the tissue-damaging, DTH response that occurs due to IFN-γ activation of macrophages as dominated by a TH1-type response. Second, we define the immune response resulting in macrophage deactivation as dominated by a TH2-type response. We are inter-

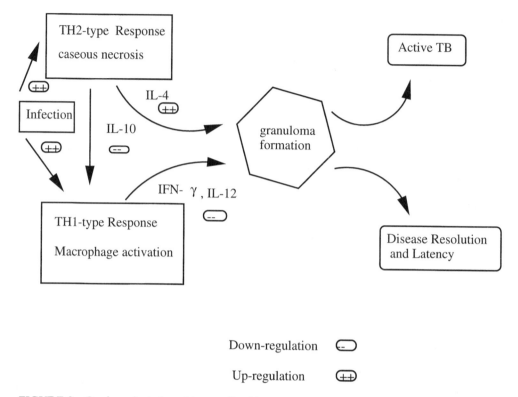

Down-regulation ⊂⁻⊃

Up-regulation ⊂⁺⁺⊃

FIGURE 9 Our hypothetical cytokine–mediated immune response network in *M. tuberculosis* infection. The progression of disease to either active or latent TB may depend on the balance of the TH1 and TH2 cytokines that are generated during the expression of disease.

ested in the interactions between these two processes and in the balance between them that allows for the establishment and maintenance of the latent state. We present a scheme for this interaction in Fig. 9.

Because we hypothesize that it is the balance between the TH2-type and the TH1-type immune responses that allows for the establishment of latency in *M. tuberculosis* infection, we developed a model of the cytokine control network during infection. In an effort to identify interactions among the immune mechanisms that are critical for the establishment of this balance, we explored the effects of perturbing different factors in the model, including cytokines, T cells, macrophages, and bacteria, and relevant interactions among these populations.

Our initial results indicate that the TH1-TH2 cytokine response is indeed a key factor in the different disease trajectories of TB. Thus, therapies that enhance or depress certain aspects of either response may have potential use for treating *M. tuberculosis* infections.

CONCLUDING REMARKS

Although mathematical-modeling approaches have been widely used in the study of virus-host interactions, they have been applied less frequently to the study of bacterium-host interactions. If we consider long-term associations between bacteria and humans a question of bacterial ecology, such as persistent infections or the homeostasis of an indigenous microflora, it becomes more logical to consider mathematical approaches to understanding these associations, as modeling has long been used by ecologists.

This chapter reviews studies which illustrate how complex problems in host-microbe interactions are unlikely to have been solved without mathematical modeling. Very often, models appear to confirm what the experimentalists may already surmise about a system. Properly understood, however, the model can be seen as a starting point for designing crucial experiments to test those assumptions. In cases when the biological system is experimentally intractable, a representative mathematical model may offer the sole means of testing key hypotheses. On other occasions, a model may illuminate testable aspects of the system that had not occurred to the experimentalist.

As we accumulate more and more detailed data, mainly on the molecular level, through experimental techniques of increasing sophistication, it is clear that there is a strong need for an integrative understanding of the complex processes of host-pathogen interactions. Mathematical modeling offers a unique method for achieving this integration and thus will be an increasingly important tool in understanding these processes.

REFERENCES

1. **Agur, Z.** 1989. Clinical trials of zidovudine in HIV infection. *Lancet* **ii:**1400–1401.
2. **Anderson, E. S.** 1975. Viability of, and transfer of a plasmid from *E. coli* K12 in the human intestine. *Nature* **255:**502–504.
3. **Anderson, R. M.** 1982. Transmission dynamics and control of infectious disease agents, p. 149–176. *In* R. M. Anderson and R. M. May (ed.), *Population Biology of Infectious Diseases.* Springer-Verlag, Berlin, Germany.
4. **Anderson, R. M., and R. M. May.** 1987. Transmission dynamics of HIV infection. *Nature* **326:**137–142.
5. **Anderson, R. W.** 1996. How adaptive antibodies facilitate the evolution of natural antibodies. *Immun. Cell Biol.* **74:**286–291.
6. **Anderson, R. W., M. S. Ascher, and H. W. Sheppard.** 1998. Direct HIV cytopathicity cannot account for CD4 decline in AIDS in the presence of homeostasis: a worst-case dynamical analysis. *J. Acquir. Immune Defic. Syndr. Hum. Retrovirol.* **17:**245–252.
7. **Antia, R., J. C. Koella, and V. Perrott.** 1996. Models of the within-host dynamics of persistent mycobacterial infections. *Proc. R. Soc. Lond.* **1:** 257–263.
8. **Antia, R., B. Levin, and R. B. May.** 1994. Within-host population dynamics and the evolution and maintenance of microparasite virulence. *Am. Nat.* **144:**457–472.
9. **Asachenkov, A., G. Marchuk, R. Mohler, and S. Zuev.** 1994. *Disease Dynamics.* Birkhauser Boston, Cambridge, Mass.
10. **Bailey, N. T. J.** 1975. *The Mathematical Theory of Infectious Diseases,* 2nd ed. Hafner, New York, N.Y.
11. **Blaser, M. J., and D. E. Kirschner.** 1999. Dynamics of Helicobacter pylori colonization of the human stomach in relation to the host immune response. *Proc. Natl. Acad. Sci. USA* **96:**8359–8364.
12. **Blaser, M. J., and J. Parsonnet.** 1994. Parasitism by the "slow" bacterium H. pylori leads to altered gastric homeostasis and neoplasia. *J. Clin. Investig.* **94:**4–8.
13. **Blower, S. M., A. R. McLean, T. C. Porco, P. M. Small, P. C. Hopewell, M. A. Sanchez, and A. R. Moss.** 1995. The intrinsic transmission dynamics of tuberculosis epidemics. *Nat. Med.* **1:** 815–821.
14. **Blower, S. M., P. M. Small, and P. C. Hopewell.** 1996. Control strategies for tuberculosis epidemics: new models for old problems. *Science* **273:** 497–500.
15. **Canetti, G.** 1955. *The Tubercle Bacillus in the Pulmonary Lesion in Man.* Springer Publishing Co., New York, N.Y.
16. **Castillo-Chavez, C., and Z. Feng.** 1997. To treat or not to treat: the case of tuberculosis. *J. Math. Biol.* **35:**629–659.
17. **Castillo-Chavez, C., and Z. Feng.** 1998. Global stability of an age-structure model for TB and its applications to optimal vaccination strategies. *Math. Biosci.* **151:**135–154.
18. **Comstock, G. W.** 1982. Epidemiology of tuberculosis. *Am. Rev. Respir. Dis.* **125:**8–16.
19. **Crabtree, J. E., J. D. Taylor, and J. L. Wyatt.** 1991. Mucosal IgA recognition of Helicobacter pylori 120 kDa protein, peptic ulceration, and gastric pathology. *Lancet* **338:**332–335.
20. **Cussac, V., R. L. Ferrero, and A. Labigne.** 1992. Expression of *Helicobacter pylori* urease genes in *Escherichia coli* grown under nitrogen-limiting conditions. *J. Bacteriol.* **174:**2466–2473.
21. **Dalton, D. K., S. Pitts-Meek, S. Keshav, I. S.**

Figari, A. Bradley, and T. A. Stewart. 1993. Multiple defects of immune cell function in mice with disrupted inteferon gamma genes. *Science* **259:**1739–1742.

22. Dooley, C. P., P. L. Fitzgibbons, H. Cohen, M. Appleman, M. Bauer, G. J. Perez-Perez, and M. J. Blaser. 1989. Prevalence of H. pylori infection and histologic gastritis in asymptomatic persons. *N. Engl. J. Med.* **321:**1562–1566.

23. Freter, R. 1983. Human intestinal microflora in health and disease, p. 33–54. *In* D. J. Hentges (ed.), *Mechanisms that Control the Microflora in the Large Intestine.* Academic Press, Inc., San Diego, Calif.

24. Freter, R. 1984. Factors affecting conjugal plasmid transfer in natural bacterial communities, p. 105–114. *In* M. J. Klug and C. A. Reddy (ed.), *Current Perspectives in Microbial Ecology.* American Society for Microbiology, Washington, D.C.

25. Freter, R., H. Brickner, and S. J. Temme. 1986. An understanding of colonization resistance of the mammalian large intestine requires mathematical analysis. *Microecol. Ther.* **16:** 147–155.

26. Freter, R., R. R. Freter, and H. Brickner. 1983. Experimental and mathematical models of *Escherichia coli* plasmid transfer in vitro and in vivo. *Infect. Immun.* **39:**60–84.

27. Gordon, D. M., and M. A. Riley. 1992. A theoretical and experimental analysis of bacterial growth in the bladder. *Mol. Microbiol.* **6:**555–562.

28. Hahn, H., and S. H. E. Kaufmann. 1981. Role of cell-mediated immunity in bacterial infections. *Rev. Infect. Dis.* **3:**1221–1250.

29. Hentschel, E., G. Brandstatter, B. Dragoisics, A. M. Hirschl, H. Nemec, K. Schutze, M. Taufer, and H. Wurzer. 1993. Effect of ranitidine and amoxicillin plus metronidazole on the eradication of H. pylori and the recurrence of duodenal ulcer. *N. Engl. J. Med.* **328:** 308–312.

30. Hessey, S. J., J. Spencer, J. Wyatt, G. Sobola, B. J. Rathbone, A. T. Axon, and M. F. Dixon. 1990. Bacterial adhesion and disease activity in H. pylori associated chronic gastritis. *Gut* **31:**134–138.

31. Hethcote, H. W., and J. A. Yorke. 1984. *Gonorrhea: Transmission, Dynamics and Control.* Springer-Verlag, Berlin, Germany.

32. Ho, D. D., A. U. Neumann, A. S. Perelson, W. Chen, J. M. Leonard, and M. Markowitz. 1995. Rapid turnover of plasma virions and CD4 lymphocytes in HIV1 infection. *Nature* **373:** 123–126.

33. Ihamaki, T., M. Kekki, P. Sipponen, and M. Siurala. 1985. The sequelae and course of chronic gastritis during a 30- to 34-year bioptic follow-up study. *Scand. J. Gastroenterol.* **20:**485–491.

34. Jorgensen, M., P. Daskalopoulos, G. Warburton, V. Mitchell, and S. L. Hazell. 1996. Multiple strain colonization and metronidazole resistance in helicobacter pylori-infected patients: identification from sequential and multiple biopsy specimens. *J. Infect. Dis.* **174:**631–635.

35. Jouanguy, E., F. Altare, S. Lamhamedi, P. Revy, J. F. Emile, M. Newport, M. Levin, S. Blanche, E. Sebourn, and A. Fischer. 1961. Interferon gamma receptor deficiency in an infant with fatal Bacille Calmette-Guerin infection. *N. Engl. J. Med.* **335:**1956–1961.

36. Karnes, W. E., Jr., I. Samloff, M. Siurala, M. Kekki, P. Sipponen, S. W. Kim, J. H. Walsh, and J. L. Casanova. 1991. Positive serum antibody and negative tissue staining for H. pylori in subjects with atrophic body gastritis. *Gastroenterology* **101:**167–174.

37. Karttunen, R. 1991. Blood lymphocyte proliferation, cytokine secretion and appearance of T cells with activation surface markers in cultures with Helicobacter pylori: comparison of the responses of subjects with and without antibodies to H. pylori. *Clin. Exp. Immunol.* **83:**396–400.

38. Kirschner, D. 1999. Dynamics of co-infection with M. tuberculosis and HIV-1. *Theor. Popul. Biol.* **55:**94–109.

39. Kirschner, D., and M. J. Blaser. 1995. The dynamics of H. pylori infection of the human stomach. *J. Theor. Biol.* **176:**281–290.

40. Kirschner, D., S. Lenhart, and S. Serbin. 1997. Optimizing chemotherapy of HIV infection: scheduling, amounts and initiation of treatment. *J. Math. Biol.* **35:**775–792.

41. Kirschner, D., R. Mehr, and A. Perelson. 1998. The role of the thymus in pediatric HIV-1 infection. *J. Acquir. Immune Defic. Syndr. Hum. Retrovirol.* **18:**95–108.

42. Kirschner, D., and A. Perelson. 1995. A model for the immune system response to HIV: AZT treatment studies. *Math. Popul. Dyn.* **1:**296–310.

43. Kirschner, D., and G. F. Webb. 1996. A model for treatment strategy in the chemotherapy of AIDS. *Bull. Math. Biol.* **58:**367–390.

44. Kirschner, D., and G. F. Webb. 1997. A mathematical model of combined drug therapy of HIV infection. *J. Theor. Med.* **1:**25–34.

45. Kirschner, D., and G. F. Webb. 1997. Qualitative differences in HIV chemotherapy between resistance and remission outcomes. *Emerg. Infect. Dis.* **3:**273–283.

46. Kirschner, D., and G. F. Webb. 1997. Understanding drug resistance in the monotherapy treatment of HIV infection. *Bull. Math. Biol.* **59:** 763–785.

47. Levin, B. R., and V. A. Rice. 1980. The kinetics of transfer of nonconjugative plasmids by mobilizing conjugative factors. *Genet. Res.* **35:** 241–259.

48. Levin, B. R., F. M. Stewart, and V. A. Rice. 1979. The kinetics of conjugative plasmid transmission: fit of a simple mass action model. *Plasmid* **2:**247–260.

49. Lipkin, M., B. Sherlock, and B. Bell. 1963. Cell proliferation kinetics in the gastrointestinal tract of man. *Gastroenterology* **46:**721–735.

50. Lipsitch, M., and B. R. Levin. 1997. The population dynamics of antimicrobial chemotherapy. *Antimicrob. Agents Chemother.* **41:**363–370.

51. Lipsitch, M., and B. R. Levin. 1998. Population dynamics of tuberculosis treatment. *Int. J. Tuberc. Lung Dis.* **2:**187–199.

52. Mai, U. E., G. Perez-Perez, J. B. Allen, S. M. Wahl, M. J. Blaser, and P. D. Smith. 1992. Surface proteins from H. pylori exhibit chemotactic activity for human leukocytes and are present in gastric mucosa. *J. Exp. Med.* **175:**517–525.

53. McDonough, K. A., Y. Kress, and B. R. Bloom. 1993. Pathogenesis of tuberculosis: interaction of M. tuberculosis with macrophages. *Infect. Immun.* **61:**2763–2773.

54. McLean, A., and M. Nowak. 1991. Interactions between HIV and other pathogens. *J. Theor. Biol.* **155:**69–86.

55. Merrill, S. J. 1987. AIDS: background and the dynamics of the decline of immunocompetence, p. 59–75. *In* A. S. Perelson (ed.), *Theoretical Immunology. Part 2.* Springer-Verlag, Berlin, Germany.

56. Mosmann, T. R. H., H. Cherwinski, and M. W. Bond. 1986. Two types of murine T cell clones. I. Definition according to profiles of lymphokine activity and secreted proteins. *J. Immunol.* **136:**2348–2357.

57. Muotiala, A., I. M. Helander, L. Pyhala, T. U. Kosunen, and A. P. Moran. 1992. Low biological activity of *Helicobacter pylori* lipopolysaccharide. *Infect. Immun.* **60:**1714–1716.

58. Murray, J. D. 1980. *Mathematical Biology.* Springer-Verlag, Berlin, Germany.

59. Myrvik, Q. N., E. S. Leake, and M. J. Wright. 1984. Disruption of phagosomal membranes of normal alveolar macrophages by the H37 Rv strain of M. tuberculosis. *Am. Rev. Respir. Dis.* **129:**322–328.

60. Nahmias, A. J., W. S. Clark, A. P. Kourtis, F. K. Lee, G. Cotsonis, C. Ibegbu, D. Thea, P. Palumbo, P. Vink, R. J. Simonds, and S. R. Nesheim. 1998. Thymic dysfunction and time of infection predict mortality in HIV-infected infants. *J. Infect. Dis.* **178:**680–685.

61. Newport, M. J., C. M. Huxley, S. Huston, C. M. Hawrylowicz, B. A. Ostra, R. Williamson, and M. Levin. 1996. A mutation in the interferon gamma receptor gene and susceptibility to mycobacterial infection. *N. Engl. J. Med.* **335:**1941–1949.

62. Nowak, J. A., B. Forouzandeh, and J. A. Nowak. 1997. Estimates of H. pylori densities in the gastric mucus layer by PCR, histological examination and CLOtest. *Anat. Pathol.* **108:** 284–288.

63. Nowak, M. A., and C. R. M. Bangham. 1996. Population dynamics of immune responses to persistent viruses. *Science* **272:**74–79.

64. Nowak, M. A., R. M. May, and R. M. Anderson. 1990. The evolutionary dynamics of HIV-1 quasispecies and the development of immunodeficiency disease. *AIDS* **4:**1095–1103.

65. Orme, I. M. 1998. The immunopathogenesis of tuberculosis: a new working hypothesis. *Trends Microbiol.* **6:**94–97.

66. Parrish, N. M., J. D. Dick, and W. R. Bishai. 1998. Mechanisms of latency in M. tuberculosis. *Trends Microbiol.* **6:**107–112.

67. Perelson, A., D. Kirschner, and R. De Boer. 1993. The dynamics of HIV infection of CD 4 + T-cells. *J. Math. Biosci.* **114:**81–125.

68. Perelson, A. S., A. U. Neumann, M. Markowitz, J. M. Leonard, and D. D. Ho. 1996. HIV-1 dynamics in vivo: virion clearance rate, infected cell life span and viral generation time. *Science* **271:**1582–1586.

69. Roos, M. T., F. Miedema, M. Koot, M. Tersmette, W. P. Schaasberg, R. A. Coutinho, and P. T. Schellekens. 1995. T cell function in vitro is an independent progression marker for AIDS in human immunodeficiency virus-infected asymptomatic subjects. *J. Infect. Dis.* **171:** 531–536.

70. Sharma, S. A., G. G. Miller, G. Perez-Perez, R. S. Gupta, and M. J. Blaser. 1994. Humoral and cellular immune recognition of H. pylori proteins are not concordant. *Clin. Exp. Immunol.* **97:** 126–130.

71. Styblo, K. 1986. Respiratory medicine. *Adv. Respir. Med.* **1:**77–108.

72. Suzuki, M., S. Miura, M. Suematsu, D. Fukumura, I. Kurose, H. Suzuki, A. Kai, Y.

Kudoh, M. Osashi, and M. Tsuchiya. *Helicobacter pylori*-associated ammonia production enhances neutrophil-dependent gastric mucosal cell injury. *Am. J. Physiol.* **263:**G719.

73. **Thomsen, L. L., J. B. Gavin, and C. T. Jones.** 1990. Relation of *H. pylori* to the human gastric mucosa in chronic gastritis of the antrum. *Gut* **31:** 1230.

74. **vanderEnde, A., E. A. Rauws, M. Feller, C.** J. J. Mulder, G. N. J. Tytgat, and J. Dankert. 1996. Heterogeneous Helicobacter pylori isolates from members of a family with a history of peptic ulcer disease. *Gastroenterology* **111:**638–647.

75. **Wei, X., S. K. Ghosh, M. E. Taylor, V. A. Johnson, E. A. Emini, P. Deutsh, J. D. Lifsoh, S. Bonhoeffer, M. A. Nowak, B. H. Hahn, et al.** 1995. Viral dynamics in HIV virus 1 infection. *Nature* **373:**117–122.

THE NATURAL HISTORY AND ECOLOGY OF COMMENSAL HUMAN FLORAS

K. A. Bettelheim

6

It has been estimated that the number of microorganisms living and thriving in or on an average human being exceeds the number of cells making up that human being by an order of magnitude. Thus, each human should be viewed as a complex ecosystem. While generally microbiologically sterile in utero, the neonate is colonized from birth, and this ecosystem is maintained, albeit modified with changing circumstances, for the rest of the individual's life. The major areas of colonization are the outer surfaces, such as skin and hair; the intestinal tract from mouth to anus; the female genital tract; and other areas with access to the outside world, such as the nasal cavities and ears. Each of these regions can be subdivided into a series of separate specific microecosystems which have different characteristics. These would be largely determined by the physico-chemical and biological nature of the environment. Thus, the oral cavity, which is mainly alkaline in pH, would have a different flora from the stomach, with its predominantly acid pH. However, even within each of these larger regions there are smaller microcosms with

unique floras. For example, the areas adjacent to the teeth have a different flora from the saliva or the regions around the tongue.

In order to gain an understanding of the complexity of the human-associated microflora it has to be seen as the complex ecosystem it is. It can be compared to a small version of a tropical rainforest, where there exist a variety of animals ranging from large mammals through smaller reptiles, birds, and amphibians to insects and smaller invertebrates, as well as a similar range of plant life. In addition, each animal and plant species is represented by a number of individuals, each with a unique genotype. Similarly, within the ecosystems inhabiting *Homo sapiens*, each species of microorganism is organized as a series of microcolonies, each derived from an individual and interacting not only with the other species but also with its conspecifics, sharing genetic information through transfer of plasmids, phages, and even naked RNA or DNA.

COMPONENTS OF THE NORMAL FLORA

The Intestinal Tract

According to Mitsuoka and Hayakawa (66), the fecal enterobacterial flora ranges from 10^8 to 10^9 CFU/g, while the total flora ranges between 10^{10} and 10^{11} CFU/g. It has been estimated that the whole gastrointestinal tract har-

K. A. Bettelheim, National *Escherichia coli* Reference Laboratory, Microbiological Diagnostic Unit, Department of Microbiology and Immunology, University of Melbourne, Melbourne, Victoria 3010, Australia.

Persistent Bacterial Infections, Edited by J. P. Nataro, M. J. Blaser, and S. Cunningham-Rundles, © 2000 ASM Press, Washington, D.C.

bors about 10^{14} microorganisms, comprising up to 500 species. Only in neonates are comparatively high levels of *Enterobacteriaceae* found. Studies of one species, *Escherichia coli*, have provided a great deal of valuable information leading to a greater understanding of the diversity of the fecal flora. This has been possible because serotyping provides a powerful tool to differentiate among clones. An extensive study was undertaken of the distribution of these organisms along the lengths of nine fecal specimens from different healthy individuals (8). From each of the fully formed stools, 10 samples taken at approximately equal distances along the length were cultured. At least 10 colonies resembling *E. coli* were selected, ensuring the greatest diversity of colonial types. In addition, from some sites up to 100 colonies were selected. Antibiotic-resistant strains were also selected separately. A total of 1,580 strains of *E. coli* were thus studied from these nine feces.

While one stool yielded only *E. coli* belonging to 1 O serogroup from all specimens, 11 different serogroups were found in another stool. The mean number of different O groups for the nine stools was 3.8. While in another stool 256 of the 270 isolates examined were from serogroup O7, there were 8 isolates of O55 found at five sites, 4 isolates of O3 in three sites, and 2 isolates of O11 in two sites. The sites yielding these rare types were not adjacent. At some sites, O serogroups which were found only in those sites were the predominant organisms. It is also noteworthy that in three specimens antibiotic-resistant variants of the O serogroups (found by nonselective means) were also found, while one specimen yielded representatives of an O group not recovered from the nonselective plates. These results should be kept in mind for the following discussions, as they are indicative of the complexity of these ecosystems.

E. coli cells colonizing the intestinal tract are generally derived from food and are able to survive the low pH of the stomach. Studies have clearly demonstrated that neonates acquire these organisms at birth from their mothers (10, 57, 82) and that adults continuously

acquire new types with their food, setting up a competitive situation with the resident flora (6).

E. coli is not normally present in the mouth, stomach, or small intestine, and even in the large intestine, it is present in comparatively low numbers, from 10^7 to 10^9 CFU/g. The predominant flora is composed of the anaerobes *Bacteroides* and *Bifidobacterium*, each with about 10^{10} to 10^{11} CFU/g, and *Eubacterium*, with 10^{10} CFU/g (21, 59). Species of *Lactobacillus* and *Streptococcus* are present at about the same levels as *E. coli*, with other enterobacteriaceae at low levels of 10^1 to 10^3 CFU/g. Yeasts are present at about 10^2 to 10^6 CFU/g, and *Clostridium* species are present at 10^6 CFU/g.

Of the members of the genus *Bacteroides*, it is the *Bacteroides fragilis* group which predominates in the human colon. Other *Bacteroides* and related species found in the colon include *Bacteroides capillosus*, *Bacteroides putredinis*, and the recently reclassified *Anaerorhabdus furcosus*, *Mitsuokella multacida*, and *Tissierella praeacuta*. It has been suggested that the facultatively anaerobic, comparatively rapidly growing bacteria, especially *E. coli* and the other enterobacteriaceae, provide the conditions which permit anaerobes to grow. While this has predominantly been demonstrated in infections such as peritonitis and in abscess formation, it is likely that the same synergistic mechanisms apply in the normal intestinal tract (90). Apart from providing the appropriate atmospheric conditions for the *Bacteroides* bacteria, *E. coli* is also believed to provide a heme-binding protein which is utilized by *Bacteroides*, and the latter consumes complement, such that insufficient quantities remain for the opsonisation of *E. coli* (89).

In estimates of the number of non-spore-forming gram-positive rods, there have often been no distinctions made between the genera *Lactobacillus* and *Bifidobacterium* and a discussion of the roles of different species of lactobacilli is complicated by the uncertain and changing taxonomy of this group. It is believed that human newborns as well as animals are rapidly colonized with the mother's vaginal and perianal flora (82, 83). As an infant's gastric acidity increases with age, lactobacilli begin to predominate in both the stomach and small intestine, while in the lower intestinal tract the strictly anaerobic *Bacteroides* and related groups predominate. These lactobacilli appear to act protectively in preventing the colonization of potentially enteropathogenic organisms, such as pathogenic *E. coli*, by producing antimicrobial factors (28). Of these lactobacilli, *Lactobacillus acidophilus* is probably the most important species present. A number of factors with bacteriocin-like properties may be produced by *L. acidophilus*. These are lactacin B (5), lactacin F (69), acidophilin (79), and possibly other agents.

Studies by Mitsuoka et al. (67) have shown that *L. acidophilus*, *Lactobacillus fermentum*, and *Lactobacillus salivarius* are present in the feces of infants at levels varying from 10^3 to 10^{10} CFU/g. *L. fermentum*, which was present in all infants tested, may not be as prevalent as the other two species. However, as a result of more recent taxonomic studies, it is thought that most strains which had previously been considered to be *L. fermentum* are probably members of the *Lactobacillus reuteri* species, which is now considered the dominant heterotrophic member of the lactobacilli in the gastrointestinal tract (45). More recent studies by Talarico et al. (84) have shown that strains of *L. reuteri* can produce a potent broad-spectrum antimicrobial agent derived from glycerol. This agent, called reuterin, may be the most important of the bacteriocins produced by lactobacilli.

The most recent study of the lactobacilli compared isolates from the tongues and rectums of 42 Swedish volunteers between 23 and 48 years of age (2). The isolates were all subjected to the same set of tests as a series of standard strains, so that the identifications were in accordance with the latest taxonomic criteria. The rectal biopsies showed a wide distribution of counts, from $<10^2$ to 10^7 CFU of lactobacilli per g of mucosa. While the median value was 10^4 CFU/g, it is noteworthy that nine individuals yielded counts below 10^2 and another nine yielded counts above 10^5. At the same time, the range of enterobacterial counts varied

from $<10^3$ to 3×10^6 (median, 2×10^4) CFU/g and the range of enterococcal counts varied from $<10^3$ to 6×10^5 (median, $<10^3$) CFU/g of mucosa.

These recent studies confirmed that lactobacilli should be considered part of the normal human intestinal flora. According to the latest taxonomic criteria, the species which were isolated most frequently from both the rectal and the oral mucosa were *Lactobacillus plantarum*, which was isolated from 52% of individuals, and *Lactobacillus rhamnosus*, which was isolated from 26% of individuals (68). These results contradict earlier findings, which showed *L. acidophilus* to be the predominant member of the genus *Lactobacillus* associated with the normal human gastrointestinal tract. The current problem with gaining a full understanding of the different lactobacilli hinges on the settlement of the taxonomic relations.

Mannose-specific adhesins may be important factors for intestinal commensals. Such adhesins were described as long ago as 1957 by Duguid and Gillies (24) and have been extensively studied in many laboratories (48, 92). A similar type of mannose-specific adhesin was shown to be present on strains of *L. plantarum* (1). In a study by Ahrne et al. (2), not only were the isolates of *L. plantarum* found to produce this mannose-specific adhesin, but another taxonomic cluster of lactobacilli, as yet unidentified, possessed an even more efficient mannose-specific adhesin.

Oral Microflora

The oral cavity may be colonized by members of more than 500 bacterial taxa at any one time. Of this wide range of taxa, the following 21 genera are considered especially important: *Actinobacillus*, *Actinomyces*, *Bacteroides*, *Campylobacter*, *Capnocytophaga*, *Corynebacterium*, *Eikenella*, *Eubacterium*, *Fusobacterium*, *Gemella*, *Haemophilus*, *Lactobacillus*, *Neisseria*, *Peptostreptococcus*, *Porphyromonas*, *Prevotella*, *Propionibacterium*, *Rothia*, *Selenomonas*, *Treponema*, and *Veillonella*.

Adherence mechanisms have been shown to play a very important role in the dynamics of oropharyngeal flora (23, 91). Following extensive cleaning of the teeth, a thin, layered host-derived pellicle develops, which consists of a variety of materials, including mucins, glycoproteins, proline- and histidine-rich proteins, and enzymes such as α-amylase, as well as phosphate-containing proteins. As bacteria adhere to this layer, they themselves become surfaces to which other bacteria may adhere. Many of these bacteria are surrounded by salivary and serum molecules which are used both for attachment and as nutrients. However, an organism may be able to adhere by itself and provide a surface for the adherence of other organisms. Growth and multiplication occur when a suitable environment is present, permitting formation of a biofilm called dental plaque (see chapter 22).

Streptococci bind to acidic proline-rich proteins, and they have been shown to be the principal early colonizers of the mouth (34, 43). Streptococci also bind to the α-amylase (78) and sialic acid (24, 43) components of the newly formed pellicle. *Actinomyces* species will also bind directly either to the pellicle (33) or to the streptococci (52). As both of these groups are facultative anaerobes, it is believed that they prepare the surface environment for the more fastidious organisms, especially obligate anaerobic groups such as *Capnocytophaga*, *Fusobacterium*, *Veillonella*, *Propionibacterium*, *Prevotella*, and *Rothia* (52). As each bacterial cell adheres and starts to metabolize, it creates new surfaces for other bacteria to adhere to, as well as changing the microenvironment around it. Whittaker et al. (91) suggest that the anaerobic *Fusobacterium* species act as bridges anchoring the environmentally more fastidious late colonizers to the streptococci (53). As part of the development of these complex microecosystems, members of different species and even genera will communicate with one another by means of nutritional end products of metabolism (37).

As the dental plaque develops, the *Fusobacterium* species gradually increase in numbers from relatively few to about 50% of either the *Actinomyces* or the streptococcal group. The *Fusobac-terium* species can coaggregate with all human oral bacterial species, which have been tested (51, 54). While many of these coaggregations are lactose inhibitable, not all of them are (50). Despite daily disruptions when the teeth are brushed, the community reforms, utilizing nutrients derived from food as well as host-derived salivary components.

A study of 22 strains of *Treponema*, including all four named human species, demonstrated that they were all capable of coagglutinating with selected strains of *Fusobacterium*, including *Fusobacterium nucleatum* and *Fusobacterium periodonticum*. They did not coagglutinate with members of nine other genera tested (54).

There are significant distinctions among the abilities of the different groups of streptococci to bind to the various sites in the oral cavity, depending on the specificities of the respective adhesins. *Streptococcus gordonii* binds to salivary α-amylase, and thus this species will congregate in areas where the protein is common, such as dental plaque (78). Similarly, the mucin-like salivary glycoprotein has been found to participate in a complex interaction with the different oral streptococci. In one way, this adherence may induce a nonimmunological means of clearing streptococci from the mouth when the mucin-like salivary glycoprotein is free. However, when it is bound to the surface of one of the oral tissues, it will induce binding of the streptococci to those tissues (12). Many specific interactions between different bacterial groups have been reported as forming the complex biofilms found on oral surfaces. *S. gordonii* coaggregates with *Actinomyces naeslundii* by means of a streptococcal adhesin which recognizes a complementary receptor on *A. naeslundii* (49). In addition, *S. gordonii* and *Streptococcus sanguis* will coaggregate with *Streptococcus oralis* and other streptococci, and a number of these will also bind to saliva-coated hydroxyapatite (70). Many more interactions have been described among the various oral bacteria, and recently specific communication mechanisms have been suggested in the development of these complex biofilms (32). As in the gastrointestinal tract, the composition of oropharyngeal flora is dynamic; however, less is known about this process in the oral cavity than in the intestine (see below).

There have been a number of suggestions aimed at intentionally modifying the oral flora, especially with reference to the possibility of reducing dental caries. One analogous approach that works in the intestine is the administration of lactulose, which is frequently given to children and the elderly in response to other medical indications. Lactulose is believed to encourage the growth of bifidobacteria (35) as well as *L. acidophilus* (77) in the intestines. As the metabolism of lactulose by oral bacteria is very slow compared to that of other carbohydrates, the release of acid is of less concern than with more readily metabolized carbohydrates.

Skin Microflora

Of the aerobic flora of the human skin, especially that on the cornified squamous epithelium, coagulase-negative members of the *Staphylococcus* group are by far the most numerous (75). However, species belonging to the genera *Corynebacterium* and *Propionibacterium* as well as other microaerophilic and even anaerobic bacterial groups are present in considerable numbers on normal human skin. As they tend to be more difficult to culture, not as much is known about them. In addition, some gram-negative bacilli and *Staphylococcus aureus* are often found transiently inhabiting the human skin. It has been suggested that organisms such as *Candida*, enterococci, and other antibiotic-resistant organisms which sometimes emerge following prophylactic antibiotic therapy are part of the normal skin flora, albeit a very small part. They are most appropriately not considered part of the normal flora, since they are typically found only upon disruption of the resident bacterial population.

The coagulase-negative members of the *Staphylococcus* group predominantly inhabit the deep layers of the squamous epithelium and are found in the dermis. They are frequently associated with sebaceous glands and hair follicles (14). While most of them are generally sensitive to antibiotics, studies have revealed

that nearly three out of four patients tested preoperatively and before any prophylactic treatment yielded methicillin-resistant coagulase-negative members of the *Staphylococcus* group from at least one sampled skin site when very sensitive isolation techniques were applied. At 61% of the sites, these methicillin-resistant coagulase-negative staphylococci emerged following perioperative prophylaxis (46). It has further been reported that following surgery many of these methicillin-resistant coagulase-negative staphylococci can acquire additional resistances, such as to gentamicin, indicating the exchange of plasmids among the normal skin flora when an appropriate selection pressure is applied (3).

The importance of being able to differentiate various clones in an investigation of the microbial ecology of a human site was amply demonstrated with the use of serotyping to study intestinal *E. coli* (8, 9). It is just as relevant in a study of the skin, where plasmid pattern profiles of coagulase-negative staphylococci were used to search for the reservoir of this resident skin flora. Glabrous skin free of dermatitis in healthy adult volunteers, who were not hospitalized and did not receive antibiotics, was investigated. After being washed with soap, rinsed with water, and air dried, the skin was sampled by means of a contact plate. The lower layers were examined by means of the tape-stripping technique (72). Using standard plasmid profile analysis techniques, the various isolated coagulase-negative staphylococci were characterized. A remarkable disparity was revealed between the surface flora and that in the underlying stratum corneum with respect to both the numbers of isolates and the strains isolated. As the sampling went below the top keratinized layers, the numbers of organisms isolated decreased by about 80%. However, no further reduction in numbers of isolates was noted following the removal of additional layers. A variety of different strains were found on the surface layers at any one site, while the number of different types was restricted to one or two in the stratum corneum underlying the surface. These results suggested that the coagulase-negative staphylococci on the skin surface are likely to be derived from a variety of sources while those found in the deeper layers should be considered the true resident flora of human skin. Indeed, in these experiments, in the deeper layers of skin, the number of types of coagulase-negative staphylococci remained relatively constant. Even following sterilization by ethanol, the same types reappeared after 18 h. The reservoir for these organisms was not found, suggesting that it might lie in deeper layers of the stratum corneum than it had been possible to sample. Others have suggested that the reservoir is in hair follicles or adjoining sebaceous glands (58) of the dermis. A few organisms have been found at these sites, but none in the sweat glands or among the living cells of the epidermis. As vellus hairs nearly completely cover the human body, these hair follicles and/or sebaceous glands could be the main reservoirs for the coagulase-negative staphylococci of the human skin.

Of the other types of bacteria found on human skin, there are a number of coryneforms, which include *Corynebacterium xerosis* and *Corynebacterium jeikeium*, as well as a number of other not yet fully named types, such as CDC group D-2. *C. xerosis* is an accepted member of the normal flora of the human skin, as well as mucocutaneous membranes such as the nasopharynx. However, this organism has also been reported from a number of different infections in immunocompromised hosts (56). *C. jeikeium*, which was originally reported under the name CDC group JK (40), is a rare inhabitant of the skins of healthy humans but frequently colonizes the skins of patients in the hospital, especially in the inguinal, perirectal, and axillary regions (55). Another species rarely found on human skin is *Corynebacterium minutissimum* (18), which is also occasionally associated with various superficial skin infections.

The status of the coryneforms now grouped among the propionibacteria, especially *Propionibacterium acnes*, as either normal inhabitants of the skin or as pathogens has always been disputed. Originally described over 100 years ago as the cause of acne vulgaris, *P. acnes* is now

accepted as a predominant member of the normal skin flora (63). *P. acnes* is found especially in areas which are rich in sebaceous glands; these include the forehead and nasolabial folds. The prominence of a strict anaerobe such as *P. acnes* growing on the human forehead clearly demonstrates how organisms can establish their own microenvironments on the human body. Of the other propionibacterial species, *Propionibacterium granulosum* is distributed on the human skin similarly to *P. acnes* but seems especially prominent in the alae nasi region. *Propionibacterium avidum* is not isolated from human skin as commonly as the other two species, apparently preferentially inhabiting moist rather than oily areas, such as the axilla, perineum, and anterior nares.

The Female Genital Tract

Propionibacteria are also commonly isolated from the human mouth, female genital tract, and intestinal tract. Bifidobacteria are commonly isolated from the female genital tract (19). The species usually encountered at this site include *Bifidobacterium bifidum*, *Bifidobacterium longum*, *Bifidobacterium infantis*, *Bifidobacterium breve*, *Bifidobacterium catenulatum*, and *Bifidobacterium dentium*. Of these, *B. bifidum* and *B. longum* are most frequently isolated. Other organisms found include *Propionibacterium propionicum* (previously *Arachnia propionica*). The predominant bacterial species found are the lactobacilli, which maintain a pH of 4.5 by their fermentative activity. It has been suggested that this low pH aids the prevention of infection by potentially pathogenic microorganisms (42).

L. acidophilus and *L. fermentum* are the most frequently described species inhabiting the human vagina, but there have also been reported isolations of other species, such as *Lactobacillus casei*, *Lactobacillus plantarum*, *Lactobacillus brevis*, *Lactobacillus delbrueckii*, *Lactobacillus lactis*, *Lactobacillus bulgaricus*, *Lactobacillus leichmannii*, *Lactobacillus salivarius*. Some of these more unusual species were first isolated in cases of vaginitis and were believed to be associated with this condition, only to be subsequently isolated from healthy individuals as well. Generally more than one species of *Lactobacillus* is present at any one time, and numbers as high as 10^5 to 10^7/ml of vaginal secretion have been reported (27). The vast majority of these lactobacilli (>95%) produce hydrogen peroxide, and this is also considered to be a nonspecific antimicrobial agent. Although only a proportion of the vaginal lactobacilli can ferment glycogen, which is the carbohydrate source present in the vagina, it is currently believed that this carbohydrate is made available to the lactobacilli by the action of a host glycogenase or possibly by the action of other microorganisms. A recent study (38) has shown an inverse relationship between the presence of hydrogen peroxide-producing lactobacilli and vaginal *E. coli* colonization in women with recurrent urinary tract infection. It has been known for many years that *E. coli*, generally derived from the fecal flora, is the most common cause of urinary tract infections in women (7). Thus, the protective effect of the vaginal lactobacilli in preventing colonization of the vagina by *E. coli* is all the more important. The hydrogen peroxide-producing lactobacilli also protect against colonization by other microorganisms (47). These studies suggest that hydrogen peroxide-producing lactobacilli might be effective probiotics for the treatment of women with recurrent urinary tract infections. However, so far only variable results have been obtained (38).

Most reports do not associate fusobacteria with the female genital tract; however, there have been some such reports. Most of these positive findings were reported many years ago, and more recent studies seem to have been less successful in isolating them. Thus, the possible role of these organisms has to be left unclarified. Similarly, whether *Actinomyces israeli* is a normal inhabitant of the female genital tract is doubtful, although it is associated with the presence of intrauterine contraceptive devices or vaginal pessaries (71). In some cases, more than one species of actinomycete can be isolated from the vagina, but whether they can colonize without the presence of a foreign body is not certain.

Other Body Sites

The occasional isolation of actinomycetes from the human eye is probably accidental. Some corynebacteria have been cultured from human eyes, especially members of CDC group F.

While there are many similarities between the nasopharyngeal flora and the oral flora, there are some differences. *C. xerosis* has occasionally been found on membranes of the nasopharynx. Another unusual inhabitant of the nasopharynx is the denitrifying *Neisseria cinerea*, which reduces nitrite to gas (5). While *Neisseria meningitidis* has been shown to colonize the healthy oro- or nasopharynx (11), other *Neisseria* and related species are more commonly encountered. These species include *Neisseria subflava*, *Neisseria mucosa*, *Neisseria cinerea*, *Neisseria lactamica*, *Branhamella catarrhalis*, and *Kingella denitrificans*. Another potentially pathogenic organism commonly found in the nasopharynx is *Haemophilus influenzae*. Up to 80% of individuals may be colonized at any one time, but mainly by the noncapsulated form, while less than 5% would be colonized by the capsulated form (86).

Specific Commensal Organisms

It is impossible here to provide a detailed account of all the various niches in which microorganisms are found on the healthy human body. Indeed, in many instances, detailed descriptions of these floras are not available. Instead, it is of greater importance to provide an understanding of the microbiological and ecological principles that underlie the distribution of bacteria on the human body.

One of the groups of organisms which has been extensively studied is the *Streptococcus milleri* group (SMG). Different taxonomic studies have given these organisms a variety of names. Some authors have also assigned them to the *Peptostreptococcus* genus, due to their status as strict anaerobes. The species defined by Guthof (39) as *S. milleri* included a narrowly defined group of nonhemolytic streptococci, but it has since been broadened to include groups previously named *S. milleri* group-intermedius and

Streptococcus anginosus-constellatus (16). Thus, the initial studies suggested that the SMG was mainly isolated from odontogenic abscesses; however, it is now apparent that they are inhabitants of the normal mouth. A Swedish study of the oral flora of 18 adults, using detailed taxonomic tests, demonstrated that members of the SMG were present in all subjects and accounted for 41% of the 220 isolated streptococci (64). In a more detailed analysis of the isolates from three of these subjects, *S. milleri* accounted for 33% of the streptococcal isolates in the gingival crevices and 11% of those in supragingival plaques; however, none of the streptococcal isolates from the saliva, the tongue, or the buccal mucosa were members of the SMG. Furthermore, extensive studies in the United States (65) demonstrated the SMG to be between 14 and 56% of all the bacteria in the gingival crevice and between 1 and 10% of those in the dental plaque. They also accounted for 1 to 10% of the salivary organisms and 5 to 10% of those on the dorsum of the tongue. This study also found none on the buccal mucosa.

Children were also found to be carrying *S. milleri*, with 6 of 24 edentulous children, 9 of 16 children with two to eight teeth, and 15 of 16 children with 20 teeth yielding SMG members (26). While *S. milleri* was widespread in the oral cavities in these and other studies, it has been regularly isolated in low numbers (about 0.5% of all cultivatable bacteria).

S. milleri has been shown to adhere to glass surfaces and is capable of forming dental plaque without other organisms on the teeth of gnotobiotic rats (93). Some strains also have peritrichously arranged fibrils and fimbriae which are probably able to initiate attachment (41). The abilities of the various oral streptococcal genera to coaggregate with each other as well as with the other plaque-forming organisms has been discussed above. The SMG has thus established itself as a common component of the dental plaque.

In addition, *S. milleri* has been isolated sporadically from throat swab specimens, with one study finding the SMG to be the third-most-common species after *Streptococcus mitis* and *S. sanguis* (62). Whether these strains were true colonizers or had merely been washed down from the dental plaque has not been established. The SMG can be cultured from fecal specimens of both adults and children in numbers which may be equivalent to those of the enterococci, up to 10^7 to 10^8 CFU/g (29). Strains of *S. milleri* have also been isolated from vaginal swabs of apparently healthy women and from other mucosal surfaces (22) and, being typical streptococci, there is no obvious reason why these organisms should not share many properties of this group, such as the expression of attachment proteins, bacteriocins, and other factors that permit these organisms to colonize humans and effectively compete with other colonizers.

Another group of organisms predominantly associated with the healthy human body are members of the genus *Bacteroides*. These are normally found to colonize the upper respiratory tract, the female genital tract, and, most importantly, the intestinal tract. In the last they are the main microbial component, and feces have been shown to contain as many as 10^{11} CFU of the *Bacteroides* group of organisms per g (20). The various species appear to be associated with different areas of the body. The main organisms in the *B. fragilis* group are predominantly found in the colon, while the *Bacteroides melaninogenicus-Bacteroides oralis* group is found in the mouth and *Bacteroides bivius* and *Bacteroides disiens* are found in the female genital tract. Of the other related species, *B. capillosus* and *B. putredinis* are found in both the mouth and the colon, *Bacteroides coagulans* is found in the intestinal and urogenital tracts, *Bacteroides forsythus* is found in dental plaque, *Bacteroides gracilis* is found in the mouth, *Bacteroides ureolyticus* is found in the respiratory, intestinal, and genital tracts, and *A. furcosus* and *T. praeacuta* are found in the intestinal tract.

The characteristics that appear to determine the sites of these various types appear quite simple. Resistance to bile salts is characteristic of the intestinal species, while the saccharolytic species are able to colonize the oral cavity. The intestinal species, such as *B. capillosus*, *B. coagulans*, *B. putredinis*, *A. furcosus*, and *T. praeacuta*, are often nonfermentative. While it is nonfermentative, *B. forsythus*, found in dental plaque, will produce α-fucosidase, trypsin, and β-galactosidase. *B. gracilis*, the main oral species, is a fermentative organism, producing acids as end products and capable of reducing nitrate to nitrite.

These observations suggest reasons why some types of *Bacteroides* group members inhabit certain parts of the human body. However, all the characteristics have not yet been elucidated. A number of suggestions were made as long as 2 decades ago (74), but there is still no resolution of this question; it is not yet clear whether these organisms have especially distinctive characteristics for an intestinal habitat or whether there are specific chemical or structural properties involved.

E. coli is the most studied bacterial species and is a normal inhabitant of the human intestinal tract. However, *E. coli* can also survive efficiently in natural waters, such as rivers, lakes, and even estuaries. Being able to survive under conditions which provide no more than a utilizable carbon source, an inorganic-nitrogen source, and a few minerals, there seems to be no good reason why it is also so successful in the human intestinal tract. The fact that it is successful, as well as able to become a pathogen, is a matter that must be addressed in order for us to gain an understanding of the true nature of the interactions between humans and microorganisms.

DYNAMICS OF THE COMMENSAL FLORA

Food provides a source of nutrients for the resident microbial flora, but it also serves as a source of new microbial flora for the gastrointestinal tract (6, 17). Humans probably ingest hundreds of species of microorganisms daily, ranging in numbers from thousands to millions (25). Changing from a normal to a sterile diet and back has a significant effect on the variety of *E. coli* found in a person's feces (6). Similarly,

travel profoundly affects the fecal *E. coli* flora (61).

Whereas it is true that *E. coli* is present in the gastrointestinal tract of virtually all humans for nearly their entire lives, the specific *E. coli* strains that are present are in a constant state of flux. Studies conducted over time suggest that each *E. coli* colonizer will be present for a limited time, generally several months (80). The factors which influence this duration are not entirely clear. Animal models and in vitro modeling suggest that the incumbent flora have a significant advantage over invading flora, most likely due to the adherence of the former to sites on the colonic mucosa (30). Indeed, substantial research has been conducted suggesting that there are ecological determinants affecting whether bacteria remain or are eliminated (30, 31). Moreover, it is clear that the normal microbial flora plays a significant role in protecting the host against colonization by enteric pathogens over and above any immune system-mediated host resistance.

The role of the immune response in the natural history of commensal intestinal bacteria is an area of intensive research. Indeed, the mucosal immune system exerts a powerful effect on bacteria at mucosal surfaces, and strikingly, these bacteria may in turn affect the immune system. Animal studies have demonstrated that the maintenance of an intestinal flora is of great importance for the very survival of the host (87, 88). The presence of the intestinal flora plays an important role in the development of germinal zones within Peyer's patches (13, 73).

The influence of thymocytes which have migrated into the gut-associated lymphoid tissues, such as the tonsils and Peyer's patches, and of intraepithelial lymphocytes on gastrointestinal colonization by microorganisms has been examined mainly in animal studies. These gut-associated lymphoid tissues are the primary sites for the induction of immunoglobulin A (IgA) precursor cells following oral administration of antigen (44, 85). The roles of secretory IgA (sIgA) include the control of the absorption of large immunogenic molecules, with which the sIgA forms complexes in the mucus.

sIgA also agglutinates bacteria and blocks the adherence properties of bacterial pili. It was noted long ago that these sIgA molecules seem to be particularly effective against intestinal pathogens such as *Vibrio cholerae* but not against the commensal flora (31). This partly explains the successful colonization and spread of such pathogens as enterohemorrhagic *E. coli*, which differ from commensal *E. coli* predominantly in their ability to form the verocytotoxins.

Yet how is it that commensal flora can persist in the face of potent mucosal immune capabilities? The answer to this question has important implications in the study of persistent bacterial infections. Investigations at several laboratories have reported that members of the commensal flora, most notably that of the gastrointestinal tract, induce a state of hyporesponsiveness to themselves (36, 73, 81). Gleeson et al. described low overall levels of sIgA in the intestinal secretions of children during the first 4 years of life (36), and Shroff et al. have reported that the commensal bacterium *Morganella morganii* induces a self-limiting humoral immune response during long-term colonization in a mouse model (81). Cole et al. have recently studied the salivary sIgA responses of infants and children to various antigens expressed by the oral commensal *A. naeslundii* and found that a very limited immune response to these antigens is engendered and that resident *A. naeslundii* strains were regularly replaced by strains of different antigenic makeup (15). However, in contrast to these observations, Marcotte and Lavoie have found that transgenic B-cell-deficient mice demonstrate acquisition and persistence of indigenous oral and intestinal microflora identical to those of normal mice (60). These data support a complex mechanism for the regulation of the commensal flora, including, in all likelihood, nonimmune factors. The confusing and in some ways contradictory evidence concerning a role for salivary IgA in the ecology of the oral flora has been extensively reviewed (60). Further discussion of the immunology of commensal floras is found in chapters 7 and 8.

CONCLUSIONS

A wide variety of microorganisms live and in many cases thrive on and in the human body. A few of these are saprophytes and even potential pathogens; however, the majority act by protecting their hosts from infection by pathogens, and some also provide forms of nutrients and other supplements. It may be purely by their presence in and successful colonization of a given site that they prevent colonization by pathogens, but probably there are many more factors involved. The production of bacteriocins, phages, and the colony incompatibility phenomena through which bacterial groups interact with each other have demonstrated that simple competition for nutrients is certainly not the only factor determining bacterial colonization. However, the very factors which permit these commensals to colonize successfully may be used by related pathogenic strains to cause disease.

One recent example may suffice as a warning to treat the commensal flora with respect. Enterohemorrhagic *E. coli*, of which only a few bacteria are required to colonize and cause disease, utilizes the colonizing abilities of the commensal *E. coli*, but with disastrous effects for the host. Recent reports by Rowbury have shown that bacteria like *E. coli* can "warn" other organisms and induce responses in them under normally noninducing conditions through the production of secreted diffusible substances which he calls "alarmones" (76). This causes the recipient bacteria to mount the appropriate stress response without specifically inducing it. As long as scientists continue to look predominantly for pathogens while ignoring the commensals, a true understanding of the role of microorganisms in health and, more importantly, in disease will not be forthcoming.

The above observations concerning the ecology and natural history of commensal flora, though obviously in the early stages of investigation, suggest that the dynamics of this flora are dependent on both ecological and immunological factors. In some instances, the presence or absence of an immune response to the microflora plays a role in the abundance and distribution of the normal flora, but especially in the gastrointestinal tract, fairly predictable mathematical models have also been developed that implicate the availability of nutrients, the rate of bacterial growth, and the presence of microbial attachment sites as important in determining what is present and for how long. In the consideration of the persistent presence of pathogenic bacteria, therefore, especially those that may inhabit the fine edge between commensalism and parasitism, it may be quite relevant to consider ecological factors in addition to immunological ones.

REFERENCES

1. **Adlerberth, I., S. Ahrné, M.-L. Johansson, G. Molin, L. Hanson, and A. E. Wold.** 1996. A mannose-specific adherence mechanism in *Lactobacillus plantarum* conferring binding to the human colonic cell line HT-29. *Appl. Environ. Microbiol.* **62:**2244–2251.
2. **Ahrné, S., S. Nobaek, B. Jeppsson, I. Adlerberth, A. E. Wold, and G. Molin.** 1998. The normal Lactobacillus flora of healthy human rectal and oral mucosa. *J. Appl. Microbiol.* **85:** 88–94.
3. **Archer, G. L., D. R. Dietrick, and J. L. Kohnston.** 1985. Molecular epidemiology of transmissible gentamicin resistance among coagulase-negative staphylococci in a cardiac surgery unit. *J. Infect. Dis.* **151:**243–251.
4. **Barefoot, S. F., and T. R. Klaenhammer.** 1983. Detection and activity of lactacin B, a bacteriocin produced by *Lactobacillus acidophilus. Appl. Environ. Microbiol.* **45:**1808–1815.
5. **Berger, U., and E. Paepcke.** 1962. Untersuchungen über die asaccharolytischen Neisserien des menschlichen Nasopharynx. *Z. Hyg. Infektionskr.* **148:**268–281.
6. **Bettelheim, K. A., E. M. Cooke, S. O'Farrell, and R. A. Shooter.** 1977. The effect of diet on intestinal Escherichia coli. *J. Hyg. Camb.* **79:** 43–45.
7. **Bettelheim, K. A., C. Dulake, and J. Taylor.** 1971. Postoperative urinary tract infections caused by Escherichia coli. *J. Clin. Pathol.* **24:**442–443.
8. **Bettelheim, K. A., M. Faiers, and R. A. Shooter.** 1972. Serotypes of Escherichia coli in normal stools. *Lancet* **ii:**1224–1226.
9. **Bettelheim, K. A., P. N. Goldwater, H. Evangelidis, J. L. Pearce, and D. L. Smith.** 1992. Distribution of toxigenic Escherichia coli

serotypes in the intestines of infants. *Comp. Immunol. Microbiol. Infect. Dis.* **15:**65–70.
10. **Bettelheim, K. A., and S. M. J. Lennox-King.** 1976. The acquisition of Escherichia coli by newborn babies. *Infection* **4:**174–179.
11. **Blakebrough, I. S., G. M. Greenwood, H. C. Whittle, A. K. Bradley, and H. M. Gilles.** 1982. The epidemiology of infections due to Neisseria meningitidis and Neisseria lactamica in a Northern Nigerian community. *J. Infect. Dis.* **146:**626–637.
12. **Brady, L. J., D. A. Piacentini, P. J. Crowley, P. C. Oyston, and A. S. Bleiweis.** 1992. Differentiation of salivary agglutinin-mediated adherence and aggregation of mutans streptococci by use of monoclonal antibodies against the major surface adhesin P1. *Infect. Immun.* **60:**1008–1017.
13. **Brockman, D. C., and M. D. Cooper.** 1973. Pinocytosis by epithelium associated with lymphoid follicles in the bursa of Fabricius, appendix and Peyer's patches. An electron microscope study. *Am. J. Anat.* **136:**455–478.
14. **Brown, E., R. P. Wenzel, and J. O. Hendley.** 1989. Exploration of the microbial anatomy of normal human skin by using plasmid pattern profiles of coagulase-negative staphylococci: search for the reservoir of resident skin flora. *J. Infect. Dis.* **160:**644–650.
15. **Cole, M. F., S. Bryan, M. K. Evans, C. L. Pearce, M. J. Sheridan, P. A. Sura, R. Weintzen, and G. H. W. Bowden.** 1998. Humoral immunity to commensal oral bacteria in human infants: salivary antibodies reactive with *Actinomyces naeslundii* genospecies 1 and 2 during colonization. *Infect. Immun.* **66:**4283–4289.
16. **Colman, G., and R. E. O. Williams.** 1972. Taxonomy of some human viridans streptococci, p. 281–299. *In* L. W. Wannamaker and J. M. Matsen (ed.), *Streptococci and Streptococcal Diseases: Recognition, Understanding, and Management.* Academic Press, New York, N.Y.
17. **Correa, C. M., A. Tibana, and P. P. Gontijo-Filho.** 1991. Vegetables as a source of infection with Pseudomonas aeruginosa in a university and oncology hospital of Rio de Janeiro. *J. Hosp. Infect.* **18:**301–306.
18. **Coyle, M. B., D. G. Hollis, and N. B. Groman.** 1985. *Corynebacterium* spp. and other coryneform organisms, p. 193–204. *In* E. H. Lennette et al. (ed.), *Manual of Clinical Microbiology,* 4th ed. American Society for Microbiology, Washington, D. C.
19. **Crociani, F., D. Matteuzzi, and H. Ghazvinizadeh.** 1973. Species of the genus Bifidobacterium found in human vagina. *Zentbl. Bakteriol. Parasitenkd. Infektkrankh. Hyg. Abt. 1 Orig. A* **223:** 298–302.

20. **Drasar, B., and M. Hill.** 1974. *Human Intestinal Flora.* Academic Press, London, United Kingdom.

21. **Drasar, B. S., M. Shiner, and G. M. McLeod.** 1969. Studies of the intestinal flora: the bacterial flora of the gastrointestinal tract in healthy and achlorhydric persons. *Gastroenterology* **56:**71–79.

22. **Drucker, D. B., and S. M. Lee.** 1983. Possible heterogeneity of Streptococcus milleri determined by DNA mol% (guanine plus cytosine) measurement and physiological characterization. *Microbios* **38:**151–157.

23. **Duan, Y., E. Fisher, D. Malamud, E. Golub, and D. R. Demuth.** 1994. Calcium-binding properties of SSP-5, the *Streptococcus gordonii* M5 receptor for salivary agglutinin. *Infect. Immun.* **62:** 5220–5226.

24. **Duguid, J. P., and R. R. Gillies.** 1957. Fimbriae and adhesive properties in dysenteric bacilli. *J. Pathol. Bacteriol.* **74:**397–411.

25. **Duncan, H. E., and S. C. Edberg.** 1995. Host-microbe interaction in the gastrointestinal tract. *Crit. Rev. Microbiol.* **21:**85–100.

26. **Edwardsson, S., and B. Mejàre.** 1975. Streptococcus milleri (Guthof) and Streptococcus mutans in the mouths of infants before and after tooth eruption. *Arch. Oral Biol.* **23:**811–814.

27. **Eschenbach, D. A., P. R. Davick, B. L. Williams, S. J. Klebanoff, K. Young-Smith, C. M. Critchlow, and K. K. Holmes.** 1989. Prevalence of hydrogen peroxide-producing *Lactobacillus* species in normal women and women with bacterial vaginitis. *J. Clin. Microbiol.* **27:**251–256.

28. **Fernandes, C. F., K. M. Shahani, and M. A. Amer.** 1987. Therapeutic role of dietary lactobacilli and lactobacillic fermented dairy products. *FEMS Microbiol. Rev.* **46:**343–356.

29. **Finegold, S. M., H. R. Atterby, and V. L. Sutter.** 1974. Effect of diet on human fecal flora: comparison of Japanese and American diets. *Am. J. Clin. Nutr.* **27:**1391–1398.

30. **Freter, R.** 1999. Continuous-flow culture models of intestinal microecology, p. 97–110. *In* L. A. Hanson and R. H. Yolken (ed.), *Probiotics, Other Nutritional Factors, and Intestinal Microflora. Nestle Nutrition Workshop Series,* vol. 42. Lippincott Williams & Wilkins, Philadelphia, Pa.

31. **Fubara, E. S., and R. Freter.** 1972. Source of protective function of coproantibodies by secretory IgA antibodies. *J. Immunol.* **111:**395–403.

32. **Fuqua, W. C., S. C. Winans, and E. P. Greenberg.** 1994. Quorum sensing in bacteria: the LuxR-LuxI family of cell density-responsive transcriptional regulators. *J. Bacteriol.* **176:** 269–275.

33. **Gibbons, R. J., D. I. Hay, J. O. Cisar, and W. B. Clark.** 1988. Adsorbed salivary proline-rich protein 1 and statherin: receptors for type 1 fimbriae of *Actinomyces viscosus* T14V-J1. *Infect. Immun.* **56:**2990–2993.

34. **Gibbons, R. J., D. I. Hay, and D. H. Schlesinger.** 1991. Delineation of a segment of adsorbed salivary acidic proline-rich proteins which promotes adhesion of *Streptococcus gordonii* to apatitic surfaces. *Infect. Immun.* **59:**2948–2954.

35. **Gibson, G. R., and M. B. Roberfroid.** 1995. Dietary modulation of the human colonic microbiota: introducing the concept of prebiotics. *J. Nutr.* **125:**1401–1412.

36. **Gleeson, M., A. W. Cripps, R. L. Clancy, J. H. Wlodarczyk, A. J. Dobson, and J. H. Hensley.** 1987. The development of IgA-specific antibodies to *Escherichia coli* O antigen in children. *Scand. J. Immunol.* **26:**639–643.

37. **Grenier, D.** 1992. Nutritional interactions between two suspected periodontopathogens, *Treponema denticola* and *Porphyromonas gingivalis. Infect. Immun.* **60:**5298–5301.

38. **Gupta, K., A. E. Stapleton, T. M. Hooton, P. L. Roberts, C. L. Fennell, and W. E. Stamm.** 1998. Inverse association of H_2O_2-producing lactobacilli and vaginal Escherichia coli colonization in women with recurrent urinary tract infections. *J. Infect. Dis.* **178:**446–450.

39. **Guthof, O.** 1956. Über pathogene "vergrünende Streptokokken"; Streptokokken-Befunde bei dentogenen Abszessen und Infiltraten im Bereich der Mundhöhle. *Zentbl. Bakteriol. Parasitenkd. Infektkrankh. Abt. 1 Orig. B* **166:**291–308.

40. **Hande, K. R., M. S. Witebsky, C. B. Brown, C. B. Shulman, S. E. Anderson, Jr., A. S. Levine, J. D. MacLowry, and B. A. Chabner.** 1976. Sepsis with a new species of Corynebacterium. *Ann. Intern. Med.* **85:**423–426.

41. **Handley, P. S., P. L. Carter, J. E. Wyatt, and L. M. Hesketh.** 1985. Surface structures (peritrichous fibrils and tufts of fibrils) found on *Streptococcus sanguis* strains may be related to their ability to coaggregate with other oral genera. *Infect. Immun.* **47:**217–227.

42. **Hill, G. B., D. A. Eschenbach, and K. K. Holmes.** 1985. Bacteriology of the vagina. *Scand. J. Urol. Nephrol. Suppl.* **86:**23–29.

43. **Hsu, S. D., J. O. Cisar, A. L. Sandberg, and M. Killian.** 1994. Adhesive properties of viridans streptococcal species. *Microb. Ecol. Health Dis.* **7:** 111–116.

44. **Kagnoff, M. F.** 1982. Oral tolerance. *Ann. N. Y. Acad. Sci.* **392:**248–264.

45. **Kandler, O., and N. Weiss.** 1986. Regular, non-sporing Gram-positive rods, p. 1208–1234. *In* P. H. Sneath, N. Mair, M. E. Sharpe, and J. G. Holt (ed.), *Bergey's Manual of Systematic Bacteri-*

ology, vol. 2. Williams and Wilkins, Baltimore, Md.

46. **Kernodle, D. S., N. L. Barg, and A. B. Kaiser.** 1988. Low-level colonization of hospitalized patients with methicillin-resistant coagulase-negative staphylococci and emergence of the organisms during surgical antimicrobial prophylaxis. *Antimicrob. Agents Chemother.* **32:**202–208.

47. **Klebanoff, S. J., S. L. Hillier, D. A. Eschenbach, and A. M. Waltersdorph.** 1991. Control of the microbial flora of the vagina by H_2O_2-generating lactobacilli. *J. Infect. Dis.* **164:**94–100.

48. **Knutton, S., D. R. Lloyd, D. C. A. Candy, and A. S. McNeish.** 1984. In vitro adhesion of enterotoxigenic *Escherichia coli* to human intestinal epithelial cells from mucosal biopsies. *Infect. Immun.* **44:**514–518.

49. **Kolenbrander, P. E., and R. N. Andersen.** 1990. Characterization of *Streptococcus gordonii* (*S. sanguis*) PK488 adhesin-mediated coaggregation with *Actinomyces naeslundii* PK606. *Infect. Immun.* **58:**3064–3072.

50. **Kolenbrander, P. E., R. N. Andersen, and N. Ganeshkumar.** 1994. Nucleotide sequence of *Streptococcus gordonii* PK488 coaggregation adhesin gene, *scaA*, and ATP-binding cassette. *Infect. Immun.* **62:**4469–4480.

51. **Kolenbrander, P. E., R. N. Andersen, and L. V. H. Moore.** 1989. Coaggregation of *Fusobacterium nucleatum, Selenomonas flueggi, Selenomonas infelix, Selenomonas noxia,* and *Selenomonas sputigena* with strains from 11 genera of oral bacteria. *Infect. Immun.* **57:**3194–3203.

52. **Kolenbrander, P. E., and J. London.** 1992. Ecological significance of coaggregation among oral bacteria. *Adv. Microb. Ecol.* **12:**183–217.

53. **Kolenbrander, P. E., and J. London.** 1993. Adhere today, here tomorrow: oral bacterial adherence. *J. Bacteriol.* **175:**3247–3252.

54. **Kolenbrander, P. E., K. D. Parrish, R. N. Andersen, and E. P. Greenberg.** 1995. Intergeneric coaggregation of oral *Treponema* spp. with *Fusobacterium* spp. and intrageneric coaggregation among *Fusobacterium* spp. *Infect. Immun.* **63:**4584–4588.

55. **Larson, E. L., K. J. McGinley, J. J. Leyden, M. E. Cooley, and G. H. Talbot.** 1986. Skin colonization with antibiotic-resistant (JK group) and antibiotic-sensitive lipophilic diphtheroids in hospitalized and normal adults. *J. Infect. Dis.* **153:**701–706.

56. **Lipsky, B. A., A. C. Goldberger, L. S. Tompkins, and J. J. Plorde.** 1982. Infections caused by nondiphtheria corynebacteria. *Rev. Infect. Dis.* **4:**1220–1235.

57. **Long, S. S., and R. M. Swenson.** 1977. Development of anaerobic fecal flora in healthy newborn infants. *J. Pediatr.* **91:**298–301.

58. **Lovell, D. L.** 1945. Skin bacteria. Their location with reference to skin sterilization. *Surg. Gynecol. Obstet.* **80:**174–177.

59. **Mackowiak, P. A.** 1982. The normal microbial flora. *N. Engl. J. Med.* **307:**83–93.

60. **Marcotte, H., and M. C. Lavoie.** 1998. Oral microbial ecology and the role of salivary immunoglobulin A. *Microbiol. Mol. Biol. Rev.* **62:**71–109.

61. **Majed, N. I., K. A. Bettelheim, R. A. Shooter, and E. Moorhouse.** 1978. The effect of travel on faecal *Escherichia coli* serotypes. *J. Hyg. Camb.* **81:**481–487.

62. **McBride, M. E., W. C. Duncan, and J. M. Knox.** 1980. Bacterial interference of *Neisseria gonorrhoeae* by α-hemolytic streptococci. *Br. J. Vener. Dis.* **56:**235–238.

63. **McGinley, K. G., G. F. Webster, and J. J. Leyden.** 1978. Regional variation of cutaneous propionibacteria. *Appl. Environ. Microbiol.* **35:**62–66.

64. **Mejàre, B., and S. Edwardsson.** 1975. Streptococcus milleri (Guthof); an indigenous organism of the human oral cavity. *Arch. Oral Biol.* **20:**757–762.

65. **Michalek, S. M., and J. R. McGhee.** 1982. Oral Streptococci with emphasis on Streptococcus mutans, p. 679–690. *In* J. R. McGhee, S. M. Michalek, and G. H. Cassel (ed.), *Dental Microbiology.* Harper & Row, Philadelphia, Pa.

66. **Mitsuoka, T., and K. Hayakawa.** 1972. Die Faecalflora bei Menschen. I. Mitteilung: die Zusammensetzung der Faecalflora der verschiedenen Altersgruppen. *Zentbl. Bakteriol. Parasitenkd. Infektkrankh. Hyg. Abt. 1 Orig. A* **223:**333–342.

67. **Mitsuoka, T., K. Hayakawa, and N. Kimura.** 1975. Die Faecalflora bei Menschen. III. Mitteilung: die Zusammensetzung der Faecalflora der verschiedenen Altersgruppen. *Zentbl. Bakteriol. Parasitenkd. Infektkrankh. Hyg. Abt. 1 Orig. A* **232:**499–511.

68. **Molin, G., B. Jeppsson, S. Ahrné, M.-L. Johansson, S. Nobaek, M. Ståhl, and S. Bengmark.** 1993. Numerical taxonomy of *Lactobacillus* spp. associated with healthy and diseased mucosa of the human intestines. *J. Appl. Microbiol.* **74:**314–323.

69. **Muriana, M. A., and T. R. Klaenhammer.** 1987. Conjugal transfer of plasmid-encoded determinants for bacteriocin production and immunity in *Lactobacillus acidophilus* 88. *Appl. Environ. Microbiol.* **53:**553–560.

70. **Oligino, L., and P. Fives-Taylor.** 1993. Overexpression and purification of a fimbria-associated

adhesin of *Streptococcus parasanguis*. *Infect. Immun.* **61:**1016–1022.

71. **Persson, E., and K. Holmberg.** 1984. Clinical evaluation of precipitin tests for genital actinomycosis. *J. Clin. Microbiol.* **20:**917–922.

72. **Pinkus, H.** 1951. Examination of the epidermis by the strip method of removing horny layers. I. Observations on thickness of the horny layer, and on mitotic activity after stripping. *J. Investig. Dermatol.* **16:**383–386.

73. **Pollard, M., and N. Sharon.** 1970. Responses of the Peyer's patches in germ-free mice to antigenic stimulation. *Infect. Immun.* **2:**96–100.

74. **Prins, R. A.** 1977. Biochemical activities of gut microorganisms, p. 73–183. *In* R. T. J. Clark and T. Bauchop (ed.), *Microbial Ecology of the Gut.* Academic Press, London, United Kingdom.

75. **Roth, R. R., and W. D. James.** 1988. Microbial ecology of the skin. *Annu. Rev. Microbiol.* **42:** 441–464.

76. **Rowbury, R. J.** 1998. Life sciences up-date. Do we need to rethink our ideas on the mechanisms of inducible processes in bacteria? *Sci. Prog.* **81:** 193–204.

77. **Salminen, S., and E. Salminen.** 1997. Lactulose, lactic acid bacteria, intestinal microecology and mucosal protection. *Scand. J. Gastroenterol.* **32**(Suppl. 222):45–48.

78. **Scannapieco, F. A., G. I. Torres, and M. J. Levin.** 1995. Salivary amylase promotes adhesion of oral streptococci to hydroxyapatite. *J. Dent. Res.* **74:**1360–1365.

79. **Shahani, K. M., J. R. Vakil, and A. Kilara.** 1977. Natural antibiotic activity of Lactobacillus acidophilus and bulgaricus. II. Isolation of acidophilin from L. acidophilus. *Cult. Dairy Prod. J.* **12:** 8–11.

80. **Shooter, R. A., K. A. Bettelheim, S. M. Lennox-King, and S. O'Farrell.** 1977. *Escherichia coli* serotypes in the faeces of healthy adults over a period of several months. *J. Hyg. Camb.* **78:** 95–98.

81. **Shroff, K. E., K. Meslin, and J. J. Cebra.** 1995. Commensal enteric bacteria engender a self-limiting humoral mucosal immune response while permanently colonizing the gut. *Infect. Immun.* **63:** 3904–3913.

82. **Smith, H. W.** 1965. The development of the flora of the alimentary tract in young animals. *J. Pathol. Bacteriol.* **90:**495–513.

83. **Smith, H. W.** 1971. The bacteriology of the alimentary tract of domestic animals suffering from Escherichia coli infection. *Ann. N. Y. Acad. Sci.* **176:**110–125.

84. **Talarico, T. L., I. A. Casas, T. C. Chung, and W. J. Dobrogosz.** 1988. Production and isolation of reuterin, a growth inhibitor produced by *Lactobacillus reuteri. Antimicrob. Agents Chemother.* **32:**1854–1858.

85. **Tomasi, T. B., L. M. Lawson, S. Challacombe, and P. McNabb.** 1980. Mucosal immunity: the origin and migration pattern of cells in the secretory system. *J. Allergy Clin. Immunol.* **65:** 12–19.

86. **Turk, D. C.** 1984. Occasional review. The pathogenicity of *Haemophilus influenzae. J. Med. Microbiol.* **18:**1–16.

87. **van der Waaij, D., T. M. Tielmans-Speltie, and A. M. de Roeck-Houben.** 1978. Relation between faecal concentration of various potentially pathogenic microorganisms and infections in individuals (mice) with severely decreased resistance to infection. *Antonie Leeuwenhoek J. Microbiol. Serol.* **44:**395–405.

88. **van der Waaij, D., and J. van der Waaij.** 1984. Spread of multiresistant gram-negative bacilli among severely immunocompromised mice during prophylactic treatment with different oral microbial drugs, p. 245–250. *In* B. S. Wostmann (ed.), *Progress in Clinical and Biological Research,* Alan R. Liss, Inc., New York, N.Y.

89. **Vel, W. A. C., F. Namavar, A. M. J. J. Verweij-van Vught, A. M. B. Pubben, and D. M. MacLaren.** 1985. Killing of *Escherichia coli* by human polymorphonucleocytes in the presence of *Bacteroides fragilis. J. Clin. Pathol.* **38:**86–91.

90. **Verweij, W. R., F. Namavir, W. T. Schouten, and D. M. MacLaren.** 1991. Early events after intra-abdominal infection with *Bacteroides fragilis* and *Escherichia coli. J. Med. Microbiol.* **35:**18–22.

91. **Whittaker, C. J., C. M. Klier, and P. E. Kolenbrander.** 1996. Mechanisms of adhesion by oral bacteria. *Annu. Rev. Microbiol.* **50:**513–552.

92. **Wold, A. E., M. Thorssen, S. Hull, and C. Svenborg-Eden.** 1988. Attachment of *Escherichia coli* via mannose- or Galα1→4Galβ-containing receptors to human colonic epithelial cells. *Infect. Immun.* **56:**2531–2537.

93. **Yoshizaki, N.** 1983. Cariogenicity of Streptococcus intermedius ATCC 27335. *Aichi Gakuin J. Dent. Sci.* **21:**371–386.

PATHOLOGICAL CONSEQUENCES OF COMMENSALISM

Agnes E. Wold and Ingegerd Adlerberth

7

The most common and long-lasting persistent infection is the colonization of different external and internal body surfaces by a microflora. Although colonization and infection are sometimes regarded as separate entities, there is no natural division between these two states. For example, most people colonized or infected with *Helicobacter pylori* do not exhibit symptoms, despite the presence of moderate mucosal inflammation. In susceptible individuals, this inflammation may lead to ulceration or malignant transformation (46).

Similarly, the normal flora of the intestine does not cause harm in most individuals, but signs of inflammation are clearly visible in the mucosa. In fact, the entire mucosal architecture and physiology are altered when microbes colonize the gut, and the functions of both the innate and acquired immune system are affected. The normal flora is likely to play an aggravating or permissive role in colon cancer, one of the most prevalent forms of malignancy. In fact, without a microflora, the life span of the host is increased (148). Intuitively foreseeing this, Metchnikoff suggested that the large bowel should be removed, in order to rid the host of the microorganisms that "appeared to be the principal cause of the short duration of human life" (22).

Several species of animals have been reared completely devoid of microbes, which requires that they be born and raised inside isolators and fed sterile food and water. This includes a boy born with severe combined immunodeficiency who lived for 12 years under germfree conditions inside a plastic bubble, eating sterilized food. In fact, he was not completely germfree, since he had low-grade colonization by poorly characterized obligately anaerobic bacteria that had been present as spores in his food (239). Germfree animals can be monocolonized with defined bacterial strains or taken out of their isolators and given a full flora by contact with other animals or by being given fecal bacteria by enema or gavage, a process termed conventionalization. Most of our knowledge of the impact of the normal microflora on the host derives from studies of germfree, monocolonized, or conventionalized animals, collectively termed gnotobiotic animals (from "gnotos," known, and "bios," life).

Thus, we shall see in this chapter that the classical distinguishing characteristics of persistent pathogens, that they elicit host responses, including inflammation, and that they have the capacity to damage the host, are increasingly

Agnes E. Wold and Ingegerd Adlerberth, Department of Clinical Immunology, Göteborg University, Guldhedsgatan 10, S-413 46 Göteborg, Sweden.

Persistent Bacterial Infections, Edited by J. P. Nataro, M. J. Blaser, and S. Cunningham-Rundles, © 2000 ASM Press, Washington, D.C.

being associated with the so-called commensal flora as well. We will focus mainly on the normal flora of the gastrointestinal tract.

THE NORMAL FLORA

All external and certain, but not all, internal body surfaces are covered by a film of microorganisms, a normal microflora. Thus, the upper respiratory tract, gastrointestinal tract, perineum, vagina, and distal urethra contain large resident bacterial populations, while the bronchi, alveolar spaces, urinary tract, and uterus are normally sterile (Fig. 1). The fact that the respiratory tract above the glottis is populated by millions of bacteria per square millimeter but is sterile below this point despite a constant

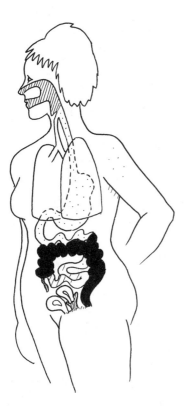

FIGURE 1 Normal floras of the human body. The bacterial population densities of different external (bacteria per square centimeter) or internal (bacteria per gram of contents) surfaces of the human body are indicated as follows: $>10^{10}$ bacteria, black; 10^8 to 10^{10}, hatched; 10^5 to 10^8, lightly hatched; 10^3 to 10^5, dotted.

seeding by airborne microbes illustrates the forceful effects of the innate defense systems, such as mucociliary transport and alveolar phagocytes.

COMPOSITION OF THE NORMAL FLORA OF THE GASTROINTESTINAL TRACT

The Stomach

Most microbes are killed by hydrochloric acid in the stomach (68). The stomach was therefore long regarded as devoid of resident bacteria. Today, it is well established that *H. pylori* is a long-term colonizer in this habitat, sometimes with detrimental consequences for the host. Acid-tolerant bacteria, like lactobacilli and streptococci, are transiently found in the stomach but are not regarded as part of a resident normal flora. In contrast to human beings, many animals have a resident lactobacillus population that colonizes the non–acid-secreting part of the stomach (158).

The Small Intestine

The proximal small intestine contains only approximately 10^2 to 10^3 bacteria per ml of intestinal fluid. This paucity of microbes is primarily due to the forceful peristalsis in the small intestine (54) and, in addition, to the effect of gastric acid (68). Since the flow of intestinal contents at this site exceeds the maximum rate of bacterial multiplication, only bacteria which adhere to the mucosa can persist (73). Further, the milieu is quite rich in oxygen, and aerobic or aerotolerant bacteria, like lactobacilli and aerobic streptococci, dominate (141).

The localized stasis proximal to the ileocecal valve permits bacteria to achieve population levels of 10^5 to 10^8/ml in the terminal ileum (132). Stasis increases anaerobiosis, and strict anaerobes, like *Bacteroides* and *Clostridium* species, as well as *Escherichia coli* and other facultative species, increase their proportions (141, 229). Still, the ileocecal valve is an effective barrier against backwash of colonic contents into the ileum and maintains a 3- to 5-log-unit difference in bacterial numbers between the terminal ileum and colon (92).

The Large Intestine

The large intestine contains huge bacterial populations, 10^{11}/g of fecal material, or 10^{14} in total, weighing approximately 1 kg. An individual adult's intestinal microflora has been estimated to comprise more than 400 species (172), but in any individual 30 to 40 species make up more than 99% of the microbial population (230). The quantitatively most important bacterial groups in the intestinal microflora are *Bacteroides*, *Fusobacterium*, *Bifidobacterium*, *Eubacterium*, *Peptostreptococcus*, and *Ruminococcus*. *Lactobacillus*, *Veillonella*, and *Clostridium* species are generally somewhat less numerous, whereas facultative bacteria, such as enterobacteria (including *E. coli*) and enterococci, constitute 0.1 to 1% of the bacterial population. More detailed reviews of the species composition of the large-intestinal normal flora have appeared previously (68, 102, 229).

Several studies have shown that the species composition of bacteria cultured from fecal samples is very similar to that obtained from culture of intestinal biopsy specimens (171, 180). However, today only between 60 and 90% of the bacterial species present in the microflora of the large intestine can be cultivated (110, 250). Molecular biological techniques to identify intestinal microbes without prior culture are rapidly being developed. Today such techniques cannot replace conventional culture, because they either detect only a few dominant groups in the microflora or require prior knowledge of the genome for specific probes or primers to be designed.

ECOLOGY OF THE LARGE-INTESTINAL MICROFLORA

Oxygen Tolerance

A majority of commensal intestinal bacteria are obligate anaerobes that cannot perform aerobic metabolism and cannot even survive in the presence of ambient oxygen because of a lack of oxygen-scavenging enzymes. Other anaerobic bacteria, sometimes termed microaerophilic, can survive and even replicate to a limited extent in air, even though their metabolisms are purely anaerobic. Lactobacilli of the groups most commonly colonizing the human gastrointestinal mucosa, *Lactobacillus plantarum*, *Lactobacillus rhamnosus*, and *Lactobacillus paracasei* (9), as well as certain bifidobacterial species, belong to this group. Facultative anaerobes, which are bacteria capable of both aerobic and anaerobic metabolism but which multiply faster in the presence of oxygen, constitute a minority of the normal intestinal microflora. However, most of the bacteria causing extraintestinal infection belong to this category, because strict anaerobes have problems surviving in the well-aerated tissues.

The degree of oxygen tolerance of various bacteria profoundly influences intestinal ecology. For example, strictly anaerobic species cannot be established alone in the intestine of a germfree animal or newborn infant because the oxygen content is too high. A facultative species must be present simultaneously to scavenge environmental oxygen in order to permit the replication of such strict anaerobes (174).

Suppression of Facultative Species by Anaerobic Floras

If an animal is monocolonized by a facultative bacterial species such as *E. coli*, the bacterium reaches 100- to 1,000-fold-higher population counts than if a full flora is present. Suppression of facultative anaerobes by anaerobes is not due to any simple competition for space but is a complex and not fully understood process (73). Anaerobes produce H_2S, organic acids, and other inhibiting substances during their metabolism. In combination with the completely anaerobic milieu prevailing in the intestine, the metabolic pathways available are limited. Only bacterial strains that can utilize available substrates under the prevailing conditions can survive, and those which do this most efficiently replicate at a higher rate than others, whose population numbers will be reduced (73). Freter et al. showed that as many as 95 anaerobic strains are needed to replicate the suppressive effect on *E. coli* of a full microflora (73). Thus, *E. coli* can retain high population numbers in the presence of a limited number of anaerobic species, such as in di- or tricolonized gnotobiotic animals (73, 104) or in infants lacking a fully developed anaerobic flora (see below).

Influence of Diet

Some poorly digestible dietary fibers avoid decomposition in the small intestine and reach the colon, where they become substrate mainly for the anaerobic bacteria. Despite this, the diet of the host has very limited influence on the composition of the large-intestinal microflora (66, 101). In general, individuals tend to have their own distinct predominant species combinations, which are not affected even by rather drastic changes in diet (170). However, the metabolic activity of intestinal bacteria may change when the diet of the host changes, even if the species composition does not (32).

The marked stability of the microflora in an individual host may suggest that many of the largest groups of intestinal bacteria in fact actually graze on the host rather than feed from the diet of the host. Approximately 1% of the colonic bacterial population, including strains of *Bifidobacterium* and *Ruminococcus*, possess carbohydrate-splitting enzymes that cut off mono- and oligosaccharides from mucin chains (114). Released saccharides may function as substrates for other bacterial species (205). In addition to the large amount of mucin produced, it is estimated that a human being sheds some 250 g of enterocytes per day (50), which ultimately will become food for the microbes. Transudated plasma proteins and micronutrients leaking out of epithelial cells may enhance bacterial growth (259). Thus, whereas crude mucus that contains all of the above components is an excellent growth substrate for bacteria, the fecal material occupying the lumen is practically devoid of metabolizable substances (94, 242).

Nevertheless, people in different geographical regions differ in the overall composition of their intestinal microfloras (169). Different types of staple food in different regions may favor certain intestinal bacteria. In addition, the food consumed in developing countries with hot climates may contain massive doses of bacteria, which is probably the reason why high levels of enterobacteria and other species are found in the small intestines of people in such countries (56). Many traditional food preservation methods employ fermentation by lactic acid bacteria, which are present in cheese, sauerkraut, yogurt, wine, olives, cured meat, etc. Such fermented foods constituted a large part of the diet for many thousands of years and still do in most parts of the world, with the United States and Great Britain as the most notable exceptions.

Colonization Resistance

It is difficult to experimentally colonize an adult individual or an animal harboring a full intestinal microflora with a new bacterial strain (45, 210). This phenomenon is termed "colonization resistance" (238) and can be attributed to the competition afforded by bacteria already present, mainly the anaerobes, for space, nutrients, adherence sites, etc. (72). This has very important implications for pathogenicity, because people or animals with a poorly developed intestinal microflora are much more likely to be colonized by pathogens than those with a full flora. For example, germfree mice are killed by 10 *Salmonella enterica* serovar Enteritidis organisms given perorally, while this requires 5×10^6 bacteria in conventional animals (41). Accordingly, human infants may be infected by as few as 40 *Salmonella* bacteria compared to 10^6 in an adult (143). Along the same lines, the oral dose of the intracellular pathogen *Listeria monocytogenes* required to kill germfree animals is 100 to 500 organisms, whereas conventional mice survive doses of 10^8 to 10^9 (35).

Although competition from anaerobes for establishment in the intestine is probably the most important mechanism of colonization resistance, other mechanisms may contribute as well, such as a nonspecific stimulation of immune effector functions by the anaerobic flora (106).

Temporal Variation in Microfloras

Despite the great difficulty in experimentally implanting new strains in the colonic microflora, such renewed colonization occurs all the time, since there is a constant appearance of new bacterial strains in the microflora of an individual while others disappear. Only for *E. coli* has the longitudinal colonization pattern of individual strains been systematically studied, but there is reason to believe that the same pattern holds true for other members of the intestinal microflora.

An individual typically harbors a few *E. coli* strains in the colonic microflora at one time. Some of these strains may persist for several months, or even years, in the microflora of an individual, while others vanish between two sampling occasions. The first type of strain is called "resident," and the second type is called "transient" (210). Tannock and coworkers studied strains of bifidobacteria using ribotyping and found the same pattern as for *E. coli*. Thus, an individual at any time carried a few bifidobacterial strains, of which some could be recovered repeatedly over long periods whereas others were gone when the next sample was taken (230).

Bacterial Factors Enabling Long-Term Persistence in the Gut Microflora

It can be anticipated that inhabiting a niche close to the mucosal surface would be advantageous for intestinal bacteria. First, bacteria sticking to the mucosa are not swept away by peristalsis and can therefore replicate at a lower rate than those which are free living (72). Secondly, substrates for bacterial growth are constantly being replenished at this site. Accordingly, the generation time of mucosally situated *E. coli* has been estimated to be 40 to 80 min, whereas lumenal bacteria do not replicate (195).

Intuitively, one could imagine that the in vitro capacity to adhere to mucosal structures would predict the capacity for long-term persistence in the gut. This seems, however, not to be the case. Instead, only adherence via certain adhesins to their reciprocal receptor structures confers colonizing capacity, whereas binding via other adhesin-receptor pairs does not. For *E. coli*, P fimbriae with adhesins recognizing

the Galα1-4Galβ disaccharide moiety found on human (5, 257) and rat (104) intestinal epithelial cells are most convincingly linked to persistence in the intestinal microflora. In epidemiological studies, resident *E. coli* strains more often than transient ones express P fimbriae (8, 236, 254) or carry the genes enabling their synthesis (F. Nowrouzian, A. E. Wold, and I. Adlerberth, unpublished data). In addition, an *E. coli* strain possessing P fimbriae colonizes much better than its isogeneic counterpart lacking these adhesins (104). Thirdly, P-fimbrial expression also seems to be retained during intestinal colonization (104, 105).

Type 1 fimbriae with mannose-specific adhesins which recognize the branching trisaccharide Manα1-3(Manα1-6)Manβ in N-linked oligosaccharide chains on various glycoproteins are almost ubiquitous among *E. coli* and other members of the family *Enterobacteriaceae* (59, 69). They confer binding to intestinal epithelial cells (257) and to the mannose-containing carbohydrate chains of secretory immunoglobulin A (IgA) (256). This binding is likely to be of ecological importance to the bacteria, since *E. coli* organisms recovered from people with selective IgA deficiency less often carry the gene for type 1 fimbriae and express less mannose-specific adhesins per cell than *E. coli* recovered from control individuals (75). A mannose-specific adhesin conferring binding to human intestinal epithelial cells was also found in *L. plantarum* (3), the lactobacillus species most frequently colonizing the gastrointestinal mucosa of healthy human beings (9). This type of adhesin was expressed by a majority of all *L. plantarum* isolates obtained from healthy human intestinal mucosa (9).

In contrast, S fimbriae and Dr hemagglutinin, two other adhesins of *E. coli* that mediate attachment to human intestinal epithelium (5), are not found more frequently among resident than transient *E. coli* (Nowrouzian et al., unpublished), and S fimbriae do not contribute to colonization in the gnotobiotic-rat model (M. V. Herías, A.-K. Robertson, T. Midtvedt, and A. E. Wold, unpublished data). Conversely, bacterial factors other than adherence may play a decisive role in the ability of bacteria to persist in the colonic microflora. Such factors include capsule formation (105), synthesis of the iron-trapping compound aerobactin (Nowrouzian et al., unpublished), and a smooth lipopolysaccharide (LPS) (140). Probably, capsules and LPS render the bacteria hydrophilic and negatively charged and thereby prevent their entrapment in mucus (42). Obviously, some traits which are traditionally seen as virulence factors for extraintestinal infections may, in fact, have evolved to increase the persistence of *E. coli* in its natural niche, the colonic microflora.

ACQUISITION OF THE NORMAL FLORA BY INFANTS

The establishment of a normal microflora commences at birth but is a process which takes several years to complete (6, 164). In general, colonization proceeds in a seemingly ordered fashion, certain bacterial groups being early colonizers while others do not become established for many months (Fig. 2). This colonization pattern results from two variables: which bacteria are available for the infant to become colonized with and which bacteria can thrive and proliferate in the intestinal milieu of the

infant. The second point is illustrated by the fact that the neonatal intestine is too rich in oxygen for obligately anaerobic bacteria to thrive during the first week(s) (222). Only after facultative bacteria have become established and consumed the oxygen may obligate anaerobes start to increase in numbers. One bacterial species may also require the metabolic action of another species in order to obtain substrate for its own growth. For example, the degradation of mucin requires the cooperation of several bacterial species, each of which can perform only a single or a few catalytic reactions (114).

Colonization of the infant occurs via the oral route—in cases of congenital bowel obstruction, bacterial colonization occurs proximal, but not distal, to the site of obstruction (23). The bacteria that colonize the infant may derive from the mother's fecal or perineal flora, from foods given the baby, or from other people in the environment, often nursing staff or other infants cared for in the same ward (6).

Mata and Urrutia studied the acquisition of the normal intestinal microflora by infants born to indigenous Indian mothers in rural Guatemala in the early 1970s. The mothers gave birth in a squatting position, commonly leading to

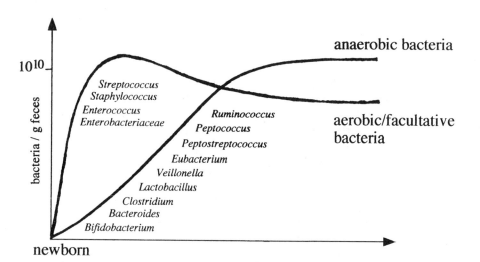

FIGURE 2 Normal pattern of acquisition of the normal intestinal microflora by the newborn infant, a process which proceeds during the first years of life.

fecal soiling of the infant. These infants were very rapidly colonized and were often culture positive for enterobacteria within a few hours after birth (153). In contrast, modern Western obstetric practice includes a supine delivery position and avoidance of fecal contamination, sometimes aggravated by giving enemas and washing the perineal area with disinfectants. As a result, colonization with enterobacteria from the mother's intestinal flora is the exception rather than the rule. Delivery by caesarean section naturally prevents the infant from being colonized by the maternal fecal or perineal flora, and colonization depends entirely on the environment.

Facultative Bacteria Colonizing the Newborn Infant

The intestinal microflora during the first days or weeks is dominated by facultative bacteria, such as enterobacteria (*E. coli, Klebsiella, Enterobacter*, and others), enterococci (*Streptococcus faecalis* or *Streptococcus faecium*), staphylococci (*Staphylococcus epidermidis* or *Staphylococcus aureus*), or aerobic streptococci (6). The absence of competition from an anaerobic flora permits *E. coli* and other facultative bacteria to reach very high population numbers, often 100 times greater than those typically found in adults (112, 222).

E. coli is traditionally one of the first colonizers of the healthy full-term newborn infant (6). As *E. coli* has no other reservoir in nature than the intestinal flora of humans and animals, its presence is a sign of fecal contamination (44). Transfer of *E. coli* from mother to infant may occur at delivery, but today this occurs in only 10 to 30% of Western infants (77, 83, 89, 178). More commonly, *E. coli* strains colonizing newborn infants are part of the "hospital flora" (77, 83, 89, 178). In the hospital "ecosystem," bacteria may be transferred between infants by the nursing staff, and strains from the infants may colonize the staff and vice versa. In this way, certain strains may persist in a maternity ward for long periods of time. A high bed occupancy and shortage of staff increase enterobacterial spread among infants (234), whereas rooming in (i.e., keeping the baby with the mother, who takes care of it) reduces such transfer (21).

Enterobacteria other than *E. coli*, i.e., *Klebsiella, Enterobacter, Proteus*, and *Citrobacter*, commonly colonize the newborn infant. These bacteria are less frequently found in the intestinal microflora of adults, where they also achieve only quite low numbers. Thus, most non-*E. coli* enterobacteria colonizing newborn infants derive from other sources. Strains may be spread between infants at the ward (76) or acquired from environmental sources, such as contaminated foods (7). The sources of enterococci and staphylococci colonizing the newborn infant have not been studied on the strain level, but staphylococci may be ingested by the infant while suckling, since these bacteria are part of the skin flora, including that of the breast and nipple (88).

Anaerobic Bacteria Colonizing the Newborn Infant

Early anaerobic colonizers of the baby include bifidobacteria, bacteroides, and clostridia (Fig. 2). The frequency of colonization by lactobacilli in the neonatal period varies very much among different studies, reflecting differences in populations or methods (6).

Little is known about the sources of anaerobic bacteria colonizing the infant. Bifidobacteria are relatively aerotolerant and can survive for some time outside the intestinal milieu, which facilitates their spread. There are indications of the transfer of bifidobacteria to the infant from both the mother and the environment (6), but only one study has employed genetic fingerprinting of bifidobacterial strains to trace their origin. In two out of five mother-infant pairs studied, the same ribotype of bifidobacteria was found in both the infant's and the mother's colonic microflora (231). Bifidobacteria, corynebacteria, propionibacteria, and lactobacilli have been found at quite high levels in human milk, probably derived from the nipple and surrounding skin and possibly even from the milk ducts (14, 244).

Bacteroides tolerates ambient oxygen very

poorly and cannot survive for a long time outside the intestine. Such bacteria are therefore not likely to be transferred between staff and infants under good hygienic conditions. Thus, infants delivered by caesarean section are colonized by *Bacteroides* much later than vaginally delivered infants (6).

Clostridial species form spores that survive boiling and disinfectants and are therefore very apt to survive and spread in the hospital environment. These bacteria are important members of the neonatal intestinal microflora, including *Clostridium difficile*, which colonizes approximately one-third of infants without causing symptoms (6).

It takes several years for the human infant to acquire the endless variety of anaerobic bacteria that characterize the adult flora (164). The successive establishment of more and more anaerobic species in the microflora is reflected by a drop in the population numbers of facultative species. The ratio of anaerobes to aerobes has been calculated to be 1.5 before the age of 4 months, 10 between 4 and 12 months, 50 between 1 and 4 years, and 200 in an adult (62).

The Intestinal Flora of Breast- and Bottle-Fed Infants

A number of differences in early colonization patterns between breast- and bottle-fed infants have been reported. They can be ascribed to two different factors: a difference in the bacterial species that infants fed different diets are exposed to and differences in the groups of bacteria favored by the intestinal milieus of infants on different diets.

We have recently summarized 23 studies of the effect of infant feeding on the intestinal colonization pattern performed between 1973 and 1995 (6). The most reliable findings are that bottle-fed infants have more enterococci and clostridia than breast-fed infants. In many studies, breast-fed infants instead have more staphylococci, especially in the early neonatal period, which could be explained by ingestion of skin bacteria from the mother's breast during suckling (88). Less frequently found differences include marginally lower counts of enterobacteria in breast-fed infants and a higher frequency of colonization with bifidobacteria in breast-fed infants. The finding of a "bifidobacterial dominance" in breast-fed infants, reported by Tissier a century ago (232), seems to have vanished in the most recent studies (6).

Intestinal Flora of High-Risk Infants

Infants delivered by caesarean section carry fewer *E. coli* organisms and more *Klebsiella* species and other types of enterobacteria than vaginally delivered infants (16). Their anaerobic flora contains fewer *Bacteroides* species and bifidobacteria than that of vaginally delivered infants, and clostridia are usually the first anaerobic colonizers (16, 182). Evidently, such differences may relate to their lack of contact with maternal perineal or fecal flora, but another important factor is that infants delivered by caesarean section are often cared for at neonatal intensive care units. These wards are characterized by a heavy use of antibiotics, leading to suppression of *E. coli* and increased colonization by *Klebsiella*, *Enterobacter*, *Citrobacter*, and *Pseudomonas* species (16). Anaerobes are often profoundly suppressed by antibiotic treatment (16). Even infants not receiving antibiotics themselves are affected, due to extensive sharing of strains within the ward (235).

Impact of Hygienic Conditions on Acquisition of the Microflora

Since many infants acquire their enterobacteria from environmental sources, the degree of hygiene will greatly affect the early enterobacterial colonization pattern. Nigerian and Pakistani infants are invariably colonized by enterobacteria after a few days, even if delivered by caesarean section, while Swedish infants are colonized much later (4, 202). Later, children in Pakistan have a neverending succession of new *E. coli* strains in their microfloras during the first 6 months (7), while Swedish infants may carry a single strain for more than a year in their microfloras, often the strain that they were first colonized with (236).

Colonization with enterococci, lactobacilli, and eubacteria is also delayed in western Europe (17, 211).

We have recently observed that in Sweden in the late 1990s, staphylococci and enterococci have become the major colonizers of newborn infants, while colonization with enterobacteria has declined greatly. Not until 1 month of age were all infants colonized by enterobacteria, and by this time only a minority were colonized by *E. coli* (I. Adlerberth, B. Åberg, N. Åberg, B. Hesselmar, R. Saalman, I.-L. Strannegård, and A. E. Wold, unpublished data). Similar findings, although not as pronounced, have been reported from France (28). The Swedish infants roomed in with their mothers, and mothers and children left the hospital within 2 days, which is likely to have profoundly reduced the possibility of acquiring enterobacteria in the hospital. Staphylococci belong to the skin flora and are probably transferred during breast-feeding and general care, and enterococci are notoriously hardy against normal hygienic routines.

In summary, when obstetricians took over and hospitalized deliveries, the natural transfer of intestinal bacteria from mother to infant decreased severely. Still, a superficially normal colonization pattern was retained because infants were cross-colonized via the staff. Today, increased adherence to hygienic measures, better-staffed wards, rooming in, and early discharge from the hospital have also stopped this chance of being colonized by normal intestinal bacteria. This has done much to reduce severe neonatal infections by virulent and often antibiotic-resistant hospital strains, but these procedures, together with the excessively hygienic habits and small family size of wealthy people in the West, have combined to produce an intestinal colonization pattern in the neonatal period not previously encountered.

BACTERIAL TRANSLOCATION FROM THE GUT

Under certain conditions, live bacteria may pass over the intestinal barrier, in which case they can be cultivated from mesenteric lymph nodes, blood, or other organs (19). Only certain bacterial species can translocate, including *E. coli* and other enterobacteria, staphylococci, enterococci, and lactobacilli, while most obligate anaerobes do not have this capacity. Translocation is highly dependent on the population level in the intestinal microflora of species which have this ability (19). For example, translocation of *E. coli* in monocolonized rats rises sharply above a colonization level of 10^9 per g of intestinal contents (103). The presence in the microflora of obligate anaerobes profoundly reduces translocation by *E. coli* and other facultative species (243). Evidently, this may result from their ability to reduce the population numbers of facultative species, but other mechanisms may also contribute, such as nonspecific stimulation of the host's defense systems (106).

It is an unresolved question whether special bacterial traits exist which favor translocation. It seems as if *E. coli* strains may differ in their capacities to translocate at a certain population level (123). P fimbriae and K5 capsule enhance translocation only indirectly, by permitting the growth of high numbers of bacteria, which in itself enhances translocation (104, 105), and S fimbriae, which are virulence factors for infant septicemia, do not seem to enhance translocation (M. V. Herias, T. Midtvedt, and A. E. Wold, unpublished data). It is also not presently known whether translocation occurs in the small or large intestine, via absorptive epithelial cells or as part of the antigen-sampling process that occurs in the Peyer's patches belonging to the gut immune system.

The defenses against translocation include intact epithelial-barrier functions and intact cell-mediated immunity (187, 188). Translocation increases when such defense mechanisms are weakened, e.g., after irradiation, hemorrhagic shock (15), burns (80), starvation (11, 99), and cortisone treatment (20). Endotoxemia greatly increases translocation, probably by inducing gut barrier leakage (167). Antibiotic treatment, which frequently suppresses the population numbers of anaerobic bacteria, predisposes for translocation (19).

EFFECT OF FLORAS ON THE IMMUNE SYSTEM

Innate Immunity and Inflammation

There is ample evidence that microbes present in the gut flora exert long-range effects on the host defense systems. Thus, peritoneal macrophages from conventional animals are better at phagocytosing C3b-opsonized particles and also possess higher levels of lysosomal enzymes than macrophages obtained from germfree animals (175). Macrophages from animals colonized by a microflora also display increased cytotoxic activity (121, 160), secrete more oxygen radicals (168), have increased levels of cyclic AMP (194), and produce more interleukin 1 (IL-1), IL-6, and tumor necrosis factor alpha in response to LPS (184, 185) than macrophages from germfree animals. A difference in LPS responsiveness between germfree and bacterium-colonized mice was also noted with macrophages derived from the culture of bone marrow precursors (185), which shows how profoundly the microbial status affects the host. Interestingly, monocolonization with *E. coli*, but not bifidobacteria, was reported to prime macrophages for cytokine production (184).

The long-range effects of the microflora on sites which are not colonized by bacteria, such as the sterile peritoneal cavity, spleen, or bone marrow, can be explained by the fact that bacterial products are taken up by macrophages in the gut wall, which then migrate, carrying their microbial components with them. Bacterial LPS may persist within macrophages in a bioactive form for very long periods of time (60). Peptidoglycans from bacterial cell walls, probably derived from the intestinal microflora, have been detected inside macrophages in the red pulp of the spleen in rats (135) and human beings (109). Breakdown products of peptidoglycans have been detected in the urine of healthy people, indicating a constant uptake, degradation, and excretion of bacteria or their components from the intestine (119).

The continuous presence of undegraded bacterial products in our lymphoid tissue may evoke a low-grade inflammation, manifested, e.g., in a slight elevation of body temperature (120) and somnolence (152). Accordingly, germfree animals have lower body temperatures than conventional animals and are more difficult to anesthetize (T. Midtvedt, personal communication).

The Gut Flora and Specific Immunity

GENERAL STRUCTURE OF THE GUT IMMUNE SYSTEM

The gut-associated immune system comprises the vast majority of lymphoid cells in the human body. The lamina propria is seeded with as many as 10^{10} antibody-producing cells/m of small intestine, most of which produce dimeric IgA (29). IgA dimers bind to secretory component exposed on the basolateral aspect of intestinal epithelial cells, and the entire complex is transported through the epithelium to the lumenal side. The transmembrane part of the secretory component is cleaved off, leaving the rest bound to IgA, together forming secretory IgA (163).

The secretory IgA molecule is specially designed to afford protection on surfaces populated by microbes. It is highly resistant to proteolysis and prevents microbial attachment to host mucosal structures (71, 228, 248) and translocation (157) without evoking inflammatory effector responses such as complement activation (204). Mucosa not regularly colonized by microbes have comparatively more IgG in their secretions, for example, the respiratory (197) and urinary (227) tracts.

The T cells found in the villus lamina propria are mainly CD4 positive and display signs of activation (52, 209). They do not respond with proliferation to mitogens and other stimuli, indicating that they are terminally differentiated cells, but they spontaneously secrete cytokines, especially gamma interferon (IFN-γ) (97, 98). Interspersed among the absorptive epithelial cells are T lymphocytes, mainly of the CD8-positive phenotype, termed intraepithelial lymphocytes. Intraepithelial lymphocytes may carry either the αβ or γδ type of antigen receptor. The exact function of the intraepithelial cells is unknown, but they can synthesize IL-2 and IFN-γ (144) and lyse virus-infected cells (36). Their T-cell receptors are oligoclonal, suggesting that the entire population derives from a limited set of T-cell clones (24).

Intestinal immune responses are mainly induced in the Peyer's patches, which are mucosal lymphoid nodules covered by a specialized epithelium, the follicle-associated epithelium. This epithelium contains specialized epithelial cells, termed M cells, which lack brush borders and the enzymatic machinery of the absorptive epithelial cell (183). M cells are specialized in transporting material from the lumen into the patches, without degrading this material. In the patches, macrophages and dendritic cells degrade and present antigenic material to specific T and B cells, which proliferate, mature, and leave the patches via the efferent lymph. Via the bloodstream, they return to the gut lamina propria and, to a certain extent, other mucosa, a process termed "homing" (49).

IMPORTANCE OF THE GUT FLORA FOR THE SPECIFIC IMMUNE SYSTEM

The majority of lymphoid cells in the gut are there because of the normal intestinal microflora. Thus, germfree animals have approximately 1/10 as many IgA-producing cells in the lamina propria and about 1/10 as many T cells as conventional animals (47, 48, 95). When germfree animals are colonized by a normal flora, their lymph nodes and Peyer's patches increase in weight and germinal centers develop, serum IgG concentration rises, and antibodies to the colonizing microorganisms appear (34). One must bear in mind that even sterilized feed given to germfree animals is contaminated by endotoxin and other bacterial components (166). Compared with the antigenic stimulation afforded by the normal flora, that of the diet is, however, very limited. Thus, serum IgA and IgG are slightly increased in germfree mice fed a commercial rat diet compared with those fed an "antigen-free," extensively hydrolyzed liquid diet but much lower than in conventional mice (95).

The "natural antibodies" directed to blood group antigens from other species, thought by Landsteiner to occur spontaneously as part of the normal physiological development, have been shown to result from immunization by gut microbes in the normal flora (207, 220, 245).

The presence and activation state of intraepithelial cells of the αβ type are strongly dependent on the presence of a normal microflora, while the γδ type is found in equal numbers in germfree and conventional animals (124). However, the γδ type of lymphocytes seems to be functionally affected by the presence of a normal microflora. In response to luminal bacteria, they start to produce IFN-γ, which in turn upregulates the expression of major histocompatibility complex class II molecules on intestinal epithelial cells (155). The oligoclonality of intraepithelial cells, however, does not seem to be determined by distinct bacterial antigens, since both germfree and conventional mice exhibit such restricted clonality (196).

THE TRANSIENT NATURE OF THE RESPONSE TO GUT BACTERIA

The capacity of a bacterial strain to induce strong immunity is linked to its ability to colonize and to invade the Peyer's patches (108). Dead bacteria may be taken up into the Peyer's patches, but the immune response they induce is much weaker, probably due to the small amounts of antigen reaching the patches.

When a bacterial strain successfully colonizes the intestine and reaches numbers high enough to permit translocation, germinal centers are formed in the Peyer's patches, B cells committed to IgA production seed the mucosa, and secretory IgA is produced in the intestinal lumen. However, this immune response is self-limiting, in that the secretory IgA produced coats the bacteria in the intestinal lumen, preventing further translocation and, hence, stimulation of the gut lymphoid tissue (215). Despite the continued presence of the microbes in the gut flora, there will be no, or only minimal, further stimulation of the gut–associated lymphoid tissue.

Because of this phenomenon, a persistent activation of the mucosal immune system requires a high turnover of bacterial strains in the microflora. Thus, Pakistani infants, who are colonized by a never-ending succession of new enterobacteria (7), have higher secretory IgA levels in their saliva and higher anti-*E. coli* antibody levels than do Swedish infants of the same age (159). Bottle-fed infants, who have a more varied and less stable microflora than breast-fed infants (6), have increased numbers of activated lymphocytes in the blood (189).

WHY ARE BACTERIA SUCH GOOD ANTIGENS?

Despite the fact that an estimated 0.01 to 0.1% of ingested food proteins are taken up into the circulation in an intact, theoretically fully immunogenic form (116, 129), these types of antigens give rise to very little stimulation of the gut immune system. The response to food proteins is dominated by serum antibodies of the IgG4 and IgG2 subclasses (115), which are poor in fixing complement and interacting with phagocytes. In laboratory animals, the feeding of high doses of protein antigens does not result in a secretory IgA antibody response but only in the formation of serum IgG antibodies (192, 255). In contrast, if the food protein ovalbumin is presented to the gut immune system by colonizing germfree rats with an *E. coli* organism transformed with an ovalbumin-producing plasmid, secretory IgA antibodies against ovalbumin are produced (51). This shows that a "microbial package" of an antigen signals a need for immune activation.

This phenomenon can be explained by considering that protein antigens must be presented by antigen-presenting cells to T cells, which in turn activate B cells to mature into antibody-producing plasma cells. In the case of whole bacteria, the chief antigen-presenting cell is the macrophage (260). In addition to presenting antigenic peptides on major histocompatibility complex class II molecules on their surfaces, antigen-presenting cells must de-

liver activating signals in the form of cytokines or membrane-bound costimulatory molecules in order for the T cell to become activated and generate an immune response. Exposure of a T cell to its specific antigen on class II molecules without the concomitant positive signals from the antigen-presenting cell leads to anergy, i.e., persistent nonreactivity of that T cell. Bacterial products stimulate macrophages to produce the T-cell-activating cytokine IL-1 (125) and to express several costimulatory molecules (96). By this mechanism, the immune system functions economically, wasting few resources on harmless substances, and minimizes the risk of evoking inflammatory reactions in response to harmless compounds.

Moreau and coworkers attempted to determine which intestinal bacteria were the best inducers of mucosal immunity. Germfree mice were colonized with a range of gram-positive and gram-negative bacteria, and the density of IgA-containing plasma cells in the intestinal lamina propria was measured. The best inducers of IgA plasma cells were *E. coli* and *Bacteroides*, while the gram-positive bacteria tested were all inferior to these species (174). Provided that high enough doses were given over long enough periods of time, killed *E. coli* or *Bacteroides* were as effective as live bacteria in inducing IgA-containing plasma cells (174).

On the other hand, Cebra and coworkers found the highest amounts of mucosal IgA to be produced after colonization of the gram-positive species *L. monocytogenes* and segmented filamentous bacteria, while the gram-negative species *Morganella morganii*, *Ochrobacterium atrophii*, and *Helicobacter muridarum* all gave less IgA stimulation (5; J. J. Cebra, personal communication).

The Gut Flora and Oral Tolerance

Not only are food antigens not very immunogenic to the gut immune system, they also induce a state of specific tolerance to themselves, termed oral (or mucosal) tolerance. Oral tolerance denotes the lack of T-cell reactivity or antibody production upon encountering an antigen which has previously been fed to the animal or human being (176). Oral tolerance may be seen as a way to avoid wasting resources on reacting to a wealth of innocuous antigens that are constantly encountered on the mucosae. Oral tolerance also protects us from exaggerated responsiveness, including inflammatory responses to antigens which are not dangerous, and thus minimizes the risk of inflammatory states in the mucosa.

Oral tolerance is chiefly mediated by suppressor, or regulatory, T cells which secrete suppressive cytokines, such as transforming growth factor-β and/or IL-10, upon encountering their specific antigens (176). These cytokines, in turn, prevent other T cells from proliferating and maturing into effector cells when they encounter their antigens.

It is difficult to achieve oral tolerance in germfree animals lacking a normal intestinal microflora (173, 225). Further, the administration of LPS together with food antigens increases the tolerance-creating effect of feeding (130), whereas cholera toxin and *E. coli* heat-labile toxin may break oral tolerance to food antigens (64, 81). Thus, it is clear that the presence of bacteria or their products not only promotes immunity to themselves but may in addition strongly influence immune responses to other antigens occurring concomitantly in a human being or experimental animal.

How is this possible? Soluble protein antigens, probably including food proteins, are mainly presented to T cells by dendritic cells, which have poor or no phagocytic capacity and therefore are not likely to present bacteria (223). A range of products secreted by macrophages in response to bacterial products have been shown to decrease the antigen-presenting capacity of dendritic cells, for example, the cytokines tumor necrosis factor alpha (111) and IL-10 (134), the prostaglandin PGE_2 (40), and nitrous oxide (111). Thus, animals from which alveolar macrophages have been removed display greatly enhanced immune responses to inhaled antigens (111). Similarly, depletion of macrophages from a preparation of dendritic cells from gut lamina propria also enhances their antigen-presenting ability (190). Thus, if

we were to lack macrophages (or if our macrophages were not activated by microbial products), it is likely that our immune systems would overreact to many harmless environmental antigens, including food proteins and airborne allergens. Accordingly, antigen-presenting cells from germfree mice are better at stimulating naive T cells than antigen-presenting cells from conventional animals, and the greatest T-cell activation is seen when the antigen-presenting cells derive from germfree animals which are fed an antigen-free sterile liquid diet (113).

EFFECT OF FLORAS ON INTESTINAL STRUCTURE AND FUNCTION

Epithelial Cells and Mucosal Architecture

The morphology of the intestinal mucosa is affected by exposure to intestinal bacteria or their products. The total mucosal surface area in the small intestine is 14 to 30% larger in conventional animals than in their germfree counterparts (87, 162), and the villi of the ileum are thicker and more numerous in conventional animals than in germfree animals (162). This may be related to an expansion of the gut immune system, since lymphoid cells occupy a large portion of the gut lamina propria.

The presence of a normal microflora stimulates the cell turnover in the intestinal epithelium. In mice reared conventionally, the ileal crypts are longer and contain more mitotic figures than those in germfree mice, and epithelial-cell renewal is speedier (1, 2). A rapid shift toward a higher epithelial turnover rate occurs following conventionalization of germfree animals (128).

Certain microorganisms may influence the host synthesis of complex oligosaccharide patterns on epithelial cells or mucin molecules. Complex carbohydrates are formed by the addition of simple sugars catalyzed by so-called glycosyl transferases, each one specific for a certain sugar and linkage. Monocolonization of mice with a *Bacteroides* strain capable of utilizing fucose as a substrate was shown to induce the production of fucosylated compounds in the host via induction of a specific fucosyl transferase (31). Colonization with a mutant strain which lacked the enzymes necessary to utilize fucose as a growth substrate could not restore production of fucosylated compounds (31).

Intestinal Motility

The presence of a normal intestinal microflora affects bowel motility. Comparisons between germfree and conventional animals show that the microflora exerts a marked stimulatory effect on intestinal motility and increases the frequency of migrating motor complexes in the small intestine (117). The bacterial species responsible for this effect have not been identified. Infusion of short-chain fatty acids into the intestinal lumen promoted motility, an effect mediated via polypeptide YY (38).

Generation of Fatty Acids

Carbohydrates cannot be combusted to CO_2 and H_2O in the large intestine, because there is no O_2 available. Instead, saccharides are anaerobically metabolized to yield acetate, propionate, and butyrate, collectively termed short-chain fatty acids. Short-chain fatty acids are absorbed by the colonic epithelial cells, which use them as fuel, especially in the distal colon (201). Other substrates for the colonocytes are glucose and glutamine, which are derived from the circulation. Butyrate is exclusively produced by anaerobic colonic bacteria. Thus, metabolism in colonocytes in germfree animals is different from that in conventional animals (39).

All three major short-chain fatty acids, acetate, propionate, and butyrate, stimulate colonic sodium and fluid absorption and enterocyte proliferation (137, 208). They also promote colonic growth (74). Short-chain fatty acids are trophic to the small-intestinal mucosa, an effect mediated via the autonomous enteric nervous system (70). Acetate increases ileal blood flow and motility (208). Butyrate may ameliorate colitis (208).

THE NORMAL MICROFLORA AS A RESERVOIR FOR INFECTIONS

Many of the bacterial species inhabiting the large intestine are potentially pathogenic, i.e., they cause disease if they spread to other sites (urinary tract infection, septicemia, or abscesses) or reach too high numbers (bacterial overgrowth).

Bacterial Overgrowth of the Small Intestine

If the mechanisms controlling bacterial proliferation in the small intestine are disturbed, bacterial populations may increase drastically. This condition is termed bacterial overgrowth and is generally defined as growth of more than 10^5 bacteria per ml of small intestinal fluid (55). Decreased gastric acid secretion, caused, for example, by chronic gastritis or iatrogenic due to acid-blocking pharmacological or surgical treatment, results in an increased seeding of the small intestine with bacteria from the food, saliva, or upper respiratory secretions (57, 203). Normally, this type of overgrowth is mainly characterized by increased numbers of gram-positive aerobic bacteria and is usually not correlated with symptoms (118).

Other important causes of bacterial overgrowth are impaired peristalsis, due to obstruction, neuropathy in diabetes mellitus, or scleroderma (85, 126), and dysfunction or lack of the ileocecal valve (131). These causes increase anaerobiosis and favor expansion of "colonic" types of microbes, i.e., enterobacteria, enterococci, and strict anaerobes, which may have serious consequences in the form of diarrhea and malnutrition (132).

Fat malabsorption may result from proliferation in the small intestine of bacterial groups that can deconjugate bile acids, which become poorly dissolved and incapable of dispensing dietary fat (132). A wide range of bacteria common in the normal colonic microflora, including *Bacteroides*, *Bifidobacterium*, *Veillonella*, *Clostridium*, and enterococci, are capable of deconjugating bile acids (217). In addition, direct toxic effects on enterocytes caused by the deconjugated bile acids or bacterial products may result in malabsorption of fat, carbohydrates, and proteins (233).

Carbohydrate malabsorption may occur due to bacterial fermentation of ingested carbohydrates (131) or from a destruction of mucosal disaccharidases by proteases secreted by the bacteria (199). Bacteria also compete with the host for available protein substrates, resulting in protein-losing enteropathy in certain cases (131). Anaerobic bacteria also consume vitamin B_{12}, and some of it is metabolized to inactive analogs, interfering with normal B_{12} absorption and leading to vitamin B_{12} deficiency and, in the worst cases, pernicious anemia (131).

The diarrhea in bacterial overgrowth may result from increased levels of osmotically active carbohydrates in the small intestine. In addition, various bacterial metabolites may function as secretagogues and contribute to the diarrhea (156).

Bacterial products and bile acids cause hyperplasia of intestinal epithelial cells with increased mitotic figures and increased crypt depth in blind loops overgrown with bacteria (161). Bacterial products are taken up in increased amounts in small-intestinal overgrowth and may cause inflammation and eventually fibrosis in the liver (142).

Chronic Diarrhea

After the invention of oral rehydration solution, mortality in acute diarrhea, which is caused by dehydration, dropped significantly. However, in 10 to 15% of cases, acute diarrhea develops into protracted diarrhea, which is today the leading cause of death among the world's children. Thus, 5% of Pakistani infants are estimated to die from diarrhea, mainly the chronic form (127). Usually no pathogen can be isolated any longer when the diarrhea has become chronic, and it is believed that the condition is caused at least in part by a deranged normal intestinal flora with overgrowth of the small intestine (90). The risk of developing chronic diarrhea is enhanced by the detrimental practice in many developing countries of "treating" acute diarrhea with antibiotics. For example, in Pakistan, 75% of infants with acute diarrhea are given antibiotics, often bought at the local market without a prescription from a medical professional (149). This is not only ineffective against acute diarrhea but also contributes to a disturbed intestinal flora by killing mainly anaerobic bacteria, contributing to decreased colonization resistance and bacterial overgrowth.

C. difficile Infection

C. difficile is detected in low numbers in the intestinal microflora of less than 4% of healthy adults (68). The detection rate and counts of C. difficile increase drastically during and after treatment with certain antibiotics (37, 67). Many, but not all, strains of C. difficile produce toxins: an enterotoxin (toxin A) that induces fluid secretion and a cytotoxin (toxin B) that causes tissue injury (146).

Most carriers of C. difficile remain asymptomatic, but depending on the toxigenicity of the strain and its population level in the intestinal flora, symptoms ranging from a mild diarrhea to pseudomembranous colitis may develop (147). In its most severe form, this disease may result in bowel perforation and death.

Abdominal Infections Caused by the Gut Flora

Intra-abdominal infections like peritonitis or abscesses may occur after perforation of the intestinal barrier, e.g., during surgery, which gives bacteria free access into the peritoneal cavity. Usually, a mixed bacterial population of facultative and anaerobic bacteria is involved. The bacterial groups most commonly isolated are E. coli and Bacteroides, followed by other enterobacteria, Clostridium spp., anaerobic cocci, and enterococci (252). The presence of facultative species permits the growth of obligate anaerobes, since they consume tissue oxygen. Bacteroides fragilis plays a dominant role in abscess formation, especially encapsulated strains (237).

Urinary Tract Infection

Urinary tract infection is caused by facultative anaerobes, most frequently E. coli, that originate in the patient's own flora (93, 241). *E. coli* alone is responsible for 85% of community-acquired urinary tract infections (218). Other common causes of urinary tract infection include enterobacteria, such as *Klebsiella*, *Proteus*, *Enterobacter*, *Pseudomonas*, enterococci, and *Staphylococcus saprophyticus* (218). Colonization of the periurethral area precedes spread to the urinary tract (26, 138) and is more common in infection-prone individuals (26, 221). Colonization of the periurethral area is very heavy before 1 year of age but decreases and is infrequent after 5 years of age, concomitant with a pronounced decline in the risk of acquiring urinary tract infection (25).

Certain *E. coli* strains are more likely than others to cause urinary tract infection. These strains possess virulence factors, such as P fimbriae, capsule, aerobactin, and hemolysin (226). Certain of these traits also confer long-term colonizing ability in the gut (see above). Intestinal carriage of P-fimbriated *E. coli* increases the risk of contracting urinary tract infection (193).

Neonatal Septicemia

Neonatal septicemia is estimated to affect about 2% of newborn infants in developing countries (127) but only 4 in 1,000, mainly the prematurely born, in highly developed societies (249).

Enterobacteria, especially *Klebsiella*, *Enterobacter*, and *E. coli*, are the most common causes of infant septicemia in developing countries and are also common in developed countries (16, 76). In enterobacterial sepsis, the infecting strain may be recovered from the infant's intestinal tract (78, 206). Direct passage of bacteria from the gastrointestinal tract could be anticipated to take place in the neonatal period, because the population counts of facultative anaerobes and aerobes are much higher during this period than later in life due to the absence of competition from anaerobes. Interestingly, transient bacteremia without accompanying symptoms has frequently been found in newborn infants at the time of intestinal colonization (10).

In developed countries gram-positive bacteria, such as *S. epidermidis*, *S. aureus*, and group B streptococci, are the most common causes of infant septicemia (18). Staphylococcal septicemia is often attributed to infections via catheters or through the umbilicus, but in fact, staphylococci are today part of the normal intestinal microflora of quite a few infants in countries with highly developed hygiene (28, 63; Adlerberth et al., unpublished).

Breast-feeding has a pronounced protective effect against neonatal septicemia (13, 251), probably related to the presence in the milk of secretory IgA antibodies which coat intestinal bacteria and prevent them from translocating across the gut barrier (157).

Sepsis with Undefined Focus and Multiple Organ Failure

Sepsis with multiple organ failure is a feared complication in major surgery, transplantation, hematologic malignancies, or patients with multiple trauma which carries a mortality of 15%. An influx of bacteria or bacterial products into the circulation, leading to massive activation of inflammatory defense systems, may be the cause of, or at least aggravate, this condition (27, 151). These patients have a number of predisposing conditions or treatments that have been shown experimentally to increase translocation of gut bacteria over the intestinal barrier, such as hemorrhage (15), starvation (99), increased plasma cortisol levels (20), immunosuppression (20), and antibiotic treatment (243). It remains a challenge to modern intensive care to develop routines that protect the gut mucosal barrier despite severe stress and to refrain from fatally altering the microbial balance of the gut.

THE GUT FLORA AND INFLAMMATORY BOWEL DISEASE

The etiology of the chronic inflammatory bowel diseases ulcerative colitis and Crohn's disease remains unknown. It is currently believed that the diseases are caused or at least aggravated by inadequately controlled immune responses to some exogenous component, possibly present in the normal gut flora. Interestingly, in practically all animal models of gut inflammation, which more or less faithfully represent human inflammatory bowel disease, the presence of a normal intestinal microflora is mandatory—animals reared under germfree conditions either remain healthy or develop much milder symptoms of disease than conventionally reared animals (12, 65). In fact, even colonization of germfree mice with fecal bacteria gives rise to a transient inflammation sharing some characteristics with ulcerative colitis, such as infiltration with polymorphonuclear cells and crypt abscesses (79). In C3H/HeJBir mice which spontaneously develop colitis, T cells reactive with gut bacterial components have been identified among the CD4 subset, and transfer of such cells into SCID mice (which lack functional B and T cells) can transfer the disease (43). Interestingly, an ileitis indistinguishable from Crohn's disease seen in children with chronic granulomatous disease or glycogen storage disease type Ib is almost certainly caused by persistent mucosal-T-cell activation by intestinal bacteria (200).

Inflammatory bowel diseases are associated with affluent and hygienic living conditions and have increased greatly during the last few decades (139, 177). It has been proposed that patients with inflammatory bowel disease have insufficiently developed tolerance towards their own microflora. Thus, intestinal lymphocytes from the lamina propria of healthy individuals have been shown to proliferate in response to sonicates of bacteria recovered from the intestinal microflora of other people but not in response to autologous flora (58). However, lamina propria lymphocytes are normally terminally differentiated and do not proliferate in response to antigen. It is possible that an increased influx of naive T cells into the inflamed bowel mucosa enhances the proliferative capacity of lamina propria lymphocytes in inflammatory bowel disease. It is difficult to envisage specific tolerance in an individual to the particular strains that individual happens to be colonized with at the moment. Considering the constant turnover of bacterial strains in the microflora of an individual, some strains must inevitably have colonized for extended periods of time whereas others are newcomers. Furthermore, there is extensive sharing of antigens between closely and more distantly related bacterial species and strains in the intestine. The immune response to intestinal bacteria must be more thoroughly studied before any firm conclusions can be drawn regarding tolerance to autologous microflora.

A human "model" for ulcerative colitis suggesting the importance of the normal microflora for mucosal inflammation is pouchitis (186). After colectomy in patients with ulcerative colitis, the management of choice today is to construct from the small intestine a continent fecal reservoir which is either emptied a few times a day via catheterization or connected to the anus, to restore almost normal bowel function. The presence of feces in the reservoir leads to a change in mucosal structure: the villi become blunted, and a more colon-like morphology is obtained. In 7 to 45% of pouch carriers, depending on the clinical center, a moderate to severe inflammation in the pouch mucosa develops, with pain, urge, and blood staining of the feces (186). This inflammation can be seen as an activation of the ulcerative colitis disease, because it occurs very seldom in patients in whom a fecal reservoir has been constructed after colectomy due to hereditary colon polyposis (133). The importance of the intestinal microflora for pouchitis is shown by the fact that inflammation does not develop in a conventional ileostomy, where the intestinal contents flow freely, but only when fecal contents are stagnant, as in a pouch. In addition, one of the most frequent treatments for pouchitis is the antibiotic metronidazole (145).

THE GUT FLORA AND CANCER

Colon cancer is one of the most common neoplastic diseases in wealthy populations but is relatively uncommon in developing countries (33). The fact that it occurs at a site with maximal bacterial load (tumors arise 100 times more often in the large intestine than in the small intestine) has naturally led to speculations that the bacteria are accomplices in the cancer development. Inflammation is a well-known predecessor of malignant transformation, as seen, e.g., in inflammatory bowel disease (198, 219). In addition, bacteria in the intestinal microflora contain a range of enzymes that are capable of converting precarcinogenic compounds to carcinogens (86, 150, 246).

Bile acids may act as promoters of the action of carcinogens in the gut (246). Bacteria modify bile acids in a number of ways, i.e., by deconjugation, dehydrogenation, or dehydroxylation (165). The secondary bile acids thus formed appear to be more active as tumor promoters than are the native bile acids (179). The synthesis of bile acids is promoted by a high-fat diet, which is also linked to colon cancer (179).

A diet high in fiber is associated with low incidence of colon cancer. It is suggested that rather than changing the microbial composition of the colonic flora, the diet may alter the metabolic properties of the microbes so that they produce fewer carcinogens or tumor promoters. In general, individuals on a mixed Western diet, rich in meat and fat, have higher levels of fecal β-glucuronidase, nitroreductase, and azoreductase but lower levels of glucosidases than do vegetarians (84, 246). On the other hand, certain short-chain fatty acids generated by intestinal anaerobic bacteria may protect colonic epithelial cells from damage (82).

Differences in Microflora in Relation to Risk of Colon Cancer Development

There might be microbial species that carry a greater risk of performing harmful metabolic processes and, conversely, bacterial species that change the intestinal milieu in a protective direction. Moore and coworkers compared the intestinal microflora of individuals with a high risk of colon cancer (polyp patients and Japanese-Hawaiians on a Western diet) with that of individuals at intermediate (U.S. Caucasians on a Western diet) and low (rural native Japanese and Africans) risk. They identified 15 bacterial species associated with high risk, e.g., Bac-

teroides vulgatus, Bacteroides stercoris, Eubacterium rectale, and Bifidobacterium longum, and 5 species associated with low risk of colon cancer, e.g., an unidentified Lactobacillus species and Eubacterium aerofaciens. Furthermore, the total concentrations of Bacteroides and Bifidobacterium species were positively correlated with increased risk of colon cancer, whereas the total Lactobacillus counts were inversely related to risk (169). Whether these differences in flora composition have any causal relations to cancer development remains to be determined.

THE GUT FLORA AND AUTOIMMUNITY

There is a well-known connection between the intestinal microflora and arthritis. Following intestinal or urogenital infections caused by, e.g., Yersinia, Campylobacter, or Neisseria gonorrhoeae, some individuals develop reactive arthritis. Bacterial components have been identified in the joints of such patients (91). Intraperitoneal injection of cell wall peptidoglycan induces joint inflammation in rats (213).

It is not known whether the gut flora plays any role in rheumatoid arthritis. Patients with rheumatoid arthritis have been reported to have more Clostridium perfringens and slightly more enterobacteria than do control individuals (214). It is difficult to know whether such differences are related to the disease or the medical treatment that such patients receive. However, a study of patients with newly diagnosed untreated rheumatoid arthritis revealed that these patients had a distinct pattern of intestinal bacterial fatty acids that differed from that of healthy control individuals (61). The differences suggested an abnormal anaerobic-microflora composition. Further, rheumatic patients randomized onto a vegan diet changed their microflora fatty acid pattern along with clinical improvement (191).

Small-intestinal overgrowth is common in rheumatoid arthritis. Although this association is very often due to loss of gastric acid production secondary to atrophic gastritis on an autoimmune basis, overgrowth in the presence of normal gastric secretion seemed to be more common in rheumatoid arthritis than among controls and was also associated with high disease activity (100).

Sulfasalazine, the first drug designed against rheumatic diseases and still in use, has both antibiotic and anti-inflammatory properties. Sulfasalazine treatment affects the composition of the gut flora, often with decreased levels of enterobacteria and anaerobes (122, 181).

THE GUT FLORA AND ALLERGY

The incidence of atopic allergy, i.e., IgE-mediated hypersensitivity, is steadily on the increase in western European countries (253). Allergies were practically nonexistent in the 19th century and afflicted a very small proportion of the population before the 1960s. The rise in allergies is not due to a rise in allergen load. On the contrary, hay fever is much more uncommon among farming than nonfarming families (30). Thus, allergies represent immunologically mediated hypersensitivity to completely harmless substances that have always been present in our immediate surroundings (food proteins, animal dandruff, pollens, etc.) and that have been tolerated before. They may thus be seen as a breakdown of normal oral tolerance mechanisms.

There is a clear epidemiological association between a highly hygienic lifestyle and the propensity to develop allergies, as shown by the high allergy incidence in modern Western countries compared with developing countries and formerly communist European countries (240, 247). Allergies are also much more common among children with no or few elder siblings (224), especially if they start late or not at all in day care (136). There is a negative association between allergic sensitization and antibodies against hepatitis A, a virus spread via the oral-fecal route and thus under conditions of poor hygiene (154). Collectively, these associations have formed the basis for "the hygiene hypothesis" (224).

It is entirely possible that the link between excessive hygiene and allergy development is mediated via changes in normal intestinal colonization patterns, especially in childhood (253).

The present composition of the normal flora may not be adequate in promoting the induction of oral tolerance, through a number of potential mechanisms. The delayed colonization with *E. coli* and other enterobacteria may result in too low an exposure of the developing immune system to LPS. The low turnover of bacterial strains in the microflora may result in an insufficient buildup of a pool of memory T cells with regulatory function. Lastly, the increased colonization with *S. aureus*, including strains secreting toxins with superantigen function (E. Lindberg, F. Nowrouzian, I. Adlerberth, and A. E. Wold, unpublished data), may result in polyclonal activation of T and/or B cells (107, 212, 216). Staphylococci have been implicated in the pathogenesis of atopic dermatitis (53, 258). Evidently, the epidemiological connection between the intestinal colonization pattern and allergy development needs to be further studied.

REFERENCES

1. **Abrams, G. D.** 1983. Impact of the intestinal microflora on intestinal structure and function, p. 291–309. *In* D. J. Hentges (ed.), *Human Intestinal Microflora in Health and Disease.* Academic Press, London, United Kingdom.
2. **Abrams, G. D., H. Bauer, and H. Sprinz.** 1963. Influence of the normal flora on mucosal morphology and cellular renewal in the ileum. A comparison of germfree and conventional mice. *Lab. Investig.* **12:**355–364.
3. **Adlerberth, I., S. Ahrné, M.-L. Johansson, G. Molin, L. Å. Hanson, and A. E. Wold.** 1996. A mannose-specific adherence mechanism in *Lactobacillus plantarum* conferring binding to the human colonic cell line HT-29. *Appl. Environ. Microbiol.* **62:**2244–2251.
4. **Adlerberth, I., B. Carlsson, P. de Man, F. Jalil, S. R. Khan, P. Larsson, L. Mellander, C. Svanborg, A. E. Wold, and L. Å. Hanson.** 1991. Intestinal colonization with *Enterobacteriaceae* in Pakistani and Swedish hospital-delivered infants. *Acta Paediatr. Scand.* **80:**602–610.
5. **Adlerberth, I., L. Å. Hanson, C. Svanborg, A.-M. Svennerholm, S. Nordgren, and A. E. Wold.** 1995. Adhesins of *Escherichia coli* associated with extraintestinal pathogenicity confer binding to colonic epithelial cells. *Microb. Pathog.* **18:**373–385.
6. **Adlerberth, I., L. Å. Hanson, and A. E. Wold.** 1999. The ontogeny of the intestinal flora,

p. 279–292. *In* I. R. Sanderson and W. A. Walker (ed.), *Development of the Gastrointestinal Tract*. B. C. Decker, Hamilton, Ontario, Canada.

7. **Adlerberth, I., F. Jalil, B. Carlsson, L. Mellander, L. Å. Hanson, P. Larsson, K. Kahlil, and A. E. Wold.** 1998. High turn-over rate of *Escherichia coli* strains in the intestinal flora of infants in Pakistan. *Epidemiol. Infect.* 121:587–598.

8. **Adlerberth, I., C. Svanborg, B. Carlsson, L. Mellander, L. Å. Hanson, F. Jalil, K. Khalil, and A. E. Wold.** 1998. P fimbriae and other adhesins enhance intestinal persistence of *Escherichia coli* in early infancy. *Epidemiol. Infect.* 121:599–608.

9. **Ahrné, S., S. Nobaek, B. Jeppsson, I. Adlerberth, A. E. Wold, and G. Molin.** 1998. The normal Lactobacillus flora of healthy human oral and rectal mucosa. *J. Appl. Microbiol.* 85:88–94.

10. **Albers, W. H., C. W. Tyler, and B. Boxerbaum.** 1966. Asymptomatic bacteremia in the newborn infant. *J. Pediatr.* 69:193–197.

11. **Alverdy, J. C., E. Aoyos, and G. S. Moss.** 1988. Total parenteral nutrition promotes bacterial translocation from the gut. *Surgery* 104:185–190.

12. **Aranda, R., B. C. Sydora, P. L. McAllister, S. W. Binder, H. Y. Yang, S. R. Targan, and M. Kronenberg.** 1997. Analysis of intestinal lymphocytes in mouse colitis mediated by transfer of CD4$^+$ CD45RB^{high} T cells into SCID recipients. *J. Immunol.* 158:3464–3473.

13. **Ashraf, R. N., F. Jalil, S. Zaman, J. Karlberg, S. R. Khan, B. S. Lindblad, and L. Å. Hanson.** 1991. Breast feeding and protection against neonatal sepsis in a high risk population. *Arch. Dis. Child.* 66:488–490.

14. **Asquith, M. T., and J. R. Harrod.** 1979. Reduction in bacterial contamination in banked human milk. *J. Pediatr.* 95:993–994.

15. **Bark, T., M. Katouli, O. Ljungqvist, R. Möllby, and T. Svenberg.** 1993. Bacterial translocation after non-lethal hemorrhage in the rat. *Circ. Shock* 41:60–65.

16. **Bennet, R.** 1987. *The Faecal Microflora of Newborn Infants During Intensive Care Management, and Its Relationship to Neonatal Sepricemia*. Karolinska Institute, Stockholm, Sweden.

17. **Bennet, R., M. Eriksson, N. Tafari, and C.-E. Nord.** 1991. Intestinal bacteria of newborn Ethiopian infants in relation to antibiotic treatment and colonization with potentially pathogenic Gram-negative bacteria. *Scand. J. Infect. Dis.* 23:63–69.

18. **Bennet, R., M. Eriksson, B. Melen, and R. Zetterström.** 1985. Changes in the incidence and spectrum of neonatal septicemia during a fifteen-year period. *Acta Paediatr. Scand.* 74:687–690.

19. **Berg, R. D.** 1983. Translocation of indigenous bacteria from the intestinal tract, p. 333–352. *In* D. J. Hentges (ed.), *Intestinal Microflora in Health and Disease*. Academic Press, New York, N.Y.

20. **Berg, R. D., E. Wommack, and E. A. Deitch.** 1988. Immunosuppression and intestinal bacterial overgrowth synergistically promote bacterial translocation. *Arch. Surg.* 123:1359–1364.

21. **Bettelheim, K. A., B. A. Peddie, and A. Cheresky.** 1983. The ecology of *Escherichia coli* in a maternity ward in Christchurch, New Zealand. *Zentbl. Bakteriol. Mikrobiol. Hyg.* 178:389–393.

22. **Bibel, D. J.** 1988. Elie Metchnikoff's bacillus of long life. *ASM News* 54:661–665.

23. **Bishop, R. F., and C. M. Anderson.** 1960. The bacterial flora of the stomach and small intestine in children with intestinal obstruction. *Arch. Dis. Child.* 35:487–491.

24. **Blumberg, R. S., C. E. Yockey, G. G. Gross, E. C. Ebert, and S. P. Balk.** 1993. Human intestinal intraepithelial lymphocytes are derived from a limited number of T cell clones that utilize multiple V beta T cell receptor genes. *J. Immunol.* 150:5144–5153.

25. **Bollgren, I., and J. Winberg.** 1976. The periurethral aerobic bacterial flora in healthy boys and girls. *Acta Paediatr. Scand.* 65:74–80.

26. **Bollgren, I., and J. Winberg.** 1976. The periurethral aerobic flora in girls highly susceptible to urinary tract infections. *Acta Paediatr. Scand.* 65:81–87.

27. **Border, J., J. Hassett, J. LaDuca, R. Seibel, S. Steinberg, B. Mills, P. Losi, and D. Border.** 1987. The gut origin septic states in blunt multiple trauma (ISS = 40) in the ICU. *Ann. Surg.* 206:427–448.

28. **Borderon, J. C., C. Lionnet, C. Rondeau, A. L. Suc, J. Laugier, and F. Gold.** 1996. Current aspects of the fecal flora of the newborn without antibiotherapy during the first seven days of life: *Enterobacteriaceae*, enterococci, staphylococci. *Pathol. Biol. Paris* 44:416–422.

29. **Brandtzaeg, P.** 1994. Distribution and characterization of mucosal immunoglobulin-producing cells, p. 251–262. *In* P. L. Ogra (ed.), *Handbook of Mucosal Immunology*. Academic Press, San Diego, Calif.

30. **Braun-Farlander, C., M. Gassner, L. Grize, U. Neu, F. H. Sennhauser, H. S. Varonier, J. C. Vuille, and B. Wütrich.** 1999. Prevalence of hay fever and allergic sensitization in farmer's children and their peers living in the same rural community. SCARPOL team. Swiss Study on Childhood Allergy and Respiratory Symptoms

with Respect to Air Pollution. *Clin. Exp. Allergy* **29:**28–34.

31. **Bry, L., P. G. Falk, T. Midtvedt, and J. I. Gordon.** 1996. A model of host-microbial interactions in an open mammalian ecosystem. *Science* **273:**1380–1383.

32. **Buddington, R. K., C. H. Williams, S. C. Chen, and S. A. Witherly.** 1996. Dietary supplementation of neosugars alters the fecal flora and decreases activities of some reductive enzymes in human subjects. *Am. J. Clin. Nutr.* **63:**709–716.

33. **Burkitt, D. P.** 1971. Epidemiology of cancer of the colon and rectum. 1971. *Dis. Colon Rectum* **36:**1071–1082.

34. **Carter, P. B., and M. Pollard.** 1971. Host responses to "normal" microbial flora in germ-free mice. *J. Reticuloendothel. Soc.* **9:**580–587.

35. **Cebra, J. J.** 1999. Influences of microbiota on intestinal immune system development. *Am. J. Clin. Nutr.* **69**(Suppl.)**:**1046S–1051S.

36. **Cebra, J. J., J. A. Cebra-Thomas, C. F. Cuff, A. George, S. I. Kost, S. D. London, and D. H. Rubin.** 1989. Reoviruses as probes of the gut mucosal T cell population. *Immunol. Investig.* **18:** 545–585.

37. **Chachaty, E., C. Depitre, N. Mario, et al.** 1992. Presence of *Clostridium difficile* and antibiotic and β-lactamase activities in feces of volunteers treated with oral cefixime, oral cefpodoxime proxetil, or placebo. *Antimicrob. Agents Chemother.* **36:**2009–2013.

38. **Cherbut, C., L. Ferrier, C. Roze, Y. Anini, H. Blottiere, G. Lecannu, and J. P. Galmiche.** 1998. Short-chain fatty acids modify colonic motility through nerves and polypeptide YY release in the rat. *Am. J. Physiol.* **275:** G1415–G1422.

39. **Cherbuy, C., B. Darcy-Vrillon, M. T. Morel, J. P. Pegorier, and P. H. Duee.** 1995. Effect of germfree state on the capacities of isolated rat colonocytes to metabolize n-butyrate, glucose, and glutamine. *Gastroenterology* **109:**1890–1899.

40. **Chouaib, S., K. Welte, R. Mertelsmann, and B. Dupont.** 1985. Prostaglandin E2 acts at two distinct pathways of lymphocyte activation: inhibition of interleukin 2 production and downregulation of transferrin receptor expression. *J. Immunol.* **135:**1172–1179.

41. **Collins, F. M., and P. B. Carter.** 1978. Growth of salmonellae in orally infected germfree mice. *Infect. Immun.* **21:**41–47.

42. **Cone, R. A.** 1999. Mucus, p. 43–64. *In* P. L. Ogra, J. Mestecky, M. E. Lamm, W. Strober, J. Bienenstock, and J. R. McGhee (ed.), *Mucosal Immunology.* Academic Press, San Diego, Calif.

43. **Cong, Y., S. L. Brandwein, R. P. McGabe, A. Lazenby, E. H. Birkenmeier, J. P. Sund-** berg, **and C. O. Elson.** 1998. CD4+ T cells reactive to enteric bacterial antigens in spontaneously colitic C3H/HeJBir mice: increased T helper cell type 1 response and ability to transfer disease. *J. Exp. Med.* **187:**855–864.

44. **Cooke, E. M.** 1974. *Escherichia coli*: distribution in nature, epidemiology, p. 13–30. *In* E. M. Cooke (ed.), Escherichia coli *and Man.* Churchill Livingstone, Edinburgh, United Kingdom.

45. **Cooke, E. M., I. G. T. Hettiaratchy, and A. C. Buck.** 1971. Fate of ingested *Escherichia coli* in normal persons. *J. Med. Microbiol.* **5:**361–369.

46. **Cover, T. L., and M. J. Blaser.** 1996. *H. pylori* infection, a paradigm for chronic mucosal inflammation: pathogenesis and implications for eradication and prevention. *Adv. Intern. Med.* **42:**85–117.

47. **Crabbé, P. A., H. Bazin, H. Eyssen, and J. F. Heremans.** 1968. The normal microbial flora as a major stimulus for proliferation of plasma cells synthesizing IgA in the gut. *Int. Arch. Allergy* **34:** 362–375.

48. **Crabbé, P. A., D. R. Nash, H. Bazin, H. Eysseb, and J. F. Heremans.** 1970. Immunohistochemical observations on lymphoid tissues from conventional and germ-free mice. *Lab. Investig.* **22:**448–457.

49. **Craig, S., and J. Cebra.** 1971. Peyer's patches: an enriched source of precursors for IgA-producing immunocytes in the rabbit. *J. Exp. Med.* **134:** 188–200.

50. **Croft, C. N., and P. B. Cotton.** 1973. Gastrointestinal cell loss in man. *Digestion* **8:**144–160.

51. **Dahlgren, U. I. H., A. E. Wold, L. Å. Hanson, and T. Midtvedt.** 1991. Expression of a dietary protein in *E. coli* renders it strongly antigenic to gut lymphoid tissue. *Immunology* **73:** 394–397.

52. **deMaria, R., S. Fais, M. Silvestri, L. Frati, F. Pallone, A. Santoni, and R. Testi.** 1993. Continuous in-vivo activation and transient hyporesponsiveness to TcR/CD3 triggering of human gut lamina propria lymphocytes. *Eur. J. Immunol.* **23:**3104–3108.

53. **Dhar, S., A. J. Kanwar, S. Kaur, P. Sharma, and N. K. Ganguly.** 1992. Role of bacterial flora in the pathogenesis and management of atopic dermatitis. *Indian J. Med. Res.* **95:**234–238.

54. **Dixon, J. M. S.** 1960. The fate of bacteria in the small intestine. *J. Pathol. Bacteriol.* **79:**131–140.

55. **Donald, I. P., G. Kitchingmam, F. Donald, and R. M. Kupfer.** 1992. The diagnosis of small bowel bacterial overgrowth in elderly patients. *J. Am. Geriatr. Soc.* **40:**692–696.

56. **Drasar, B. S.** 1974. Some factors associated with geographical variations in the intestinal microflora, p. 187–196. *In* F. A. Skinner and F. A. Carr (ed.),

The Normal Microbial Flora of Man. Academic Press, London, United Kingdom.

57. **Drasar, B. S., M. Shiner, and G. M. McLeod.** 1969. Studies on the intestinal flora. I. The bacterial flora of the gastrointestinal tract in healthy and achlorhydric persons. *Gastroenterology* **56:**71–79.

58. **Duchmann, R., I. Kaiser, E. Hermann, W. Mayet, K. Ewe, and K.-H. Meyer Zum.** 1995. Tolerance exists towards resident intestinal flora but is broken in active inflammatory bowel disease (IBD). *Clin. Exp. Immunol.* **102:**448.

59. **Duguid, J. P., and D. C. Old.** 1980. Adhesive properties of *Enterobacteriaceae*, p. 185–217. *In* E. C. Beachey (ed.), *Bacterial Adherence, Receptors and Recognition.* Chapman & Hall, London, United Kingdom.

60. **Duncan, R. L. J., and D. C. Morrison.** 1984. The fate of *E. coli* lipopolysaccharide after the uptake of *E. coli* by murine macrophages *in vitro. J. Immunol.* **132:**1416–1424.

61. **Eerola, E., T. Mottonen, P. Hannonen, L. R. I. Kantola, K. Vuori, J. Tuominen, and P. Toivanen.** 1994. Intestinal flora in early rheumatoid arthritis. *Br. J. Rheumatol.* **33:**1030–1038.

62. **Ellis-Pegler, R. B., C. Crabtree, and H. P. Lambert.** 1975. The fecal flora of children in the United Kingdom. *J. Hyg. Camb.* **75:**135–142.

63. **El Mohandes, A. E., J. F. Keiser, L. A. Johnson, M. Refat, and B. J. Jackson.** 1993. Aerobes isolated in fecal microflora of infants in the intensive care nursery: relationship to human milk use and systemic sepsis. *Am. J. Infect. Control* **21:**231–234.

64. **Elson, C. O., and W. Ealding.** 1984. Cholera toxin feeding did not induce oral tolerance in mice and abrogated oral tolerance to an unrelated protein antigen. *J. Immunol.* **133:**2892–2897.

65. **Elson, C. O., R. B. Sartor, G. S. Tennyson, and R. H. Riddell.** 1995. Experimental models of inflammatory bowel disease. *Gastroenterology* **109:**1344–1367.

66. **Finegold, S. M., H. R. Attebery, and V. L. Sutter.** 1974. Effect of diet on human fecal flora: comparison of Japanese and American diets. *Am. J. Clin. Nutr.* **27:**1456.

67. **Finegold, S. M., L. Ingram-Drake, R. Gee, J. Reinhardt, M. A. Edelstein, K. MacDonald, and H. Wexler.** 1987. Bowel flora changes in humans receiving cefixime (CL 284,635) or cefaclor. *Antimicrob. Agents Chemother.* **31:**443–446.

68. **Finegold, S. M., V. L. Sutter, and G. E. Mathiesen.** 1983. Normal indigenous intestinal flora, p. 3–31. *In* D. J. Hentges (ed.), *Human Intestinal Microflora in Health and Disease.* Academic Press, London, United Kingdom.

69. **Firon, N., I. Ofek, and N. Sharon.** 1983. Carbohydrate specificity of the surface lectins of *Escherichia coli, Klebsiella pneumoniae* and *Salmonella typhimurium. Carbohydr. Res.* **120:**235–249.

70. **Frankel, W. L., W. Zhang, A. Singh, D. M. Klurfeld, S. Don, S. Sakata, I. Modlin, and J. L. Rombeau.** 1994. Mediation of the trophic effects of short-chain fatty acids on the rat jejunum and colon. *Gastroenterology* **106:**375–380.

71. **Freter, R.** 1969. Studies on the mechanism of action of intestinal antibody in experimental cholera. *Texas Rep. Biol. Med.* **27**(Suppl.):299–316.

72. **Freter, R.** 1983. Mechanisms that control the microflora of the large intestine, p. 33–54. *In* D. J. Hentges (ed.), *Human Intestinal Microflora in Health and Disease.* Academic Press, New York, N.Y.

73. **Freter, R., E. Stauffer, D. Cleven, L. V. Holdeman, and W. E. C. Moore.** 1983. Continuous-flow cultures as in vitro models of the ecology of large intestinal flora. *Infect. Immun.* **39:**666–675.

74. **Friedel, D., and G. M. Levine.** 1992. Effect of short-chain fatty acid on colonic function and structure. *J. Parenter. Enteral Nutr.* **16:**1–4.

75. **Friman, V., I. Adlerberth, H. Connell, C. Svanborg, L. Å. Hanson, and A. E. Wold.** 1996. Decreased expression of mannose-specific adhesins by *Escherichia coli* in the colonic microflora of IgA-deficient individuals. *Infect. Immun.* **64:**2794–2798.

76. **Fryklund, B.** 1994. *Epidemiology of Enterobacteria and Risk Factors for Invasive Gram-Negative Bacterial Infection in Neonatal Special-Care Units.* Stockholm University, Stockholm, Sweden.

77. **Fryklund, B., K. Tullus, B. Berglund, and L. G. Burman.** 1992. Importance of the environment and the faecal flora of infants, nursing staff and parents as sources of Gram-negative bacteria colonizing newborns in three neonatal wards. *Infection* **20:**253–257.

78. **Fryklund, B., K. Tullus, and L. G. Burman.** 1994. Epidemiology and attack index of gram-negative bacteria causing invasive infection in three special-care neonatal units and risk factors for infection. *Infection* **23:**76–80.

79. **Fukushima, K., I. Sasaki, H. Ogawa, H. Naito, Y. Funayama, and S. Matsuno.** 1999. Colonization of microflora in mice: mucosal defense against luminal bacteria. *J. Gastroenterol.* **34:**54–60.

80. **Fukushima, R., L. Gianotti, J. W. Alexander, and T. Pyles.** 1992. The degree of bacterial translocation is a determinant factor for mortality after burn injury and is improved by prostaglandin analogs. *Ann. Surg.* **216:**438–445.

81. **Gaborieau-Routhiau, V., and M.-C. Moreau.** 1996. Gut flora allows recovery of oral tolerance to ovalbumin in mice after transient break-

down mediated by cholera toxin or *Escherichia coli* heat-labile enterotoxin. *Pediatr. Res.* **39**:625–629.

82. **Gamet, L., D. Daviaud, C. Denis-Pouxviel, C. Remesy, and J. C. Murat.** 1992. Effects of short-chain fatty acids on growth and differentiation of the human colon-cancer cell line HT-29. *Int. J. Cancer* **52**:286–289.

83. **Gareau, F. E., D. C. Mackel, J. Boring III, F. J. Payne, and F. L. Hammet.** 1959. The acquisition of fecal flora by infants from their mothers during birth. *J. Pediatr.* **54**:313–318.

84. **Goldin, B. R.** 1990. Intestinal microflora: metabolism of drugs and carcinogens. *Ann. Med.* **22**: 43–48.

85. **Goldstein, F., C. W. Wirts, and O. D. Kowlessar.** 1970. Diabetic diarrhea and steatorrhea. Microbiologic and clinical observations. *Ann. Intern. Med.* **72**:215–218.

86. **Gorbach, S. L., and B. R. Goldin.** 1990. The intestinal microflora and the colon cancer connection. *Rev. Infect. Dis.* **12**(Suppl. 2):S252–S261.

87. **Gordon, H. A., and E. Bruckner-Kardoss.** 1961. Effect of normal microbial flora on intestinal surface area. *Am. J. Physiol.* **201**:175–178.

88. **Gothefors, L.** 1975. *Studies of Antimicrobial Factors in Human Milk and Bacterial Colonization of the Newborn.* Umeå University, Umeå, Sweden.

89. **Gothefors, L., B. Carlsson, S. Ahlstedt, L. Å, Hanson, and J. Winberg.** 1976. Influence of maternal gut flora and colostral and cord serum antibodies on presence of *Escherichia coli* in faeces of the newborn infant. *Acta Paediatr. Scand.* **65**: 225–232.

90. **Gracey, M.** 1984. The intestinal microflora in malnutrition and protracted diarrhoea in infancy, p. 223–236. *In* E. Lebenthal (ed.), *Chronic Diarrhea in Children.* Raven Press, New York, N.Y.

91. **Granfors, K., S. Jalkanen, A. A. Lindberg, O. Maki-Ikola, R. von Essen, R. Lahesmaa-Rantala, H. Isomaki, R. Saario, W. J. Arnold, and A. Toivanen.** 1990. Salmonella lipopolysaccharide in synovial cells from patients with reactive arthritis. *Lancet* **335**:685–688.

92. **Griffin, W. O., Jr., J. D. Richardson, and E. S. Medley.** 1971. Prevention of small bowel contamination by ileocecal valve. *South. Med. J.* **64**: 1056–1058.

93. **Grüneberg, R. N.** 1969. Relationship of infecting urinary organisms to the faecal flora in patients with symptomatic urinary infections. *Lancet* **ii**:766–768.

94. **Guiot, H. F. L.** 1982. Role of competition for substrate in bacterial antagonism in the gut. *Infect. Immun.* **38**:887–892.

95. **Hashimoto, K., H. Handa, K. Umehara, and S. Sasaki.** 1978. Germfree mice reared on an "antigen free" diet. *Lab. Anim. Sci.* **28**:38–45.

96. **Hathcock, K. S., G. Laszlo, C. Pucillo, P. Linsley, and R. J. Hodes.** 1994. Comparative analysis of B7-1 and B7-2 costimulatory ligands: expression and function. *J. Exp. Med.* **180**: 631–640.

97. **Hauer, A. C., M. Bajaj-Elliot, C. B. Williams, J. A. Walker-Smith, and T. T. MacDonald.** 1998. An analysis of interferon gamma, IL-4, IL-5 and IL-10 production by ELISPOT and quantitative reverse transcriptase-PCR in human Peyer's patches. *Cytokine* **10**:627–634.

98. **Hauer, A. C., E. J. Breese, J. A. Walker-Smith, and T. T. MacDonald.** 1997. The frequency of cells secreting interferon-gamma and interleukin-4, -5, and -10 in the blood and duodenal mucosa of children with cow's milk hypersensitivity. *Pediatr. Res.* **42**:629–638.

99. **Hendrickson, B. A., J. Guo, R. Laughlin, Y. M. Chen, and J. C. Alverdy.** 1999. Increased type 1 fimbrial expression among commensal *Escherichia coli* isolates in the murine cecum following catabolic stress. *Infect. Immun.* **67**:745–753.

100. **Henriksson, A. E., L. Blomquist, C. E. Nord, T. Midtvedt, and A. Uribe.** 1993. Small intestinal bacterial overgrowth in patients with rheumatoid arthritis. *Ann. Rheum. Dis.* **52**: 503–510.

101. **Hentges, D. J.** 1978. Fecal flora of volunteers on controlled diets. *Am. J. Clin. Nutr.* **31**: S123–S124.

102. **Hentges, D. J.** 1993. The anaerobic microflora of the human body. *Clin. Infect. Dis.* **16**(Suppl. 4):175–180.

103. **Herías, M. V.** 1998. *Colonization, Translocation and Immune Responses in a Gnotobiotic Rat Model.* Göteborg University, Göteborg, Sweden.

104. **Herías, M. V., T. Midtvedt, L. Å. Hanson, and A. E. Wold.** 1995. Role of *Escherichia coli* P fimbriae in intestinal colonization in gnotobiotic rats. *Infect. Immun.* **63**:4781–4789.

105. **Herías, M. V., T. Midtvedt, L. Å. Hanson, and A. E. Wold.** 1997. *Escherichia coli* K5 capsule expression enhances colonization of the large intestine in the gnotobiotic rat. *Infect. Immun.* **65**:531–536.

106. **Herías, M. V., T. Midtvedt, L. Å. Hanson, and A. E. Wold.** 1998. Increased antibody production against gut-colonizing *Escherichia coli* in the presence of the anaerobic bacterium *Peptostreptococcus. Scand. J. Immunol.* **48**:277–282.

107. **Herman, A., J. Kappler, P. Marrack, and A. Pullen.** 1991. Superantigens: mechanism of T-cell stimulation and role in immune responses. *Annu. Rev. Immunol.* **9**:745–772.

108. **Hohmann, A., G. Schmidt, and D. Rowley.** 1979. Intestinal and serum antibody responses in mice after oral immunization with *Salmonella,*

Escherichia coli, and *Salmonella-Escherichia coli* hybrid strains. *Infect. Immun.* 25:27–33.

109. **Hoijer, M. A., M.-J. Melief, C. G. van Helden-Meeuwsen, F. Eulderink, and M. Hazenberg.** 1995. Detection of muramic acid in a carbohydrate fraction of human spleen. *Infect. Immun.* 63:1652–1657.

110. **Holdeman, L. V., I. J. Good, and W. E. C. Moore.** 1976. Human fecal flora: variation in bacterial composition within individuals and a possible effect of emotional stress. *Appl. Environ. Microbiol.* 31:359–375.

111. **Holt, P. G., J. Oliver, N. Bilyk, C. McMenamin, P. G. McMenamin, G. Kraal, and T. Thepen.** 1993. Downregulation of the antigen presenting cell function(s) of pulmonary dendritic cells in vivo by resident alveolar macrophages. *J. Exp. Med.* 177:397–407.

112. **Hoogkamp-Korstanje, J. A. A., J. G. E. M. Lindner, J. H. Marcells, H. den Daas-Slagt, and N. M. de Vos.** 1979. Composition and ecology of the human intestinal flora. *Antonie Leeuwenhoek* 45:335–340.

113. **Hooper, D. C., E. H. Molowitz, N. A. Bos, V. A. Ploplis, and J. J. Cebra.** 1995. Spleen cells from antigen-minimized mice are superior to spleen cells from germ-free and conventional mice in the stimulation of primary *in vitro* proliferative responses to nominal antigens. *Eur. J. Immunol.* 25:212–217.

114. **Hoskins, L. C.** 1993. Mucin degradation in the human gastrointestinal tract and its significance to enteric microbial ecology. *Eur. J. Gastroenterol. Hepatol.* 5:205–213.

115. **Husby, S., J. C. Jensenius, and S.-E. Svehag.** 1985. ELISA quantitation of IgG subclass antibodies to dietary antigens. *J. Immunol. Methods* 82:321–331.

116. **Husby, S., J. C. Jensenius, and S.-E. Svehag.** 1985. Passage of undegraded dietary antigen into the blood of healthy adults. Quantification, estimation of size distribution and relation of uptake to levels of specific antibodies. *Scand. J. Immunol.* 22:83–92.

117. **Husebye, E., P. M. Hellström, and T. Midtvedt.** 1992. Introduction of conventional microbial flora to germfree rats increases the frequency of migrating myoelectric complexes. *J. Gastrointest. Motil.* 4:39–45.

118. **Husebye, E., V. Skar, T. Hoverstad, and K. Melby.** 1992. Fasting hypochlorhydria with gram positive gastric flora is highly prevalent in healthy old people. *Gut* 33:1331–1337.

119. **Johannsen, L., and J. M. Krueger.** 1988. Quantitation of diaminopimelic acid in human urine. *Adv. Biosci.* 68:445–449.

120. **Johannsen, L., J. Wecke, F. Obal, and J. Krueger.** 1991. Macrophages produce somnogenic and pyrogenic muramyl peptides during digestion of staphylococci. *Am. J. Physiol.* 260:R126–R133.

121. **Johnson, W. J., and E. Balish.** 1980. Macrophage function in germ-free, athymic (nu/nu) and conventional flora (nu +) mice. *J. Reticuloendothel. Soc.* 28:55–66.

122. **Kanerud, L., A. Scheynius, C. E. Nord, and I. Hafström.** 1994. Effect of sulphasalazine on gastrointestinal microflora and on mucosal heat shock protein expression in patients with rheumatoid arthritis. *Br. J. Rheumatol.* 33:1039–1048.

123. **Katouli, M., C. G. Nettlebladt, V. Muratov, O. Ljungqvist, T. Bark, T. Svenberg, and R. Möllby.** 1997. Selective translocation of coliform bacteria adhering to caecal epithelium of rats during catabolic stress. *J. Med. Microbiol.* 46:1–8.

124. **Kawaguchi, M., M. Nanno, Y. Umesaki, S. Matsumoto, Y. Okada, Z. Cai, T. Shimamura, Y. Matsuoka, M. Ohwaki, and H. Ishikawa.** 1993. Cytolytic activity of intestinal intraepithelial lymphocytes in germ-free mice is strain dependent and determined by T cells expressing gamma delta T-cell antigen receptors. *Proc. Natl. Acad. Sci. USA* 90:8591–8594.

125. **Keller, R., R. Gehri, and R. Keist.** 1994. Macrophage response to viruses, protozoa, and fungi: secretory and cellular activities induced in resting unprimed bone marrow-derived mononuclear phagocytes. *Cell. Immunol.* 159:323–330.

126. **Khan, I. J., G. H. Jeffries, and M. H. Sleisenger.** 1966. Malabsorption in intestinal scleroderma: correction by antibiotics. *N. Engl. J. Med.* 274:1339–1344.

127. **Khan, S. R., F. Jalil, S. Zaman, B. S. Lindblad, and J. Karlberg.** 1993. Early child health in Lahore, Pakistan. X. Mortality. *Acta Paediatr. Suppl.* 390:109–117.

128. **Khoury, K. A., M. H. Floch, and T. Hersh.** 1969. Small intestinal mucosal cell proliferation and bacterial flora in conventionalization of the germfree mouse. *J. Exp. Med.* 130:659–670.

129. **Kilshaw, P. J., and A. J. Cant.** 1984. The passage of maternal dietary proteins into human breast milk. *Int. Arch. Allergy Appl. Immunol.* 75:8–15.

130. **Kim, J. H., and M. Ohsawa.** 1995. Oral tolerance to ovalbumin in mice as a model for detecting modulators of the immunologic tolerance to a specific antigen. *Biol. Pharm. Bull.* 18:854–858.

131. **King, C. E.** 1979. Small intestine bacterial overgrowth. *Gastroenterology* 76:1035–1055.

132. **Kirsch, M.** 1990. Bacterial overgrowth. *Am. J. Gastroenterol.* 85:231–237.

133. **Kmiot, W. A., M. R. Williams, and M. R. B. Keighley.** 1990. Pouchitis following colectomy and ileal reservoir construction for familial adenomatous polyposis. *Br. J. Surg.* **77:**1283.

134. **Koch, F., U. Stanzl, P. Jennewein, K. Janke, C. Heufler, E. Kampgen, N. Romani, and G. Schuler.** 1996. High level IL-12 production by murine dendritic cells: upregulation via MHC class II and CD40 molecules and downregulation by IL-4 and IL-10. *J. Exp. Med.* **184:**741–746.

135. **Kool, J., H. de Visser, M. Y. Gerritsboeye, I. S. Klasen, M. J. Melief, C. G. van Heiden-Meeuwsen, L. M. van Lieshout, W. B. Ruseler-van Embden, W. B. van den Berg, G. M. Bahr, and M. P. Hazenberg.** 1994. Detection of intestinal flora-derived bacterial-antigen complexes in splenic macrophages of rats. *J. Histochem. Cytochem.* **11:**1435–1441.

136. **Kramer, U., J. Heinrich, M. Wijst, and H. E. Wichman.** 1999. Age of entry to day nursery and allergy in later childhood. *Lancet* **353:**450–454.

137. **Kripke, S. A., A. D. Fox, J. M. Berman, R. G. Settle, and J. L. Rombeau.** 1989. Stimulation of intestinal mucosal growth with intracolonic infusion of short-chain fatty acids. *J. Parenter. Enteral Nutr.* **13:**109–116.

138. **Kunin, C. M., F. Polyak, and E. Postel.** 1980. Periurethral bacterial flora in women. Prolonged intermittent colonization with *Escherichia coli. JAMA* **243:**134–139.

139. **Langholtz, E., P. Munkholm, O. Haagen Nielsen, S. Kreiner, and V. Binder.** 1991. Incidence and prevalence of ulcerative colitis in Copenhagen County from 1962 to 1987. *Scand. J. Gastroenterol.* **26:**1247–1256.

140. **Licht, T. R., K. A. Krogfelt, P. S. Cohen, L. K. Poulsen, J. Urbance, and S. Molin.** 1996. Role of lipopolysaccharide in colonization of the mouse intestine by *Salmonella typhimurium* studied by in situ hybridization. *Infect. Immun.* **64:**3811–3817.

141. **Lichtenstein, A. H., and B. R. Goldin.** 1993. Lactic acid bacteria and intestinal drug and cholesterol metabolism, p. 227–236. *In* S. Salminen and A. von Wright (ed.), *Lactic Acid Bacteria.* Marcel Dekker Inc., New York, N.Y.

142. **Lichtman, S. N., R. B. Sartor, J. Keku, and J. H. Schwab.** 1990. Hepatic inflammation in rats with experimental small intestinal bacterial overgrowth. *Gastroenterology* **98:**414–423.

143. **Lipson, A.** 1976. Infectious dose of *Salmonella. Lancet* **i:**969.

144. **Lundqvist, C., S. Melgar, M. M. Yeung, S. Hammarström, and M.-L. Hammarström.** 1996. Intraepithelial lymphocytes in human gut have lytic potential and a cytokine profile that suggest T helper 1 and cytotoxic functions. *J. Immunol.* **157:**1926–1934.

145. **Luukonen, P., V. Valtonen, A. Sivonen, P. Sipponen, and H. Jarvinen.** 1988. Fecal bacteriology and reservoir ileitis in patients operated for ulcerative colitis. *Dis. Colon Rectum* **31:**864–867.

146. **Lyerly, D. M., D. E. Lockwood, S. H. Richardson, and T. D. Wilkins.** 1982. Biological activities of toxins A and B of *Clostridium difficile. Infect. Immun.* **35:**1147–1150.

147. **Lyerly, D. M., D. E. Lockwood, S. H. Richardson, and T. D. Wilkins.** 1988. *Clostridium difficile:* its disease and toxins. *Clin. Microbiol. Rev.* **1:**1–18.

148. **Mackowiak, P. A.** 1982. The normal microbial flora. *N. Engl. J. Med.* **307:**83–93.

149. **Mahmud, A., F. Jalil, J. Karlberg, and B. S. Lindblad.** 1993. Early child health in Lahore, Pakistan. VII. Diarrhoea. *Acta Paediatr. Suppl.* **390:**79–85.

150. **Mallett, A. K., and I. R. Rowland.** 1990. Bacterial enzymes: their role in the formation of mutagens and carcinogens in the intestine. *Dig. Dis.* **8:**71–79.

151. **Marshall, J. C., N. V. Christou, and J. L. Meakins.** 1993. The gastro-intestinal tract. The "undrained abscess" of multiple organ failure. *Arch. Surg.* **218:**111–119.

152. **Martin, S. A., J. L. Karnovsky, J. M. Krueger, J. R. Pappenheimer, and K. Biemann.** 1984. Peptidoglycans as promoters of slow wave sleep. 1. Structure of the sleep-promoting factor isolated from human urine. *J. Biol. Chem.* **259:**7514–7522.

153. **Mata, L. J., and J. J. Urrutia.** 1971. Intestinal colonization of breast-fed children in a rural area of low socioeconomic level. *Ann. N. Y. Acad. Sci.* **176:**93–109.

154. **Matricardi, P. M., F. Rosmini, L. Ferrigno, R. Nisini, M. Rapicetta, P. Chionne, T. Stroffolini, P. Pasquini, and R. D'Amelio.** 1997. Cross sectional retrospective study of prevalence of atopy among Italian military students with antibodies against hepatitis A virus. *BMJ* **314:**999–1003.

155. **Matsumoto, S., M. Nanno, N. Watanabe, M. Miyashita, H. Amasaki, K. Suzuki, and Y. Umesaki.** 1999. Physiological roles of γδ T-cell receptor intraepithelial lymphocytes in cytoproliferation and differentiation of mouse intestinal epithelial cells. *Immunology* **97:**18–25.

156. **Mattias, J. R., and M. H. Clench.** 1985. Review: pathophysiology of diarrhea caused by bacterial overgrowth of the small intestine. *Am. J. Med. Sci.* **289:**243–248.

157. **Maxson, R. T., R. J. Jackson, and S. D.**

Smith. 1995. The protective role of enteral IgA supplementation in neonatal gut origin sepsis. *J. Pediatr. Surg.* **30**:231–233.

158. **McCracken, V. J., and P. D. Cranwell.** 1992. Anaerobic microflora associated with the pars oesophaga of the pig. *Res. Vet. Sci.* **53**:110–115.

159. **Mellander, L., B. Carlsson, F. Jalil, T. Söderström, and L. Å. Hanson.** 1985. Secretory IgA antibody response against *Escherichia coli* antigens in infants in relation to exposure. *J. Pediatr.* **107**:430–433.

160. **Meltzer, M. S.** 1976. Tumoricidal responses in vitro of peritoneal macrophages from conventionally housed and germ-free nude mice. *Cell. Immunol.* **22**:176–181.

161. **Menge, H., R. Kohn, K. H. Dietermann, H. Lorenz-Meyer, E. O. Riecken, and J. W. Robinson.** 1979. Structural and functional alterations in the mucosa of self-filling intestinal blind loops in rats. *Clin. Sci.* **56**:121–131.

162. **Meslin, J. C., E. Sacquet, and J. L. Guenet.** 1973. Action de la flore bactérienne sur la morphologie et la surface de la muqueuse de l'intestine grèle du rat. *Ann. Biol. Anim. Biochim. Biophys.* **13**:203–214.

163. **Mestecky, J., I. Moro, and B. J. Underdown.** 1999. Mucosal immunoglobulins, p. 133–152. *In* P. L. Ogra, J. Mestecky, M. E. Lamm, W. Strober, J. Bienenstock, and J. R. McGhee (ed.), *Mucosal Immunology.* Academic Press, San Diego, Calif.

164. **Midtvedt, A.-C.** 1994. *The Establishment and Development of Some Metabolic Activities Associated with the Intestinal Microflora in Healthy Children.* Karolinska Institute, Stockholm, Sweden.

165. **Midtvedt, T.** 1999. Microbial functional activities, p. 79–96. *In* L. Å. Hanson and R. H. Yolken (ed.), *Probiotics, Other Nutritional Factors, and Intestinal Microflora.* Vevey/Lipincott-Raven Publishers, Philadelphia, Pa.

166. **Midtvedt, T., and B. E. Gustafsson.** 1981. Digestion of dead bacteria by germ-free rats. *Curr. Microbiol.* **6**:13–15.

167. **Mishima, S., D. Xu, Q. Lu, and E. A. Deitch.** 1998. The relationship among nitric oxide production, bacterial translocation, and intestinal injury after endotoxin challenge in vivo. *J. Trauma* **44**:175–182.

168. **Mitsuyama, M., R. Ohara, K. Amako, K. Nomoto, and T. Yokokura.** 1986. Ontogeny of macrophage function to release superoxide anion in conventional and germfree mice. *Infect. Immun.* **52**:236–239.

169. **Moore, W. E., and L. H. Moore.** 1995. Intestinal floras of populations that have a high risk of colon cancer. *Appl. Environ. Microbiol.* **61**:3202–3207.

170. **Moore, W. E. C., E. P. Cato, I. J. Good, and L. V. Holdeman.** 1981. The effect of diet on the human fecal flora, p. 11–24. *In* W. R. Bruce, P. Correa, M. Lipkin, S. R. Tannenbaum, and T. D. Wilkins (ed.), *Gastrointestinal Cancer: Endogenous Factors.* Cold Spring Harbor Laboratory, Cold Spring Harbor, N.Y.

171. **Moore, W. E. C., E. P. Cato, and L. V. Holdeman.** 1978. Some current concepts in intestinal bacteriology. *Am. J. Clin. Nutr.* **31**:S33–S42.

172. **Moore, W. E. C., and L. V. Holdeman.** 1974. Human fecal flora: the normal flora of 20 Japanese-Hawaiians. *Appl. Microbiol.* **27**:961–979.

173. **Moreau, M. C., and G. Corthier.** 1988. Effect of gastrointestinal microflora on induction and maintenance of oral tolerance to ovalbumin in C3H/HeJ mice. *Infect. Immun.* **56**:2766–2768.

174. **Moreau, M. C., R. Ducluzeau, D. Guy-Grand, and M. C. Muller.** 1978. Increase in the population of duodenal immunoglobulin A plasmocytes in axenic mice associated with different living or dead bacterial strains of intestinal origin. *Infect. Immun.* **21**:532–539.

175. **Morland, B., and T. Midtvedt.** 1984. Phagocytosis, peritoneal influx and enzyme activities in peritoneal macrophages from germ-free, conventional, and ex-germ-free mice. *Infect. Immun.* **44**:750–752.

176. **Mowat, A. M., and H. L. Weiner.** 1999. Oral tolerance: physiological basis and clinical applications, p. 587–618. *In* P. L. Ogra, J. Mestecky, M. E. Lamm, W. Strober, J. Bienenstock, and J. R. McGhee (ed.), *Mucosal Immunology.* Academic Press, San Diego, Calif.

177. **Munkholm, P., E. Langholtz, O. Haagen Nielsen, S. Kreiner, and V. Binder.** 1992. Incidence and prevalence of Crohn's disease in the County of Copenhagen, 1962–87: a sixfold increase in incidence. *Scand. J. Gastroenterol.* **27**:609–614.

178. **Murono, K., K. Fujita, M. Yoshikawa, M. Saijo, F. Inyaku, H. Kakehashi, and T. Tsukamoto.** 1993. Acquisition of nonmaternal *Enterobacteriaceae* by infants delivered in hospitals. *J. Pediatr.* **122**:120–125.

179. **Nagengast, F. M., M. J. Grubben, and I. P. van Munster.** 1995. Role of bile acids in colorectal carcinogenesis. *Eur. J. Cancer* **31A**:1067–1070.

180. **Nelson, D. P., and L. J. Mata.** 1970. Bacterial flora associated with the human gastrointestinal mucosa. *Gastroenterology* **58**:56–61.

181. **Neumann, V. C., R. Shinebaum, E. M. Cooke, and V. Wright.** 1987. Effects of sulphasalazine on faecal flora in patients with rheu-

matoid arthritis: a comparison with penicilla-mine. *Br. J. Rheumatol.* **26:**334–337.

182. **Neut, C., E. Bezirtzoglou, C. Romond, H. Beerens, M. Delcroix, and A. M. Noel.** 1987. Bacterial colonization of the large intestine in newborns delivered by caesarean section. *Zentbl. Bakteriol. Microbiol. Hyg. A* **266:**330–337.

183. **Neutra, M. R., A. Frey, and J. P. Kraehen-buhl.** 1996. M-cells: gateways for mucosal infection and immunization. *Cell* **86:**345–348.

184. **Nicaise, P., A. Gleizes, F. Forestier, A. M. Quero, and C. Labarre.** 1993. Influence of intestinal bacterial flora on cytokine (IL1, IL6 and TNFα) production by mouse peritoneal macrophages. *Eur. Cytokine Netw.* **4:**133–139.

185. **Nicaise, P., A. Gleizes, F. Forestier, C. Sandre, A. M. Quero, and C. Labarre.** 1995. The influence of *E. coli* implantation in axenic mice on cytokine production by peritoneal and bone marrow-derived macrophages. *Cytokine* **7:**713–719.

186. **Oresland, T., S. Fasth, S. Nordgren, and L. Hultén.** 1989. The clinical and functional outcome after restorative protocolectomy. A prospective study in 100 patients. *Int. J. Colorect. Dis.* **4:**50–56.

187. **Owens, W. E., and R. D. Berg.** 1980. Bacterial translocation from the gastrointestinal tract of athymic (*nu/nu*) mice. *Infect. Immun.* **27:**461–467.

188. **Owens, W. E., and R. D. Berg.** 1982. Bacterial translocation from the gastrointestinal tracts of thymectomized mice. *Curr. Microbiol.* **7:**169–174.

189. **Pabst, H. F., D. W. Spady, L. M. Pilarski, M. M. Carson, J. A. Beeler, and M. P. Krez-olek.** 1997. Differential modulation of the immune response by breast- or formula-feeding of infants. *Acta Pediatr.* **86:**1291–1297.

190. **Pavli, P., C. E. Woodhams, W. F. Doe, and D. A. Hume.** 1990. Isolation and characterization of antigen-presenting dendritic cells from the mouse intestinal lamina propria. *Immunology* **70:**40–47.

191. **Peltonen, R., M. Nenonen, T. Helve, O. Hanninen, P. Toivanen, and E. Eerola.** 1997. Fecal microbial flora and disease activity in rheumatoid arthritis during a vegan diet. *Br. J. Rheumatol.* **36:**64–68.

192. **Peri, B. A., C. M. Theodore, G. A. Loson-sky, J. M. Fishaut, R. M. Rothberg, and P. L. Ogra.** 1982. Antibody content of rabbit milk and serum following inhalation or ingestion of respiratory syncytial virus and bovine serum albumin. *Clin. Exp. Immunol.* **48:**91–101.

193. **Plos, K., H. Connell, U. Jodal, B. I. Mark-lund, S. Mårild, B. Wettergren, and C. Svanborg.** 1995. Intestinal carriage of P-fimbriated *Escherichia coli* and the susceptibility to urinary tract infection in young children. *J. Infect. Dis.* **171:**625–631.

194. **Podroprigera, G. I., J. Hoffman, J. Janecek, and J. Naprstka.** 1980. Cyclic AMP in macrophages, intestinal mucosa and blood plasma of germfree and ordinary animals. *Bull. Exp. Biol. Med.* **89:**878–880.

195. **Poulsen, L. K., T. R. Licht, C. Rang, K. A. Krogfeldt, and S. Molin.** 1995. Physiological state of *Escherichia coli* BJ4 growing in the large intestines of streptomycin-treated mice. *J. Bacteriol.* **177:**5840–5845.

196. **Regnault, A., J. P. Levraud, A. Lim, A. Six, C. Moreau, A. Cumano, and P. Kourilsky.** 1996. The expansion and selection of T cell receptor αβ intestinal intraepithelial T cell clones. *Eur. J. Immunol.* **26:**914–921.

197. **Reynolds, H. Y.** 1988. Immunoglobulin G and its function in the human respiratory tract. *Mayo Clin. Proc.* **63:**161–174.

198. **Riegler, G., T. Carratu, M. Tartaglione, F. Morace, R. Manzione, and A. Arimoli.** 1998. Prevalence and relative risk of malignancy in relatives of inflammatory bowel disease patients and control subjects. *J. Clin. Gastroenterol.* **27:**211–214.

199. **Riepe, S. P., J. Goldstein, and D. H. Alpers.** 1980. Effect of secreted *Bacteroides* proteases on human intestinal brush border hydrolases. *J. Clin. Investig.* **66:**314–322.

200. **Roe, T. F., T. D. Coates, D. W. Thomas, J. H. Miller, and V. Gilsanz.** 1992. Treatment of chronic inflammatory bowel disease in glycogen storage disease type Ib with colony-stimulating factors. *N. Engl. J. Med.* **326:**1666–1669.

201. **Roediger, W. E.** 1980. Role of anaerobic bacteria in the metabolic welfare of the colonic mucosa in man. *Gut* **21:**793–798.

202. **Rotimi, V. O., S. A. Olowe, and I. Ahmed.** 1985. The development of bacterial flora of premature neonates. *J. Hyg. Camb.* **94:**309–318.

203. **Ruddell, W. S., and M. S. Losowsky.** 1980. Severe diarrhoea due to small intestinal colonisation during cimetidine treatment. *Br. Med. J.* **281:**273.

204. **Russell, M. W., D. A. Sibley, E. B. Niko-lova, M. Tomana, and J. Mestecky.** 1997. IgA antibody as a non-inflammatory regulator of immunity. *Biochem. Soc. Trans.* **25:**466–470.

205. **Salyers, A. A., J. R. Vercellotti, S. E. H. West, and T. D. Wilkins.** 1977. Fermentation of mucin and plant polysaccharides by strains of *Bacteroides* from the human colon. *Appl. Environ. Microbiol.* **33:**319–322.

206. Sarff, L. D., G. H. McCracken, Jr., M. S. Schiffer, M. P. Glode, J. B. Robbins, I. Orskov, and F. Orskov. 1975. Epidemiology of *Escherichia coli* K1 in healthy and diseased newborns. *Lancet* i:1099–1104.

207. Scheffel, J. W., and Y. B. Kim. 1979. Role of environment in the development of "natural" hemagglutinins in Minnesota miniature swine. *Infect. Immun.* 26:202–210.

208. Scheppach, W. 1994. Effects of short chain fatty acids on gut morphology and function. *Gut* 35(Suppl. 1):S35–S38.

209. Schieferdecker, H. L., R. Ullrich, H. Hirseland, and M. Zeitz. 1992. T cell differentiation antigens on lymphocytes in the human intestinal lamina propria. *J. Immunol.* 149:2816–2822.

210. Sears, H. J., and I. Brownlee. 1951. Further observations on the persistence of individual strains of *Escherichia coli* in the intestinal tract of man. *J. Bacteriol.* 63:47–57.

211. Sepp, E., K. Julge, M. Vasar, P. Naaber, B. Björkstén, and M. Mikkelsaar. 1997. Intestinal microflora of Estonian and Swedish infants. *Acta Pediatr.* 86:956–961.

212. Seppälä, I., M. Kaartinen, S. Ibrahim, and O. Mäkelä. 1990. Mouse Ig coded by V_H families S107 or J606 bind to protein A. *J. Immunol.* 145:2989–2993.

213. Severijnen, A. J., R. van Kleef, M. P. Hazenberg, and J. P. van der Merwe. 1989. Cell wall fragments from major residents of the human intestinal flora induce chronic arthritis in rats. *J. Rheumatol.* 16:1061–1068.

214. Shinebaum, R., V. C. Neumann, E. M. Cooke, and V. Wright. 1987. Comparison of fecal florae in patients with rheumatoid arthritis and controls. *Br. J. Rheumatol.* 26:329–333.

215. Shroff, K. E., K. Meslin, and J. J. Cebra. 1995. Commensal enteric bacteria engender a self-limiting humoral mucosal immune response while permanently colonizing the gut. *Infect. Immun.* 63:3904–3913.

216. Silverman, G. J. 1992. Human antibody responses to bacterial antigens: studies of a model conventional antigen and a proposed model B cell superantigen. *Int. Rev. Immunol.* 9:57–78.

217. Simon, G. L., and S. L. Gorbach. 1986. The human intestinal microflora. *Dig. Dis. Sci.* 31(Suppl. 9):147S–162S.

218. Sobel, J. D. 1991. Bacterial etiologic agents in the pathogenesis of urinary tract infection. *Med. Clin. N. Am.* 75:253–273.

219. Solomon, M. J., and M. Schnitzler. 1998. Cancer and inflammatory bowel disease: bias, epidemiology, surveillance, and treatment. *World J. Surg.* 22:352–358.

220. Springer, G. F., and R. E. Horton. 1969. Blood group isoantibody stimulation in man by feeding blood group-reactive bacteria. *J. Clin. Investig.* 48:1280–1291.

221. Stamey, T. A., M. Timothy, M. Millar, and G. Mihara. 1971. Recurrent urinary infections in adult women. The role of introital enterobacteria. *Calif. Med.* 115:1.

222. Stark, P. L., and A. Lee. 1982. The microbial ecology of the large bowel of breast-fed and formula-fed infants during the first year of life. *J. Med. Microbiol.* 15:189–203.

223. Steinman, R. M. 1991. The dendritic cell system and its role in immunogenicity. *Annu. Rev. Immunol.* 9:271–296.

224. Strachan, D. P. 1989. Hay fever, hygiene and household size. *Br. Med. J.* 289:1259–1260.

225. Sudo, N., S. Sawamura, K. Tanaka, Y. Aiba, C. Kubo, and Y. Koga. 1997. The requirement of intestinal bacterial flora for the development of an IgE production system fully susceptible to oral tolerance induction. *J. Immunol.* 159:1739–1745.

226. Svanborg Edén, C., L. Hagberg, R. Hull, S. Hull, K.-E. Magnusson, and L. Öhman. 1987. Bacterial virulence versus host resistance in the urinary tracts of mice. *Infect. Immun.* 55:1224–1232.

227. Svanborg Edén, C., R. Kulhavy, S. Mårild, S. J. Prince, and J. Mestecky. 1985. Urinary immunoglobulins in healthy individuals and children with acute pyelonephritis. *Scand. J. Immunol.* 21:305–313.

228. Svanborg Edén, C., and A.-M. Svennerholm. 1978. Secretory immunoglobulin A and G antibodies prevent adhesion of *Escherichia coli* to human urinary tract epithelial cells. *Infect. Immun.* 22:790–797.

229. Tannock, G. V. 1995. *Normal Microflora. An Introduction to Microbes Inhabiting the Human Body.* Chapman and Hall, London, United Kingdom.

230. Tannock, G. W. 1999. Microecology of lactobacilli and bifidobacteria inhabiting the digestive tract: essential knowledge for successful probiotic research, p. 17–31. *In* L. Å. Hanson and R. H. Yolken (ed.), *Probiotics, Other Nutritional Factors, and Intestinal Microflora.* Vevey/Lipincott-Raven Publishers, Philadelphia, Pa.

231. Tannock, G. W., R. Fuller, S. L. Smith, and M. A. Hall. 1990. Plasmid profiling of members of the family *Enterobacteriaceae*, lactobacilli, and bifidobacteria from mother to infant. *J. Clin. Microbiol.* 28:1225–1228.

232. Tissier, H. 1900. *Recherches sur la Flore Intestinale des Nourrissons (État Normal et Pathologique).* Paris, France.

233. Toskes, P. P., R. A. Giannella, H. R. Jervis, W. R. Rout, and A. Takeuchi. 1975. Small

intestinal mucosal injury in the experimental blind loop syndrome. Light- and electron-microscopic and histochemical studies. *Gastroenterology* **68:**193–203.

234. **Tullus, K.** 1987. Fecal colonization with P-fimbriated *Escherichia coli* in newborn children and relation to development of extraintestinal *E. coli* infections. *Acta Paediatr. Scand.* **334:**(Suppl): 1–35.

235. **Tullus, K., and L. G. Burman.** 1989. Ecological impact of ampicillin and cefuroxime in neonatal units. *Lancet* **i:**1405–1407.

236. **Tullus, K., I. Kühn, I. Ørskov, F. Ørskov, and R. Möllby.** 1992. The importance of P and type 1 fimbriae for the persistence of *Escherichia coli* in the human gut. *Epidemiol. Infect* **108:** 415–421.

237. **Tzianabos, A. O., A. B. Onderdonk, B. Rosner, R. L. Cisneros, and D. L. Kasper.** 1993. Structural features of polysaccharides that induce intra-abdominal abscesses. *Science* **262:** 416–419.

238. **van der Waaij, D.** 1989. The ecology of the human intestine and its consequences for overgrowth by pathogens such as *Clostridium difficile*. *Annu. Rev. Microbiol.* **43:**69–87.

239. **van der Waaij, D.** 1999. Microbial ecology of the intestinal microflora: influence of interactions with the host organism, p. 1–16. *In* L. Å. Hanson and R. H. Yolken (ed.), *Probiotics, Other Nutritional Factors, and Intestinal Microflora*. Vevey/Lippincott-Raven Publishers, Philadelphia, Pa.

240. **von Mutius, E., F. D. Martinez, C. Fritzsch, T. Nicolai, G. Roell, and H. H. Thiemann.** 1994. Prevalence of asthma and atopy in two areas of West and East Germany. *Am. J. Respir. Crit. Care Med.* **149:**358–364.

241. **Vosti, K. L., L. M. Goldberg, A. S. Monto, and L. A. Rantz.** 1964. Host-parasite interaction in patients with infections due to *Escherichia coli*. I. The serogrouping of *E. coli* from intestinal and extraintestinal sources. *J. Clin. Investig.* **43:** 2377–2385.

242. **Wadolkowski, E. A., D. C. Laux, and P. S. Cohen.** 1988. Colonization of the streptomycin-treated mouse large intestine by a human fecal *Escherichia coli* strain: role of growth in mucus. *Infect. Immun.* **56:**1030–1035.

243. **Wells, C. L., M. A. Maddaus, C. M. Reynolds, R. P. Jechorek, and R. L. Simmons.** 1987. Role of anaerobic flora in the translocation of aerobic and facultatively anaerobic intestinal bacteria. *Infect. Immun.* **55:**2689–2694.

244. **West, P. A., J. H. Hewitt, and O. M. Murphy.** 1979. The influence of methods of collec-

tion and storage on the bacteriology of human milk. *J. Appl. Bacteriol.* **46:**269–277.

245. **Wiener, A. S.** 1951. Origin of naturally occurring hemagglutinins and hemolysins: a review. *J. Immunol.* **66:**287–295.

246. **Wilkins, T. D., and R. L. van Tassell.** 1983. Production of intestinal mutagens, p. 265–288. *In* D. J. Hentges (ed.), *Human Intestinal Microflora in Health and Disease*. Academic Press, New York, N.Y.

247. **Williams, H. C., D. P. Strachan, and R. J. Hay.** 1994. Childhood eczema: disease of the advantaged? *BMJ* **308:**1132–1135.

248. **Williams, R. C., and R. J. Gibbons.** 1972. Inhibition of bacterial adherence by secretory immunoglobulin A: a mechanism of antigen disposal. *Science* **177:**697–699.

249. **Wilson, H. D., and H. F. Eichenwald.** 1974. Sepsis neonatorum. *Pediatr. Clin. N. Am.* **21:** 571–582.

250. **Wilson, K. H.** 1997. Biota in the human gastrointestinal tract, p. 39–58. *In* R. I. Mackie, B. A. White, and R. E. Isaacson (ed.), *Gastrointestinal Microbiology*. Chapman & Hall, Ltd., London, United Kingdom.

251. **Winberg, J., and G. Wessner.** 1971. Does breast milk protect against septicemia in the newborn? *Lancet* **i:**1091–1094.

252. **Wittman, D. H.** 1985. Die Bedeutung der Infektionserreger für die Therapie der eitrigen Peritonitis. *Chirurg* **56:**363–370.

253. **Wold, A. E.** 1998. The hygiene hypothesis revised: is the rising frequency of allergy due to changes in the intestinal flora? *Allergy* **53:**20–25.

254. **Wold, A. E., D. A. Caugant, G. Lidin-Janson, P. de Man, and C. Svanborg.** 1992. Resident colonic *Escherichia coli* strains frequently display uropathogenic characteristics. *J. Infect. Dis.* **165:**46–52.

255. **Wold, A. E., U. I. H. Dahlgren, L. Å, Hanson, I. Mattsby-Baltzer, and T. Midtvedt.** 1989. Difference between bacterial and food antigens in mucosal immunogenicity. *Infect. Immun.* **57:**2666–2673.

256. **Wold, A. E., J. Mestecky, M. Tomana, A. Kobata, H. Ohbayashi, T. Endo, and C. Svanborg Edén.** 1990. Secretory immunoglobulin A carries oligosaccharide receptors for *Escherichia coli* type 1 fimbrial lectin. *Infect. Immun.* **58:** 3073–3077.

257. **Wold, A. E., M. Thorssén, S. Hull, and C. Svanborg Edén.** 1988. Attachment of *Escherichia coli* via mannose or Galα1-4Galβ-containing receptors to human colonic epithelial cells. *Infect. Immun.* **56:**2531–2537.

258. **Yudate, T., H. Yamada, and T. Tezuka.**

1996. Role of staphylococcal enterotoxins in pathogenesis of atopic dermatitis: growth and expression of T cell receptor V beta of peripheral blood mononuclear cells stimulated by entero-toxins A and B. *J. Dermatol. Sci.* **13:**63–70.

259. **Zafriri, D., Y. Oron, B. Eisenstein, and I. Ofek.** 1987. Growth advantage and enhanced toxicity of *Escherichia coli* adherent to tissue cul-ture cells due to restricted diffusion of products secreted by the cells. *J. Clin. Investig.* **79:** 1210–1216.

260. **Ziegler, H. K., C. A. Orlin, and C. W. Cluff.** 1987. Differential requirements for the process-ing and presentation of soluble and particulate bacterial antigens by macrophages. *Eur. J. Immu-nol.* **17:**1287–1296.

BACTERIAL INFECTIONS IN THE IMMUNOCOMPROMISED HOST

Susanna Cunningham-Rundles and Mirjana Nesin

8

A primary function of the immune system is to provide host defense against invasion by microorganisms and viruses. After birth, bacteria are always present in great abundance on the skin and in the gastrointestinal tract, and critical development of immune function occurs in early neonatal life in response to microbial colonization (103). The normal flora in the gut and on the skin are made up of commensals that carry out key functions, for example, as the gut flora does, by producing vitamins (60) and fermenting complex fibers and proteins (7). Maintaining this balance requires intact anatomical barriers, host secretions, and the flexible interacting processes of immune recognition and response, which lead to the containment and elimination of potentially harmful pathogens. The role of commensal bacteria in this process is now being recognized and studied (32, 66).

In a very real sense, the immune system metabolizes microbes and viruses. The aspect of

the immune system that adapts to newly encountered antigens by means of antibody responses of thymus-derived T cells and bone marrow-derived B cells is central to this activity. Adaptive immune response develops and retains a kind of memory, which can be built up in response to successive encounters with microbial or other antigens. This memory, which exists as specific T-cell clones, B-cell memory, and specific antibodies, is affected by the normal bacterial flora, has a vital function in regulating microbial activity, and is also crucial for protection against pathogenesis. In addition to this system, there is a fundamental native or natural (constitutive) aspect of immune response which is essentially nonadaptive. The nonadaptive, or natural, immune system is centered in phagocytic cells, such as monocytes and neutrophils, and includes the natural killer (NK) lymphocyte. NK cells, unlike T cells or B cells, do not require specific antigenic presentation, processing, or recognition to be active. The nonadaptive immune system offers the first line of defense against microbes.

While altered immune response to microbes is directly associated with susceptibility to infection, less is known about how bacteria affect and mold immune response in the healthy or the persistently infected host. This chapter will

Susanna Cunningham-Rundles, Immunology Research Laboratory, Division of Hematology and Oncology, Department of Pediatrics, Cornell University Weill Medical College-The New York Presbyterian Hospital, New York, NY 10021. *Mirjana Nesin*, Perinatology Center, Division of Neonatology, Department of Pediatrics, Cornell University Weill Medical College-The New York Presbyterian Hospital, New York, NY 10021.

Persistent Bacterial Infections, Edited by J. P. Nataro, M. J. Blaser, and S. Cunningham-Rundles, © 2000 ASM Press, Washington, D.C.

focus on bacterial infections in specific settings where fundamental relationships relevant to the persistence of bacterial infections in the human host may be observed and studied. These settings are the following: (i) neonatal susceptibility to infection, (ii) primary immune deficiency, and (iii) acquired immune deficiency.

Since the neonate is born with an immature immune system, there is a critical period when encounters with microbes may cause serious infection. Exposure to pathogens in association with prematurity adds significant stress that can alter the development of the normal immune response. Study of the premature infant may help to illuminate the normal process through which commensal relationships are established, initially at birth, and to characterize how regulation of immune response through interaction with bacteria informs the evolving immune system.

In addition to developmental sensitivity to potential pathogens, vulnerability to microbial pathogenesis accompanies the defined primary immune deficiency diseases, which confer generalized susceptibility to specific types of microbes depending upon the type of underlying immune deficiency. Furthermore, since primary immune deficiency increases the risk of cancer (21), fundamental relationships between altered response to microbes and carcinogenesis may be observable. This is relevant to chapter 7, where the interaction between commensals and cancer is explored.

There is current interest in the emergence of new infections and the increase in occurrence of established infections due to enhanced exposure or changes in host susceptibility associated with changes in world conditions (93). The AIDS pandemic has had a major impact on world health and has fundamentally altered our understanding of the continuing relationship between immune response and the lives of microbes and viruses (121). With the intention of clarifying how the immune system affects and is affected by persistent bacterial infection, this chapter addresses what is currently known about clinically significant bacterial infections when immune response is immature or deregulated in specific ways.

NEONATAL SUSCEPTIBILITY TO BACTERIAL INFECTIONS

Antigen-specific humoral and cellular immunities are central to immune response generated in the adult host. In contrast, neonates and young infants rely primarily on innate immunity, circulating mediators of inflammation, and phagocytosis. However, many of the components of innate immunity are not as functional in neonates as in adults, and an encounter with potential pathogens may overwhelm these resources.

Neonates usually acquire bacterial pathogens transplacentally through the umbilical vein or by aspiration from amniotic fluid or cervical secretions (72). The most common bacterial pathogens specific for the neonate are group B beta-hemolytic streptococci (GBBS) and gram-negative bacteria, usually *Escherichia coli*, and *Listeria monocytogenes* (46). Premature neonates often acquire nosocomial infections and develop staphylococcal, enterococcal, and *Pseudomonas aeruginosa* infections (3, 116). The bacterial factors that characterize these interactions are presented in detail in other chapters. While virulence of each type of microorganism is related to its serotype and toxin production, it is also known that bacterial products can actually inactivate the host immune response. Examples include the observation that GBBS strains expressing the alpha component of C protein resist phagocytosis, that C5a-ase has been shown to inactivate complement, and that phage-type *Staphylococcus aureus* type 2 modulates the immune response while causing scalded-skin syndrome (11, 45, 84).

Although many bacteria colonize the skin and mucous membranes, the overall incidence of congenital bacterial infections is approximately 1 to 3 per 1,000 births (71). Thus, invasion is rather rare. Intrapartum maternal infection, prematurity, perinatal hypoxia, and restricted intrauterine growth are predisposing factors. The integrity of the mucous membranes is crucial for some, but not all, bacterial species. Some microorganisms, like coagulase-negative staphylococci, rarely can penetrate the uninterrupted mucosal barrier but can colonize it (70, 89). Others, like GBBS, do not require disruption of the mucosal barrier and are transferred into the cytoplasm of respiratory epithelial cells by an actin microfilament-dependent process (109).

Mucosal secretions in adults contain secretory immunoglobulin A (IgA) antibodies against common colonizing bacteria. For example, the cervical secretions of healthy women colonized with GBBS contain protective IgA antibodies (13), but these pathogen-specific antibodies are absent or decreased in the mucosal secretions during the first 2 weeks of life, even in a full-term baby (88). Therefore, neonates depend on complement and acute-phase reactants as the most important circulating nonadaptive specific mediators against bacterial infections, since acquired maternal IgG antibodies drop in the first days of life.

The Neonatal Innate Immune Response to Bacteria

The complement system is able directly to lyse some gram-negative bacteria even in the absence of specific antibodies, but circulating levels of complement in the sera of neonates are lower than those in adults (31). Even full-term infants are born with approximately 50% of adult levels of complement. There is no transplacental passage of complement components, but both the fetus and the newborn child are able to synthesize them. In general, synthesis increases with gestational age. However, even full-term neonates are not able to increase component production in response to bacterial antigens. For example, neonatal monocytes do not increase production of C3 after stimulation with lipopolysaccharide (LPS) during *E. coli* sepsis (37), leading to decreased opsonizing activity. Activation of either the classic or alternate complement cascade is slower in neonates than in adults (125).

The innate immune system is activated by endotoxins from gram-negative bacteria and *S. aureus*, as well as encapsulated and nonencapsulated type III beta-hemolytic streptococci (120). This leads to production of tumor necrosis factor alpha (TNF-α), interleukin 1 (IL-1), and IL-6. As in adults, bacterial invasion activates tissue macrophages rapidly to produce TNF and IL-1, stimulating endothelial cells to express adhesion molecules and to initiate the cytokine cascade towards increasing production of IL-6, IL-8, and chemokines (8). As inflammation progresses, other humoral mediators of infection are activated, such as complement, platelet-activating factor, C-reactive protein, and prostaglandins (126). Anti-inflammatory mediators (IL-4, IL-10, and IL-13) regulate this process (38, 97). In general, stimulated monocytes from the cord blood of full-term infants produce levels of TNF, IL-6, and IL-8 similar to or slightly lower than those of adults (64). Premature neonates produce much less of these but show levels of IL-1 similar to those of full-term infants and adults as part of the acute-phase response. Serum TNF levels have been correlated to morbidity during septic shock (26). Acute-phase reactants play a significant role in the neonatal response to infections. The most important are C-reactive protein, which is produced in large amounts and acts as an opsonin; LPS-binding protein, which facilitates the binding of LPS to CD14 receptors on monocytes; and surfactant proteins, the collectins surfactant protein A (SP-A) and SP-D (129). SP-A binds to the Fc portion of immunoglobulin and facilitates phagocytosis. SP-D is able to bind to the LPSs of gram-negative bacteria (75).

Several aspects of neonatal phagocytosis seem inadequate compared to those of adults. The most important are a decreased neutrophil pool in the bone marrow and diminished ability of neonatal neutrophils to adhere to the endothelium and migrate to the site of infection. Both full-term and premature neonates show several major deficiencies in phagocytosis and the number of tissue macrophages. This is especially evident in the lungs of a newborn suffering from respiratory distress (2).

The neutrophil storage pool in fetal and neonatal bone marrow is limited and does not efficiently respond to infection by increasing production of neutrophils. The number of circulating neutrophils is low in the fetus and rises at birth, even in a healthy full-term neonate (86). Although neonates produce circulating granulocyte colony-stimulating factor and granulocyte-macrophage colony-stimulating factor and the cells express receptors, the increase in production is inadequate. This deficiency may be partially a consequence of a decreased neutrophil pool in neonatal bone marrow. It is likely that neonates are near their maximal production of neutrophils and have a limited ability to increase the number of circulating neutrophils in response to infection (78).

Migration of neutrophils through the endothelium to the site of infection is slower in neonates than in infected adults. Neonatal neutrophils express less L-selectin and seem not to upregulate expression of β_2 integrins (Mac-1 and LFA-1) in response to chemotactic factors (15). Once neutrophils adhere to the activated endothelium, they respond to chemotaxis and enter tissues through junctions between endothelial cells (42). Some studies indicate that neonatal neutrophils seem to be less deformable in entering tissues, perhaps because of differences in neutrophil cell membrane fluidity (104). Chemotaxis is slower in neonates than in adults (90, 108). Lower levels of chemotaxins, such as C5a, are produced, and neonatal neutrophils may have fewer receptors (98).

Full-term healthy neonates who received protective IgG antibodies from the mother are able to successfully opsonize bacteria and have enough Fc receptors on their neutrophils to bind and phagocytose bacteria, but premature neonates have received fewer antibodies and express fewer Fc receptors (100). These infants depend on endogenous production of IgM and complement activation. In contrast to IgG antibodies, if bacteria are coated by IgM, the presence of C3b is essential, since phagocytes lack the Fc receptor for IgM. The process of phagocytosis and killing is normal in both full-term and premature healthy infants (41), but mono-

cyte migration is delayed and the number of monocytes entering the infected site is diminished (132).

The lymphocyte mediating innate immune response is the NK cell. The NK cell is characterized by the spontaneous ability to kill a tumor cell or virus-infected cell. In addition, NK cells produce cytokines, which regulate the host defense against bacteria and may kill bacteria. Neonatal NK cells show decreased or even absent cytolytic activity against the reference erythroleukemia tumor cell target K562, perhaps as a developmental consequence of the need to maintain maternal-fetal tolerance (23). Interestingly, as shown in Fig. 1, activation of the neonatal NK cell system may occur in response to certain bacteria. The immature immune system may lack this activity because of deficient production of gamma interferon (IFN-γ) (81), a key cytokine for the regulation of NK cell activity (79). However, as shown in Fig. 2, neonatal IFN-γ production can be induced by some bacteria. Both preparations of bacteria used in these studies, ImuVert (ribosomal vesicles from *Serratia marcescens*) and OK432 (whole inactivated *Streptococcus pyogenes*), have immunoadjuvant properties (24, 76). These bacteria and certain others may influence immune response, and they hold clues to the formation of microbial immune relationships. However, both of these bacteria in their native states and others, such as *L. monocytogenes*, can pose a threat to the immature immune system. In an immunocompetent adult, the clearing of *Listeria* requires the function of NK cells (122). Therefore, it is not surprising that *L. monocytogenes* is the third most common neonatal bacterial pathogen, with an incidence of 13 per 100,000 births (44).

The Neonatal Adaptive Immune Response to Bacteria

Both the infected fetus and the neonate are able to produce protective IgM antibodies in response to bacterial antigens, but the levels in serum are lower than those in adults. Neonates can respond to these bacteria in the presence of the complement component C3, but since

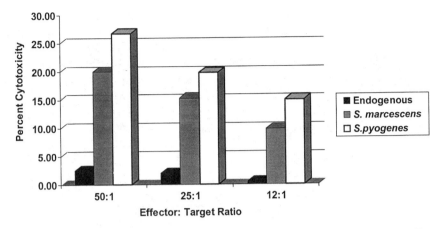

FIGURE 1 Neonatal NK cell activity in response to bacteria. The data show the effect of *S. marcescens*, prepared as ribosomal vesicles, and *S. pyogenes*, prepared as whole inactivated cells, on neonatal NK effector cell function against the K562 target in the 4-h short-term ^{51}Cr release assay following 18 h of pretreatment compared to endogenous activity at different effector-to-target ratios.

IgM and complement levels are lower, gram-negative sepsis is common (117). Adequate antibody production against capsular polysaccharides is delayed until the second, or even third, year of life, with the appearance of special lymph node-derived B lymphocytes (114).

The infant derives protective IgG antibodies from the mother; all subclasses cross the placenta. Transplacental transfer of antibodies increases with gestation and after 34 weeks of gestation is similar to or even higher than maternal levels (61). However, infants of mothers who have no antibodies to a particular pathogen are not protected. Attempts to increase maternal antibody production have led to the development of antistreptococcal and antistaphylococcal vaccines (83). Although some of these vaccines have shown promising results in pregnant women, immunization carries special risks and warrants special consideration. There is essentially no currently recognized comparable, significant T-cell-specific immunity transferred from the mother to the fetus.

Although cord blood monocytes express fewer major histocompatibility complex (MHC) class II antigens, bacterial antigen presentation, for example, to tetanus or *E. coli*, is normal (62, 135). Most cord blood T cells express receptors specific for naive T cells (64). Due to a lack of memory T cells, there is a

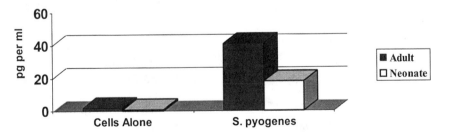

FIGURE 2 Production of IFN-γ in response to *S. pyogenes*. The data show the production of IFN-γ by adult and neonatal mononuclear cells in response to *S. pyogenes* after 18 h of culture.

delayed T-cell-dependent antigen-specific response, decreased cytokine production by the T cells, and diminished T-cell help for B-cell differentiation in response to antigen (64). Since T cells control the isotype switching from IgM to IgG, neonates produce mainly IgM antibodies. In response to antigen, the naive T cells switch and start expressing CD45RO receptors specific for memory T cells. With the acquisition of memory T cells, neonates become capable of response to bacterial protein antigens.

Neonatal T-cell response assessed as proliferative response in vitro is surprisingly strong at birth, and, interestingly, we have found that the response of the premature infant to *Haemophilus influenzae*, *Staphylococcus epidermidis*, and *Staphylococcus* protein A is stronger than that of the full-term infant or adult (123). This does not imply resistance to infection, since effector cell functions are likely to be deficient. There are significant differences in neonatal cytokine responses to bacterial antigen. As noted above, IFN-γ is not made at birth. This is because of altered regulation of IL-2 production (56). These deficiencies tend to allow prolonged intracellular survival of bacteria. Once antigen-specific memory T cells are generated, neonates become less susceptible to infections.

BACTERIAL DEFENSE IN PRIMARY IMMUNE DEFICIENCY

Primary immune deficiency appears to occur fairly consistently across all populations, although many of these disorders are probably underdiagnosed. Study of the immune disorders due to genetic alterations, some of which have been characterized at the molecular level, is very informative as to how specific alterations in immune response actually affect the response to particular microbes and how these lesions support opportunistic infections or confer unusual vulnerability to greater severity of infections.

Bacterial Pathogens in Primary Immune Deficiency

Selective IgA deficiency is the most commonly detected primary immune deficiency disorder and is often accompanied by IgG subclass deficiency (14, 91). Diarrhea and infections with the protozoon *Giardia lamblia* are relatively increased. The severity of respiratory tract infections with *Streptococcus pneumoniae* and *H. influenzae* in IgA deficiency has been linked to associated IgG2 and IgG4 deficiencies rather than to IgA levels (40). Low levels of specific pneumococcal antibodies have been observed, suggesting a defect in affinity maturation.

Most of the primary immunodeficiency diseases are diagnosed in childhood (9). Those which include antibody deficiency confer susceptibility to pyogenic bacterial infections. Fevers of unknown origin without localizing signs may suggest occult bacteremia with *S. pneumoniae*, *H. influenzae*, *Neisseria meningitidis*, *Salmonella*, or *S. aureus*. For reasons discussed in the previous section, especially in early infancy, children may display susceptibility to bacterial infections unrelated to primary immunodeficiency. This may spring from delayed ability to make specific IgG antibodies, which can even appear as a transient hypogammaglobulinemia of infancy.

Quantitative development of antibodies, in response to *S. pneumoniae* vaccine, for example, is gradually acquired over a relatively long period of time into adolescence (115). Interestingly, adults with a history of invasive pneumococcal infections, but who are otherwise healthy, have been shown to have a higher incidence of poor response to immunization with pneumococcus, often in association with IgG1-IgG2 deficiency (34). While IgG is essential for host defense against bacteria, absence of natural IgM has been shown experimentally to cause a lack of immediate defense against bacterial infection (10). The relationships between primary immune deficiency disorders and clinically significant bacterial infections are presented in Table 1.

Pulmonary disease, including persistent pneumonitis, is a common presenting feature or complication of many T-cell immunodeficiency diseases, especially the severe combined immune deficiency (SCID) disorders and DiGeorge syndrome, which frequently includes

TABLE 1 Bacterial infections in primary immune deficiency

Type of deficiency	Bacterial infections	Basis
X-linked agammaglobulinemia	Encapsulated bacteria, *H. influenzae,* staphylococci, streptococci	No gamma globulin; no antibodies
IgG subclass deficiency	IgG1 deficiency is like CVI; encapsulated bacterial infections if deficient IgG2 or IgG3 as well	Antibody deficiency
Selective IgA deficiency	Pyogenic bacteria if IgG2 subclass deficiency	Reduced or absent IgA; often IgG subclass deficiency
Common variable immunodeficiency (CVI)	Susceptibility to pyogenic infections	All Igs are reduced; reduced or nonfunctional antibodies
Hyper-IgM syndrome	Susceptibility to pyogenic infections	Defect in switch to IgG antibodies with CD40L deficiency
Severe combined immune deficiency	Highly susceptible to many infections, including with *E. coli* and *Salmonella*	Reduced or absent T and B cells; general immune deficiency
MHC class II deficiency	Variable, but can include infections with encapsulated bacteria or *E. coli.*	May include low MHC class I; poor antibody formation
Wiskott-Aldrich disease	*S. aureus* infection	Monogenic effect on signal transduction
Ataxia telangiectasia	Sinopulmonary infections; often bacterial	Chromosomal breaks
Chronic granulomatous disease	*S. aureus, Salmonella enterica* serovar Typhimurium, *Mycobacterium fortuitum, S. marcescens* infections	Phagocytic defect
Leukocyte adhesion deficiency	Recurrent infections with bacteria, including pyogenic bacteria; nonresolving abscesses	Adhesion molecule deficiency; affects migration, phagocytosis, and killing
Hyper-IgE syndrome	*S. aureus, H. influenzae, S. pneumoniae* infections	T-cell regulatory defects; altered IFN-γ, IL-4 regulation
Complement deficiency	*S. pneumoniae* infection	Defective opsonization and clearance
Congenital neutropenia	*S. epidermidis, S. marcescens* infections	Inadequate number of neutrophils
Chediak-Higashi disease	Pyogenic infections	Defective bacterial killing
IFN-γ receptor 1 deficiency	Myobacterial infections; also with nonpathogenic strains	Th1 defect
DiGeorge anomaly	Rarely may include bacterial infections	Thymic absence

recurrent bacterial as well as viral infections (28).

The primary T-cell deficiencies produce defects in the cytokine production that is required to activate macrophages to kill intracellular bacteria. These deficiencies may lead to persistent and recurrent bacterial infections, limit or block the production of specific antibodies, or fail to support the development of functionally effective antibodies. Studies of immune response to mycobacterial antigens have led to an understanding of lipid and glycolipid antigen presentation to T cells by proteins coding outside the MHC in the CD1 gene family expressed on Langerhans cells, certain dendritic cells, B cells, thymocytes (102), and certain stem cells (19). These observations reflect the role of bacteria, perhaps particularly intracellular bacteria, in the evolution of immune response.

T-cell receptor (TCR) $\gamma\delta$ T cells are currently recognized as the subset of T cells which respond to intracellular infection, as discussed in chapter 9. Peripheral blood $\gamma\delta$ T cells, normally present in very small numbers in healthy persons, have been shown to proliferate in response to the nonpeptide antigen isopentenyl pyrophosphate and to produce IFN-γ (43), consistent with the postulated role of these cells for host defense against intracellular pathogens. Defects in IFN-γ interactions are closely associated with immune deficiency and susceptibility to persistent bacterial infections (65), including those caused by normally nonpathogenic strains of bacteria (67). For example, disseminated *Mycobacterium smegmatis* has been reported in a child with an inherited IFN-γ receptor 1 defect that caused a lingering infectious course that never resolved, despite optimal therapy, and was ultimately fatal (101).

Growing evidence supports the concept that cytokine patterns are crucial to immune response to a wide range of pathogens and that favorable response is associated with key cytokines (107). Specific cytokine profiles have been identified that relate to the severity of several types of infections. The Th1 cytokines (IFN-γ, IL-2, and IL-12) enhance cell-mediated immunity, inhibit humoral immunity, and result in protective action towards often-persistent pathogens that are controlled primarily through cell-mediated immunity (*Mycobacterium tuberculosis*, *Mycobacterium leprae*, and *Leishmania*). The Th2 cytokines (IL-4, IL-5, IL-10, and IL-13) enhance humoral immunity and inhibit cell-mediated immunity and result in protective effects for pathogens controlled primarily through humoral mechanisms.

As an example, IL-10-deficient mice have been found to become highly resistant to *L. monocytogenes* (27). Absence of IL-10 production was associated with a dramatically enhanced proinflammatory cytokine response (IL-12, IFN-γ, TNF-α, IL-1α, and IL-6). Furthermore, these studies indicated that the innate immune system was strengthened by the absence of IL-10 as well, since the bacterial burden was reduced very soon after infection compared with control mice. Although *Listeria* is controlled mainly by macrophages activated by T cells, there is evidence that CD8$^+$ T cells may be important in controlling secondary infection through cytotoxicity (68). The role of $\gamma\delta$ T cells in controlling this type of bacterial infection is discussed in chapter 9.

Interactive Aspects of Innate and Adaptive Immune Deficiencies

There are primary immune deficiencies, which involve the innate immune system. Thus, complement-mediated bacteriolysis is important for protection against neisserial infections, such as meningococcus, and primary deficiency of C5-C9 is associated with susceptibility to these bacteria (30). A primary defect of superoxide synthesis or adhesion of neutrophils is related to severe infection with pyogenic bacteria (63).

Even a selective defect in the ability to generate the oxygen burst can be sufficient to cause persistent infections. As shown in Fig. 3, such defects can be specific for a phagocytic cell type. Neutrophils, and by implication altered neutrophil activity, may also affect cytokine production. Recent data suggest that bacterial LPS binding to CD14 on neutrophils may lead to release of TNF-α, showing that polymor-

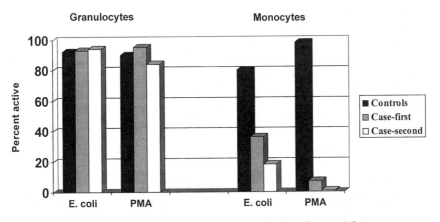

FIGURE 3 Superoxide production in phagocytes. The data show a deficient monocyte respiratory burst in response to *E. coli* and phorbol myristate acetate in a child on two test dates compared with normal controls. The data are shown as percent activated cells detected by flow cytometry.

phonuclear leukocyte response may actually act to regulate cytokine patterns and influence the expression of Th1 or Th2 cytokines (57).

Although specific immune deficiencies are associated with particular patterns of susceptibility, the interactions are actually rather complex. Host defense against bacteria includes both innate and adaptive elements, and interactions between T-lymphocyte activation and B-cell response are required to prevent bacterial sepsis. Targeted gene disruptions have uncovered new findings relevant to pathogenesis. Thus, mucosal immune defense against *Bordetella pertussis* appears to involve both IFN-γ and B-cell functions (85). In some instances, B cells may be required for T-cell priming, as shown in recent studies of gene knockout B-cell-deficient mice in response to *Chlamydia trachomatis* (130). Conversely, the same organism infects the genital mucosa of mice, and in this setting, disruption of the IFN-γ receptor was associated with IL-4 dominance, leading to highly increased local production of specific IgA antibodies, but this was not sufficient to prevent infection (65). Recent studies of the role of TNF-α showed that mice with genes for this cytokine deleted succumbed to *L. monocytogenes* infection, lacked splenic primary B-cell follicles, and could not form follicular dendritic

cell networks and germinal centers, but that Ig class switching still occurred despite deregulated antibody response (99).

In most infections, cooperation among components of the immune response is likely to be essential for host defense (51). For example, a lack of CD40L (ligand) on T cells prevents interaction with CD40 on B cells and has been demonstrated as a cause of the failure to switch from IgM to IgG in the hyper-IgM syndrome (1); therefore, it was postulated as the cause of susceptibility to infections. However, recent studies showed that mice made genetically deficient in CD40L (CD40LKO) were resistant to intravenous infection with *M. tuberculosis* (16). Infected CD40LKO mice developed granulomas, and CD4[+] T cells produced high levels of IFN-γ but not IL-4, showing that protective Th1 immunity could be achieved independently of CD40L.

Taken as a whole, these studies suggest that there are overlapping pathways which characterize immune regulation such that alternate pathways may be inducible in response to threat. Knowledge of the alternate pathways may provide crucial basic information about how the immune system has developed and how specific pathogens may condition immune response.

BACTERIAL INFECTION IN ACQUIRED IMMUNE DEFICIENCY

With the advent of technological advances, it has become possible to pinpoint consistent defects in individual immune response to specific types of bacterial infection. In some cases these are not obviously part of a known primary immune deficiency disorder but may have developed following an illness, such as a viral infection. This may lead to an acquired chronic immune deficiency that may be limited in scope but nonetheless persistent. The immune system may remain altered over a long period of time even when the original infecting agent is no longer detectable, such as in the chronic fatigue syndrome or idiopathic CD4 T-cell deficiency (77, 80). Malnutrition also produces acquired immune deficiency (25). Severe or chronic moderate malnutrition leads to susceptibility to infection and morbidity from normally sustainable infections.

The extreme example of acquired immune deficiency is human immunodeficiency virus (HIV) infection, which produces AIDS. Since HIV generally continues to infect the host, the lesion widens and, despite host defense, produces an evolving immune deficiency that requires therapeutic intervention at several levels to prevent morbidity from opportunistic infections or rare tumors. Although the development and improved use of highly active antiretroviral therapy have greatly reduced the HIV burden in the responding host, immune response is not fully restored (128). While HIV infection is being gradually transformed into a chronic illness, persistent bacterial infections continue to threaten the immune equilibrium.

Bacterial Infections in the HIV⁺ Host

The HIV⁺ host has an altered immune system, which is associated with enhanced vulnerability to opportunistic infections and rare tumors. Chapter 10 explores the possibility that a virally encoded gene product, Nef, is a superantigen which can induce T-cell proliferation as bacterial superantigens do.

Immune deficiency in HIV disease is associated with opportunistic infections and severe bacterial infections. At least in part, defective response to pathogens may be attributable to altered antigen presentation by antigen-presenting cells, affecting the antigen-presenting cell-CD4 interaction (36). Effector functions are also affected (55). Mycobacteria represent a particular threat to the HIV-infected host and have been a leading cause of serious morbidity in both adults and children. Infection with *M. tuberculosis* depends upon exposure of the vulnerable host, and adequate response depends upon cytotoxic and memory CD4⁺ T-cell function, leading to granuloma formation and immune destruction. CD1-restricted T cells, which lack CD4 but produce IFN-γ in response to nonpeptide mycobacterial antigens, are central to host defense. Response to nonpeptide antigens is compromised in the course of HIV disease (4). Studies of response to phosphoantigens showed that while HIV-infected responders could produce Th1 cytokines, IFN-γ, and TNF-α, anergic nonresponders could not produce either Th1 or Th2 cytokines. Neither IL-12 nor IL-15 could reverse this anergy (12). A novel approach to restoration of response to *M. tuberculosis* antigen has been attempted using expansion of CD1-restricted T cells from HIV⁺ persons. IFN-γ production was enhanced by adding anti-transforming growth factor-β or IL-15, and these CD4-negative cells continued to be resistant to HIV infection (48).

HIV infection has been observed to cause a polyclonal decrease of peripheral Vγ9/Vδ2 T cells, the main γδ T-cell population in peripheral blood. The residual population was frequently found to be anergic to stimulation with *M. tuberculosis*. These changes provide a probable basis for increased vulnerability to intracellular infection in general and failure to mount an adequate response in HIV infection. Further, *M. tuberculosis* has been found to enhance HIV type 1 (HIV-1) replication by transcriptional activation at the long terminal repeat (134). Correlation has been noted between increase of viral replication and onset of *M. tuberculosis* disease (47). A general consequence of mycobacterial infection appears to be production of IL-10, which downregulates IFN-γ production, CTLA-4 (cytotoxic T-lymphocyte antigen 4) expression, and monocyte production of IL-12 (49). This may explain why priming with IFN-γ has been found to restore mononuclear cell production of IL-12 in vitro in response to several opportunistic infections, including *M. tuberculosis* infection (54).

Since HIV infection causes altered immune response at multiple levels and is associated with abnormal cytokine production, infection with *M. tuberculosis* in HIV$^+$ adults is more frequent due to increased exposure and is often more virulent. Association with multidrug-resistant *M. tuberculosis* has been widely reported (94). Since household contact is increased in the urban New York multiethnic populations, we assessed whether children with congenital HIV infection were more vulnerable to *M. tuberculosis*. We found that 30% of children ($n = 29$) who presented at the New York Presbyterian Hospital (Cornell) clinic with possible *M. tuberculosis* infection were HIV$^+$ and that 60% had a family member who was *M. tuberculosis* positive. Seventy percent of the household contacts were known to be HIV$^+$. However, only about 10% of the children were found to be culture positive for *M. tuberculosis*, which did not suggest enhanced vulnerability.

Mycobacterium avium complex bacteria are the cause of a major opportunistic infection in HIV disease (6). Early mycobacterial bacteremia is accompanied by increased levels of IL-6 (53). Studies have shown that *M. avium* infection is associated with higher levels of HIV burden and that immune response to HIV-1 antigen is reduced in *M. avium* coinfection (29), while IL-6 and TNF-α release is enhanced. Conversely, when monocytes from HIV-negative persons were exposed to HIV, production of TNF-α was reduced even in the absence of productive HIV infection, suggesting that *M. avium* infection can be a cofactor for progression in HIV-1 disease (133). Response to *M. avium* may be upregulated by addition of IL-12 in vitro in patients with low CD4 T-cell numbers (95). In contrast, response to *M. leprae* in coinfected HIV$^+$ persons does

not prevent granuloma formation or cytokine activation to *M. leprae* antigens even in CD4$^+$ T-cell-deficient persons (110).

Invasive pneumococcal disease is also relatively common in HIV infection (59). In addition to *Pneumococcus pneumoniae*, respiratory infection with *H. influenzae* is more frequent and often severe. Nosocomial pneumonias from aerobic gram-negative bacilli and from *S. aureus* and *P. aeruginosa* have been observed (92). *S. aureus* appears to have increased pathogenicity in the HIV-infected host. The risk of infection shows a relationship to decline in CD4$^+$ T-cell numbers, and *S. aureus* infection may induce additional HIV production (20). This increased pathogenicity may be associated with deficient IL-12 production and at least in one study was reversible by priming with IFN-γ. Non-Typhi *Salmonella* may be increased in HIV-infected persons (52). Other infections that have been observed include *Campylobacter jejuni* infection, which produces a severe and debilitating febrile illness that may include pulmonary involvement (119), bacterial vaginosis (50), *Listeria* infection (35), and *Yersinia enterocolitica* infection (5). Correlation between neutropenia and bacterial infections in HIV infection has now been established in HIV disease (69). In a large retrospective study, the effect of neutropenia was strongest for *E. coli*, *Klebsiella pneumoniae*, and *P. aeruginosa* (17). Although HIV infection does not preclude response to immunization to pneumococcal polysaccharides, nonresponders are unlikely to respond to revaccination, indicating failure of the immune response (105). Normal response to pneumococcal immunization elicits IgM, IgG2, and IgG2A response. IgG2 levels appear to be lower before immunization in HIV infection, and the IgM response appears to be reduced postimmunization (18). Passive administration of intravenous gamma globulin has proven useful as a prophylactic measure against this type of infection in HIV disease (131).

As described above, susceptibility to bacterial infections is linked to defects in the innate immune system. Recent studies have suggested that monocytes and neutrophils from HIV$^+$

persons, whether symptomatic or not, have relatively diminished numbers of oxygen radical-producing cells compared with the number of phagocytic cells (111). Deficiency was associated with a decline in CD4$^+$ T cells. An interesting recent study investigating the effect of LPS activation on HIV replication in the monocyte-derived macrophage showed that activation stimulated virus entry but also led to protection from infection by inhibition of synthesis of late reverse transcription products and repression of nuclear import of viral RNA (136).

Therefore, susceptibility to bacterial infection in the HIV$^+$ host involves both innate and adaptive immune responses and altered regulation of both TCR-$\alpha\beta$ CD4$^+$ T cells and TCR-$\gamma\delta$ CD4$^-$ cells. Mycobacterial infections in HIV infection provide a model for persistent bacterial infection in the immunocompromised host.

Immune Response to Commensals in the HIV$^+$ Host

The normal bacterial flora is altered in HIV infection, as shown by the frequency of bacteremia (82, 96), in association with altered gastrointestinal function, diarrhea, and malabsorption (74). These conditions are characterized by intestinal damage, enterocyte injury, partial villus atrophy, crypt hyperplasia, and enteropathy associated with opportunistic infections (73). Enteral nutrition is important for the ecology of the gastrointestinal tract and protection of the surface by surfactants, mucus, and fiber. This can be compromised by the loss of commensal bacteria for fermentation of fibers and complex proteins. When mucosal atrophy ensues, this also promotes the translocation of potential pathogens. General alteration in the bacterial flora in HIV disease may be reflected in bacterial vaginosis, which has recently been shown to be a risk factor for the acquisition of HIV infection perinatally (118). This finding suggests the potential importance of the altered flora in susceptibility to infection.

Immune response towards resident gastrointestinal commensals is thought to be regulated

towards tolerance (113), a concept that is supported by studies in inflammatory bowel disease where lamina propria lymphocytes from the inflamed intestine proliferated in response to bacteria but those from uninflamed areas or from peripheral blood did not (33). Even in HIV infection, commensal bacteria rarely produce infection (106). In other experimental studies, IgA response to *Morganella morganii*, a murine commensal, was examined in the germ-free mouse. IgA response both attenuated germinal center response to *M. morganii* and reduced translocation, suggesting that commensals may induce this self-attenuating response as a feature of evolutionary adaptation (113). While some commensals may become pathogenic in the immune-deficient athymic neonatal beige mouse (124), a recent study in which *Lactobacillus reuteri* was given to HIV$^+$ persons showed that fecal levels of *L. reuteri* and total *Lactobacillus* species were lower than levels previously observed in healthy male adults and that there were no safety or tolerance problems (127).

HIV-associated failure to thrive is relatively common in congenital HIV infection and, although multifactorial, may be linked to altered gastrointestinal function. We have been studying the effect of *Lactobacillus plantarum* 299v (65) in the HIV$^+$ child for impact on growth and on specific systemic immune response following oral supplementation. Preliminary studies of immune response in vitro showed that the HIV$^+$ children had a level of cross-reacting immune response to *L. plantarum* 299v that was equal to that of adult controls despite their much poorer immune response to other activators (22). Surprisingly, the level of response was essentially independent of the percentage of CD4$^+$ T cells, which is also unlike the response to any other activator, where the level of response was associated with the CD4$^+$ T-cell level. The data are shown in Fig. 4. The supplementation study also showed that the growth of the growth-impaired children was significantly improved and that deficient immune response to other activators was significantly augmented. Colonization was tempo-

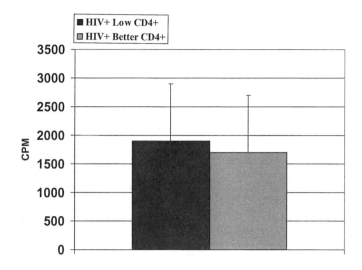

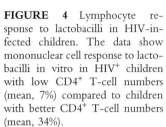

FIGURE 4 Lymphocyte response to lactobacilli in HIV-infected children. The data show mononuclear cell response to lactobacilli in vitro in HIV$^+$ children with low CD4$^+$ T-cell numbers (mean, 7%) compared to children with better CD4$^+$ T-cell numbers (mean, 34%).

rary, and there were no side effects. Other studies also suggest that lactobacilli given orally are capable of stimulating peripheral immune response (112). Furthermore, a recent study suggests that there may be strain differences among lactobacilli with respect to the type of cytokine response elicited (58). These studies support the current interest in commensal bacteria as antigen delivery vehicles as well as potential adjuvants, perhaps especially if given intermittently (39, 87).

SUMMARY

In summary, bacterial infections tend to be recurrent or persistent in the immunocompromised host. Persistent infections modulate all aspects of immune response, including both adaptive and natural immune functions, and have long-term consequences for immune defense. Although encounters with bacteria are a normal aspect of neonatal life, infants are also more susceptible to bacterial infections than are adults. Despite these deficiencies, the neonate is potentially highly responsive to bacteria, and the neonatal immune system may be modulated very rapidly through these encounters such that immune regulation, which may have formerly favored preservation of maternal fetal tolerance, is permanently altered. In contrast, both primary immune deficiency disease and

acquired immune deficiency are characterized by a fundamentally weakened response to bacteria and a tendency towards loss of containment leading to bacterial overgrowth. Efforts to maintain balance in primary immune deficiency have been based on strategies to compensate for immunoglobulin and cytokine deficiencies as well as therapeutic replacement of the immune system through bone marrow transplantation and evolving genetic transfer approaches. However, in AIDS, bacterial infection is secondary to HIV-associated immune deficiency, leads to further deregulation of immune response, and is often associated with increased HIV production as well. While current antiretroviral therapies are far more effective than formerly, reduction of viral load does not provide immune reconstitution. Present efforts are directed towards understanding and treatment of the altered immune system. While the role of commensal bacteria in the development of the normal immune system is poorly understood, it is likely that future approaches to immune reconstitution will include living bacteria or be modeled on the principles intrinsic to this fundamental biological interaction.

ACKNOWLEDGMENTS

The work described in this chapter is supported in part by NIH grants R01 AI35517 and IK08 AI01422-

01 and by ConAgra, Probi, the Helena Rubinstein Foundation, and the Children's Blood Foundation.

REFERENCES

1. **Agematsu, K., H. Nagumo, K. Shinozaki, S. Hokibara, K. Yasui, K. Terada, N. Kawamura, T. Toba, S. Nonoyama, H. D. Ochs, and A. Komiyama.** 1998. Absence of IgD-CD27(+) memory B cell population in X-linked hyper-IgM syndrome. *J. Clin. Investig.* **102:** 853–860.
2. **Alenghat, E. E., and J. R. Sterly.** 1984. Alveolar macrophages in perinatal infants. *Pediatrics* **74:** 221–223.
3. **Baltimore, R. S.** 1998. Neonatal nosocomial infections. *Semin. Perinatol.* **22:**25–32.
4. **Barnes, P. F., and R. L. Modlin.** 1996. Human cellular immune responses to Mycobacterium tuberculosis. *Curr. Top. Microbiol. Immunol.* **215:** 197–219.
5. **Beaugerie, L., B. Salauze, A. Bure, A. M. Deluol, N. Hoyeau-Idrissi, F. Carbonnel, Y. Ngo, J. Cosnes, W. Rozenbaum, J. C. Nicolas, and J. Gendre.** 1996. Results of culture from colonoscopically obtained specimens for bacteria and fungi in HIV-infected patients with diarrhea. *Gastrointest. Endosc.* **44:**663–666.
6. **Benator, D. A., and F. M. Gordin.** 1996. Nontuberculous mycobacteria in patients with human immunodeficiency virus infection. *Semin. Respir. Infect.* **11:**285–300.
7. **Bengmark, S., and B. Jeppsson.** 1995. Gastrointestinal surface protection and mucosa reconditioning. *J. Parenter. Enteral Nutr.* **19:**410–415.
8. **Berner, R., C. M. Niemeyer, J. U. Leititis, A. Funke, C. Schwab, U. Rau, K. Richter, M. S. Tawfeek, M. Clad, and M. Brandis.** 1998. Plasma levels and gene expression of G-CSF, TNF-alpha, IL-1beta, IL-6, IL-8 and soluble intercellular adhesion molecule in neonatal early onset sepsis. *Pediatr. Res.* **44:**469–477.
9. **Berthet, F., F. Le Deist, A. M. Duliege, and C. Griscelli.** 1994. Clinical consequences and treatment of primary immunodeficiency syndromes characterized by functional T and B lymphocyte anomalies (combined immune deficiency). *Pediatrics* **93:**265–270.
10. **Boes, M., A. P. Prodeus, T. Schmidt, M. C. Carroll, and J. Chen.** 1998. A critical role of natural immunoglobulin M in immediate defense against systemic bacterial infection. *J. Exp. Med.* **188:**2381–2386.
11. **Bohnsack, J. F., K. Vidjaja, S. Ghazizadeh, C. E. Rubens, D. R. Hilhyard, C. J. Parker, K. H. Ablertne, and H. R. Hill.** 1997. A role for C5a and C5-ase in the acute neutrophil re-sponse to group B streptococcal infections. *J. Infect. Dis.* **175:**847–855.
12. **Boullierin, S., Y. Poquet, T. Debord, J. J. Fournie, and M. L. Gougeon,** 1999. Regulation by cytokines (IL-12, IL-15, IL-4 and IL-10) of the V gamma9Vdelta2 T cell response to mycobacterial phosphoantigens in responder and anergic HIV-infected persons. *Eur. J. Immunol.* **29:** 90–99.
13. **Brown, T. A., R. Jonsson, and B. Haneberg.** 1998. Cervical secretions in pregnant women colonized rectally with group B streptococci have high levels of antibodies to serotype III polysaccharide capsular antigen and protein R. *Scand. J. Immunol.* **47:**179–188.
14. **Buckley, R. H.** 1996. Primary immunodeficiency disease, p. 1401–1408. *In* J. C. Bennett and F. Plum (ed.), *Cecil Textbook of Medicine.* W. B. Saunders Co., Philadelphia, Pa.
15. **Buhrer, C., J. Graulich, D. Stibenz, J. W. Dudenhousen, and M. Obladen.** 1994. L-selection is down-regulated in umbilical cord blood granulocytes and monocytes of newborn infants with acute bacterial infection. *Pediatr. Res.* **36:** 799–804.
16. **Campos-Neto, A., P. Ovendale, T. Bement, T. A. Koppi, W. C. Fanslow, M. A. Rossi, and M. R. Alderson.** 1998. CD40 ligand is not essential for the development of cell-mediated immunity and resistance to Mycobacterium tuberculosis. *J. Immunol.* **160:**2037–2041.
17. **Caperna, J., R. E. Barber, J. G. Toerner, and W. C. Mathews.** 1998. Estimation of the effect of neutropenia on rates of clinical bacteraemia in HIV-infected patients. *Epidemiol. Infect.* **120:** 71–80.
18. **Carson, P. J., R. L. Schut, M. L. Simpson, J. O'Brien, and E. N. Janoff.** 1995. Antibody class and subclass responses to pneumococcal polysaccharides following immunization of human immunodeficiency virus-infected patients. *J. Infect. Dis.* **172:**340–345.
19. **Caux, C., C. Dezutter-Dambuyant, D. Schmitt, and J. Banchereau.** 1992. GM-CSF and TNF-α cooperate in the generation of dendritic Langerhans cells. *Nature* **360:**258–261.
20. **Craven, D. E.** 1995. Staphylococcus aureus colonisation and bacteraemia in persons infected with human immunodeficiency virus: a dynamic interaction with the host. *J. Chemother.* **7**(Suppl. 3):19–28.
21. **Cunningham-Rundles, C., F. P. Siegal, S. Cunningham-Rundles, and P. Lieberman.** 1987. Incidence of cancer in 98 patients with common varied immunodeficiency in the United States. *Clin. Immunol.* **7:**294–303.
22. **Cunningham-Rundles, S., S. Arne, S. Beng-**

mark, R. Johann-Liang, F. Marshall, L. Metakis, C. Califano, A. M. Dun, C. Grassey, G. Hinds, and J. Cervia. Probiotics and immune response. *J. Gastroenterol.*, in press.

23. **Cunningham-Rundles, S., C. Chen, J. B. Bussel, C. Blankenship, M. B. Veber, D. Sanders-Laufer, T. Hinds, J. S. Cervia, and P. Edelson.** 1995. Human immune development: implications for congenital HIV infection. *Ann. N.Y. Acad. Sci.* **693:**70–84.

24. **Cunningham-Rundles, S., and F. P. Pearson.** 1990. ImuVert activation of natural killer cytotoxicity and interferon gamma production via CD16 triggering. *Int. J. Immunopharmacol.* **12:**589–598.

25. **Cunningham-Rundles, S.** 1994. Malnutrition and gut immune function. *Curr. Opin. Gastroenterol.* **10:**664–670.

26. **Cusumano, V., V. Mancuso, F. Genovese, M. Cuzzola, M. Carbone, J. A. Cook, J. B. Cochran, and G. Teti.** 1997. Neonatal hypersusceptibility to endotoxin correlates with increased TNF production in mice. *J. Infect. Dis.* **176:**168–176.

27. **Dai, W. J., G. Kohler, and F. Brombacher.** 1997. Both innate and acquired immunity to Listeria monocytogenes infection are increased in IL-10-deficient mice. *J. Immunol.* **158:**2259–2267.

28. **Deerojanawong, J., A. B. Chang, P. A. Eng, C. F. Robertson, and A. S. Kemp.** 1997. Pulmonary diseases in children with severe combined immune deficiency and DiGeorge syndrome. *Pediatr. Pulmonol.* **24:**324–330.

29. **Denis, M., and E. Ghadirian.** 1994. Mycobacterium avium infection in HIV-1-infected subjects increases monokine secretion and is associated with enhanced viral load and diminished immune response to viral antigens. *Clin. Exp. Immunol.* **97:**76–82.

30. **Derkx, H. H., E. I. Kuijper, C. A. Fijen, M. Jak, J. Dankert, and S. J. van Deventer.** 1995. Inherited complement deficiency in children surviving fulminant meningococcal septic shock. *Eur. J. Pediatr.* **154:**735–738.

31. **Devis, C. A., E. H. Vallota, and J. Forristal.** 1979. Serum complement level in infancy; age related changes. *Pediatr. Res.* **13:**1043–1046.

32. **Drago, L., M. R. Gismondo, A. Lombardi, C. de Haen, and L. Gozzini.** 1997. Inhibition of in vitro growth of enteropathogens by new Lactobacillus isolates of human intestinal origin. *FEMS Microbiol. Lett.* **153:**455–463.

33. **Duchmann, R., I. Kaiser, E. Hermann, W. Mayet, K. Ewe, and K. H. Meyer zum Buschenfelde.** 1995. Tolerance exists towards resident intestinal flora but is broken in active inflammatory bowel disease (IBD). *Clin. Exp. Immunol.* **102:**448–455.

34. **Ekdahl, K., J. H. Braconier, and C. Svanborg.** 1997. Impaired antibody response to pneumococcal capsular polysaccharides and phosphorylcholine in adult patients with a history of bacteremic pneumococcal infection. *Clin. Infect. Dis.* **25:**654–660.

35. **Ewert, D. P., L. Lieb, P. S. Hayes, M. W. Reeves, and L. T. I. Mascola.** 1995. Listeria monocytogenes infection and serotype distribution among HIV-infected persons in Los Angeles County, 1985–1992. *J. Acquir. Immune Defic. Syndr. Hum. Retrovirol.* **8:**461–465.

36. **Fidler, S. J., I. Dorrell, S. Ball, G. Lombardi, J. Weber, C. Hawrylowicz, and A. D. Rees.** 1996. An early antigen-presenting cell defect in HIV-1-infected patients correlates with CD4 dependency in human T-cell clones. *Immunology* **89:**46–53.

37. **Figueroa, J. E., and P. Densen.** 1991. Infectious disease associated with complement deficiencies. *Clin. Microbiol. Rev.* **4:**359–395.

38. **Fiorentino, D. F., A. Zlotnik, T. R. Mosman, M. Howard, and A. O'Garra.** 1991. IL-10 inhibits cytokine production by activated macrophages. *J. Immunol.* **147:**3815–3822.

39. **Fischetti, V. A., D. Medaglini, and G. Pozzi.** 1996. Gram-positive commensal bacteria for mucosal vaccine delivery. *Curr. Opin. Biotechnol.* **7:**659–666.

40. **French, M. A., K. A. Denis, R. Dawkins, and J. B. Peter.** 1995. Severity of infections in IgA deficiency: correlation with decreased serum antibodies to pneumococcal polysaccharides and decreased serum IgG2 and/or IgG4. *Clin. Exp. Immunol.* **100:**47–53.

41. **Fujiwara, T., T. Kobayashi, J. Takaya, S. Taniuchi, and J. Kobayashi.** 1997. Plasma effects on phagocytic activity and hydrogen peroxide production by PMNs in neonates. *Clin. Immunol. Immunopathol.* **85:**67–72.

42. **Gao, J. X., and A. C. Issekutz.** 1995. PMN migration through human dermal fibroblast monolayers is dependent on beta 2 integrin and beta 1 integrin mechanisms. *Immunology* **85:**485–494.

43. **Garcia, V. E., P. A. Sieling, J. Gong, P. F. Barnes, K. Uyemura, Y. Tanaka, B. R. Bloom, C. T. Morita, and R. L. Modlin.** 1997. Single-cell cytokine analysis of gamma delta T cell responses to nonpeptide mycobacterial antigens. *J. Immunol.* **159:**1328–1335.

44. **Gellin, B. G., C. V. Broome, and W. F. Bilb.** 1991. The epidemiology of listeriosis in the United States–1986. *Am. J. Epidemiol.* **133:**392–401.

45. **Gemmell, C. G.** 1995. Staphylococcal scalded skin syndrome. *J. Med. Microbiol.* **43:**318–322.

46. **Gladstone, I. M., R. A. Ehenkranz, S. C. Edberg, and R. S. Baltimore.** 1990. A ten-year review of neonatal sepsis and comparison with the previous fifty-year experience. *Pediatr. Infect. Dis. J.* **9:**819–825.

47. **Goletti, D., D. Weissman, R. W. Jackson, N. M. Graham, D. Vlahov, R. S. Klein, S. S. Munsiff, L. Ortona, R. Cauda, and A. S. Fauci.** 1996. Effect of Mycobacterium tuberculosis on HIV replication. Role of immune activation. *J. Immunol.* **157:**1271–1278.

48. **Gong, J., S. Stenger, J. A. Zack, B. E. Jones, G. C. Bristol, R. L. Modlin, P. J. Morrissey, and P. F. Barnes.** 1998. Isolation of mycobacterium-reactive CD1-restricted T cells from patients with human immunodeficiency virus infection. *J. Clin. Investig.* **101:**383–389.

49. **Gong, J. H., M. Zhang, R. L. Modlin, P. S. Linsley, D. Iyer, Y. Lin, and P. F. Barnes.** 1996. Interleukin-10 downregulates *Mycobacterium tuberculosis*-induced Th1 responses and CTLA-4 expression. *Infect. Immun.* **64:**913–918.

50. **Gray, R. H., M. J. Wawer, N. Sewankambo, and D. Serwadda.** 1997. HIV-1 infection associated with abnormal vaginal flora morphology and bacterial vaginosis. *Lancet* **350:**1780.

51. **Grewal, I. S., and R. A. Flavell.** 1997. The CD40 ligand. At the center of the immune universe? *Immunol. Res.* **16:**59–70.

52. **Gruenewald, R., S. Blum, and J. Chan.** Relationship between human immunodeficiency virus infection and salmonellosis in 20- to 59-year-old residents of New York City. *Clin. Infect. Dis.* **18:**358–363.

53. **Haas, D. W., M. M. Lederman, L. A. Clough, R. S. Wallis, D. Chernoff, and S. L. Crampton.** 1998. Proinflammatory cytokine and human immunodeficiency virus RNA levels during early Mycobacterium avium complex bacteremia in advanced AIDS. *J. Infect. Dis.* **177:**1746–1749.

54. **Harrison, T. S., and S. M. Levitz.** 1997. Priming with IFN-gamma restores deficient IL-12 production by peripheral blood mononuclear cells from HIV-seropositive donors. *J. Immunol.* **158:**459–463.

55. **Harrison, T. S., and S. M. Levitz.** 1995. Interaction with human immunodeficiency virus type 1 modulates innate effector functions of human monocytes. *J. Infect. Dis.* **172:**1598–1601.

56. **Hassan, J., and D. J. Reen.** 1996. Reduced primary antigen-specific T-cell precursor frequencies in neonates is associated with deficient interleukin-2 production. *Immunology* **87:**604–608.

57. **Haziot, A., B. Z. Tsuberi, and S. M. Goyert.** 1993. Neutrophil CD14: biochemical properties and role in the secretion of tumor necrosis factor-alpha in response to lipopolysaccharide. *J. Immunol.* **150:**5556–5565.

58. **Hessle, C., L. Å. Hanson, and A. E. Wold.** 1999. Lactobacilli from human gastro-intestinal mucosa are strong stimulators of IL-12 production. *Clin. Exp. Immunol.* **116:** 276–282.

59. **Hibbs, J. R., J. M. Douglas, Jr., F. N. Judson, W. L. McGill, C. A. Rietmeijer, and E. N. Janoff.** 1997. Prevalence of human immunodeficiency virus infection, mortality rate, and serogroup distribution among patients with pneumococcal bacteremia at Denver General Hospital, 1984–1994. *Clin. Infect. Dis.* **25:**195–199.

60. **Hill, M. J.** 1997. Intestinal flora and endogenous vitamin synthesis. *Eur. J. Cancer Prev.* **6**(Suppl. 1): S43–S45.

61. **Hobbs, J. R., and J. A. Davis.** 1967. Serum gamma globulin levels and gestational age in premature babies. *Lancet* **i:**757–759.

62. **Hoffman, A. A.** 1981. Presentation of antigen by human newborn monocytes to maternal tetanus toxoid-specific T cells. *J. Clin. Investig.* **1:**127.

63. **Hogg, N., M. P. Stewart, S. L. Scarth, R. Newton, J. M. Shaw, S. K. Law, and N. Klein.** 1999. A novel leukocyte adhesion deficiency caused by expressed but nonfunctional beta2 integrins Mac-1 and LFA-1. *J. Clin. Investig.* **103:**97–106.

64. **Howard, A. M., and M. Cosyns.** 1994. Proliferative and cytokine responses by human newborn T cells stimulated with staphylococcal enterotoxins. *Pediatr. Res.* **35:**293–298.

65. **Johansson, M., K. Schon, M. Ward, and N. Lycke.** 1997. Genital tract infection with *Chlamydia trachomatis* fails to induce protective immunity in gamma interferon receptor-deficient mice despite a strong local immunoglobulin A response. *Infect. Immun.* **65:**1032–1044.

66. **Johansson, M. L., G. Molin, B. Jeppsson, S. Nobaek, S. Ahrne, and S. Bengmark.** 1993. Administration of different *Lactobacillus* strains in fermented oatmeal soup: in vivo colonization of human intestinal mucosa and effect on the indigenous flora. *Appl. Environ. Microbiol.* **59:**15–20.

67. **Jouanguy, E., F. Altare, S. Lamhamedi-Cherradi, and J. L. Casanova.** 1997. Infections in IFNGR-1-deficient children. *J. Interferon Cytokine Res.* **17:**583–587.

68. **Kagi, D., B. Ledermann, K. Burki, H. Hengartner, and R. M. Zinkernagel.** 1994. CD8 + T cell-mediated protection against an intracellular bacterium by perforin-dependent cytotoxicity. *Eur. J. Immunol.* **24:**3068–3072.

69. **Keiser, P., E. Higgs, and J. Smith.** 1996. Neutropenia is associated with bacteremia in patients

infected with the human immunodeficiency virus. *Am. J. Med. Sci.* **312**:118–122.

70. **Klein, J. O.** 1990. From harmless commensal to invasive pathogen: coagulase negative staphylococci. *N. Engl. J. Med.* **323**:1–3.

71. **Klein, J. O., and S. M. Marcy.** 1995. Bacterial sepsis and meningitis, p. 847. *In* J. S. Remington and J. O. Klein (ed.), *Infectious Diseases of the Fetus and Newborn Infant,* 4th ed. W. B. Saunders Co., Philadelphia, Pa.

72. **Klein, J. O., and J. S. Remington.** 1995. Current concepts of infections of the fetus and newborn infant, p. 11–13. *In* J. S. Remington and J. O. Klein (ed.), *Infectious Diseases of the Fetus and Newborn Infant,* 4th ed. W. B. Saunders Co., Philadelphia, Pa.

73. **Kotler, D. P.** 1998. Intestinal disease associated with HIV infection: characterization and response to antiretroviral therapy. *Pathobiology* **66**:183–188.

74. **Kotler, D. P.** 1998. Human immunodeficiency virus-related wasting: malabsorption syndromes. *Semin. Oncol.* **25**(Suppl. 6):70–75.

75. **Kuan, S. F.** 1992. Interactions of surfactant protein D with bacterial lipopolysaccharides. Surfactant protein D is an *Escherichia coli*-binding protein in bronchoalveolar lavage. *J. Clin. Investig.* **90**:97–106.

76. **Kurosawa, S., M. Harada, Y. Shinomiya, H. Terao, and K. Nomoto.** 1996. The concurrent administration of OK432 augments the antitumor vaccination effect with tumor cells by sustaining locally infiltrating natural killer cells. *Cancer Immunol. Immunother.* **43**:31–38.

77. **Laurence, J., D. Mitra, M. Steiner, D. H. Lynch, F. P. Siegal, and L. Staiano-Coico.** 1996. Apoptotic depletion of CD4+ T cells in idiopathic CD4+ T lymphocytopenia. *J. Clin. Investig.* **97**:672–680.

78. **Laver, J., E. Duncan, and M. Abboud.** 1990. High levels of granulocyte and GM-CSF in cord blood of normal full term neonates. *J. Pediatr.* **116**:627–632.

79. **Lee, S. M., Y. Suen, L. Chang, V. Bruner, J. Qian, J. Indes, E. Knoppel, C. van de Ven, and M. S. Cairo.** 1996. Decreased interleukin-12 (IL-12) from activated cord versus adult peripheral blood mononuclear cells and upregulation of interferon-gamma, natural killer, and lymphokine-activated killer activity by IL-12 in cord blood mononuclear cells. *Blood* **88**:945–954.

80. **Levy, J. A.** 1994. Viral studies of chronic fatigue syndrome. *Clin. Infect. Dis.* **18**(Suppl. 1):S117–S120.

81. **Lewis, D. A., A. Larsen, and C. B. Wilson.** 1986. Reduced interferon gamma mRNA levels in human neonates. *J. Exp. Med.* **163**:1018–1023.

82. **Lichenstein, R., J. C. King, Jr., J. J. Farley,** P. Su, P. Nair, and P. E. Vink. 1998. Bacteremia in febrile human immunodeficiency virus-infected children presenting to ambulatory care settings. *Pediatr. Infect. Dis. J.* **17**:381–385.

83. **Madoff, L. C.** 1994. Maternal immunization of mice with group B streptococcal type III polysaccharide beta C protein conjugate elicits protective antibodies to multiple serotypes. *J. Clin. Investig.* **94**:286–292.

84. **Madoff, L. C., J. L. Michel, E. W. Gong, D. E. Kling, and D. L. Kager.** 1996. Group B streptococci escape host immunity by deletion of tandem repeat elements of the alpha C protein. *Proc. Natl. Acad. Sci. USA* **93**:4131–4136.

85. **Mahon, B. P., B. J. Sheahan, F. Griffin, G. Murphy, and K. H. Mills.** 1997. Atypical disease after Bordetella pertussis respiratory infection of mice with targeted disruptions of interferon-gamma receptor or immunoglobulin mu chain genes. *J. Exp. Med.* **186**:1843–1851.

86. **Manroe, B. L., A. G. Weinberg, and C. R. Rosenfeld.** 1979. The neonatal blood count in health and disease. *J. Pediatr.* **95**:89–98.

87. **Medaglini, D., G. Pozzi, T. P. King, V. A. Fischetti.** 1995. Mucosal and systemic immune responses to a recombinant protein expressed on the surface of the oral commensal bacterium Streptococcus gordonii after oral colonization. *Proc. Natl. Acad. Sci. USA* **92**:6868–6872.

88. **Mellander, L., B. Carlsson, F. Jelil, T. Soderstrom, and L. A. Hanson.** 1985. Secretory IgA antibody response against *E. coli* antigens in infants in relation to exposure. *J. Pediatr.* **107**:430–433.

89. **Menzies, B. E., and I. Kourteva.** 1998. Internalization of *Staphylococcus aureus* by endothelial cells induces apoptosis. *Infect. Immun.* **66**:5994–5998.

90. **Merry, C., P. Puri, and D. J. Reen.** 1998. Phosphorylation and the actin cytoskeleton in defective newborn neutrophil chemotaxis. *Pediatr. Res.* **44**:259–264.

91. **Morell, A.** 1994. Clinical relevance of IgG subclass deficiencies. *Ann. Biol. Clin.* (Paris). **52**:49–52.

92. **Moroni, M., and F. Franzetti.** 1995. Bacterial pneumonia in adult patients with HIV infection. *J. Chemother.* **7**:292–306.

93. **Morris, J. G., Jr., and M. Potter.** 1997. Emergence of new pathogens as a function of changes in host susceptibility. *Emerg. Infect. Dis.* **3**:435–440.

94. **Murray, J. F.** 1998. Tuberculosis and HIV infection: a global perspective. *Respiration* **65**:335–342.

95. **Newman, G. W., J. R. Guarnaccia, E. A. Vance III, J. Y. Wu, H. G. Remold, and P. H. Kazanjian, Jr.** 1994. Interleukin-12 enhances antigen-specific proliferation of peripheral blood mononuclear cells from HIV-positive and neg-

ative donors in response to Mycobacterium avium. *AIDS* **8:**1413–1419.

96. **Nguyen, M. H., C. A. Kauffman, R. P. Goodman, C. Squier, R. D. Arbeit, N. Singh, M. M. Wagener, and V. L. Yu.** 1999. Nasal carriage of and infection with Staphylococcus aureus in HIV-infected patients. *Ann. Intern. Med.* **130:**221–225.

97. **Nicoletti, F., G. Mancuso, V. Cusumano, R. DiMarco, P. Zaccone, K. Benndtzen, and G. Teti.** 1997. Prevention of endotoxin induced lethality in neonatal mice by IL-13. *Eur. J. Immunol.* **27:**1580–1583.

98. **Nybo, M., O. Soversen, R. Leslie, and P. Wang.** 1998. Reduced expression of C5a receptors on neutrophils from cord blood. *Arch. Dis. Child. Fetal Neonatal Ed.* **78:**129–132.

99. **Pasparakis, M., L. Alexopoulou, V. Episkopou, and G. Kollias.** 1996. Immune and inflammatory responses in TNF alpha-deficient mice: a critical requirement for TNF alpha in the formation of primary B cell follicles, follicular dendritic cell networks and germinal centers, and in the maturation of the humoral immune response. *J. Exp. Med.* **184:**1397–1411.

100. **Payne, N. R., and H. B. Fleit.** 1996. Extremely low birth weight infants have lower Fc gamma RIII plasma levels and their PMN produce less Fc gamma compared to adults. *Biol. Neonate* **69:**235–242.

101. **Pierre-Audigier, C., E. Jouanguy, S. Lamhamedi, F. Altare, J. Rauzier, V. Vincent, D. Canioni, J. F. Emile, A. Fischer, S. Blanche, J. L. Gaillard, and J. L. Casanova.** 1997. Fatal disseminated Mycobacterium smegmatis infection in a child with inherited interferon gamma receptor deficiency. *Clin. Infect. Dis.* **24:**982–984.

102. **Porcelli, S., C. T. Morita, and M. B. Brenner.** 1992. CD1b restricts the response of human CD4-8-T lymphocytes to a microbial antigen. *Nature* **360:**593–597.

103. **Prindull, G., and M. Ahmad.** 1993. The ontogeny of the gut mucosal immune system and the susceptibility to infections in infants of developing countries. *Eur. J. Pediatr.* **152:**786–792.

104. **Rebuck, N.** 1995. Neutrophil adhesion molecules in term and preterm infants: normal or enhanced leukocyte integrins but defective L selectin expression and shedding. *Clin. Exp. Immunol.* **101:**183–189.

105. **Rodriguez-Barradas, M. C., J. E. Groover, C. E. Lacke, D. W. Gump, C. I. Lahart, J. P. Pandey, and D. M. Musher.** 1996. IgG antibody to pneumococcal capsular polysaccharide in human immunodeficiency virus-infected subjects: persistence of antibody in responders,

revaccination in nonresponders, and relationship of immunoglobulin allotype to response. *J. Infect. Dis.* **173:**1347–1353.

106. **Rogasi, P. G., S. Vigano, P. Pecile, and F. Leoncini.** 1998. Lactobacillus casei pneumonia and sepsis in a patient with AIDS. Case report and review of the literature. *Ann. Ital. Med. Int.* **13:**180–182.

107. **Romagnani, S.** 1995. Biology of human TH1 and TH2 cells. *J. Clin. Immunol.* **15:**121–129.

108. **Rowen, J. L., C. W. Smith, and M. S. Edwards.** 1995. Group B streptococci elicit leukotriene B4 and IL-8 from human monocytes: neonates exhibit a diminished response. *J. Infect. Dis.* **172:**420–426.

109. **Rubens, C. E.** 1992. Epithelial cell invasion by group B streptococci. *Infect. Immun.* **60:** 5157–5161.

110. **Sampaio, E. P., J. R. Caneshi, J. A. Nery, N. C. Duppre, G. M. Pereira, L. M. Vieira, A. L. Moreira, G. Kaplan, and E. N. Sarno.** 1995. Cellular immune response to *Mycobacterium leprae* infection in human immunodeficiency virus-infected individuals. *Infect. Immun.* **63:** 1848–1854.

111. **Schaumann, R., J. Krosing, and P. M. Shah.** 1998. Phagocytosis of Escherichia coli and Staphylococcus aureus by neutrophils of human immunodeficiency virus-infected patients. *Eur. J. Med. Res.* **3:**546–548.

112. **Schiffrin, E. J., F. Rochat, H. Link-Amster, J. M. Aeschlimann, and A. Donnet-Hughes.** 1995. Immunomodulation of human blood cells following the ingestion of lactic acid bacteria. *J. Dairy Sci.* **78:**491–497.

113. **Shroff, K. E., K. Meslin, and J. J. Cebra.** 1995. Commensal enteric bacteria engender a self-limiting humoral mucosal immune response while permanently colonizing the gut. *Infect. Immun.* **63:**3904–3913.

114. **Smith, D. H., G. Peter, and D. L. Ingram.** 1973. Responses of children immunized with capsular polysaccharides of *Haemophilus influenzae*. *Pediatrics* **52:**637–644.

115. **Sorensen, R. U., L. E. Leiva, F. C. Javier III, D. M. Sacerdote, N. Bradford, B. Butler, P. A. Giangrosso, and C. Moore.** 1998. Influence of age on the response to Streptococcus pneumoniae vaccine in patients with recurrent infections and normal immunoglobulin concentrations. *J. Allergy Clin. Immunol.* **102:**215–221.

116. **Stoll, B. J., T. Gordon, S. B. Korones, S. Shankaron, J. E. Tyson, C. R. Bauer, A. A. Fanaroff, J. A. Lemons, E. F. Donovan, W. Oh, D. K. Stevenson, R. A. Ehrenkanz, L. A. Papile, J. Verter, and L. L. Wright.** 1996. Late onset sepsis in very low birth weight neo-

nates: a report from the National Institute of Child Health and Human Development Neonatal Research Network. *J. Pediatr.* **129:**63–71.

117. **Stoll, B. J., T. Gordon, S. B. Korones, S. Shankaron, J. E. Tyson, C. R. Bauer, A. A. Fanaroff, J. A. Lemons, E. F. Donovan, W. Oh, D. K. Stevenson, R. A. Ehrenkanz, L. A. Papile, J. Verter, and L. L. Wright.** 1996. Early onset sepsis in very low birth weight neonates: a report from the National Institute of Child Health and Human Development Neonatal Research Network. *J. Pediatr.* **129:**72–80.

118. **Taha, T. E., D. R. Hoover, G. A. Dallabetta, and N. I. Kumwenda.** 1998. Bacterial vaginosis and disturbances of vaginal flora: association with increased acquisition of HIV. *AIDS* **12:**1699–1706.

119. **Tee, W., and A. Mijch.** 1998. Campylobacter jejuni bacteremia in human immunodeficiency virus (HIV)-infected and non-HIV-infected patients: comparison of clinical features and review. *Clin. Infect. Dis.* **26:**91–96.

120. **Teti, G., G. Mancuso, and F. Tomasello.** 1993. Cytokine appearance and effects of anti-TNF alpha antibodies in a neonatal rat model of group B streptococcal infection. *Infect. Immun.* **61:**227–235.

121. **Tossing, G.** 1996. Immunodeficiency and its relation to lymphoid and other malignancies. *Ann. Hematol.* **73:**163–167.

122. **Tsukada, H., I. Kawamura, and M. Arakawa.** 1991. Dissociated development of T cells mediating delayed-type hypersensitivity and protective T cells against *Listeria monocytogenes* and their functional difference in lymphokine production. *Infect. Immun.* **59:**3589–3595.

123. **Veber, M. B., S. Cunningham-Rundles, M. Schulman, F. Mandel, and P. A. M. Auld.** 1991. Acute shift in immune response to microbial activators in very low birthweight infants. *Clin. Exp. Immunol.* **83:**391–395.

124. **Wagner, R. D., T. Warner, L. Roberts, J. Farmer, and E. Balish.** 1997. Colonization of congenitally immunodeficient mice with probiotic bacteria. *Infect. Immun.* **65:**3345–3351.

125. **Winkelstein, J. A.** 1998. The complement system in the fetus and newborn, p. 1964–1967. *In* R. A. Polin and W. W. Fox (ed.), *Fetal and Neonatal Physiology*, 2nd ed. W.B. Saunders Co., Philadelphia, Pa.

126. **Wolbink, G. J., A. W. Bossink, A. B. Groneweld, M. C. de Grott, L. G. Thijs, and C. E. Hack.** 1998. Complement activation in patients with sepsis is in part mediated by C-reactive protein. *J. Infect. Dis.* **177:**81–87.

127. **Wolf, B. W., K. B. Wheeler, D. G. Ataya, and K. A. Garleb.** 1998. Safety and tolerance of Lactobacillus reuteri supplementation to a population infected with the human immunodeficiency virus. *Food Chem. Toxicol.* **36:**1085–1094.

128. **Woods, M. L., II, R. MacGinley, D. P. Eisen, and A. M. Allworth.** 1998. HIV combination therapy: partial immune restitution unmasking latent cryptococcal infection. *AIDS* **12:**1491–1494.

129. **Wright, J. R., and D. C. Youmansi.** 1993. Pulmonary surfactant protein A stimulates chemotaxis of alveolar macrophage. *Am. J. Physiol.* **264:**L338–L344.

130. **Yang, X., and R. C. Brunham.** 1998. Gene knockout B cell-deficient mice demonstrate that B cells play an important role in the initiation of T cell responses to Chlamydia trachomatis (mouse pneumonitis) lung infection. *J. Immunol.* **161:**1439–1446.

131. **Yap, P. L.** 1994. Does intravenous immune globulin have a role in HIV-infected patients? *Clin. Exp. Immunol.* **97**(Suppl. 1)**:**59–67.

132. **Yegin, O.** 1983. Chemotaxis in childhood. *Pediatr. Res.* **17:**183–187.

133. **Zerlauth, G., E. Maier, H. Chehadeh, K. Zimmermann, M. M. Eibl, and J. W. Mannhalter.** 1995. Interaction with human immunodeficiency virus type 1 modulates innate effector functions of human monocytes. *J. Infect. Dis.* **172:**1598–1601.

134. **Zhang, Y., K. Nakata, M. Weiden, and W. N. Rom.** 1995. Mycobacterium tuberculosis enhances human immunodeficiency virus-1 replication by transcriptional activation at the long terminal repeat. *J. Clin. Investig.* **95:**2324–2331.

135. **Zlabinger, G. J.** 1983. Cord blood macrophages present bacterial antigen (E. coli) to paternal T cells. *Clin. Immunol. Immunopathol.* **28:**405–412.

136. **Zybarth, G., N. Reiling, H. Schmidtmayerova, B. Sherry, and M. Bukrinsky.** 1999. Activation-induced resistance of human macrophages to HIV-1 infection in vitro. *J. Immunol.* **162:**400–406.

INFLUENCE OF γδ T CELLS ON THE DEVELOPMENT OF CHRONIC DISEASE AND PERSISTENT BACTERIAL INFECTIONS

Paul J. Egan and Simon R. Carding

9

The discovery of γδ T cells originally occurred as an unexpected result of attempts to identify and clone the T-cell receptor (TCR). The search for genes coding for the TCR used the approach of identifying DNA rearrangements expressed exclusively by T cells. This strategy resulted in the identification of the TCR α- and β-chains, which together code for the TCR expressed by the majority of T cells. Unexpectedly, however, other T-cell-specific gene rearrangements were also discovered, which were designated the TCR γ- and δ-chains. These chains formed a distinct TCR expressed by a minority population of T cells whose existence had not been predicted on the basis of any known functional activity. Since the initial description of these cells, now known as γδ T cells, a great deal of research has been devoted to answering two key questions: what is the nature of the antigen or antigens recognized by the γδ TCR and what are the specific functions carried out by γδ T cells? Although these questions have still not been definitively answered, considerable evidence suggests that γδ T cells are active participants in

the host response to environmental pathogens. Here, we will present evidence that γδ T cells are required in order to prevent the development of chronic disease, which in turn may be a contributing factor in determining whether a microbial pathogen is eradicated or becomes persistent. First, however, some general features of γδ T cells will be briefly reviewed. For more extensive reviews, see the articles by Haas et al. (43) and Egan et al. (34).

DISTRIBUTION AND RECEPTOR USAGE

In humans and mice, γδ T cells form a small subset of lymphocytes circulating in the blood and peripheral lymphoid organs and making up approximately 1 to 5% of lymphocytes (Table 1). In other animals, such as ruminants and birds, γδ T cells are more widespread and can compose up to 70% of peripheral lymphocytes (49). In all species, however, γδ T cells are more commonly found within epithelial surfaces, such as the skin, the intestinal epithelium, or the mucosa of the reproductive tract, where they may compose up to 50% of T cells. All populations of γδ T cells are derived from the thymus, with the exception of intestinal intraepithelial γδ T cells of the gut, which are thought to develop locally (see below). In the mouse, development of the γδ TCR repertoire

Paul J. Egan, Department of Clinical Studies, School of Veterinary Medicine, University of Pennsylvania, Philadelphia, PA 19104. *Simon R. Carding*, School of Biological Sciences, University of Leeds, Leeds LS2 9JT, England.

Persistent Bacterial Infections, Edited by J. P. Nataro, M. J. Blaser, and S. Cunningham-Rundles, © 2000 ASM Press, Washington, D.C.

TABLE 1 Contrasting features and properties of γδ T cells and other lymphocyte lineages[a]

Property	Value for the following lymphocyte lineage:		
	αβ T cells	γδ T cells	B cells
Antigen receptor	CD3-αβ	CD3-γδ	Ig
Receptor diversity (no.)			
V-segments	52 (α), ~70 (β)	14 (γ), 7 (δ)	~51 (H), ~69 (L)
D-segments	2 (β)	3 (δ)	~30 (H)
J-segments	61 (α), 13 (β)	5 (γ), 2 (δ)	6 (H), 9 (L)
C-segments	1 (α), 2 (β)	2 (γ), 1 (δ)	9 (H), 5 (L)
No. of functional combinations	~10^{16}	~10^{20}	~10^{16}
Antigen recognition	Peptide + MHC	MHC alone MHC-like (e.g., CD1, MICA) Protein (e.g., hsp60) Nonprotein (e.g., prenyl pyrophosphate)	Protein Nonprotein
MHC restriction	Yes	No	No
Development	Thymus dependent	Thymus dependent Thymus independent (Vγ7$^+$)	Bone marrow
Phenotype	CD4$^+$ or CD8$^+$	Majority CD4$^-$, CD8$^-$	CD19$^+$, CD20$^+$
Distribution			
Blood	65–75%	1–5% (>80% Vγ9/Vδ2$^+$)	5–10%
Periphery	Lymphoid tissue	1–5% thymus (Vδ1$^+$) 10% intestine (Vδ1$^+$)	Lymphoid tissue
Function	Cytotoxicity Lymphokine release	Cytotoxicity Lymphokine release Immunoregulation	Ig secretion Lymphokine secretion Antigen presentation

[a] Properties refer to human lymphocyte populations; data were compiled from references 28 and 57.

occurs in distinct waves throughout ontogeny and is characterized by migration of cells bearing distinct receptors into specific tissues (1). For instance, γδ T cells expressing the Vγ5 (the TCR Vγ gene nomenclature used is that of Heilig and Tonegawa [48]) receptor chain are the first γδ T-cell population to arise during gestation, and they migrate to the skin epithelium around day 14 of gestation. The Vγ6 population is the next wave of γδ T cells to develop, and these cells are predominantly localized in the female reproductive tract and the tongue. γδ T cells that arise later in ontogeny, such as the Vγ1 or Vγ4 populations, are mainly found circulating through the blood

and peripheral lymphoid organs. γδ T cells of the intestinal epithelium predominantly express the Vγ7 receptor and first appear during the week after birth. These cells are thought to be generated within the gut, independently of the thymus (80, 91). In view of this epithelial tropism, it has been proposed that γδ T cells perform an immune-surveillance-type function (58), providing an immediate response to infection.

In addition to tissue-specific localization, γδ T cells expressing different TCR Vγ and Vδ chains also differ markedly in the extent of junctional diversity of the rearranged receptor genes (reviewed in reference 43). TCR junctional diversity is generated through the insertion of germ line-encoded diversity (D) elements, which can be read in all three reading frames, as well as through the addition of non-germ line-encoded nucleotides at the V-D-J junctions during gene rearrangement. Following rearrangement, receptors expressed by γδ T cells of the skin or reproductive tract are monomorphic and contain no junctional diversity, forming an essentially oligoclonal population of γδ T cells that theoretically can respond to a very limited repertoire of antigens. In contrast, receptors expressed by peripheral lymphoid γδ T cells or by intestinal intraepithelial γδ T cells express a variable repertoire of junctional sequences. This diversity is particularly evident in the Vδ chain, while the Vγ chain is more conserved. The junctional diversity of these subpopulations of γδ TCRs is so great that there are potentially more γδ TCR rearrangements possible than those of αβ TCRs or immunoglobulin (Ig) molecules combined, even though the number of variable gene segments coding for the γδ TCR is limited (Table 1). This diversity suggests that γδ T cells have the ability to respond to a diverse array of antigens, perhaps within the context of a conserved antigen-presenting molecule.

ANTIGEN RECOGNITION BY γδ T CELLS

It is now clear that γδ T cells recognize and respond to antigen in a fundamentally different way than do αβ T cells (Table 1). Unlike CD8[+] and CD4[+] αβ T cells, which bind to processed antigenic peptides presented by major histocompatibility complex (MHC) class I or class II molecules, respectively, MHC molecules do not play a role in antigen recognition by the majority of γδ TCRs and antigen processing is not required for γδ T-cell activation (97). The vast majority of γδ T cells do not express CD4 or CD8, and analysis of the γδ TCR has demonstrated similarities in the CDR3 length and crystal structure between the δ chain and the heavy and light chains of Ig molecules (69, 94). These observations suggest that antigen recognition by γδ T cells may instead occur through direct binding of the receptor to its

ligand, in a manner similar to that of antibodies binding to their antigens. As with the αβ TCR, however, signal transduction following γδ TCR engagement occurs through the CD3 complex.

Unlike αβ T cells that recognize peptide antigens, γδ T cells can recognize nonprotein antigens (reviewed in reference 78). Among these, the low-molecular-mass (100 to 600 Da) nonpeptide prenyl pyrophosphate antigens isolated from lysates or culture supernatants of *Mycobacterium tuberculosis* have received a great deal of attention. In humans these antigens preferentially activate Vγ9/Vδ2 γδ T cells, which are the major γδ T-cell population in the peripheral blood (Table 1). These antigens are produced in many biosynthetic pathways in both prokaryotic and eukaryotic cells, allowing for γδ T-cell recognition of a broad range of infections with bacteria and parasites (78). Accordingly, γδ T cells could potentially recognize and respond to phosphorylated metabolites produced by infecting microorganisms or even to antigens released from host cells following local cellular necrosis after infection. Recognition of these antigens requires cell-to-cell contact and occurs in a γδ TCR-dependent fashion (79), and the γ-chain has been shown to be required for recognition of these antigens (19). However, direct binding of these antigens to the TCR has not yet been demonstrated. These compounds may, therefore, be acting as haptens that need to be associated with other proteins for γδ TCR recognition to occur. As yet, no surface molecule has been identified that has the ability to present pyrophosphate antigens to γδ T cells, although there appears to be no requirement for MHC class I or class II or CD1a, 1b, or 1c for γδ T-cell stimulation to occur (79).

A second group of antigens recognized by γδ T cells are those upregulated as a result of cellular stress. The best-characterized antigen of this type is a member of the heat shock protein (Hsp) family, Hsp60 (16, 83). This protein is able to stimulate a large percentage of murine γδ T cells, although its ability to stimulate human γδ T cells is more controversial. Hsp60 is a highly conserved protein, and significant homology occurs between mammalian and bacterial Hsp60s (115). γδ T-cell activation can be induced following stimulation with both mycobacterium derived and autologous Hsp60 (15). Cells that respond to stimulation with Hsp60 invariably express the Vγ1 receptor chain, in conjunction with the Vδ6 or Vδ4 chain, which together are expressed by the majority (>90%) of γδ T cells present in the blood and secondary lymphoid organs of mice (83). Since the δ-chains of these cells have highly variable junctional sequences, there is a paradox in which γδ T cells expressing diverse receptors are capable of responding to the same antigen. One possible explanation for this paradox lies with the function of Hsp60 as a chaperonin to refold proteins (46). Hsp60 has the ability to form stable complexes with a wide variety of proteins (112), so it is possible that γδ T cells respond to a complex of Hsp60 and another protein in association with it. Hsp60 is normally localized in the mitochondria, but it has also been detected on the plasma membranes of cells taken from inflammatory lesions associated with both infectious disease (8) and autoimmunity (11, 102). Plasma membrane expression of Hsp60 would allow for recognition of this molecule by the γδ TCR, although the signals responsible for inducing the expression of Hsp60 to the plasma membrane are not known.

FUNCTIONAL PROPERTIES OF γδ T CELLS

Activated γδ T cells recovered from sites of infection produce immunoregulatory cytokines, such as gamma interferon (IFN-γ), interleukin 2 (IL-2), IL-4, and IL-10 (21, 54, 96), suggesting that they are able to regulate the activities of other cell populations during the course of an immune response via cytokine release. In addition, some populations of γδ T cells, such as the Vγ7+ population of γδ T cells present in the murine intestinal epithelium (6, 42, 66, 113) or γδ T cells present in human peripheral blood (12, 18, 64), have potent cytotoxic activity. Cytotoxicity is mediated

through the production of the pore-forming protein, perforin, and granzyme molecules, which induce apoptosis in target cells. In addition, γδ T cells can express Fas ligand following stimulation, enabling them to kill Fas-expressing cells, generated during an immune response. However, without more detailed knowledge of the ligands recognized by γδ T cells and when they are induced within the context of inflammatory responses, it is difficult to make definitive statements about the functions carried out by γδ T cells. Potential activities of γδ T cells are summarized in Fig. 1A. It is important to note, however, that the specific activities carried out by each γδ T-cell subpopulation probably vary, depending on the type of receptor the cell expresses and its tissue localization. It is important to specify, therefore, which population of γδ T cells is involved when discussing their functions.

A HYPOTHESIS

Based upon the studies of γδ T cells in infectious disease published to date, we would argue that γδ T cells are not directly responsible for pathogen eradication. In published models of γδ T-cell activation following infection, such as with *Listeria monocytogenes* or influenza virus, the expansion of γδ T cells at the site of infection occurs after the peak of the infection, at a time when the pathogen load is in decline or has been eliminated (9, 21) (Fig. 1B). Instead, γδ T cells may serve to regulate and coordinate the cell-mediated immune response to infection, and in particular, the resolution phase of pathogen-induced immune responses. Their absence or dysfunction, therefore, is likely to contribute to ineffective immune responses and chronic disease, conditions favoring pathogen persistence. As we will discuss here, evidence in support of this proposed role for γδ T cells comes primarily from two lines of experimentation: (i) demonstrating their presence and accumulation at the site of infection in mice or humans and (ii) comparing the course of infection in mice that lack γδ T cells, either by depletion with anti-TCR-γδ monoclonal antibodies or by a targeted mutation in the

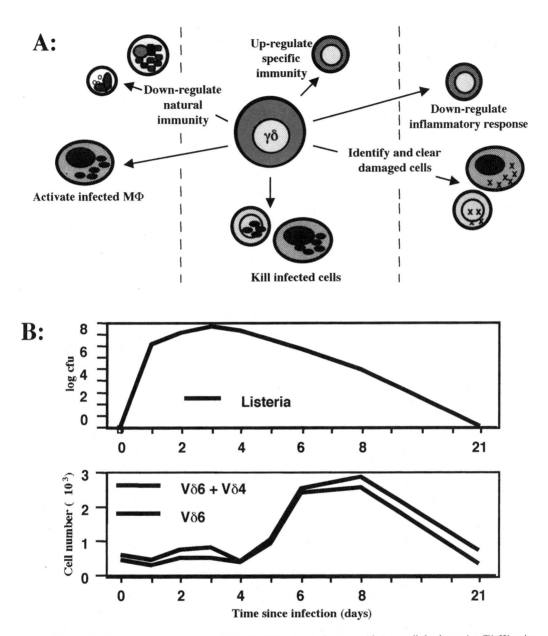

FIGURE 1 (A) Proposed functions for γδ T cells following infection with intracellular bacteria. (B) Kinetics of the growth of *L. monocytogenes* and the expansion of γδ T cells in the spleens of mice following infection. Mice were infected with 2×10^4 CFU of *Listeria*, and the spleens were harvested on the indicated days. Bacterial numbers were determined by plating dilutions of organ homogenates on Luria-Bertani agar plates. γδ T-cell numbers were determined by flow cytometry. The expansion of Vδ6 and Vδ4 γδ T cells, which are the predominant populations that respond to infection with *Listeria*, occurs when the bacterial numbers are in decline (9). MΦ, macrophage.

TCR-δ locus. Using these approaches, γδ T-cell involvement in the responses to infection with bacteria such as *L. monocytogenes*, *M. tuberculosis*, *Mycobacterium leprae*, *Borrelia*, and *Salmonella* has been demonstrated.

The immunoregulatory role of γδ T cells that we have outlined is not necessarily incompatible with the immune surveillance function originally proposed by Janeway and colleagues over 10 years ago (58). The predominance of γδ T cells in epithelium-rich tissues and their ability to respond to antigens associated with stress or infection make them ideally suited to initiating and orchestrating the host response to infection. At first consideration, the numerous accounts of large numbers of γδ T cells within the inflammatory lesions associated with autoimmune diseases, such as rheumatoid arthritis and multiple sclerosis and its mouse model, experimental autoimmune encephalitis, would appear to indicate a pathogenic rather than immunoregulatory role for γδ T cells. However, rather than being an indication of involvement in the pathogenesis of these disorders, we would argue that the presence of γδ T cells is an attempt to downregulate the extent of inflammation associated with these diseases. This model is supported by the finding that autoimmune *lpr* mice depleted of γδ T cells have more extensive inflammatory lesions and higher levels of serum autoantibodies (88).

We will use two populations of γδ T cells, one that is localized to the epithelium of the intestine and one that is predominant among peripheral γδ T cells and that resides in secondary lymphoid organs, as examples of how γδ T cells can influence the immune response to both commensal and pathogenic bacteria.

INVOLVEMENT OF γδ T CELLS IN MUCOSAL IMMUNITY TO COMMENSAL OR PATHOGENIC BACTERIA IN THE GUT

Oral Tolerance

The intestinal epithelium represents one of the largest physical barriers to microbial invasion. It is continuously exposed to a complex bacterial microflora that comprises as many as 400 different species (76) and can reach concentrations of 10^8 organisms per gram of tissue (86). These resident, or autochthonous, bacteria are in close proximity to a large number of specialized intestinal lymphocytes in the lamina propria. The observation that this lymphocyte infiltration is reduced in gnotobiotic (germfree) mice but resumes its normal appearance after bacterial colonization suggests that bacterial antigens maintain a chronic and immunologically balanced intestinal inflammatory response. In support of this proposal are the findings that the mammalian host responds to each individual gut bacterial colonizer (10, 22, 77, 90) but that this response may ordinarily be self-limiting and may forestall contributions of that organism to continuing gut inflammation (100). Clearly then, the mucosal immune system does interact with autochthonous bacteria, and yet it retains its ability to mount a rapid and potent response to pathogenic organisms while remaining tolerant ("oral tolerance") to the resident microflora. Tolerance to enteric bacteria appears to be restricted to, or specific for, the flora present in each individual. Although T cells of one individual fail to respond to the individual's own enteric bacteria, they can be activated by preparations of colonic bacteria obtained from other individuals (33). The advantage for the host of oral tolerance is that inappropriate immune responses to innocuous antigens secreted by commensal bacteria or present in food will not be generated. Oral tolerance is not necessarily permanent or irreversible, and a breakdown in tolerance to enteric bacteria is associated with inflammatory bowel disease (IBD) and immune-cell-mediated tissue injury (32, 33, 89). In addition, the ability to "protect" or prevent the development of intestinal lesions in rodents that spontaneously develop IBD by maintaining them under gnotobiotic or germfree conditions (25, 29, 105) also illustrates the importance of tightly regulating and suppressing mucosal T-cell responses to enteric bacteria.

How then is mucosal T-cell tolerance established? It appears to involve multiple mechanisms, including the induction of hyporesponsiveness or anergy in antigen-specific T cells, deletion of responsive T cells, and the production of regulatory T cells that produce inhibitory cytokines, such as transforming growth factor β, following activation (reviewed in reference 41). However, it is important to note that the identity(s) of the mucosal T cells that are the targets or mediators of these mechanisms is not known. In view of their unique distribution within the intestine and their intimate association with the intestinal epithelium, much attention has focused on the possibility that TCR-γδ⁺ intraepithelial lymphocytes (IELs) contribute to the development and/or maintenance of oral tolerance.

TCR-γδ⁺ IELs

In rodents γδ T cells compose the largest IEL population (reviewed in reference 65). γδ, as well as αβ, IELs can be distinguished based on their expression of the accessory molecules CD4 and CD8. Most IELs also express the CD8αα homodimer instead of the CD8αβ heterodimer, which is expressed on peripheral CD8 T cells. CD8αα IELs are thought to be generated locally in the gut from bone marrow-derived precursors rather than in the thymus, although thymus-derived IEL populations are also present. In mice, gut-derived γδ IELs uniformly express the Vγ7 receptor chain, although the TCR repertoire of this population is characterized by multiple δ-chains, which express high junctional diversity. In rodents, the γδ IEL population is generated perinatally, before weaning and the establishment of a conventional luminal microflora (51). Environmental stimuli do, however, determine the magnitude of the accumulation of IELs, as shown by their rapid postnatal expansion in humans (23, 71) and in conventionalized germfree rodents (50, 109). Human IELs are first generated during fetal life in the first trimester prior to or coincident with thymic development and prior to bacterial colonization (73). Although the signals driving development of the γδ IEL compartment have not been characterized, a requirement for the cytokines IL-2 and IL-7 has been demonstrated.

IL-2$^{-/-}$ (25) and IL-2 receptor β-chain$^{-/-}$ (104) mice show reduced numbers of γδ T cells in the IEL compartment, and IL-2$^{-/-}$ bone marrow is not able to reconstitute the γδ T-cell compartment of IELs when transferred into irradiated wild-type hosts (25). On the other hand, IL-7$^{-/-}$ mice lack γδ IELs altogether (41).

In vitro, γδ IELs have been shown to constitutively express potent cytotoxic activity against tumor targets. This ability seems to be acquired following exposure of the IELs to gut bacteria, as γδ IELs isolated from mice raised under germfree conditions were not cytotoxic (66). These cells are also capable of secreting cytokines, such as IL-2, IL-3, and IFN-γ (6). The ability of these cells to proliferate, however, is limited. The ability of enteric bacterial pathogens to modulate γδ IEL cytokine (IFN-γ) release and cytotoxicity in vivo following oral infection of mice with the intracellular bacterium *L. monocytogenes* (114) suggests that γδ IELs have the potential to interact with enteric bacteria.

γδ IELs and Oral Tolerance

Studies of γδ IELs and oral tolerance have relied on analyzing their response to model protein or cellular antigens in mice that have an established enteric bacterial flora. The choice of this experimental approach is less than ideal, considering the difficulties inherent in attempting to analyze the hosts' immune response to enteric bacteria. The intestinal flora is vast, and the colonic flora alone may comprise as many as 400 different species, the vast majority of which are obligate anaerobes that have been identified only morphologically, since obtaining them as pure cultures has proven very difficult, if not impossible. In addition, experimentation with gnotobiotic animals requires the use of specialized equipment and technical expertise that is not widely available. The less-than-optimal choice of antigens and animals with which to study γδ IELs and oral tolerance may explain at least in part the conflicting findings obtained from such studies. For example, it has been reported that adoptive transfer of γδ T cells into tolerized hosts results in the abrogation of tolerance to sheep red blood cells (40). Other reports, however, have demonstrated that treatment of mice with an antibody to the γδ TCR prior to feeding the mice with the model antigen ovalbumin (OVA) abolished the induction of oral tolerance to OVA and that tolerance was unable to be generated in TCR-δ$^{-/-}$ mice (61, 74). In addition, systemic tolerance could be induced following administration of antigen to the mucosal tissues of the lung as a result of inhalation of aerosolized antigen. Inhalation of OVA was shown to result in the generation of a population of regulatory γδ T cells that could suppress IgE responses to OVA (72), while administration of aerosolized proinsulin induced the production of a population of CD8αα$^+$ γδ T cells that was able to prevent the development of insulin-dependent diabetes in susceptible mice (45). In summary, therefore, although γδ T cells do seem to play a role in the development of mucosal tolerance, the exact mechanisms by which this occurs remain unknown.

One clue as to how γδ IELs might contribute to oral tolerance has been obtained from studies using TCR-δ$^{-/-}$ mice. In the absence of γδ T cells, the turnover rate of the intestinal epithelium is lower than that in wild-type mice (62), suggesting that γδ IELs may be responsible for maintaining the integrity of the epithelial-cell layer in the gut. Although these mice do not develop IBD or other intestinal pathology under specific-pathogen-free conditions (62), following infection with the intestinal parasite Eimeria vermiformis, the epithelial-cell layer is badly damaged (93). In spite of this tissue damage, however, the number of parasite oocysts recovered from TCR-δ$^{-/-}$ mice did not differ from that in wild-type mice. Similar experiments comparing the extent of intestinal epithelial-cell damage in wild-type and TCR-δ$^{-/-}$ mice to that in mice with bacterial infections now need to be done in order to determine the significance of the results obtained with Eimeria infection and whether disruption of epithelial-cell function is peculiar to parasite infection. In contrast to γδ-deficient mice,

TCR-β$^{-/-}$ mice lacking all αβ T cells develop spontaneous IBD. Collectively, these findings suggest that αβ IELs are required to maintain normal intestinal physiology, while γδ IELs are required for host defense and/or tissue repair once the gut epithelium has been damaged.

PERIPHERAL (Vγ1/Vδ6) γδ T CELLS IN ACUTE AND PERSISTENT INFECTIONS

The second population of γδ T cells we will discuss is one that is commonly associated with cellular immune responses to microbial pathogens, particularly intracellular bacteria that cause systemic infection. Two of the most extensively studied models of intracellular bacterial infection and γδ T-cell activation are L. monocytogenes and Mycobacterium species, such as M. tuberculosis and M. leprae. Whereas Listeria induces an acute infection that is rapidly cleared following the activation of antigen-specific T cells, Mycobacterium resists the development of an immune response and persists in the infected host for many months or years. The studies we will discuss provide compelling evidence in support of the immunoregulatory function of γδ T cells (outlined above) and that these T cells, by preventing the development of chronic disease, may be a determining factor in preventing bacterial persistence.

L. monocytogenes

Listeria is infectious in the mouse and has been widely used as a model intracellular pathogen (reviewed in references 110 and 111). Many of the paradigms of infection and cell-mediated immunity have been established using the mouse model of listeriosis (111). It was also one of the first experimental systems in which the involvement of γδ T cells in antibacterial immune responses was demonstrated (52, 84).

The immune response to Listeria infection can be divided into three distinct phases characterized by the involvement of different immune-cell populations. During the early phase of infection, bacteria are phagocytosed by resident macrophages in target organs such as the liver, and within 24 h after infection there is an influx of granulocytes into the infected organs, forming microabscesses around the bacteria. This stage is essential for the containment of bacterial growth, since mice depleted of granulocytes prior to infection fail to control bacterial growth and rapidly die from an overwhelming bacterial infection. During the second phase of infection, occurring after 2 to 4 days, granulomas form around the site of infection as blood-borne monocytes are recruited to the site of infection and differentiate into mature macrophages. This phase is characterized by an innate immune response in which NK cells are stimulated to produce IFN-γ in response to macrophage-derived IL-12 and is necessary for controlling bacterial growth prior to the generation of specific αβ T cells. Listeria-specific CD8 αβ T cells are generated from 4 to 5 days after infection and are responsible for the lysis of Listeria-infected cells and sterilizing immunity. Generation of Listeria-specific CD4 αβ T cells of the T-helper 1 (Th1) type that produce high levels of IFN-γ is also a crucial requirement for the resolution of infection with Listeria, as demonstrated by the extreme sensitivity of IFN-γ or IFN-γ receptor knockout mice to infection with Listeria (35, 55).

A requirement for γδ T cells in the immune response to Listeria has been demonstrated by a number of groups (9, 52, 84, 101). Activation and expansion of γδ T cells have been shown to occur at the sites of infection with Listeria, such as in the liver, spleen, or peritoneal cavity. Expansion has been shown to occur in both the early stages of infection, before the activation of αβ T cells, and at the late stage of infection, when the number of bacteria present in the infected host is falling. Differences in the kinetics of the γδ T-cell response may be related to the receptor specificity of the γδ T-cell population that is induced. The γδ T cells that arise early (24 h) in the response to Listeria preferentially express the Vδ1 receptor chain, while the cells that respond during the late phase of infection, when bacterial clearance is being effected, predominantly express the Vδ6 or Vδ4 receptor chains (9). Similar populations of γδ T cells are induced in the late phase of the

inflammatory response in mice infected with influenza virus (20) or Sendai virus (53), at a time when the virus has been cleared. Together, these findings are consistent with a role for these subsets in the resolution of the inflammatory response and in returning the animal to normal homeostasis.

γδ T cells do not seem to play a direct role in antibacterial immunity but are involved in regulating the extent of the inflammatory response induced following infection. This has been most clearly shown following infection of mice deficient in γδ T cells (39, 75). The kinetics of bacterial growth and clearance in these mice are either the same or only slightly exacerbated compared with those in wild-type mice, and TCR-δ$^{-/-}$ mice do not show increased mortality from infection, except when infected with high doses of bacteria. However, TCR-δ$^{-/-}$ mice show a distinctive pathology in the liver, characterized by localized regions of tissue necrosis, resulting in secondary inflammation (39, 75). The increased susceptibility of TCR-δ$^{-/-}$ mice to Listeria, when infected with high doses of bacteria, may therefore be due to liver failure as a result of tissue necrosis rather than as a result of uncontrolled bacterial growth (39) (Fig. 2). The exact mechanisms by which these lesions are formed, however, are not known, although this question would have obvious bearing on the in vivo functions of γδ T cells during infection. It has been suggested, however, that γδ T cells promote the influx of macrophages into the site of infection, resulting in the generation of granulomas, which are essential for bacterial clearance (31). This hypothesis is based on the finding that the production of macrophage-specific chemokines, such as macrophage inflammatory protein-1α (MIP-1α), MIP-1β, MIP-2, and methyl-accepting chemotaxis protein 1, is reduced in TCR-δ$^{-/-}$ mice following infection.

Results from our laboratory, however, suggest that γδ T cells may be cytotoxic to inflammatory macrophages and therefore act to downregulate the inflammatory response. We have found that a subset of activated peritoneal

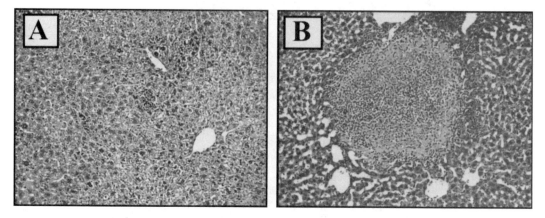

FIGURE 2 TCR-$\delta^{-/-}$ mice develop necrotic liver abscesses following infection with *Listeria*. Wild-type (A) and TCR-$\delta^{-/-}$ (B) mice were infected for 6 days with 2×10^4 CFU of *Listeria*, and liver sections were stained with hematoxylin and eosin. Magnification, $\times 352$.

macrophages isolated from *Listeria*-infected mice on day 6 postinfection, which was the peak of the γδ T-cell response, was stimulatory for γδ T-cell hybridomas derived from *Listeria*-infected spleen cells (P. J. Egan and S. R. Carding, unpublished data). In addition, there was reduced cellular death in this subset of macrophages isolated from TCR-$\delta^{-/-}$ mice compared to that in wild-type mice, indicating a role for γδ T cells in the downregulation of inflammation through the removal of activated macrophages. According to this model (Fig. 3), in the absence of γδ T cells, macrophages accumulate at the site of infection, resulting in uncontrolled production of inflammatory mediators and the necrotic death of hepatocytes. This model is consistent with the kinetics of the γδ T-cell response to both *Listeria* and influenza virus infections. In both cases, expansion and activation of Vγ1/Vδ6 γδ T cells at the site of infection occur when the pathogen has been eliminated (9, 20), arguing against a direct antimicrobial function and suggesting a role for γδ T cells in the negative regulation of inflammation.

Mycobacteria

M. tuberculosis is another intracellular bacterium that induces a Th1-type cellular immune response in the infected host. *M. tuberculosis* is

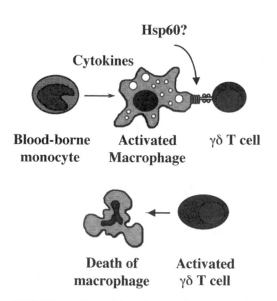

FIGURE 3 Proposed modulatory function of γδ T cells during the inflammatory response to infection with intracellular bacteria. According to this model, γδ T cells respond to stimulatory ligands, such as Hsp60, expressed by activated macrophages at the conclusion of an immune response to infection. Activated γδ T cells then acquire cytotoxic activity to kill the macrophage. In the absence of γδ T cells, activated macrophages accumulate in the animal, resulting in tissue necrosis as a result of overproduction of inflammatory mediators.

the etiological agent of pulmonary tuberculosis (TB), which remains the leading cause of morbidity and mortality due to infectious disease. It is estimated that a third of the world's population is currently infected (92), that there are over 8 million new cases of TB each year, accounting for 3 million deaths annually, and that more people will die this year of TB than at any other time in history (113a).

In contrast to the importance of CD8 αβ T cells in the development of protective immunity to *Listeria* infection, the bulk of experimental and clinical evidence favors a dominant but not exclusive role for CD4 αβ T cells in the immune defense against TB (reviewed in references 4, 5, and 24). This is made strikingly apparent by the susceptibility of human immunodeficiency virus–infected individuals to TB (99). There are, however, many similarities in the effector mechanisms employed by the cell-mediated immune response to infection with *Listeria* and *Mycobacterium*. Phagocytosis of the bacterium by macrophages results in the production of inflammatory cytokines, such as tumor necrosis factor alpha (TNF-α) and IL-12. These cytokines promote the differentiation of effector CD4 T cells into Th1-type cells, characterized by the production of IFN-γ. As is the case with *Listeria*, this is the key cytokine that must be produced for resolution of the disease. Production of IFN-γ by CD4 Th1 cells leads to macrophage activation and destruction of the bacteria (reviewed in reference 5). The importance of IFN-γ in the host response to infection is demonstrated in murine models of infection, in which infected IFN-γ$^{-/-}$ mice were unable to contain bacterial growth and rapidly succumbed to infection (30, 35). Macrophage activation in response to IFN-γ is therefore critical to the resolution of infection. In addition, cytotoxic T cells, such as MHC class I-restricted CD8 cells (36) and CD1-restricted T cells, also play a role in the elimination of the bacteria in mice by killing cells infected with bacteria. Cytolytic proteins, such as granulysin, produced by CD8 T cells, are also directly toxic to the bacteria and are important mediators of bacterial clearance

(103). In contrast, human CD4 T cells are cytolytic for *M. tuberculosis*-infected macrophages (12, 63, 70). Another important cytokine in the immune response to infection with *M. tuberculosis* is TNF-α, although this cytokine can have both beneficial and detrimental effects on the development of disease. The production of TNF-α during the course of infection is essential for survival, since mice treated with antibodies to TNF-α over the course of infection or mice that lacked the 55-kDa TNF-α receptor died of the infection (37). These mice showed delayed granuloma formation, increased tissue necrosis at the site of infection, and reduced production of reactive nitrogen intermediates by macrophages. In contrast, overproduction of TNF-α and other inflammatory cytokines, such as IL-1, has also been implicated in the pathology of TB as being responsible for the tissue necrosis and cachexia seen during the disease (7, 95).

Unlike *Listeria*, the immune response to *M. tuberculosis* infection is insufficient to eliminate the bacteria from the infected host, and a persistent infection may result. Although the initial infection with *M. tuberculosis* can be cleared by the immune system, the bacteria can also enter a latent phase within macrophages in the lungs of infected individuals. The majority of people with latent infection remain asymptomatic, although they will show a delayed–type hypersensitivity reaction to purified protein derivative from *M. tuberculosis*. In other cases, however, the bacteria can be reactivated and cause clinical disease (98). Of interest, therefore, is knowing what immune-cell factors, in addition to the mechanisms employed by *M. tuberculosis* to evade killing by activated macrophages, are responsible for the failure to eradicate mycobacteria and for subsequently reactivating them and if γδ T cells are involved or required for these processes.

In humans, γδ T cells represent the largest population of mycobacterium-reactive T cells in the blood (60, 87), and the vast majority (>85%) express a TCR encoded by the Vγ9 and Vδ2 gene subunits (28, 59, 85). This subset of human γδ T cells proliferates vigorously and releases cytokines in vitro in response to live, intact *M. tuberculosis* and to cell-associated protein (13, 14, 38, 44, 60, 82) and nonprotein, phosphorylated compounds, such as isopentenyl pyrophosphate (78). Depletion of Vγ9/Vδ2 T cells from peripheral blood lymphocytes abolishes the proliferative response of all γδ T cells to *M. tuberculosis* (59). In contrast, γδ T cells respond poorly to soluble secreted mycobacterial antigens, such as the purified protein derivative of *M. tuberculosis* (2, 60).

Although increases in γδ T-cell numbers in patients infected with *M. tuberculosis* have been reported (4, 56, 108), other studies have failed to detect any change in γδ T-cell numbers in the blood or granulomatous lymph node lesions of TB patients (3, 106, 107). Although the reasons for these contradictory findings are not known, none of these patient studies included analyses of the *M. tuberculosis*-reactive Vγ9/Vδ2 T-cell population. Since this subset of γδ T cells has been shown to be cytotoxic to a variety of tumor cell lines, such as the Daudi B-cell lymphoma line, it is possible that Vγ9/Vδ2 T cells may be acting to eliminate infected or stressed cells at the site of infection. Since both peripheral-blood-derived macrophages (14) and alveolar macrophages (2) have been shown to act as accessory cells for γδ T-cell activation in response to mycobacterial antigens, it is conceivable that activated and/or infected macrophages may be the target cells for γδ T cells in vivo. γδ T cells have been shown to lyse human peripheral blood monocytes infected in vitro with *M. tuberculosis* (81), and similar cytotoxicity is likely to be occurring in vivo. Under these circumstances, the γδ T cells would be acting as regulatory cells, modulating the extent of the inflammatory response by the elimination of activated macrophages. Although this model remains speculative, this scenario would agree with data obtained from mice with the *Listeria* system, in which activated macrophages preferentially stimulate γδ T cells.

More compelling evidence for the requirement for intact and functional Vγ9/Vδ2 T cells in order to prevent chronic and debilitating disease has been obtained from our own studies of γδ T cells in patients with pulmonary TB. Patients with active TB show a progressive loss of Vγ9/Vδ2 T cells accompanied by hyporesponsiveness of the remaining γδ T cells to stimulation with mycobacterial antigens in vitro (68). This loss or absence of Vγ9/Vδ2 T cells is seen both in the blood and in bronchoalveolar lavage and is most severe in patients with TB who have had persistent positive cultures for *M. tuberculosis*. Interestingly, the number of Vγ9/Vδ2 T cells returns to near-normal values in patients successfully treated with chemotherapy. In the more than 50 patients with active TB that we have analyzed to date, persistent infection, chronic disease, and/or poor clinical prognosis is correlative with an absence of functional *M. tuberculosis*-reactive γδ T cells (67). We have also shown that the loss of Vγ9/Vδ2 T cells is due to Fas-FasL-mediated apoptotic death as a result of chronic exposure to, and stimulation by, *M. tuberculosis* antigens (67). These findings suggest that the conditions under which γδ T cells are exposed to *M. tuberculosis* antigens are an important factor in determining their response and fate. In view of the immunoregulatory role for γδ T cells that we have proposed, the absence of immunoregulatory γδ (Vγ9/Vδ2) T cells in patients with TB and the inability to effectively downmodulate inflammatory immune responses could be an important factor in determining the outcome of infection. A loss of Vγ9/Vδ2 would favor disease progression, cell and tissue necrosis, and bacterial persistence rather than bacterial clearance and protective immunity. Although our studies of patients with TB cannot, by their very nature, establish whether the loss of functional *M. tuberculosis*-reactive γδ T cells is causally related to disease, a role for γδ T cells in the prevention or amelioration of immunopathology is attractive in view of the exaggerated pathology seen in *M. tuberculosis*-infected TCR-$\delta^{-/-}$ mice (31).

CONCLUSIONS

Although the existence of γδ T cells has been known for over a decade, information about the nature of antigen recognition by the γδ TCR and the functions carried out by these cells is only now beginning to emerge. It is clear that γδ T cells are fundamentally different from αβ T cells in terms of their antigen recognition and the conditions under which they are stimulated following infection. Although γδ T cells do not appear to have direct antimicrobial activity, there is now convincing evidence that they act to regulate the extent of inflammation following infection and that they are probably performing the same function during autoimmune diseases. The mechanisms by which γδ T cells regulate the inflammatory response are now an active area of research and will be of great interest for understanding the pathogenesis of both acute and chronic infectious disease.

ACKNOWLEDGMENTS

The work carried out in our laboratory that has been discussed in this chapter was supported by Public Health Service grants AI-31972, AI-45993, and HL-51749 from the National Institutes of Health; by grant RPG-97-027 from the American Cancer Society; and by a grant from the University of Pennsylvania Research Foundation.

We thank members of the Carding laboratory for their helpful discussions and review of the manuscript.

REFERENCES

1. **Allison, J. P. A., and W. L. Havran.** 1991. The immunobiology of T cells with invariant γδ antigen receptors. *Annu. Rev. Immunol.* **9:** 679–705.

2. **Balaji, K., S. K. Schwander, E. A. Rich, and W. H. Boom.** 1995. Alveolar macrophages as accessory cells for human γδ T cells activated by *Mycobacterium tuberculosis. J. Immunol.* **154:** 5959–5968.

3. **Balbi, B., M. T. Valle, S. Oddera, D. Giunti, F. Manca, G. A. Rossi, and L. Allegra.** 1993. T-lymphocytes with γδ+ Vδ2+ antigen receptors are present in increased proportions in a fraction of patients with tuberculosis or with sarcoidosis. *Am. Rev. Respir. Dis.* **148:**1685–1691.

4. **Barnes, P. E., C. L. Grisso, J. S. Abrams, H. Band, T. H. Rea, and R. L. Modlin.** 1992. γδ T lymphocytes in human tuberculosis. *J. Infect. Dis.* **165:**506–512.

5. **Barnes, P. F., R. L. Modlin, and J. J. Ellner.** 1994. T-cell responses and cytokines, p. 417–436. *In* B. R. Bloom (ed.), *Tuberculosis. Pathogenesis, Protection, and Control.* ASM Press, Washington, D.C.

6. **Barrett, T. R., T. F. Gajewski, D. Danielpour, E. B. Chang, K. W. Beagley, and J. A. Bluestone.** 1992. Differential function of intestinal intraepithelial lymphocyte subsets. *J. Immunol.* **149:**1124–1130.

7. **Bekker, L. G., G. Maartens, L. Steyn, and G. Kaplan.** 1998. Selective increase in plasma tumor necrosis factor-alpha and concomitant clinical deterioration after initiating therapy in patients with severe tuberculosis. *J. Infect. Dis.* **178:**580–584.

8. **Belles, C., A. Kuhl, R. Nosheny, and S. R. Carding.** 1999. Plasma membrane expression of heat shock protein 60 in vivo in response to infection. *Infect. Immun.* **67:**4191–4200.

9. **Belles, C., A. L. Kuhl, A. J. Donoghue, Y. Sano, R. L. O'Brien, W. Born, K. Bottomly, and S. R. Carding.** 1996. Bias in the γδ T cell response to *Listeria monocytogenes:* Vδ6.3+ cells are a major component of the γδ T cell response to *Listeria monocytogenes. J. Immunol.* **156:**4280–4289.

10. **Berg, R., and D. Savage.** 1975. Immune responses of specific-pathogen-free and gnotobiotic mice to antigens of indigenous and nonindigenous microorganisms. *Infect. Immun.* **11:**320–329.

11. **Boog, C. J. P., E. R. de Graeff-Meeder, M. A. Lucassen, R. van der Zee, M. M. Voorhorst-Ogink, J. S. van Kooten, H. J. Geuze, and W. van Eden.** 1992. Two monoclonal antibodies generated against human HSP60 show reactivity with synovial membranes of patients with juvenile chronic arthritis. *J. Exp. Med.* **175:** 1805–1810.

12. **Boom, W. H., R. S. Wallis, and K. A. Chervenak.** 1991. Human *Mycobacterium tuberculosis*-reactive CD4+-T-cell clones: heterogeneity in antigen recognition, cytokine production, and cytotoxicity for mononuclear phagocytes. *Infect. Immun.* **59:**2737–2743.

13. **Boom, W. H., K. N. Balaji, R. Nayak, K. Tsukaguchi, and K. A. Chervenak.** 1994. Characterization of a 10- to 14-kilodalton protease-sensitive *Mycobacterium tuberculosis* H37Ra antigen that stimulates human γδ T cells. *Infect. Immun.* **62:**5511–5518.

14. **Boom, W. H., K. A. Chervenak, M. A. Mincek, and J. J. Ellner.** 1992. Role of the mononuclear phagocyte as an antigen-presenting cell for human γδ T cells activated by live *Mycobacterium tuberculosis. Infect. Immun.* **60:**3480–3487.

15. **Born, W., L. Hall, A. Dallas, J. Boymel, T. Shinnick, D. Young, P. Brennan, and R. O'Brien.** 1990. Recognition of a peptide antigen by heat shock-reactive γδ T lymphocytes. *Science* **249:**67–69.

16. **Born, W. K., P. Happ, A. Dallas, C. Reardon, R. Kubo, T. Shinnick, P. Brennan, and R. L. O'Brien.** 1990. Recognition of heat

shock proteins and γδ cell function. *Immunol. Today* **11**:40.

17. Borst, J., R. J. van de Griend, J. W. van Oostveen, S.-L. Ang, C. Melief, J. G. Seidman, and R. L. H. Bolhuis. 1987. A T cell-receptor γ/CD3 complex found on cloned functional lymphocytes. *Nature* **325**:683–688.

18. Brenner, M. B., J. McLean, H. Scheft, J. Riberdy, S.-L. Ang, J. G. Seidman, P. Devlin, and M. S. Krangel. 1987. Two forms of the T cell-receptor γ protein found on peripheral blood cytotoxic T lymphocytes. *Nature* **325**:689–694.

19. Bukowski, J. F., C. T. Morita, H. Band, and M. B. Brenner. 1998. Crucial role of TCRγ chain junctional region in prenyl pyrophosphate antigen recognition by γδ T cells. *J. Immunol.* **161**: 286–293.

20. Carding, S. R., W. Allan, S. Kyes, A. Hayday, K. Bottomly, and P. C. Doherty. 1990. Late dominance of the inflammatory process in murine influenza by γ/δ⁺ T cells. *J. Exp. Med.* **172**:1225–1231.

21. Carding, S. R., W. Allan, A. McMickle, and P. C. Doherty. 1993. Activation of cytokine genes in T cells during primary and secondary murine influenza pneumonia. *J. Exp. Med.* **177**: 475–482.

22. Carter, P., and M. Pollard. 1971. Host responses to normal microbial flora in germfree mice. *J. Reticuloendothel. Soc.* **9**:580–587.

23. Cerf-Bensussan, N., and D. Guy-Grand. 1991. Intestinal intraepithelial lymphocytes. *Gastroenterol. Clin. N. Am.* **20**:549–576.

24. Chan, J., and S. H. E. Kaufmann. 1994. Immune mechanisms of protection, p. 389–416. *In* B. R. Bloom (ed.), *Tuberculosis. Pathogenesis, Protection, and Control.* ASM Press, Washington, D.C.

25. Contractor, N. V., H. Bassiri, T. Reya, A. V. Park, D. C. Baumgart, M. Wasik, S. G. Emerson, and S. R. Carding. 1998. Lymphoid hyperplasia, autoimmunity and compromised intestinal intraepithelial lymphocyte development in colitis-free gnotobiotic interleukin 2-deficient mice. *J. Immunol.* **160**:385–394.

26. Cooper, A. M., D. K. Dalton, T. A. Stewart, J. P. Griffin, D. G. Russell, and I. M. Orme. 1993. Disseminated tuberculosis in interferon-γ gene-disrupted mice. *J. Exp. Med.* **178**: 2243–2247.

27. Davis, M. M. 1991. T-cell receptors for antigen, p. 44–61. *In* B. D. Schwartz (ed.), *Immunology.* The Upjohn Company, Kalamazoo, Mich.

28. De Libero, G., G. Casorati, C. Giachino, C. Carbonara, N. Migone, P. Matzinger, and A. Lanzavecchia. 1991. Selection by two powerful antigens may account for the presence of the major

29. Dianda, L., A. M. Hanby, N. A. Wright, A. Sebesteny, A. C. Hayday, and M. J. Owen. 1997. T cell receptor-αβ-deficient mice fail to develop colitis in the absence of a microbial environment. *Am. J. Pathol.* **150**:91–97.

30. DiTirro, J., E. R. Rhodes, A. D. Roberts, J. M. Burke, A. Mukasa, A. M. Cooper, A. A. Frank, W. K. Born, and I. M. Orme. 1998. Disruption of cellular inflammatory response to *Listeria monocytogenes* infection in mice with disruptions in targeted genes. *Infect. Immun.* **66**: 2284–2289.

31. D'Souza, C. D., A. M. Cooper, A. A. Frank, R. J. Mazzaccaro, B. R. Bloom, and I. M. Orme. 1997. An anti-inflammatory role for γδ T lymphocytes in acquired immunity to *Mycobacterium tuberculosis. J. Immunol.* **158**:1217–1221.

32. Duchmann, R., E. Marker-Hermann, and K. H. Meyer zum Buschenfelde. 1996. Bacteria-specific T cell-clones are selective in their reactivity towards different enterobacteria or *H. pylori* and increased in inflammatory bowel disease. *Scand. J. Immunol.* **44**:71–79.

33. Duchmann, R., I. Kaiser, E. Hermann, W. Mayet, K. Ewe, and K.-H. Meyer Zum Büschenfelde. 1995. Tolerance exists towards resident intestinal flora but is broken in active inflammatory bowel disease (IBD). *Clin. Exp. Med.* **102**:448–455.

34. Egan, P., C. Belles, and S. R. Carding. 1998. The properties of γδ T-cells. *Biochemist* **20**:29–33.

35. Flynn, J. L., J. Chan, K. J. Triebold, D. K. Dalton, T. A. Stewart, and B. R. Bloom. 1993. An essential role for IFN-γ in resistance to *Mycobacterium tuberculosis* infection. *J. Exp. Med.* **178**:2249–2254.

36. Flynn, J. L., M. A. Goldstein, K. J. Triebold, B. Koller, and B. R. Bloom. 1992. Major histocompatibility complex class I-restricted T cells are required for resistance to *Mycobacterium tuberculosis* infection. *Proc. Natl. Acad. Sci. USA* **89**:12013–12017.

37. Flynn, J. L., M. M. Goldstein, J. Chan, K. J. Triebold, K. Pfeffer, C. J. Lowenstein, R. Schreiber, T. W. Mak, and B. R. Bloom. 1995. Tumor necrosis factor-α is required in the protective immune response against *Mycobacterium tuberculosis* in mice. *Immunity* **2**:561–572.

38. Follows, G. A., M. E. Munk, A. J. Gatrill, P. Conradt, and S. H. E. Kaufmann. 1992. Gamma interferon and interleukin-2, but not interleukin-4, are detected in gamma-delta T-cell cultures after activation with bacteria. *Infect. Immun.* **60**:1229–1231.

39. Fu, Y.-X., C. E. Roark, K. Kelly, D. Drevets,

P. Campbell, R. O'Brien, and W. Born. 1994. Immune protection and control of inflammatory tissue necrosis by γδ T cells. *J. Immunol.* **153**:3101–3115.

40. Fujihashi, K., T. Taguchi, W. K. Aicher, J. R. McGhee, J. A. Bluestone, J. H. Eldridge, and H. Kiyono. 1992. Immunoregulatory functions for murine intraepithelial lymphocytes: γδ T cell receptor positive (TCR+) T cells abrogate oral tolerance, while αβ TCR+ T cells provide B cell help. *J. Exp. Med.* **175**:695–707.

41. Garside, P., and A. M. Mowat. 1997. Mechanisms of oral tolerance. *Crit. Rev. Immunol.* **17**: 119–137.

42. Guy-Grand, D., M. Malassis-Seris, C. Briottet, and P. Vassalli. 1991. Cytotoxic differentiation of mouse gut thymodependent and independent intraepithelial lymphocytes is induced locally. Correlation between functional assays, presence of perforin and granzyme transcripts and cytoplasmic granules. *J. Exp. Med.* **173**:1549–1552.

43. Haas, W., P. Pereira, and S. Tonegawa. 1993. Gamma/delta cells. *Annu. Rev. Immunol.* **11**: 637–685.

44. Haregewoin, A., G. Soman, R. C. Hom, and R. W. Finberg. 1989. Human γδ T cells respond to mycobacterial heat shock protein. *Nature* **340**: 309–311.

45. Harrison, L. C., M. Dempsey-Collier, D. R. Kramer, and K. Takahashi. 1996. Aerosol insulin induces regulatory CD8 γδ T cells that prevent murine insulin-dependent diabetes. *J. Exp. Med.* **184**:2167–2174.

46. Hartl, F. U., J. Martin, and W. Neupert. 1992. Protein folding in the cell: the role of molecular chaperones Hsp70 and Hsp60. *Annu. Rev. Biophys. Biomol. Struct.* **21**:293–322.

47. Havlir, D. V., J. J. Ellner, K. A. Chervenak, and W. H. Boom. 1991. Selective expansion of human γδ T cells by *Mycobacterium tuberculosis*-infected macrophages. *J. Clin. Investig.* **87**: 729–737.

48. Heilig, J. S., and S. Tonegawa. 1986. Diversity of murine gamma genes and expression in fetal and adult lymphocytes. *Nature* **322**:836.

49. Hein, W. R., and C. R. MacKay. 1991. Prominence of γδ T cells in the ruminant immune system. *Immunol. Today* **12**:30–34.

50. Helgeland, L., J. T. Vaage, B. Rolstad, T. Midtvedt, and P. Brandtzaeg. 1996. Microbial colonization influences composition and T cell-receptor Vβ repertoire of intraepithelial lymphocytes in rat intestine. *Immunology* **89**:494–501.

51. Helgeland, L., P. Brandtzaeg, B. Rolstad, and J. T. Vaage. 1997. Sequential development of intraepithelial γδ and αβ T lymphocytes expressing CD8αβ in neonatal rat intestine; requirement for the thymus. *Immunology* **92**:447–456.

52. Hiromatsu, K., Y. Yoshikai, G. Matsuzaki, S. Ohga, K. Muramori, K. Matsumoto, J. A. Bluestone, and K. Nomoto. 1992. A protective role of γδ T cells in primary infection with *Listeria monocytogenes* in mice. *J. Exp. Med.* **175**:49–56.

53. Hou, S., P. C. D. J. Katz, and S. R. Carding. 1992. Extent of γδ T cell involvement in the pneumonia caused by Sendai virus. *Cell. Immunol.* **143**:183–188.

54. Hsieh, B., M. D. Schrenzel, T. Mulvania, H. D. Lepper, L. DiMolfetto-Landon, and D. A. Ferrick. 1996. *In vivo* cytokine production in murine listeriosis: evidence for immunoregulation by γδ+ T cells. *J. Immunol.* **156**:232–237.

55. Huang, S., W. Hendricks, A. Althage, S. Hemmi, H. Bluethmann, R. Kamijo, J. Vilcek, R. M. Zinkernagel, and M. Aguet. 1993. Immune responses in mice that lack the interferon-gamma receptor. *Science* **259**:1742–1745.

56. Ito, M., N. Kojiro, T. Ikeda, T. Ito, J. Funada, and T. Kokubu. 1992. Increased proportions of peripheral blood γδ T cells in patients with pulmonary tuberculosis. *Chest* **102**:195–199.

57. Janeway, C. A. J., and P. Travers. 1997. *Immunobiology. The Immune System in Health and Disease*, 3rd ed. Garland Publishing Inc., New York, N.Y.

58. Janeway, C. A. J., B. Jones, and A. C. Hayday. 1988. Specificity and function of T cells bearing γδ receptors. *Immunol. Today* **9**:73–76.

59. Kabelitz, D., A. Bender, T. Prospero, S. Wesselborg, O. Janssen, and K. Pechold. 1991. The primary response of human γδ T cells to *Mycobacterium tuberculosis* is restricted to Vγ9-bearing cells. *J. Exp. Med.* **173**:1331–1337.

60. Kabelitz, D., A. Bender, S. Schondelmaier, B. Schoel, and S. H. E. Kaufmann. 1990. A large fraction of human peripheral blood γδ+ T cells is activated by *Mycobacterium tuberculosis* but not by its 65-kDa heat shock protein. *J. Exp. Med.* **171**:667–674.

61. Ke, Y., K. Pearce, J. P. Lake, H. K. Ziegler, and J. A. Kapp. 1997. γδ T lymphocytes regulate the induction and maintenance of oral tolerance. *J. Immunol.* **158**:3610–3618.

62. Komano, H., Y. Fujiura, M. Kawaguchi, S. Matsumoto, Y. Hashimoto, S. Obana, P. Mombaerts, S. Tonegawa, H. Yamamoto, S. Itohara, M. Nanno, and H. Ishikawa. 1995. Homeostatic regulation of intestinal epithelia by intraepithelial γδ T cells. *Proc. Natl. Acad. Sci. USA* **92**:6147–6151.

63. Kumaratne, D. S., A. S. Pitkie, P. Drysdale, J. S. H. Gaston, R. Kiessling, P. B. Iles, C. J. Ellis, J. Innes, and R. Wise. 1990. Specific lysis of mycobacterial antigen-bearing macro-

phages by class II MHC-restricted polyclonal T cell lines in healthy donors or patients with tuberculosis. *Clin. Exp. Immunol.* **80**:314–323.

64. **Lanier, L. L., J. J. Ruitenberg, and J. H. Phillips.** 1986. CD3[+] T lymphocytes that express neither CD4 nor CD8 antigens. *J. Exp. Med.* **164**:339–344.

65. **Lefrancois, L.** 1991. Phenotypic complexity of intraepithelial lymphocytes of the small intestine. *Immunol. Today* **147**:1746–1750.

66. **Lefrancois, L., and T. Goodman.** 1989. In vivo modulation of cytolytic activity and Thy-1 expression in TCR-γδ+ intraepithelial lymphocytes. *Science* **243**:1716–1718.

67. **Li, B., H. Bassiri, M. D. Rossman, P. Kramer, A. F.-S. Eyuboglu, M. Torres, E. Sada, T. Imir, and S. R. Carding.** 1998. Involvement of Fas/Fas-ligand pathway in activation-induced cell death of mycobacteria-reactive human γδ T cells: a mechanism for the loss of γδ T cells in patients with pulmonary tuberculosis. *J. Immunol.* **161**:1558–1567.

68. **Li, B., M. D. Rossman, T. Imir, A. F. Oner-Eyuboglu, C. W. Lee, R. Biancaniello, and S. R. Carding.** 1996. Disease-specific changes in γδ T cell repertoire and function in patients with pulmonary tuberculosis. *J. Immunol.* **157**:4222–4229.

69. **Li, H., M. I. Lebedeva, A. S. Llera, B. A. Fields, M. B. Brenner, and R. A. Mariuzza.** 1998. Structure of the Vδ domain of a human γδ T cell antigen receptor. *Nature* **391**:502–506.

70. **Lorgat, F., M. M. Keraan, P. T. Lukey, and S. R. Rees.** 1992. Evidence for in vivo generation of cytotoxic T cells: PPD-stimulated lymphocytes from tuberculous pleural effusions demonstrate enhanced cytotoxicity with accelerated kinetics of induction. *Am. Rev. Respir. Dis.* **145**:418–423.

71. **Machado, C. S. M., M. A. M. Rodrigues, and H. V. L. Maffei.** 1994. Gut intraepithelial lymphocyte counts in neonates, infants and children. *Acta Pediatr.* **83**:1264–1267.

72. **McMenamin, C., C. Pimm, M. McKersey, and P. G. Holt.** 1994. Modulation of IgE responses to inhaled antigen in mice by antigen-specific γδ T cells. *Science* **265**:1869–1871.

73. **McVay, L. D., S. S. Jaswal, C. Kennedy, A. Hayday, and S. R. Carding.** 1998. The generation of human γδ T cell repertoires during fetal development. *J. Immunol.* **160**:5851–5860.

74. **Mengel, J., F. Cardillo, L. S. Aroeira, O. Williams, M. Russo, and N. M. Vaz.** 1995. Anti-γδ T cell antibody blocks the induction of oral tolerance to ovalbumin in mice. *Immunol. Lett.* **48**:97–100.

75. **Mombaerts, P., J. Arnoldi, F. Russ, S. Tonegawa, and S. H. E. Kaufmann.** 1993. Different roles of αβ and γδ T cells in immunity against an intracellular bacterial pathogen. *Nature* **365**:53–56.

76. **Moore, W., and L. Hodeman.** 1975. Discussion of current bacteriologic investigations of the relationship between intestinal flora, diet and colon cancer. *Cancer Res.* **35**:3418–3420.

77. **Moreau, M., D. Ducuzeau, D. Guy-Grand, and M. Muller.** 1978. Increase in the population of duodenal immunoglobulin A plasmocytes in axenic mice associated with different living or dead bacterial strains of intestinal origin. *Infect. Immun.* **21**:532–539.

78. **Morita, C. T., H. K. Lee, D. S. Leslie, Y. Tanaka, J. F. Bukowski, and E. Marker-Hermann.** 1999. Recognition of nonpeptide prenyl pyrophosphate antigens by human γδ T cells. *Microbes Infect.* **1**:175–186.

79. **Morita, C. T., E. M. Beckman, J. F. Bukowski, Y. Tanaka, H. Band, B. R. Bloom, D. E. Golan, and M. B. Brenner.** 1995. Direct presentation of nonpeptide prenyl pyrophosphate antigens to human γδ T cells. *Immunity* **3**:495–507.

80. **Mosely, R. L., D. Styre, and J. R. Klein.** 1990. Differentiation and functional maturation of bone marrow derived intestinal epithelial T cells expressing membrane T cell receptor in athymic radiation chimeras. *J. Immunol.* **145**:1369–1375.

81. **Munk, M. E., A. J. Gatrill, and S. H. E. Kaufmann.** 1991. In vitro activation of human γδ T cells by bacteria: evidence for specific interleukin secretion and target cell lysis. *Curr. Top. Microbiol. Immunol.* **173**:159–165.

82. **Munk, M. E., B. Schoel, S. Modrow, R. W. Karr, R. A. Young, and S. H. E. Kaufmann.** 1989. T lymphocytes from healthy individuals with specificity to self-epitopes shared by mycobacterial and human 65-kilodalton heat shock protein. *J. Immunol.* **143**:2844–2850.

83. **O'Brien, R. L., Y.-X. Fu, R. Cranfill, A. Dallas, C. Ellis, C. Reardon, J. Lang, S. R. Carding, R. Kubo, and W. Born.** 1992. Heat shock protein Hsp60-reactive γδ cells: a large, diversified T-lymphocyte subset with highly focused specificity. *Proc. Natl. Acad. Sci. USA* **89**:4348–4352.

84. **Ohga, S., Y. Yoshikai, Y. Takeda, K. Muramori, and K. Nomoto.** 1990. Sequential appearance of γδ and αβ-bearing T cells in the peritoneal cavity during i.p infection with *Listeria monocytogenes*. *Eur. J. Immunol.* **20**:533–540.

85. **Panchamoorthy, G., J. McLean, R. L. Modlin, C. T. Morita, S. Ishikawa, M. B. Brenner, and H. Band.** 1991. A predominance of the T cell receptor Vγ2/Vδ2 subset in human mycobac-

teria-responsive T cells suggests germline gene encoded recognition. *J. Immunol.* **147:**3360–3366.

86. **Peach, S., M. Lock, D. Katz, I. Todd, and S. Tabaqchali.** 1978. Mucosal-associated bacterial flora of the intestine in patients with Crohn's disease and in a control group. *Gut* **19:**1034–1042.

87. **Peffer, K., B. Schoel, H. Gulle, S. H. E. Kaufmann, and H. Wanger.** 1990. Primary responses of human T cells to mycobacteria: a frequent set of γδ T cells are stimulated by protease-resistant ligands. *Eur. J. Immunol.* **20:**1175–1184.

88. **Peng, S. L., M. P. Madaio, A. C. Hayday, and J. Craft.** 1996. Propagation and regulation of systemic autoimmunity by γδ T cells. *J. Immunol.* **157:**5689–5698.

89. **Pirzer, U., A. Schonhaar, B. Fleischer, E. Hermann, K. Hermann, and K. H. Meyer zum Buschenfelde.** 1991. Reactivity of infiltrating T lymphocytes with microbial antigens in Crohn's disease. *Lancet* **338:**1238–1239.

90. **Pollard, M., and N. Sharon.** 1970. Response of the Peyer's patches in germfree mice to antigenic stimulation. *Infect. Immun.* **2:**96–100.

91. **Poussier, P., P. Edouard, C. Lee, M. Binnie, and M. Julius.** 1992. Thymus-independent development and negative selection of T cells expressing T cell receptor α/β in the intestinal epithelium: evidence for distinct circulation patterns of gut- and thymus-derived T lymphocytes. *J. Exp. Med.* **176:**187–199.

92. **Raviglione, M. C., D. E. Snider, and A. Kochi.** 1995. Global epidemiology of tuberculosis: morbidity and mortality of a worldwide epidemic. *JAMA* **273:**220–226.

93. **Roberts, S. J., A. L. Smith, A. B. West, L. Wen, R. C. Findly, M. J. Owen, and A. C. Hayday.** 1996. T-cell αβ+ and γδ+ deficient mice display abnormal but distinct phenotypes towards a natural, widespread infection of the intestinal epithelium. *Proc. Natl. Acad. Sci. USA* **93:**11774–11779.

94. **Rock, E. P., P. R. Sibbald, M. M. Davis, and Y.-H. Chien.** 1994. CDR3 length in antigen-specific immune receptors. *J. Exp. Med.* **179:**323–328.

95. **Rook, G. A. W., J. Taverne, C. Leveton, and J. Steele.** 1987. The role of gamma-interferon, vitamin D3 metabolites and tumour necrosis factor in the pathogenesis of tuberculosis. *Immunology* **62:**229–234.

96. **Sarawar, S., S. R. Carding, W. Allan, A. McMickle, K. Fujihashi, H. Kiyono, J. R. McGhee, and P. C. Doherty.** 1993. Cytokine profiles in bronchoalveolar lavage cells from mice with influenza pneumonia: consequences of CD4+ and CD8+ T cell depletion. *Reg. Immunol.* **5:**142–150.

97. **Schild, H., N. Matvaddat, C. Litzenberger, E. W. Ehrich, M. M. Davis, J. A. Bluestone, L. Matis, R. K. Draper, and Y. Chien.** 1994. The nature of major histocompatibility complex recognition by γδ T cells. *Cell* **76:**29–37.

98. **Schluger, N. W., and W. N. Rom.** 1998. The host immune response to tuberculosis. *Am. J. Respir. Crit. Care Med.* **157:**679–691.

99. **Selwyn, P., D. Hartel, V. A. Lewis, E. E. Schoenbaum, S. H. Vermund, R. S. Klein, A. T. Walker, and G. H. Friedland.** 1989. A prospective study of the risk of tuberculosis among intravenous drug users with human immunodeficiency virus infection. *N. Engl. J. Med.* **320:**545–549.

100. **Shroff, K., K. Meslin, and J. J. Cebra.** 1995. Commensal enteric bacteria engender a self-limiting humoral mucosal immune response while permanently colonizing the gut. *Infect. Immun.* **63:**3904–3913.

101. **Skeen, M. J., and H. K. Ziegler.** 1993. Induction of murine peritoneal γ/δ T cells and their role in resistance to bacterial infection. *J. Exp. Med.* **178:**971–984.

102. **Soltys, B. J., and R. S. Gupta.** 1996. Immunoelectron microscopic localization of the 60-kDa heat shock chaperonin protein (Hsp60) in mammalian cells. *Exp. Cell Res.* **222:**16–27.

103. **Stenger, S., D. A. Hanson, R. Teitelbaum, P. Dewan, K. R. Niazi, C. J. Froelich, T. Ganz, S. Thoma-Uszynski, A. Melian, C. Bogdan, S. A. Porcelli, B. R. Bloom, A. M. Krensky, and R. L. Modlin.** 1998. An antimicrobial activity of cytolytic T cells mediated by granulysin. *Science* **282:**121–125.

104. **Suzuki, H., G. S. Duncan, H. Takimoto, and T. W. Mak.** 1997. Abnormal development of intestinal intraepithelial lymphocytes and peripheral natural killer cells in mice lacking the IL2-receptor β chain. *J. Exp. Med.* **185:**499–505.

105. **Taurog, J. D., J. A. Richardson, J. T. Croft, W. A. Simmons, M. Zhou, J. L. Fernández-Sueiro, E. Balish, and R. E. Hammer.** 1994. The germfree state prevents development of gut and joint inflammatory disease in HLA-B27 transgenic rats. *J. Exp. Med.* **180:**2359–2364.

106. **Tazi, A., F. Bouchonnet, D. Valeyre, J. Cadranel, J. P. Battesti, and A. J. Hance.** 1992. Characterization of γδ T lymphocytes in the peripheral blood of patients with active tuberculosis. *Am. Rev. Respir. Dis.* **146:**1216–1220.

107. **Tazi, A., I. Fajac, D. Soler, D. Valeyre, J. P. Battesti, and A. J. Hance.** 1991. Gamma/delta T-lymphocytes are not increased in number in granulomatous lesions of patients

with tuberculosis and sarcoidosis. *Am. Rev. Respir. Dis.* **144**:1373–1376.

108. **Ueta, C., I. Tsuyuguchi, H. Kawasumi, T. Takashima, H. Toba, and S. Kishimoto.** 1994. Increase in γδ T cells in hospital workers who are in close contact with tuberculosis patients. *Infect. Immun.* **62**:5434–5440.

109. **Umesaki, Y., Y. Okada, S. Matsumoto, A. Imaoka, and H. Setoyama.** 1995. Segmented filamentous bacteria are indigenous intestinal bacteria that activate intraepithelial lymphocytes and induce MHC class II molecules and fucosyl asialo GM1 glycolipids on the small intestinal epithelial cells in the ex-germfree mouse. *Immunology* **39**:555–562.

110. **Unanue, E. R.** 1997. Studies in listeriosis show the strong symbiosis between the innate and cellular system and the T cell response. *Immunol. Rev.* **158**:11–25.

111. **Unanue, E. R.** 1997. Why listeriosis? A perspective on cellular immunity to infection. *Immunol. Rev.* **158**:5–9.

112. **Viitanen, P. V., A. A. Gatenby, and G. H. Lorimer.** 1992. Purified chaperonin 60 (groEL) interacts with the nonnative states of a multitude of *Escherichia coli* proteins. *Protein Sci.* **1**:363–369.

113. **Viney, J. L., P. J. Kilshaw, and T. T. MacDonald.** 1990. Cytotoxic α/β+ and γ/δ+ T cells in the murine intestinal epithelium. *Eur. J. Immunol.* **20**:1623–1626.

113a.**World Health Organization.** 1998. Fact sheet no. 19. World Health Organization, Geneva, Switzerland.

114. **Yamamoto, S., F. Russ, H. C. Teixeira, P. Conradt, and S. H. E. Kaufmann.** 1993. *Listeria monocytogenes*-induced gamma interferon secretion by intestinal intraepithelial γδ T lymphocytes. *Infect. Immun.* **61**:2154–2161.

115. **Zeilstra-Ryalls, J., O. Fayet, and C. Georgopoulos.** 1991. The universally conserved GroE (Hsp60) chaperonins. *Annu. Rev. Microbiol.* **45**:301–325.

MICROBIAL SUPERANTIGENS AND IMMUNOLOGICAL DEREGULATION

Barbara A. Torres, Jeanne M. Soos, George Q. Perrin, and Howard M. Johnson

10

Superantigens are potent activators of CD4$^+$ T cells; such activation typically involves a large number of T cells, thereby causing the production of high levels of cytokines. These cytokines may, in part, be responsible for the superantigen's toxic effects. A spectrum of pathogenic bacteria and viruses have been found to produce superantigens (Table 1), which may act as virulence factors by subverting normal immune responses and causing delays in the establishment of pathogen-specific immunity; it is noteworthy that all of the bacteria listed in Table 1 (with the exception of *Streptococcus*) are established persistent pathogens. Superantigens have been implicated in a wide array of human disorders, including acute diseases, such as food poisoning and toxic shock syndrome (4), and chronic diseases, such as atopic allergy (26), periodontal disease (K. Leung and B. A. Torres, unpublished data), and Tourette's syndrome (T. Murphy, B. A. Torres, and W. Goodman, unpublished data). Furthermore superantigens can cause deregulation of immune responses, resulting in autoimmunity or immunodeficiency.

Superantigens interact with T cells in a manner that significantly differs from that of conventional antigens (Fig. 1). Conventional antigens are taken up or are endogenously produced by antigen-presenting cells and are processed into discrete peptides. These peptide antigens are then presented to antigen-specific T cells in the antigen-binding groove of either major histocompatibility complex (MHC) class I or class II molecules on the surface of the antigen-presenting cell. Superantigens, on the other hand, function as intact molecules and bind directly to MHC class II molecules on the surfaces of antigen-presenting cells (49). Superantigens can be presented to T cells by many types of immunologic class II-bearing cells, including monocytes/macrophages, B cells, and natural killer cells (14). Binding to class II molecules occurs at a site outside the antigen-binding groove (62, 63). This complex of superantigen MHC class II interacts directly with the variable region of the β-chain (Vβ) of the T-cell receptor (TCR) on T cells, thereby causing T-cell activation (6).

Approximately 60 different Vβ elements of human TCRs have been identified. The subsets of Vβ-bearing T cells that are activated by one superantigen may differ from those activated by another superantigen. Two toxins produced by *Staphylococcus aureus* can be used

Barbara A. Torres, George Q. Perrin, and Howard M. Johnson, Department of Microbiology and Cell Science, University of Florida, Gainesville, FL 32611. *Jeanne M. Soos,* Clinical Immunology, SmithKline Beecham Pharmaceuticals, King of Prussia, PA 19406.

Persistent Bacterial Infections, Edited by J. P. Nataro, M. J. Blaser, and S. Cunningham-Rundles, © 2000 ASM Press, Washington, D.C.

TABLE 1 Human diseases associated with bacterial and viral superantigens

Organism	Protein or gene	Disease	Reference(s)
Bacterium			
S. aureus	Enterotoxins[a]	Food poisoning	4
		Toxic shock syndrome	4
		MS	65, 72
		Kawasaki's disease	1, 35
		Atopic allergy	26
Group A streptococci	Pyrogenic exotoxins	Psoriasis	35, 43
		Rheumatic heart disease	35
		Obsessive/compulsive disorder	Murphy et al., unpublished
M. arthritidis	T-cell mitogen	Arthritis	10
Mycobacterium tuberculosis	Not identified	Tuberculosis	54
Yersinia	Not identified	Reiter's syndrome	83
Prevotella intermedia	Not identified	Periodontal disease	Leung and Torres, unpublished
Virus			
MMTV	vSAg gene[a]	Mammary tumors	25
Murine leukemia virus	Gag protein	Murine AIDS	27
IDDMK$_{1,2}$22	pPOL-ENV-U3	IDDM	11, 12
HIV	Nef	AIDS	82
Rabies virus	Nucleocapsid protein	Rabies	38, 39
Epstein-Barr virus	Not identified	B-ceil lymphoma	79

[a] Prototype for either bacterial or viral superantigens.

as examples. Toxic shock syndrome toxin 1 (TSST-1) interacts with human T cells bearing Vβ2, whereas staphylococcal enterotoxin B (SEB) activates human T cells expressing Vβ3, Vβ12, Vβ14, Vβ15, Vβ17, and Vβ20 (46). Thus, superantigens induce expansion of unique subsets of Vβ-specific T cells independent of antigen specificity and can activate as

many as 20% of the cells in a given T-cell population.

T-cell stimulation by superantigens causes proliferation and the prodigious production of cytokines, primarily from CD4+ cells (7, 31, 40, 56). The predominant cytokines produced and released during superantigen activation are interleukin-2 (IL-2) and gamma interferon

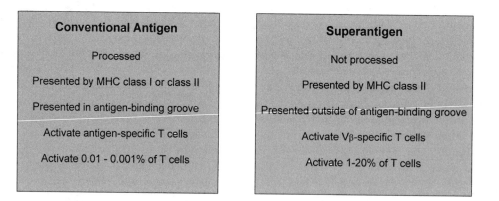

FIGURE 1 Differences between conventional antigens and superantigens.

(IFN-γ), both of which are intimately involved in the cascade of cytokines produced during immune responses. The levels of cytokines produced are higher than those normally achieved during conventional antigen-induced T-cell activation, presumably due to the potency of superantigens in activating large numbers of cells. Cytokines may be responsible for the toxic effects seen in food poisoning by SEs, the prototypic superantigens produced by *S. aureus*. Superantigen-induced cytokine production is also directly involved in the symptoms of toxic shock syndrome, where active staphylococcal infection produces TSST-1 (4).

The activation of Vβ-specific T cells by superantigens is independent of the antigen specificity of those cells. A possible ramification of such T-cell activation is the proliferation of T cells which may be autoreactive. Superantigen-producing pathogens are ubiquitous. Approximately 45% of food poisoning incidents, for example, are caused by staphylococcal superantigens (4). Thus, superantigen-producing pathogens may play a role in the establishment and/or exacerbation of autoimmune disorders, such as multiple sclerosis (MS), rheumatoid arthritis, psoriasis, and diabetes.

Persistent bacterial infections occur frequently among human populations and therefore have played a strongly modulating role in the evolution of immune response. In contrast, superantigens are usually regarded as potent inducers of an overwhelming (unmodulated) immune response that manifests as a rare event, such as toxic shock syndrome or food poisoning. So do these molecules truly play an adaptive role in the development of persistent pathogens? Whereas this role is currently only speculative, this chapter presents evidence that response to superantigens may well trigger or exacerbate autoimmunity. Autoimmunity is based on chronic immune activation and has an effect on the host defense system that is analogous to immune activation in persistent bacterial infection.

While the continuing presence of bacteria is central to persistent infection, the continuing response to autoantigen may, as shown here, be strongly modulated by bacterial superantigens. In both cases the ultimate effect is chronic immune activation and dysregulated immune response. Little is known about how persistent bacterial infections affect host defense against a new microbial or viral challenge or how they affect reactivation of other potential pathogens or opportunistic infections. The study of how superantigens modulate or even induce autoimmune states may provide a model of microbial interaction in chronic immune activation. Interactive events such as these must be common in the normal host and yet not lead to disease. The study of how normal immune response may be restored may shed light on the fundamental requirements for a stable commensal relationship.

SUPERANTIGENS IN AUTOIMMUNITY

Neurologic Inflammatory Disease

MS is an inflammatory demyelinating autoimmune disease of the central nervous system (CNS) that causes paralysis and affects speech, motor functions, and vision. MS symptomology can often be observed to occur in a relapsing-remitting manner. This form of MS consists of presentation with clinical symptoms of MS followed by periods of remission. How relapses and exacerbations occur and what causes the reactivation of autoimmune disease have been the topic of much speculation. It has been suggested that environmental influences may contribute to or even be responsible for exacerbations of autoimmune disease (66). Such influences from the environment potentially include exposure to infectious agents as well as factors possessing immunostimulatory activity. As indicated previously, microbial superantigens are ubiquitous in our environment.

An animal model useful for the study of MS is experimental allergic encephalomyelitis (EAE) (89). In the EAE model of disease, components of the myelin sheath, including myelin basic protein (MBP), proteolipid protein, and myelin oligodendrocyte protein, serve as CNS antigens for the induction of autoimmunity. Upon immunization with MBP, PL/J mice develop clinically observable tail and limb paralysis due to lymphocytic infiltration into the CNS accompanied by acute demyelination.

Exacerbation evidenced by a clinical relapse of EAE was first demonstrated by the administration of a microbial superantigen. In the PL/J mouse, acute episodes of EAE usually resolve and clinical relapses have been shown not to occur (22). After resolution of all clinical signs of EAE induced by immunization with MBP, administration of either of the SE superantigens, SEB or SEA, was shown to cause reactivation of disease (65). These results were confirmed by studies of SEB in mice (5) and SED in rats (48). Studies by our group revealed several interesting features of superantigen-induced EAE. In addition to reactivation of a single episode of disease, SEB could also induce clinical disease in mice immunized with MBP but which never developed clinical signs of EAE (65). In this case, superantigens were able to initiate the development of disease in immunized but asymptomatic animals bearing autoreactive T cells. Multiple injections of SEB also resulted in multiple relapses of EAE over a 3-month period, suggesting that upon superantigen activation these autoreactive T cells were resistant to anergy and deletion.

SEB can also prevent EAE when administered prior to immunization with MBP (32, 75). Anergy and/or deletion of the $V\beta8^+$-T-cell subset that is responsible for the initial induction of EAE appears to be the mechanism for this protection. Naïve T cells appear to be susceptible to superantigen-induced anergy and/or deletion, while activated T cells are not susceptible. Targeting of a $V\beta$-specific T-cell population does not, however, provide absolute protection from development of EAE. When mice protected from development of EAE by SEB pretreatment are exposed to SEA (which has a $V\beta$ T-cell specificity different from that of SEB), induction of EAE does occur (72). This SEA-induced EAE is characterized by severe paralysis and the accelerated onset of clinical symptoms. Thus, the effects of microbial superantigens introduce a profound complexity to autoimmune disease models

such as EAE, akin to the complexity of the pathogenesis observed in MS (Fig. 2).

It has been demonstrated that an event known as epitope spreading occurs during the course of disease in the EAE model (42, 70). At later time points after immunization of mice with a specific autoantigen, T-cell proliferative responses to other previously cryptic epitopes can be detected. Epitope spreading includes both intramolecular (spreading of T-cell responsiveness to other epitopes within the same autoantigen) and intermolecular (spreading of T-cell responsiveness to other, separate autoantigens) spreading. It has been suggested that induction of epitope spreading may be linked to disease relapse and the development of chronic disease.

We hypothesized that superantigen reactivation of EAE may result in the spreading of T-cell specificities for other epitopes of MBP. PL/J mice which had resolved an initial episode of EAE were treated with SEA and developed a second episode of paralysis. At the onset of symptoms, the mice were sacrificed and their splenocytes were stimulated in vitro with a panel of MBP peptides. EAE reactivation by SEA resulted in the spreading of T-cell specificities from the immunodominant epitope Ac1-17 to residues 100 to 120 of MBP (J. M. Soos, M. G. Mujtaba, J. Schiffenbauer, and H. M. Johnson, submitted for publication). While intramolecular spreading did occur, spreading to other antigens did not, as evidenced by the lack of response to a proteolipid protein peptide and heat shock protein 60. To further characterize the epitope MBP 100-120, PL/J mice were immunized with MBP 100-120. No initial development of disease was observed. However, administration of SEA 2 weeks after MBP 100-120 immunization resulted in the onset of paralysis. In addition to a proliferative response to MBP 100-120, these mice also exhibited a proliferative response to the flanking MBP peptides 81-100 and 120-140. Thus, SEA is able to induce intramolecular epitope spreading in PL/J mice after the reactivation of EAE.

These results suggest that superantigen in-

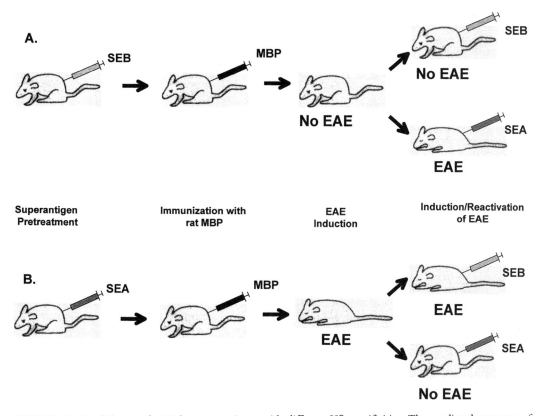

FIGURE 2 Modulation of EAE by superantigens with different Vβ specificities. The predicted outcome of the hypothesis proposed is denoted by "EAE" (induction of disease) and "No EAE" (absence of disease). The predicted outcome was confirmed by studies of the development of EAE after administration of either SEA or SEB. (A) In the first group, SEB pretreatment prevented development of EAE following injection of MBP, and while mice administered a second dose of SEB were refractory to development of disease, mice administered SEA exhibited accelerated onset of EAE. (B) In the second group, SEA pretreatment did not prevent EAE. After resolution of clinical symptoms, administration of a second dose of SEA did not reactivate disease. SEB administration, however, did reactivate EAE in the SEA-pretreated mice.

volvement may increase the complexity of disease in the EAE model. In strains of mice which are able to develop a chronic form of EAE it has been demonstrated that the spreading of T-cell responses from a dominant autoantigen epitope to other subdominant or cryptic epitopes can occur (42, 70). Likewise, reactivation of EAE by superantigen can lead to the spreading of T-cell responses to other autoantigen epitopes in the PL/J strain, which normally only develops an acute episode of disease after immunization for induction of EAE (22). Thus, a contributing mechanism for development of clinical disease in the EAE model by

superantigen administration may be the spreading of T-cell responses to other subdominant but pathogenic autoantigen epitopes.

Rheumatoid Arthritis

Superantigens have also been implicated in rheumatoid arthritis, a chronic autoimmune disease. Superantigen effects are suggested by studies of peripheral and synovial Vβ14+ T cells from patients with rheumatoid arthritis versus those from controls (55) and of B-cell production of rheumatoid factor upon stimulation with SED (24). Furthermore, recent studies suggest that the staphylococcal superantigens increase the cellular cytotoxic activity of T cells, with synovial fibroblasts being the targets of this cytoxicity (36).

Animal studies also suggest that superantigens may be involved in rheumatoid arthritis. Superantigens have been shown to reactivate bacterial-wall-induced arthritis (69) and collagen-induced arthritis (10). In these models, reactivation was induced by immunization with autoantigen prior to superantigen exposure. Mice immunized with a cell wall preparation of *Streptococcus pyogenes* were administered TSST-1, resulting in rapid reactivation characterized by multiple episodes of inflammation lasting as long as 6 weeks (69). In collagen-induced arthritis, mice which had undergone and resolved an episode of arthritis were subsequently challenged with *Mycoplasma arthritidis* mitogen. These mice showed reactivation of disease in 5 to 10 days (10). In another collagen-induced-arthritis study, treatment with SEB prior to the induction of disease by collagen administration resulted in significant protection against arthritis (37). Furthermore, administration of SEB after immunization with collagen caused increased severity of arthritis (53). Infection with a superantigen-producing microorganism may also lead to autoimmunity after the initial infection has resolved. Examples include scarlet fever caused by *Streptococcus*, which can lead to rheumatic heart disease (35, 67), and *Yersinia enterocolitica* infection, leading to reactive arthritis and Reiter's syndrome (71). These findings are similar to those concerning the role of superantigens in EAE.

Psoriasis

Psoriasis is a cutaneous inflammatory disorder characterized by epidermal keratinocyte hyperproliferation in association with inflammatory infiltrates (84). Increases in the numbers of $V\beta2$ and $V\beta5.1$ T cells have been seen in the dermis and epidermis of patients with guttate and chronic plaque psoriasis compared to T-cell populations in peripheral blood (43). Skin lesion eruptions in guttate psoriasis have been linked with throat infections and increased antibody titers to streptococcal antigens

(85). T cells specific for group A streptococcal antigens have been isolated from psoriatic lesions. The group A streptococci produce multiple superantigens, including streptococcal pyrogenic exotoxins (SPEs) A, B, and C. Significantly, $V\beta2$ T cells are stimulated by SPE-A and SPE-C while $V\beta15$ T cells are stimulated by SPE-C (86). Such results appear to further substantiate the hypothesis that superantigens are involved in the etiology and/or exacerbation of psoriasis.

Diabetes

Insulin-dependent diabetes mellitus (IDDM) is an autoimmune disorder in which pancreatic β cells are destroyed. There is evidence that autoreactive $V\beta7^+$ T cells are responsible for the destruction of pancreatic cells (11), suggesting that the disease may involve a superantigen. An endogenous human retrovirus has recently been isolated from patients with IDDM that induces the proliferation of $V\beta7^+$ T cells, the same subset of T cells thought to be involved in destruction of the pancreas (12). Thus, initial evidence suggests that a virus-encoded superantigen may modulate autoimmune disease.

IMMUNODEFICIENCY

Following the intense activation by superantigens, $V\beta$-specific T cells may become anergic or even be deleted (33, 44), possibly resulting in a state of immunodeficiency in an individual. One mechanism by which anergy may be induced in T cells by superantigens is $V\beta$-specific internalization of TCRs (45).

Human immunodeficiency virus (HIV) causes a loss of $CD4^+$ T cells over the course of the disease, resulting in the inability to effectively combat infections by other microbial agents. Other immunologic perturbations seen in HIV-infected individuals include polyclonal activation of B cells with increased immunoglobulin production, reduced antigen and mitogen responses, and increased natural killer cell activity (17).

It has been speculated that the immunologic perturbations observed during the course of infection may be due to an HIV-encoded superantigen. Several pieces of evidence implicate the involvement of an HIV superantigen (68). Initial studies suggested that HIV-infected patients had deletions in the Vβ repertoire (30), although later studies disagreed with this finding (41). Of all the Vβ T-cell subsets tested, Vβ12$^+$ cells were shown to support enhanced HIV replication and proliferation in response to HIV-infected cells (41). Another study in which the T-cell subsets of monozygotic twins discordant for HIV infection were analyzed showed perturbations in several Vβ subsets (61).

An HIV-encoded superantigen has recently been identified (82). Nef, a regulatory protein expressed early in the infection of CD4$^+$ T cells, was shown to induce Vβ-specific-T-cell proliferation in the absence of processing (80, 81). T-cell proliferation required the presence of antigen-presenting cells. Cytokine production, in particular, that of IL-2 and IFN-γ, was induced by Nef. More importantly, Nef-stimulated T cells were capable of supporting HIV replication. Antibodies to two regions of Nef, the carboxyl terminus and an internal site, blocked Nef-induced proliferation and the ability of cells to support virus replication. Furthermore, HIV-infected cells caused proliferation and activation of autologous T cells that were then capable of supporting HIV replication. Anti-Nef antibodies blocked both of these events. Thus, data suggest that Nef may be involved in the establishment of HIV infection by causing the expansion of T-cell subsets that may act as cellular reservoirs for viral replication.

Nef has been shown to induce the differentiation of human B cells to immunoglobulin-secreting cells, probably as a result of T-cell activation and the release of cytokines that aid in B-cell activation and differentiation (8). Antibodies to MHC class II antigens abrogated differentiation. B-cell differentiation required the presence of T cells and monocytes (8). Interestingly, superantigens such as the SEs have also been shown to cause B-cell differentiation (77). These data show that Nef superantigen can result in both T- and B-cell activation in

a manner reminiscent of the staphylococcal superantigens.

A model for the hypothetical role of Nef in the pathogenesis of HIV is presented in Fig. 3. Nef may be released in a soluble form as the result of lysis of infected cells and presented by antigen-presenting cells and/or may be expressed on the surfaces of infected T cells. Interaction of T cells with Nef in either of these ways activates T cells to proliferate and produce cytokines, such as IFN-γ and IL-2. An outcome of Nef stimulation is the establishment of a cellular reservoir of activated CD4$^+$ T cells for virus production, with eventual depletion of T cells via virus replication, anergy, and/or apoptosis. B-cell differentiation can be seen as the result of CD4$^+$ cells providing help and producing cytokines that aid in B-cell maturation. Nef activation may also explain, in part, the increased spontaneous immunoglobulin levels seen throughout the course of HIV infection (17). Thus, the outcome of Nef-induced immune activation may include increased virus yield with T-cell anergy and/or apoptosis and polyclonal-B-cell activation, the latter resulting in hypergammaglobulinemia and possibly autoimmune-like sequelae.

MMTV AND CANCER

The prototype for viral superantigens is produced by mouse mammary tumor virus (MMTV), a type B retrovirus that causes mammary tumors (15, 21, 47, 88). Although MMTV superantigens were recognized in the 1990s, they were originally described by Festenstein in 1973 as minor lymphocyte-stimulating (Mls) antigens (19). These antigens were identified by their abilities to induce proliferation in studies using lymphocytes from strains of MHC-identical mice. Mls antigens were determined to be the products of endogenous superantigens from germ line-encoded MMTV provirus (2, 9).

Initial studies of the infectivity of MMTV indicated that an intact immune system was required for infection (25). Although MMTV ultimately infects mammary gland tissue, it is ingested and initially infects B cells and T cells in the mucosa-associated lymphoid tissue. Both

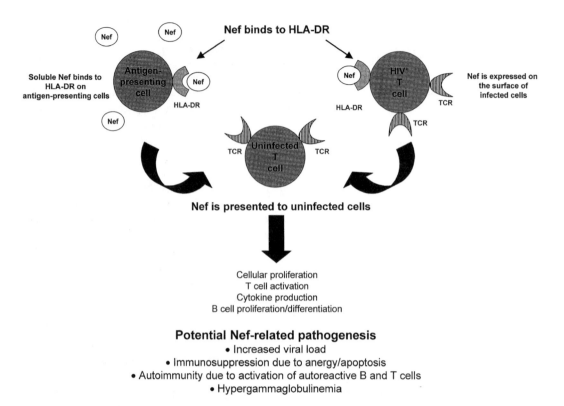

FIGURE 3 Model for the role of Nef in the pathogenesis of HIV. Soluble Nef released by lysed infected cells binds to HLA-DR on antigen-presenting cells or is an integral component of the cell membranes of infected T cells. Nef is then presented to uninfected T cells, causing proliferation and activation of T cells with concomitant cytokine production. Such proliferation results in a cellular reservoir for virus replication. Differentiation of B cells may possibly be mediated by release of T-cell cytokines.

B cells and T cells produce infectious virions (16). It has been speculated that MMTV superantigen is required for the amplification of virus replication by causing Vβ-specific-T-cell expansion, which enhances the further infection of immune cells (25).

Recently, MMTV superantigen has been implicated in the migration of infected immune cells to the mammary gland and in the subsequent efficient infection of mammary tissue (23). Low or undetectable levels of virus were found in the mammary tissue of transgenic mice expressing endogenous MMTV superantigen (and thus lacking superantigen-reactive T cells) when high virus doses were introduced directly into the mammary gland. These data indicate that immune cells are essential for the infection of mammary tissue,

which is the site for transmission of virus via milk to suckling pups. Furthermore, fewer of these transgenic mice had incidences of mammary tumors compared to nontransgenic mice, probably as a consequence of significantly lower virus levels in these animals (23). Thus, MMTV superantigen acts as a virulence factor, not only in the establishment of infection in immune cells and mammary tissue but also in the tumorigenesis of the virus.

IMMUNE-BASED THERAPIES THAT AMELIORATE SUPERANTIGEN EFFECTS

Type I IFNs

In spite of their undesirable side effects, IFNs, in particular the type I IFNs, are well established as useful drugs, and their application is likely to expand as research continues. IFN-β was approved in 1993 by the Food and Drug Administration for the treatment of the relapsing-remitting form of MS and is currently being used in that capacity (28). Despite its positive effects in ameliorating the symptomology of MS, IFN-β has undesirable side effects, including bone marrow suppression and weight loss (13, 18).

A unique type I IFN, IFN-τ, has been used in the EAE animal model (51, 52, 73, 74, 76). IFN-τ was initially identified as a pregnancy recognition hormone in sheep (3). Cloning of its cDNA and comparison with other genes showed strong homology with IFN-α (29). This led to the characterization of the antiviral activity of ovine IFN-τ, which resulted in the demonstration of some very interesting biological properties (58, 60). Ovine IFN-τ possesses antiviral activity similar to that of IFN-α across several species, including humans (60). However, unlike IFN-α and IFN-β, IFN-τ lacks toxicity for cells at high concentrations (34, 60) and does not induce weight loss or bone marrow suppression in animal models (52, 74, 76). This is a very important observation for the use of type I IFNs as therapeutics, particularly for treatment of MS.

IFN-τ, administered both intraperitoneally (i.p.) and orally, was shown to induce remission in SJL/J mice that had ongoing chronic active EAE disease and protected the mice against secondary relapses (52, 74). Treatment with IFN-τ reversed lymphocyte infiltration and microglial activation in the CNS. Lower anti-MBP antibody levels were found in IFN-τ-treated mice than in untreated mice in both the acute and chronic forms of EAE. MBP induced the proliferation of B cells in mice with EAE, but activation was blocked by either in vivo or in vitro treatment with IFN-τ. Furthermore, IFN-τ inhibited MBP activation of T cells from mice with EAE. Thus, IFN-τ inhibited both cellular and humoral immunity in EAE, possibly explaining the effectiveness of type I IFNs in the treatment of MS.

IFN-τ was shown to prevent EAE by the induction of suppressor cells and suppressor factors (51). Specifically, the protective effects

of IFN-τ are mediated, at least in part, by CD4+ Th2 suppressor cells and by the induction of suppressor factors consisting of IL-10 and transforming growth factor β by these cells (51, 74). IL-10 and transforming growth factor β were found to act synergistically to inhibit the proliferation of autoreactive T cells from mice with EAE in response to autoantigen. Furthermore, administration of IFN-τ to mice having either the chronic or relapsing-remitting form of EAE resulted in IL-10 production in vivo.

Structure studies have shown that the N terminus of IFN-τ is involved in its lack of toxicity (59, 78). After the identification of this region, a "humanized" chimera has recently been constructed, consisting of human IFN-α and the N terminus of IFN-τ. This chimeric IFN possesses potent biological activity in tissue culture but, like ovine IFN-τ, lacks the toxicity associated with IFN-α (50). This chimera has been constructed because a human IFN-τ with the properties of ovine IFN-τ has not yet been identified. A previous report of a human IFN-τ has not held up or been confirmed (87). The chimeric IFN is currently being tested in animal models.

IL-10

Studies have shown that one mechanism for the protection of mice against antigen induction of EAE and superantigen reactivation of relapses is the induction of IL-10 by type I IFNs in treated mice (51, 74). IL-10 is a Th2 cytokine that suppresses the activity of CD4+ Th1 cells (20). Antibodies to IL-10 block the protective effects of IL-10 against EAE. Focusing on cell cycle events, we have determined the effects of IL-10 on the entry of quiescent CD4+ T cells into the cell cycle upon stimulation with the staphylococcal superantigen SEB (57). IL-10 blocked cells at the G_0/G_1 phase of the cell cycle. IL-10 treatment prevented the down-regulation of $p27^{KIP1}$, an inhibitor protein that controls progression out of the G_0 phase of the cell cycle. IL-10 also prevented the upregulation of the G_1 cyclins D2 and D3, proteins necessary for entry and progression through the G_1 phase of the cell cycle. Associated with the inhibition of the cell cycle, IL-10 suppressed

SEB induction of IL-2 (57). Addition of exogenous IL-2 to IL-10-treated cells significantly reversed the antiproliferative effects of IL-10. Moreover, IL-10 effects on the early G_1 proteins p27^{KIP1} and cyclin D2 were similarly reversed by exogenous IL-2. Although this reversal by IL-2 was pronounced, it was not complete, suggesting that IL-10 may have some effects not directly related to the suppression of IL-2 production.

Cell separation experiments suggest that IL-10 can affect purified CD4$^+$ T cells directly, providing functional evidence for the presence of IL-10 receptors on these cells. Furthermore, IL-10 inhibited expression of the IL-2 transcription regulators c-fos and c-jun, which also inhibit other cell functions. The studies show that the mechanism of IL-10 regulation of quiescent CD4$^+$ T-cell activation consists mainly of blocking the induction of IL-2 that is central to down-regulation of p27^{KIP1} and up-regulation of D cyclins in T-cell activation and entry into the cell cycle (57).

The mitogen-activated protein (MAP) kinase pathway involving the kinase cascade Ras → Raf → Mek → Erk → Elk-1 is important for gene activation in T cells (64). IL-10 blocks the phosphorylation of Raf and Erk, thus inhibiting signal transduction via the MAP kinase pathway of T-cell activation (G. Q. Perrin, P. S. Subramaniam, and H. M. Johnson, unpublished data). Blockage of the MAP kinase pathway is one possible mechanism by which IL-10 blocks IL-2 induction by SEB and blocks the direct effects of SEB on T-cell activation.

POTENTIAL USE OF SUPERANTIGENS IN THE TREATMENT OF CANCER

As shown in the case of activation or reactivation of EAE, superantigens are capable of expanding populations of antigen-specific T cells. This property of superantigens can potentially be exploited in the custom treatment of some forms of cancer, specifically, in cancers where tumor-specific antigens are involved in conferring protection on the host.

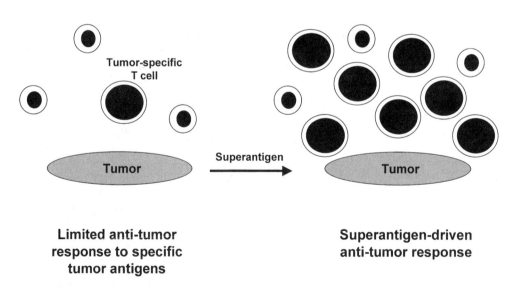

Limited anti-tumor response to specific tumor antigens

Superantigen-driven anti-tumor response

FIGURE 4 Antitumor responses in the absence and presence of superantigens. Limited antitumor responses are elicited by poorly immunogenic tumors even after vaccination with inactivated tumor cells. However, administration of superantigens after vaccination with inactivated tumor cells stimulates amplified antitumor responses, augmenting specific antitumor immunity.

Hypothetically, patients could be immunized to cancer, either naturally through the early course of the disease itself or through induction by actual injection of inactivated cancer cells. The patients could be monitored for the establishment of a pool of tumor-specific T cells. Once tumor-specific T cells were detected, superantigens could be used to expand these cells to enhance their activity with the expectation of protection against the tumor (Fig. 4). Tumor-specific T cells should not become anergized in this situation because they would already have been activated by tumor-specific antigens prior to encountering superantigens.

The above scenario has been tested with a mouse melanoma model (A. C. Hobeika, S. L. Kominsky, B. Torres, and H. M. Johnson, unpublished data). Initially, mice were administered inactivated B16F10 mouse melanoma cells and injected 4 days later with a combination of SEA and SEB or sham injected. After 24 h, the mice were challenged with live melanoma cells. The mice were evaluated for metastases to the lung. Preliminary data indicate that mice administered superantigens did not have lung metastases, whereas all control mice were positive (Table 2). These results are encouraging and suggest that the immune activation properties of superantigens can be used to amplify immune responses in a host to combat tumors and, possibly, infectious agents, including persistent bacterial pathogens.

CONCLUSIONS

During the course of infection with a superantigen-elaborating microbe, the host immune system can be activated in a polyclonal fashion, resulting in massive cytokine production. The long-term effects of superantigen activation of T cells can include the induction of autoreactive cells, leading to an autoimmune state. Superantigens can also cause relapses into disease in patients with remission. Another ramification of superantigen activation of the immune system is anergy or deletion of specific subsets of T cells, resulting in an immunodeficient state.

Current immunologic therapies for autoimmune disorders include the type I IFNs. Evidence indicates that the IFNs function by establishing a network of suppressor cells that produce factors that dampen the activity of autoreactive immune cells. Both cellular and humoral autoimmune responses are reduced. Furthermore, IFN-τ, a novel IFN that possesses the beneficial features of other type I IFNs but lacks the toxicity associated with them, ameliorates both the chronic and relapsing-remitting forms of EAE, the animal models

TABLE 2 Effect of staphylococcal superantigens on B16F10 melanoma tumor growth

Treatment group	Vaccination dosage (no. of B16F10 cells)	No. of mice positive for lung metastases/total	Day of death (mean ± SD)	No. of survivors/total (% survival)
Expt 1[a]				
PBS[b] (control)	10^6	4/4		
SEA–SEB	10^6	0/4		
Expt 2[c]				
PBS	0		16.1 ± 1.4	2/4 (50)
PBS	10^6		16.0 ± 1.0	3/6 (50)
SEA–SEB	10^6			6/6 (100)

[a] C57BL/6 mice were vaccinated i.p. with 10^6 inactivated B16F10 melanoma cells 4 days prior to treatment with PBS (control) or 25 μg each of SEA and SEB. The mice were then challenged the following day with 5×10^5 live B16F10 cells via tail vein injection. The mice were killed 16 days later for evaluation of lung metastases.
[b] PBS, phosphate-buffered saline.
[c] C57BL/6 mice were vaccinated with 0 or 10^6 inactivated B16F10 melanoma cells 5 days prior to i.p. challenge with 5×10^5 live cells. The mice in the last group were administered SEA and SEB (25 μg each) 1 day prior to live-cell challenge. The mice were monitored over the course of 18 days for death, which is the expected outcome of i.p. administration of live-cell challenge.

of MS. IFN-τ is being tested in phase I clinical trials. Also, studies of a humanized form of IFN-τ are under way.

The profound activation of the immune system by superantigens can be exploited to increase beneficial antitumor immune responses. Such studies could be expanded to determine the possible benefits of using superantigens in vaccination protocols against pathogens, particularly in those instances where vaccines elicit mediocre immune responses. Ongoing studies on cancer are preliminary in nature but may help in establishing novel therapies for human diseases.

REFERENCES

1. **Abe, J., B. L. Kotzin, K. Jujo, M. E. Melish, M. P. Glode, T. Kohsaka, and D. Y. M. Leung.** 1992. Selective expansion of T cells expressing T cell receptor variable region Vβ2 and Vβ8 in Kawasaki's disease. *Proc. Natl. Acad. Sci. USA* **89**:4066–4070.

2. **Acha-Orbea, H., A. N. Shakhov, L. Scarpellino, E. Kolb, V. Muller, A. Vessaz-Shaw, R. Fuchs, K. Blochinger, P. Rollini, J. Billote, M. Sarafidou, and H. R. MacDonald.** 1992. Clonal deletion of Vβ14-bearing T cells in mice transgenic for mouse mammary tumor virus. *Nature* **350**:207–211.

3. **Bazer, F. W., J. L. Vallet, R. M. Roberts, D. C. Sharp, and W. W. Thatcher.** 1986. Role of conceptus secretory products in establishment of pregnancy. *J. Reprod. Fertil.* **76**:841–850.

4. **Bergdoll, M. S.** 1985. The staphylococcal enterotoxins—an update, p. 247–266. *In* J. Jelaszewics (ed.), *The Staphylococci.* Gustav Fisher Verlag, New York, N.Y.

5. **Brocke, S., A. Gaur, C. Piercy, A. Gautam, K. Gijbels, C. G. Fathman, and L. Steinman.** 1993. Induction of relapsing paralysis in experimental allergic encephalomyelitis by bacterial superantigen. *Nature* **365**:642–644.

6. **Callahan, J. E., A. Herman, J. Kappler, and P. Marrack.** 1990. Stimulation of B110.BR T cells with superantigenic staphylococcal enterotoxins. *J. Immunol.* **144**:2473–2479.

7. **Carlsson, R., and H. O. Sjogren.** 1985. Kinetics of IL-2 and IFNγ production, expression of IL-2 receptors, and cell proliferation in human mononuclear cells exposed to SEA. *Cell. Immunol.* **96**:175–183.

8. **Chirmule, N., N. Oyaizu, C. Saxinger, and S. Pahwa.** 1994. Nef protein of HIV-1 has B cell stimulatory activity. *AIDS* **8**:733–739.

9. **Choi, Y., J. W. Kappler, and P. Marrack.** 1992. A superantigen encoded in the open reading frame of the 3′ long terminal repeat of mouse mammary tumor virus. *Nature* **350**:203–207.

10. **Cole, B. C., and M. M. Griffiths.** 1993. Triggering and exacerbation of autoimmune arthritis by the *Mycoplasma arthritidis* superantigen MAM. *Arthritis Rheum.* **36**:994–1002.

11. **Conrad, B., E. Weldmann, G. Trucco, W. A. Rudert, R. Behboo, C. Ricordi, H. Rodriquez-Rilo, D. Finegold, and M. Trucco.** 1994. Evidence for superantigen involvement in insulin-dependent diabetes mellitus aetiology. *Nature* **371**:351–355.

12. **Conrad, B., R. N. Weissmahr, J. Boni, R. Arcari, J. Schupbach, and B. Mach.** 1997. A human endogenous retroviral superantigen as candidate autoimmune gene in type I diabetes. *Cell* **90**:303–313.

13. **Degre, M.** 1974. Influence of exogenous interferon on the peripheral white blood cell count in mice. *Int. J. Cancer* **14**:699–703.

14. **D'Orazio, J. A., and J. Stein-Streilein.** 1996. Human natural killer (NK) cells present staphylococcal enterotoxin B (SEB) to T lymphocytes. *Clin. Exp. Immunol.* **104**:366–373.

15. **Dyson, P. J., A. M. Knight, S. Fairchild, E. Simpson, and K. Tomonari.** 1991. Genes encoding ligands for deletion of Vβ11 T cells cosegregate with mouse mammary tumour virus genomes. *Nature* **349**:531–532.

16. **Dzuris, J. L., T. V. Golovkina, and S. R. Ross.** 1997. Both T and B cells shed infectious mouse mammary tumor virus. *J. Virol.* **71**:6044–6048.

17. **Edelman, A. S., and S. Zolla-Pazner.** 1989. AIDS: a syndrome of immune dysregulation, dysfunction, and deficiency. *FASEB J.* **3**:22–29.

18. **Fent, K., and G. Zbinden.** 1987. Toxicity of interferon and interleukin. *Trends Pharmacol. Sci.* **8**:100–105.

19. **Festenstein, H.** 1973. Immunogenetic and biological aspects of in vitro lymphocyte allotransformation (MLR) in the mouse. *Transplant. Rev.* **15**:62–88.

20. **Fiorentino, D. F., M. W. Bond, and T. R. Mosmann.** 1989. Two types of mouse T helper cell. IV. Th2 clones secrete a factor that inhibits cytokine production by Th1 clones. *J. Exp. Med.* **170**:2081–2095.

21. **Frankel, W. N., C. Rudy, J. M. Coffin, and B. T. Huber.** Linkage of Mls genes to endogenous mammary tumor viruses of inbred mice. *Nature* **349**:526–528.

22. **Fritz, R. B., C. H. Chou, and D. E. McFarlin.** 1983. Relapsing murine experimental allergic encephalomyelitis induced by myelin basic protein. *J. Immunol.* **130**:1024–1026.

23. **Golovkina, T. V., J. P. Dudley, and S. R. Ross.** 1998. Superantigen activity is needed for mouse mammary tumor virus spread within the mammary gland. *J. Immunol.* **161:**2375–2382.

24. **He, X., J. J. Goronzy, and C. M. Weyand.** 1993. The repertoire of rheumatoid factor producing B cells in normal subjects and patients with rheumatoid arthritis. *Arthritis Rheum.* **36:** 1061–1069.

25. **Held, W., H. Acha-Orbea, H. R. MacDonald, and G. A. Waanders.** 1994. Superantigens and retroviral infection: insights from mouse mammary tumor virus. *Immunol. Today* **15:** 184–190.

26. **Hofer, M. F., R. J. Harbeck, P. M. Schlievert, and D. Y. M. Leung.** 1999. Staphylococcal toxins augment specific IgE responses by atopic patients exposed to allergen. *J. Investig. Dermatol.* **112:**171–176.

27. **Hugin, A. W., M. S. Vacchio, and H. C. Morse III.** 1991. A virus-encoded "superantigen" in a retrovirus-induced immunodeficiency syndrome of mice. *Science* **252:**424–427.

28. **IFNβ Multiple Sclerosis Study Group.** 1993. IFNβ-1b is effective in relapsing-remitting multiple sclerosis. I. Clinical results of a multicenter, randomized, double-blind, placebo-controlled trial. *Neurology* **43:**655–661.

29. **Imakawa, K., R. V. Anthony, M. Kezemi, K. R. Marotti, H. G. Polites, and R. M. Roberts.** 1987. Interferon-like sequence of ovine trophoblast protein secreted by embryonic trophectoderm. *Nature* **330:**377–379.

30. **Imberti, L., A. Sottini, A. Bettinardi, M. Puoti, and D. Primi.** 1991. Selective depletion in HIV infection of T cells that bear specific T cell receptor V beta sequences. *Science* **254:**860–862.

31. **Johnson, H. M., and H. I. Magazine.** 1988. Potent mitogenic activity of staphylococcal enterotoxin A requires induction of interleukin 2. *Int. Arch. Allergy Appl. Immunol.* **87:**87–90.

32. **Kalman, B., F. D. Lublin, E. Lattime, J. Joseph, and R. L. Knobler.** 1993. Effects of staphylococcal enterotoxin B on T cell receptor Vβ utilization and clinical manifestations of experimental allergic encephalomyelitis. *J. Neuroimmunol.* **45:**83–88.

33. **Kawabe, Y., and A. Ochi.** 1990. Selective anergy of V beta 8⁺, CD4⁺ T cells in Staphylococcus enterotoxin B-primed mice. *J. Exp. Med.* **172:** 1065–1070.

34. **Khan, O. A., H. Jiang, P. S. Subramaniam, H. M. Johnson, and S. S. Dhib-Jalbut.** 1998. Immunomodulating functions of recombinant ovine interferon tau: potential for therapy in multiple sclerosis and autoimmune disorders. *Mult. Scler.* **4:**63–69.

35. **Kotzin, B. L., D. Y. M. Leung, J. Kappler, and P. Marrack.** 1993. Superantigens and their potential role in human disease. *Adv. Immunol.* **54:** 99–166.

36. **Kraft, M., S. Filsinger, K. L. Kramer, D. Kabelitz, G. M. Hansch, and M. Schoels.** 1998. Synovial fibroblasts as target cells for staphylococcal enterotoxin-induced T-cell cytotoxicity. *Immunology* **93:**20–25.

37. **Kumar, V., F. Aziz, E. Sercarz, and A. Miller.** 1997. Regulatory T cells specific for the same framework 3 region of the Vbeta 8.2 chain are involved in the control of collagen II-induced arthritis and experimental allergic encephalomyelitis. *J. Exp. Med.* **185:**1725–1733.

38. **Lafon, M., and A. Galleli.** 1996. Superantigen related to rabies. *Springer Semin. Immunopathol.* **17:** 307–318.

39. **Lafon, M., M. Lafarge, A. Martinez-Arends, R. Ramirez, F. Vuiller, D. Charron, V. Lotteau, and D. Scott-Algara.** 1992. Evidence for a viral superantigen in humans. *Nature* **358:** 507–510.

40. **Langford, M. P., G. J. Stanton, and H. M. Johnson.** 1978. Biological effects of staphylococcal enterotoxin A on human peripheral lymphocytes. *Infect. Immun.* **22:**62–68.

41. **Laurence, J., A. S. Hodstev, and D. N. Posnett.** 1992. Superantigen implicated in dependence of HIV-1 replication in T cells on TCR Vβ expression. *Nature* **358:**255–258.

42. **Lehmann, P. V., T. Forsthuber, A. Miller, and E. E. Sercarz.** 1992. Spreading of T cell autoimmunity to cryptic determinants of an autoantigen. *Nature* **358:**155–157.

43. **Leung, D. Y., J. B. Travers, R. Giorno, D. A. Norris, R. Skinner, J. Aelion, L. V. Kazemi, M. H. Kim, A. E. Trumble, M. Kotb, and P. M. Schlievert.** 1995. Evidence for a streptococcal superantigen-driven process in acute guttate psoriasis. *J. Clin. Investig.* **96:**2106–2112.

44. **Mahlknecht, U., M. Herter, M. K. Hoffmann, D. Niethammer, and G. E. Dannecker.** 1996. The toxic shock syndrome toxin-1 induces anergy in human T cells in vivo. *Hum. Immunol.* **45:**42–45.

45. **Makida, R., M. F. Hofer, K. Takase, J. C. Cambier, and D. Y. Leung.** 1996. Bacterial superantigens induce Vβ-specific T cell receptor internalization. *Mol. Immunol.* **33:**891–900.

46. **Marrack, P., and J. Kappler.** 1990. The staphylococcal enterotoxins and their relatives. *Science* **248:**705–711.

47. **Marrack, P., E. Kushnir, and J. Kappler.** 1991. A maternally inherited superantigen encoded by a mammary tumor virus. *Nature* **349:** 524–526.

48. **Matsumoto, Y., and M. Fujiwara.** 1993. Immunomodulation of experimental autoimmune encephalomyelitis by staphylococcal enterotoxin D. *Cell. Immunol.* **149:**268–278.

49. **Mollick, J. A., R. G. Cook, and R. R. Rich.** 1989. Class II MHC molecules are specific receptors for staphylococcal enterotoxin A. *Science* **244:** 817–820.

50. **Mujtaba, M. G., and H. M. Johnson.** 1999. IFNτ inhibits IgE production in a murine model of allergy and in an IgE-producing human myeloma cell line. *J. Allergy Clin. Immunol.* **104:** 1037–1044.

51. **Mujtaba, M. G., J. M. Soos, and H. M. Johnson.** 1997. CD4 T suppressor cells mediate interferon tau protection against experimental allergic encephalomyelitis. *J. Neuroimmunol.* **75:**35–42.

52. **Mujtaba, M. G., W. J. Streit, and H. M. Johnson.** 1998. IFN-tau suppresses both the autoreactive humoral and cellular immune responses and induces stable remission in mice with chronic experimental allergic encephalomyelitis. *Cell. Immunol.* **186:**94–102.

53. **Nagai, H., Y. Takoka, H. Kamada, and H. Mori.** 1994. The model of arthritis induced by superantigen in mice. *Life Sci.* **55:**PL233–PL237.

54. **Ohmen, J. D., P. F. Barnes, C. L. Grisso, B. R. Bloom, and R. L. Modlin.** 1994. Evidence for a superantigen in human tuberculosis. *Immunity* **1:**35–43.

55. **Paliard, X., S. G. West, J. A. Lafferty, J. R. Clements, J. W. Kappler, P. Marrack, and B. L. Kotzin.** 1991. Evidence for the effects of a superantigen in rheumatoid arthritis. *Science* **253:** 325–329.

56. **Peavy, D. L., W. H. Adler, and R. T. Smith.** 1970. Mitogenic effects of endotoxin and SEB on mouse spleen cells and human lymphocytes. *J. Immunol.* **105:**1453–1458.

57. **Perrin, G. Q., H. M. Johnson, and P. S. Subramaniam.** 1999. Mechanism of interleukin-10 inhibition of T-helper cell activation by superantigen at the level of the cell cycle. *Blood* **93:** 208–216.

58. **Pontzer, C. H., F. W. Bazer, and H. M. Johnson.** 1991. Antiproliferative activity of a pregnancy recognition hormone, ovine trophoblast protein-1. *Cancer Res.* **51:**5304–5307.

59. **Pontzer, C. H., T. L. Ott, F. W. Bazer, and H. M. Johnson.** 1994. Structure/function studies with IFN tau: evidence for multiple active sites. *J. Interferon Res.* **14:**133–141.

60. **Pontzer, C. H., B. A. Torres, J. L. Vallet, F. W. Bazer, and H. M. Johnson.** 1988. Antiviral activity of the pregnancy recognition hormone ovine trophoblast protein-1. *Biochem. Biophys. Res. Commun.* **152:**801–807.

61. **Rebai, N., G. Pantaleo, J. F. Demarest, C. Ciuril, H. Soudeyns, J. W. Adelsberger, M. Vaccarezza, R. E. Walker, R. P. Sekaly, and A. S. Fauci.** 1994. Analysis of the TCR Vβ repertoire in monozygotic twins discordant for HIV. *Proc. Natl. Acad. Sci. USA* **91:**1529–1533.

62. **Russell, J. K., C. H. Pontzer, and H. M. Johnson.** 1990. The I-Aβb region (65–85) is a binding site for the superantigen staphylococcal enterotoxin A. *Biochem. Biophys. Res. Commun.* **168:**696–701.

63. **Russell, J. K., C. H. Pontzer, and H. M. Johnson.** 1991. Both α-helices along the major histocompatibility complex binding cleft are required for staphylococcal enterotoxin A function. *Proc. Natl. Acad. Sci. USA* **88:**7228–7232.

64. **Schaeffer, H. J., and M. J. Weber.** 1999. Mitogen-activated protein kinases: specific messages from ubiquitous messengers. *Mol. Cell. Biol.* **19:** 2435–2444.

65. **Schiffenbauer, J., H. M. Johnson, E. Butfiloski, L. Wegrzyn, and J. M. Soos.** 1993. Staphylococcal enterotoxins reactivate experimental allergic encephalomyelitis. *Proc. Natl. Acad. Sci. USA* **90:**8543–8546.

66. **Schiffenbauer, J., J. M. Soos, and H. M. Johnson.** 1998. The possible role of bacterial superantigens in the pathogenesis of autoimmune disorders. *Immunol. Today* **19:**117–120.

67. **Schlievert, P. M.** 1993. Role of superantigens in human disease. *J. Infect. Dis.* **167:**997–1002.

68. **Schnittman, S. M., and A. C. Fauci.** 1994. Human immunodeficiency virus and acquired immunodeficiency syndrome: an update. *Adv. Intern. Med.* **39:**305–355.

69. **Schwab, J. H., R. R. Brown, S. K. Anderle, and P. M. Schlievert.** 1993. Superantigen can reactivate bacterial cell wall-induced arthritis. *J. Immunol.* **150:**4151–4159.

70. **Sercarz, E. E., P. V. Lehman, A. Ametani, G. Benichou, A. Miller, and K. Moudgil.** 1993. Dominance and crypticity of T cell antigenic determinants. *Annu. Rev. Immunol.* **11:** 729–766.

71. **Solem, J. H., and J. Lassen.** 1971. Reiter's disease following *Yersinia enterocolitica* infection. *Scand. J. Infect. Dis.* **3:**83–85.

72. **Soos, J. M., A. C. Hobeika, E. J. Butfiloski, J. Schiffenbauer, and H. M. Johnson.** 1995. Accelerated induction of experimental allergic encephalomyelitis in PL/J mice by a non-Vβ8-specific superantigen. *Proc. Natl. Acad. Sci. USA* **92:** 6082–6086.

73. **Soos, J. M., and H. M. Johnson.** 1995. Type I IFN inhibition of superantigen stimulation: implications for treatment of superantigen associated disease. *J. Interferon Res.* **15:**39–45.

74. Soos, J. M., M. G. Mujtaba, P. S. Subramaniam, W. J. Streit, and H. M. Johnson. 1997. Oral feeding of interferon τ can prevent the acute and relapsing forms of experimental allergic encephalomyelitis. *J. Neuroimmunol.* **75**:43–50.

75. Soos, J. M., J. Schiffenbauer, and H. M. Johnson. 1993. Treatment of PL/J mice with the superantigen, staphylococcal enterotoxin B, prevents development of experimental allergic encephalomyelitis. *J. Neuroimmunol.* **43**:39–43.

76. Soos, J. M., P. S. Subramanlam, A. C. Hobeika, J. Schiffenbauer, and H. M. Johnson. 1995. The pregnancy recognition hormone, IFN tau, blocks both development and superantigen reactivation of experimental allergic encephalomyelitis without associated toxicity. *J. Immunol.* **155**:2747–2753.

77. Stohl, W., J. E. Elliot, and P. S. Linsley. 1994. Human T cell-dependent B cell differentiation induced by staphylococcal superantigens. *J. Immunol.* **153**:117–127.

78. Subramaniam, P. S., S. A. Khan, C. H. Pontzer, and H. M. Johnson. 1995. Differential recognition of the type I interferon receptor by interferons τ and α is responsible for their disparate cytotoxicities. *Proc. Natl. Acad. Sci. USA* **92**:12270–12274.

79. Sutkowski, N., T. Palkama, C. Ciurli, R.-P. Sekaly, D. A. Thorley-Lawson, and B. T. Huber. 1996. An Epstein-Barr virus-associated superantigen. *J. Exp. Med.* **184**:971–980.

80. Tanabe, T., B. A. Torres, P. S. Subramaniam, and H. M. Johnson. 1997. Vβ activation by HIV Nef protein: detection by a simple amplification procedure. *Biochem. Biophys. Res. Commun.* **230**:509–513.

81. Torres, B. A., T. Tanabe, and H. M. Johnson. 1996. Characterization of Nef-induced CD4 T cell proliferation. *Biochem. Biophys. Res. Commun.* **225**:54–61.

82. Torres, B. A., T. Tanabe, J. K. Yamamoto, and H. M. Johnson. 1996. HIV encodes for its own CD4 T cell superantigen mitogen. *Biochem. Biophys. Res. Commun.* **225**:672–678.

83. Uchiyama, T., T. Miyoshi-Akiyama, H. Kato, W. Fujimaki, K. Imanishi, and X. Yan. 1993. Superantigenic properties of a novel mitogenic substance produced by *Yersinia pseudotuberculosis* isolated from patients manifesting acute and systemic symptoms. *J. Immunol.* **151**:4407–4413.

84. Valdimarsson, H., B. S. Baker, I. Jonsdottir, A. Powles, and L. Fry. 1995. Psoriasis: a T-cell-mediated autoimmune disease induced by streptococcal superantigens? *Immunol. Today* **16**:145–149.

85. Valdimarsson, H., H. Sigmundsdottir, and I. Jonsdottir. 1997. Is psoriasis induced by streptococcal superantigens and maintained by M-protein-specific T cells that cross-react with keratin? *Clin. Exp. Immunol.* **107**(Suppl. 1):21–24.

86. Watanabe-Ohnishi, R., J. Aelion, L. LeGros, M. A. Tomai, E. V. Sokurenko, D. Newton, J. Takahara, S. Irino, S. Rashed, and M. Kotb. 1994. Characterization of unique human TCR V beta specificities for a family of streptococcal superantigens represented by rheumatogenic serotypes of M protein. *J. Immunol.* **152**:2066–2073.

87. Whaley, A. E., C. S. Meka, L. A. Harbison, J. S. Hunt, and K. Imakawa. 1994. Identification and cellular localization of unique interferon mRNA from human placenta. *J. Biol. Chem.* **269**:10864–10868.

88. Woodland, D. L., M. P. Happ, K. J. Gollub, and E. Palmer. 1991. An endogenous retrovirus mediating deletion of αβ T cells? *Nature* **349**:529–530.

89. Zamvil, S. S., and L. Steinman. 1990. The T lymphocyte in experimental allergic encephalomyelitis. *Annu. Rev. Immunol.* **8**:579–621.

PERSISTENT
BACTERIAL
PATHOGENS

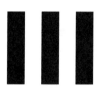

NEISSERIA GONORRHOEAE: ADAPTATION AND SURVIVAL IN THE UROGENITAL TRACT

Ann E. Jerse

11

OVERVIEW OF GONOCOCCAL PATHOGENESIS

Colonization of the Lower Urogenital Tract

Uncomplicated gonorrhea is most commonly an acute urogenital infection involving the urethra in men and the endocervix in women of reproductive age. The female urethra may also be infected, and rectal and pharyngeal gonococcal infection can occur in either sex (29, 99). In prepubescent girls (128, 205) and postmenopausal women (119), gonorrhea often manifests as vaginitis rather than cervicitis, most likely due to age-related differences in the histology of the endocervical region and the more hospitable vaginal pH of females that are not under the influence of estrogen (22). Upon entering the urogenital tract, *Neisseria gonorrhoeae* adheres to columnar epithelial cells, a step that presumably enables the gonococcus to withstand the flushing force of urine and the constant shedding of cervical mucus (Fig. 1). Adherence to human epithelial cells is mediated by colonization pili (139, 173, 189, 220) and a family of antigenically variable outer membrane proteins called opacity (Opa) proteins (14, 124, 209). The human membrane cofactor protein (CD46) serves as the receptor for gonococcal pili (111), and interestingly, this molecule also serves as the host cell receptor for the measles virus (58). Gonococcal Opa proteins bind to host CD66 glycoproteins, a subset of the carcinoembryonic antigen family (40, 234, 235). Opa-mediated adherence can induce bacterial uptake by both epithelial cells and neutrophils (reviewed in reference 55). Evidence that *N. gonorrhoeae* invades epithelial cells during infection is based on the visualization of gonococci within urethral and cervical cells from infected patients (4, 239, 240) and within the subepithelium of endometrial tissue excised from an infected woman during the 10th week of the disease (86). The identification of *N. gonorrhoeae* as a facultatively intracellular pathogen of nonprofessional phagocytes is further supported by tissue culture invasion assays (14, 88, 153, 186, 206, 209). Studies with polarized epithelial cell monolayers (101, 147, 153, 237) suggest that intracellular gonococci invade the subepithelium via traversal through epithelial cells. Entry into the subepithelial space may promote access to the bloodstream, resulting in disseminated gonococcal infection (DGI).

Ann E. Jerse, Department of Microbiology and Immunology, Uniformed Services University of the Health Sciences, Bethesda, MD 20814.

Persistent Bacterial Infections, Edited by J. P. Nataro, M. J. Blaser, and S. Cunningham-Rundles, © 2000 ASM Press, Washington, D.C.

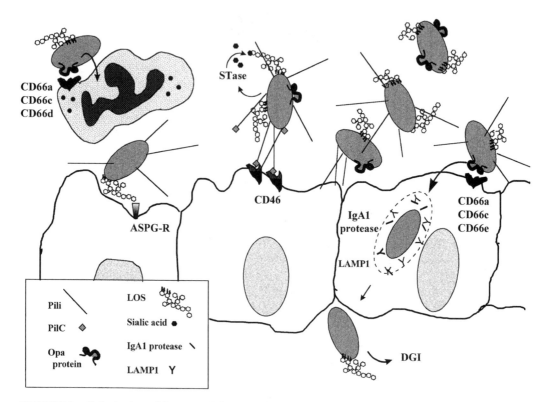

FIGURE 1 Colonization of the urogenital mucosa by *N. gonorrhoeae*. Initial bacterial adherence to the urethral or cervical mucosa is mediated by gonococcal pili. Gonococcal pili are composed of the antigenically variable pilin subunit PilE and several pilin-associated proteins, including the tip-associated adhesin PilC (reviewed in reference 228). Adherence to the CD46 receptor via the tip-associated PilC adhesin is depicted, although it has not yet been reported if the PilC adhesin binds to this receptor. Adherence capabilities are also inherent in the PilE subunit (194). Binding between Opa proteins and members of the CD66 family expressed on epithelial cells can occur with or without uptake, depending on the particular Opa protein and CD66 receptor involved. Opa-mediated adherence to CD66 receptors on neutrophils can result in nonopsonic uptake. Opa proteins differ in the capacity to bind to various members of the CD66 family, thereby conferring tropism for different cells. Some Opa proteins utilize heparin sulfate molecules to mediate invasion of epithelial cells; entry via Opa protein-heparin sulfate-vitronectin interactions has also been reported (reviewed in reference 55). Expression of gonococcal pili, Opa proteins, and LOS undergoes phase and antigenic variation. This characteristic is represented by gonococci having different combinations of these molecules and expressing LOSs of different lengths. Binding of a gonococcal LOS variant expressing a terminal lacto-*N*-neotetraose molecule to the asialoglycoprotein receptor (ASPG-R) is also shown (172). Sialylation of the terminal galactose in this tetrasaccharide, an event that is catalyzed by the gonococcal sialyltransferase (STase) (137), blocks gonococcal epithelial cell invasion by an unknown mechanism (233). Intracellular replication and survival are enhanced by the cleavage of LAMP1, a late endosomal maturation protein, by IgA1 protease (132). A nonpiliated gonococcus is shown traversing the cell, based on reports that piliation impedes traversal (147) or is lost (101) during this process. Passage of the gonococcus to the subepithelium may ultimately provide access to the bloodstream, leading to DGI.

Locally Disseminated (Ascended) Infection

Ascension of *N. gonorrhoeae* from the lower to the upper genital tract can lead to epididymitis in males and endometritis, salpingitis, and pelvic peritonitis in females. The general term for any combination of these upper reproductive tract infections in females is pelvic inflammatory disease (PID) (243). Gonococci selectively adhere to nonciliated secretory cells of the fallopian tubes, as opposed to ciliated cells, and invade the subepithelium via passage through epithelial cells and between neighboring cells. Exfoliation of ciliated cells and decreased ciliary activity occur due to the toxic effects of gonococcal lipooligosaccharide (LOS) and peptidoglycan fragments (reviewed in reference 216). Infertility may result from irreversible damage to the tissues of the upper reproductive tract. Other postinfection complications include chronic pelvic pain and ectopic pregnancy, a life-threatening condition that results from scarring of the fallopian tubes (99). Gonococcal PID often occurs within a week after menses (168, 223). It is not known how this nonmotile pathogen ascends to the upper reproductive tract; avenues such as refluxed menstrual blood or travel attached to spermatozoa have been hypothesized (29). Ascended infection in females is relatively common, occurring in 10 to 20% of women with acute gonococcal cervicitis (99).

Systemically Disseminated Gonococcal Infection

DGI occurs in 0.5 to 3.0% of patients with untreated mucosal infection. Hematogenous spread of *N. gonorrhoeae* to the joints and/or skin results in acute arthritis and dermatitis, respectively (52, 96, 115). Endocarditis is an uncommon but serious manifestation of DGI (227), and gonococcal meningitis is rare (193). Interestingly, as with PID, a high percentage of DGI in women occurs within a week after menstruation (96).

PERSISTENT INFECTION

The first laboratory advance towards a clearer understanding of gonorrhea was Albert Neisser's 1879 description of diplococci that "lie in the outer layers of leukocytes" in clinical exudates and were "separated by a space about a diameter of a coccus" (112). An increased awareness of the proportions of the gonorrhea epidemic soon followed. As described in *No Magic Bullet*, Allan M. Brandt's excellent chronology of the social history of venereal disease in the United States, the impact of latent gonococcal infections on society through increased sterility rates, the devastation to women's health, and the threat to the institution of marriage was increasingly appreciated by physicians at the turn of the century (25). Today, despite an enormous body of knowledge concerning the pathogenesis of *N. gonorrhoeae*, gonorrhea remains highly prevalent: it is the second most common reportable infectious disease in the United States (37) and has a high incidence in the developing world (5). *N. gonorrhoeae* continues to take a high toll on society in terms of public cost and the degree of morbidity and mortality it inflicts upon women (232, 241).

The capacity of *N. gonorrhoeae* to persist within an individual and within a community is truly a major strength of this organism as a pathogen. Although a specific immune response is induced during gonococcal urogenital infection (reviewed in reference 32), the response lacks effectiveness, as evidenced by the high incidence of repeated infections with the same serovar (31, 69, 95) or strain (66). The high rate of asymptomatic gonococcal infection suggests that *N. gonorrhoeae* has also evolved mechanisms for avoiding the induction of inflammation and for coexisting with the host commensal flora. Although the presence of discharge does not promote abstinence from sexual activity in a high percentage of infected individuals (231), long-term asymptomatic colonization by *N. gonorrhoeae* is the primary obstacle to controlling the spread of gonorrhea.

Men with symptomatic gonococcal urethritis develop symptoms within 1 to 14 days following exposure, with an average incubation time of 2 to 5 days. Women typically develop symptomatic infection within 10 days after exposure (29, 99). The diagnosis of gonorrhea in women is often difficult because the symptoms are not always distinct from those of other sexually transmitted infections or of the many causes of vaginitis. Reported rates of asymptomatic infection in females range from 19 to 80% (15, 142, 167). It is estimated that 1 to 3% of urethral infections in men are asymptomatic (99), although rates as high as 10 to 68% have been reported (85, 161, 207). Many infected men develop only minimal discharge (207). The wide variation in the reported rates of asymptomatic gonorrhea reflects a bias in the populations being studied. Rates of asymptomatic infection derived from the screening of outpatients tend to be higher than those based on patients in acute-care settings, since the latter group is often in search of treatment in response to signs of infection (99). The incidence of asymptomatic infection may also be influenced by the genetic makeup of the predominant strains within a community being surveyed. For example, gonococcal strains of the $A^-H^-U^-$ auxotype (requiring arginine, hypoxanthine, and uracil for in vitro growth) and the PorA (P.IA) serovar were implicated as being commonly associated with asymptomatic urethritis in men and with DGI (51, 211). Interestingly, a decline in the prevalence of this auxotype and serovar is associated with a decrease in the incidence of DGI in some regions (187).

Spontaneous cure of symptomatic infection in men occurs after several weeks; however, asymptomatic carriage of N. gonorrhoeae may persist for longer periods of time. In the often-cited study of gonococcal urethritis by Handsfield et al. (85), asymptomatic males were colonized for as long as 6 months and those that developed symptoms were colonized for as long as 90 days, with a median of 3 weeks reported for each group. Others have reported urethral colonization in males for as long as 56 days (161). A caveat in interpreting data regarding persistent gonococcal infection is that long duration of colonization may in fact reflect re-infection rather than sustained infection from a single exposure. This is particularly true for

data in which the date and frequency of potential exposures are based on patient interviews. Among men in whom the risk of re-exposure to N. gonorrhoeae was minimized, 97% of 81 men developed symptoms within 3 days following exposure while the remaining man developed symptoms 14 days following exposure (87). Urogenital infections in women lasting at least 13 to 21 days following treatment failure have been documented (134). Longer episodes of persistent infection may also occur in women, based on descriptions of women with gonococcal salpingitis for 10 months due to inadequate treatment or for 8 weeks following delivery of a child with gonococcal conjunctivitis (179). Gonococcal infections of nongenital mucosa are noteworthy for both the tendency to be asymptomatic and the duration of colonization. It is estimated that the majority (79 to 100%) of pharyngeal infections (30, 236) and 18 to 40% of rectal infections (54, 130, 175, 245) are asymptomatic and that pharyngeal infections can last for at least 10 weeks if left untreated (236). Although persistent gonococcal infections are not associated with immunopathology or neoplasia, an increased risk of DGI is associated with asymptomatic urethritis in men and with asymptomatic cervicitis (96) and pharyngeal infections (96, 245). Case studies of both men and women in whom gonococcal arthritis developed several months following urogenital gonococcal infection have also been described (215).

MECHANISMS OF PERSISTENCE

General Overview

N. gonorrhoeae is well equipped to avoid and/or capitalize on host factors encountered during urogenital infection. Transcriptional regulation of genes in response to environmental stimuli in the mucus layer may coordinate adaptation of this pathogen to nutritionally different microenvironments and to physiological stress induced by nonspecific host defenses. Iron limitation is the best-studied stimulus for gonococcal gene expression, as discussed below. Oxygen- and pH-regulated proteins have also been identified (41, 42, 165, 166), but other environmental stimuli remain largely unexplored. Taha et al. (224) reported that a two-component system (*pilA*-*pilB*) regulates the expression of pilin. Arvidson et al. (8), however, were unable to detect regulation of pilin expression by *pilA* and instead demonstrated that *pilA* (which is highly homologous to the *ftsY* gene of *Escherichia coli*) is involved in protein maturation. Multiple sigma factors exist in *N. gonorrhoeae* (120), and promoter regions that contain sigma factor consensus sequences have been described for several genes (20, 72, 129, 163). However, with the exception of oxygen limitation (100), the environmental conditions that trigger regulation by sigma factors are not well defined.

A second means by which *N. gonorrhoeae* survives within the host is through its remarkable capacity to exhibit high-frequency, reversible-phase, and antigenic variation of surface molecules. Early clues as to the resourcefulness of *N. gonorrhoeae* in this respect were revealed in the 1960s by Douglas Kellogg and his colleagues at the Communicable Disease Center in Atlanta, Ga. In two landmark papers published in the *Journal of Bacteriology* Kellogg et al. (113, 114) documented the occurrence of reversible changes in gonococcal colony morphology and demonstrated an association between particular colony phenotypes and virulence through experimental inoculation of male volunteers. Kellogg's careful scrutiny of colony morphology inspired an exciting period of discovery during which the genetic basis of antigenic and phase variation of gonococcal surface phenotypes was explored. Through this mechanism, *N. gonorrhoeae* maintains subpopulations of antigenically different variants that may facilitate immune evasion within an individual, as well as ensuring that each new host will be immunologically naïve. A reservoir of functionally different phenotypes is also perpetuated by this mechanism, the biological implications of which continue to be revealed as we learn more about the function of these factors. The propensity of *N. gonorrhoeae* to utilize phase variation of gene expression to promote

diversity within a population may not yet be fully realized, as evidenced by the recent discoveries of the phase-variable *pilC* gene (110), the *hpuAB* operon (39), and several LOS biosynthesis genes (10, 35, 53, 80, 249).

Antigenic and phase variation of gonococcal pili is a complicated scenario involving several unlinked loci on the gonococcal chromosome. The major pilin subunit, PilE, is encoded by one or two expression loci (*pilE*) on the chromosome. Antigenic variation of PilE arises from genetic recombination between regions of the *pilE* sequence and homologous regions within one of several promoterless partial loci called "silent" or "storage" loci (*pilS*). The *pilS* loci consist of a number of variable "minicassettes" corresponding to variable regions in the center and C-terminal end of the pilin molecule. The minicassettes are separated by short conserved regions that provide homology for recombination with the expressed gene. The recombination event is unidirectional and may occur via intragenic recombination or with exogenous DNA taken up from lysed gonococci (reviewed in references 148 and 201). The theoretical number of pilin variants that can be produced by a single strain through these recombination events is staggering (ca. 17^6 different variants per strain); however, the actual number is probably fewer due to structural constraints (83). Phase variation of gonococcal pilin expression resulting in changes from piliated to nonpiliated phenotypes occurs at a high rate in vitro (10^{-3} to 10^{-4}/cell/generation). A variety of mechanisms can lead to pilus phase variation, including posttranslational modification of pilin to produce a soluble, unassembled form (S pilin) and the inadvertent production of longer versions of pilin incapable of correct assembly through inexact recombination between the *pilE* and *pilS* loci (reviewed in reference 201). Phase variation of the *pilC* gene can also cause decreased piliation; *pilC* phase variation occurs by way of a frame-shift mechanism stemming from changes in the number of bases in a polyguanine region of the *pilC* coding sequence during replication (110).

Antigenic variation of the Opa protein phenotype arises from phase variation of individual *opa* genes on the chromosome. *N. gonorrhoeae* expresses 9 to 11 antigenically distinct Opa proteins, ranging from 25 to 30 kDa in molecular mass. A separate chromosomal gene consisting of both conserved and highly variable regions encodes each individual Opa protein. Phase variation of gonococcal *opa* genes occurs by virtue of a frame-shift mechanism which results in changes in the number of a pentameric repeated unit (CTCTT) in the signal sequence-encoding region of an *opa* gene. This event, which takes place during replication, is hypothesized to occur via a mechanism known as slipped-strand mispairing. The resultant translational reading frame can be in or out of frame, depending on the number of repeated units that are lost or added from the newly synthesized strand. The rate of phase variation of *opa* genes is relatively high (10^{-3}/cell/generation), and an individual variant can produce none, one, or more than one Opa protein at a time (reviewed in references 55 and 148). Different Opa proteins within a strain confer different degrees of photo-opacity on a colony, ranging from transparent to highly opaque (126, 219). The Opa repertoire differs among strains, although some strains share some hypervariable sequences (33).

The LOS of *Neisseria* spp. differs from the lipopolysaccharide of enteric gram-negative bacteria in that the repeating O antigen is absent. Instead, gonococcal LOS consists of a lipid A moiety attached to a branched carbohydrate core that varies in length and sugar composition (81). Several glycosyltransferases play a role in the stepwise addition of carbohydrates to the LOS chain. Phase variation of individual glycosyltransferase genes occurs via high-frequency, reversible frame shifts within a stretch of guanines (35, 53, 80, 249) or cytosines (10) in the coding sequences of these genes. The result of phase variation of glycosyltransferase genes is the production of LOS molecules that differ in length and carbohydrate composition. These variant forms of LOS can be distinguished by differences in molecular weight and recognition by monoclonal antibodies (2, 136,

197). Some LOS species have a terminal lactose-*N*-tetraose moiety that is similar to the asialo-GM$_1$ ganglioside found on human cells. Posttranslational sialylation of the terminal galactose residue of this tetrasaccharide is an interesting modification that is catalyzed by gonococcal sialytransferase using host-derived cytidine monophosphate neuraminic acid (CMP-NANA) as the substrate (reviewed in references 138 and 212). A high percentage of gonococci in urethral exudates are sialylated (3), and as will be discussed, the biological impact of this LOS modification is impressive with respect to the survival advantage it confers upon a gonococcus.

Evasion of Nonspecific Host Factors

Several excellent reviews of the adaptation of *N. gonorrhoeae* to the host have been published (45, 203, 212, 213); this chapter will focus on the survival mechanisms utilized by the gonococcus specifically in the context of the urogenital mucosa. A number of nonspecific host defenses function to maintain a healthy urogenital mucosa, including pH, sequestration of free iron, the constant shedding of mucus, and the presence of inhibitory commensal flora. Additionally, surveillance by neutrophils and complement is a frontline defense against bacterial infection. In women, the dynamics of several host factors fluctuate over the course of the menstrual cycle due to the cyclical influence of reproductive hormones (Fig. 2).

LOCAL pH

Gonococci present in the urethra are subjected to local pH changes resulting from exposure to urine of varying pH. Growth of *N. gonorrhoeae* on solid agar is inhibited at a pH of less than 5.8 in vitro (166), and studies examining the bactericidal activity of urine for *N. gonorrhoeae* identified low pH as the major inhibitory factor (144). The average pH of urethral exudates from infected men ranged from 6.2 to 8.4 (91). Although the average pH of endocervical mucus is relatively neutral (6.1 to 6.8) (210), variation among infected donors ranged from a pH of less than 5.0 to 7.6 (122). The pH of

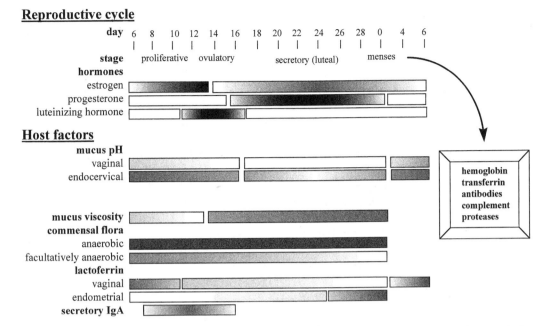

FIGURE 2 Cyclical fluctuation of host factors that may challenge the survival of *N. gonorrhoeae* during infection of the female genital tract. Shading is used to illustrate relative differences in mucus viscosity (248), commensal flora (11, 246), and local concentrations of reproductive hormones (230), lactoferrin (43, 140), and secretory IgA (125). Light shading is used to represent a pH of <7; moderate shading represents neutral pH. The pH of vaginal mucus is based on a reported pH value of 4.6 (range, 3.3 to 7.4) on days 9 and 10 and 4.4 (range, 3.6 to 6.0) on days 22 to 24 of the cycle. Cervical mucus pH is based on a reported average of 6.8 (range, 5.5 to 8.0) on days 9 and 10 and 6.1 (range, 5.1 to 8.4) on days 22 and 24 (210). In a study of 50 women with cervical gonorrhea, the cervical mucus pH ranged from 6.8 to 7.6 during the proliferative stage (days 6 to 12), 5.2 to 6.6 during the secretory phase (days 20 to 25), and 4.8 to 7.4 just prior to and during menses (days 26 to 5) (122).

vaginal mucus is lower than that of endocervical mucus (210, 248), a feature that may restrict the gonococcus from colonizing the vaginas of females of reproductive age. *N. gonorrhoeae* may tolerate conditions of low pH through the induction of a stress response, as evidenced by the expression of the 63-kDa analog (Hsp63) of the heat shock protein GroEL during growth at pH 5.8 (165). Acidic culture also induced the expression of several high-molecular-weight outer membrane proteins that were recognized by convalescent-serum antibody from women with gonococcal PID (166). Changes in LOS phenotype (164) and repression of the restriction-modifiable protein RmpA (P.III) (165) also occurred at low pH. Antibodies to RmpA block the bactericidal activity of antiporin antibodies in vitro (184); therefore, one might hypothesize that bacteria in niches of low pH are more susceptible to the host immune response. The low pH optimum of gonococcal sialyltransferase (pH 5.8) (137), however, suggests that higher numbers of serum-resistant bacteria may be present at low pH, resulting from more efficient LOS sialylation (138, 212). An additional effect that pH might have on the behavior of the gonococcus is an alteration of adherence capabilities via pH-related changes in bacterial surface charge (135).

IRON

Sequestration of free Fe^{3+} on mucosal surfaces and in serum by host lactoferrin and transferrin qualifies as a nonspecific host defense because iron is an essential element for microbial growth (242). *N. gonorrhoeae* gains access to extracellular iron stores by expressing receptors that can obtain iron directly from human transferrin (1, 49, 131), lactoferrin (17, 18, 131), and hemoglobin (38, 39). The iron-binding proteins of N. gonorrhoeae are expressed under conditions of iron starvation in vitro. Transferrin is primarily found in serum; however, it may also be introduced onto mucosal surfaces in serum exudates formed during inflammation. Cornelissen et al. (50) reported that a transferrin-binding protein mutant of N. gonorrhoeae was noninfectious in male volunteers compared to an equivalent dose of the wild-type parent strain. This result suggests that transferrin is a critical source of iron on mucosal surfaces; whether lactoferrin can substitute for the loss of transferrin utilization is not yet known, as the strain used in the volunteer trial described above does not express lactoferrin-binding protein. Although all strains of N. gonorrhoeae are capable of utilizing human transferrin as an iron source, only ca. 50% of gonococcal strains can obtain iron from lactoferrin (150). The amount of lactoferrin present on mucosal surfaces appears to be hormonally regulated in women; the concentration of lactoferrin is highest on endometrial tissue during the secretory phase of the cycle (140) and in vaginal mucus just after menses (43) (Fig. 2). It is not known if changes in the abundance of lactoferrin influence infection in women. Lactoferrin is also released from primary granules in neutrophils as part of their defense, and N. gonorrhoeae can perhaps capitalize upon this burst of a usable iron source to proliferate during periods of inflammation (45).

The gonococcal hemoglobin binding proteins (HpuA and HpuB) are interesting in that the hpuAB operon undergoes both transcriptional regulation in response to iron availability and phase variation via frame shifts within a stretch of guanines in the hpuA gene (39). It is tempting to speculate that the association between menses and locally and systemically disseminated infection may be due in part to the increased proliferation of variants capable of utilizing hemoglobin and hemoglobin-haptoglobin complexes as iron sources (38, 60). N. gonorrhoeae can also use free heme and soluble compounds in which iron is complexed to citrate, oxalacetate, pyrophosphate, and nitrilotriacetate for in vitro growth (149). The relevance of these iron sources to gonococcal survival in various body sites is not known.

An iron uptake regulator (Fur) that is functionally homologous to that of E. coli (13) regulates the expression of gonococcal receptors involved in iron uptake and transport (226). The isolation of a gonococcal fur mutant by Thomas and Sparling (226) facilitated the identification of numerous fur-dependent iron-induced (Fip) and iron-repressed (Frp) proteins by two-dimensional electrophoresis; from this work one might predict the existence of gonococcal virulence genes that are regulated by iron but not involved in iron uptake.

COMMENSAL FLORA

The cervical, pharyngeal, and rectal mucosae are a mixed ecosystem of commensal flora that defend their turf either by direct inhibition of other microbes or by competition for nutrients and colonization receptors. This host defense may play less of a role during gonococcal urethritis, since the commensal flora only resides in the anterior segment of the urethra and N. gonorrhoeae colonizes more distally (27). The composition of commensal vaginal flora fluctuates over the course of the menstrual cycle. Fewer facultatively anaerobic bacteria are isolated during the secretory phase; however, the anaerobic flora remains constant throughout the cycle (11, 246) (Fig. 2). It is not known how N. gonorrhoeae adjusts to this dynamic ecosystem. Although N. gonorrhoeae is considered an aerobic organism, it can grow anaerobically in vitro if nitrite is supplied as a terminal electron acceptor (121). The nitrite that is produced during the normal metabolism of anaerobes may facilitate the coexistence of N. gonorrhoeae with anaerobes in vivo. Indeed, recognition of anaerobically induced gonococcal outer membrane proteins by convalescent serum antibody from women with gonococcal PID suggests that anaerobic growth of N. gonorrhoeae occurs in vivo (42).

A variety of members of the commensal flora inhibit *N. gonorrhoeae* in vitro, including other *Neisseria* spp. (26, 94, 190, 208). Lactobacilli are the most common facultatively anaerobic bacteria of the vagina (178) and endocervix (76). The potential of commensal *Lactobacillus* spp. to inhibit *N. gonorrhoeae* is of particular interest due to the focus on lactobacilli as probiotic agents to combat urinary tract infections (180) and bacterial vaginosis (36; M. Antonio and S. L. Hillier, *Abstr. 97th Gen. Meet. Am. Soc. Microbiol. 1997*, p. 126, 1997). The production of organic acids, bacteriocins, and hydrogen peroxide by *Lactobacillus* spp. may ward off pathogenic bacteria as well as maintain the normal ecosystem of the vagina. Clinical data suggest that lactobacilli may protect women from gonorrhea (190). Theoretically, gonococcal catalase may defend against H_2O_2-producing lactobacilli; this defense may not be effective during times of low pH, however, based on the evidence that other factors produced by lactobacilli at low pH either decrease the effectiveness of gonococcal catalase or directly inhibit *N. gonorrhoeae* (251).

In addition to the resident commensals of the female lower genital tract, *N. gonorrhoeae* often shares this niche with other sexually transmitted agents, such as *Chlamydia trachomatis* and *Trichomonas vaginalis*. Whether coinfection has a synergistic effect on the pathogenesis of each individual pathogen is not known. The demonstration that *T. vaginalis* phagocytizes *N. gonorrhoeae* in vitro suggests that trichomonads are antagonistic to gonococcal infection (70). The detection of a higher serum proinflammatory cytokine response in women who were coinfected with *N. gonorrhoeae* and either *C. trachomatis* or *T. vaginalis* compared to women infected with any single agent suggests that sexually transmitted pathogens may alter host-parasite dynamics (93).

REPRODUCTIVE HORMONES

N. gonorrhoeae is inhibited by progesterone in vitro (123, 152), and endogenous progesterone may therefore directly challenge the viability of gonococci during infection of women. In 1947 Koch (122) reported that *N. gonorrhoeae* was more frequently isolated from infected women during the proliferative phase of the menstrual cycle than during the secretory phase and that the return of culture positivity coincided with transition back to the proliferative stage in hospitalized subjects. This investigator hypothesized that the low pH of cervical mucus and higher levels of progesterone were responsible for the latency of infection observed during the secretory phase. After this initial report, others made similar observations (102, 107, 143), although no association between the culture result and the phase of the menstrual cycle was reported in some studies (65, 133). Data concerning the incidence of gonorrhea with regard to oral contraceptive use do not support the hypothesis that progesterone decreases susceptibility to lower genital tract infection (102, 133, 143), although it may protect against PID (64). Interestingly, sera from uninfected women on oral contraceptives were more bactericidal against *N. gonorrhoeae* than were sera from women not using this birth control method (26).

Studies with female mice also support the hypothesis that the secretory stage is inhospitable to *N. gonorrhoeae*. Short-term recovery of gonococci was reported from mice that were inoculated intravaginally or intrauterinally during the proestrus (high-estrogen) stage but not the postovulatory (high-progesterone) stages of the estrus cycle (26, 106, 117, 217). Also, estradiol promotes long-term vaginal colonization of mice (105, 225). Kita et al. (118) reported that estradiol-treated mice developed a lethal bacteremia following intraperitoneal inoculation with *N. gonorrhoeae* in contrast to progesterone-treated mice, which developed a short-term bacteremia that was rapidly cleared. Another indication that factors present during the secretory stage challenge the survival of *N. gonorrhoeae* may be furnished by the gonococcus itself. In a survey of 176 cervical isolates, James and Swanson (102, 103) found that isolates from women in the preovulatory phase of the menstrual cycle expressed one or more Opa proteins while those cultured from women postovulation or during menses were Opa negative. This intriguing observation suggests that phase variation of Opa protein expression provides a reservoir of variants that can persist during the secretory phase of the reproductive cycle. Host factors that may select against Opa protein-expressing variants include proteases and antibody (102, 103) and progesterone itself, based on in vitro evidence that opaque gonococcal variants are more sensitive to progesterone than are transparent variants (191).

In addition to fluctuations in pH, commensal flora, and the availability of lactoferrin as already discussed, other hormonally driven factors that might indirectly affect gonococcal survival include the relative abundance of sialic acid substrate needed for LOS modification. The sialic acid content of endometrial glycolipids was reported to fluctuate over the course of the menstrual cycle (177); in contrast, however, no differences in the sialic acid content of cervical mucus were detected with respect to the menstrual cycle, although differences between individuals were found (247). Finally, and perhaps most importantly, fluctuations in reproductive hormones may also influence the type and degree of immune response to gonococcal infection. For example, cyclical changes in the concentration of immunoglobulin A (IgA) in cervical mucus (125) may influence the survival of N. gonorrhoeae during different phases of the menstrual cycle. This exciting area has not yet been tapped in gonococcal research.

PHAGOCYTE SURVEILLANCE

The surveillance of mucosal surfaces by phagocytes constitutes an important facet of the host innate immune response. While some aspects of the interaction of phagocytes with bacteria have a host-specific component, such as the opsonic uptake of bacteria coated with specific antibodies directed towards bacterial surface antigens, neutrophils, and later macrophages, are recruited to the scene as a first-line nonspecific defense against foreign invaders (151). The host inflammatory response can be induced during gonococcal infection by bacterial prod-

ucts such as peptidoglycan and by the deposition of the C5a chemoattractant component on bacterial surfaces. Differences in any or all of these modes of inducing inflammation may be responsible for the occurrence of asymptomatic infection in some individuals. Complement-derived chemoattractants are generated more efficiently by serum-sensitive strains than by serum-resistant strains, suggesting that strain-related differences may determine the degree of inflammation produced during a gonococcal infection (reviewed in reference 203). Recruitment of neutrophils can also be signaled by proinflammatory cytokines and chemokines. Naumann et al. (157) showed that N. gonorrhoeae induced interleukin 1 (IL-1), IL-6, IL-8, tumor necrosis factor alpha, granulocyte/macrophage colony-stimulating factor, transforming growth factor β, and methyl-accepting chemotaxis protein 1 in tissue culture cells, and that invasion was not required for induction. Consistent with this report was the detection of elevated levels of proinflammatory cytokines (IL-6, IL-8, and tumor necrosis factor alpha) in the urine of experimentally infected male volunteers before the onset of acute symptoms and of IL-1β upon the development of urethral discharge (176). In contrast, Hedges et al. (93) detected no significant differences in the levels of IL-1, IL-6, and IL-8 in cervical mucus and vaginal washes from women naturally infected with N. gonorrhoeae versus those of uninfected women. This interesting result may be a clue as to why gonococcal infection in women often occurs with minimal or no symptoms. Continued characterization of the cytokines produced by patients with and without symptomatic infection may elucidate the cellular basis behind the generation of an inflammatory response by N. gonorrhoeae.

Once neutrophils arrive upon the scene, phagocytosis can occur in the absence of opsonins through the interaction between Opa proteins and the CD66 receptors of neutrophils (reviewed in reference 55) (Fig. 3A). Phase variation of gonococcal Opa protein expression may play a critical role in avoiding nonopsonic phagocytosis by maintaining populations

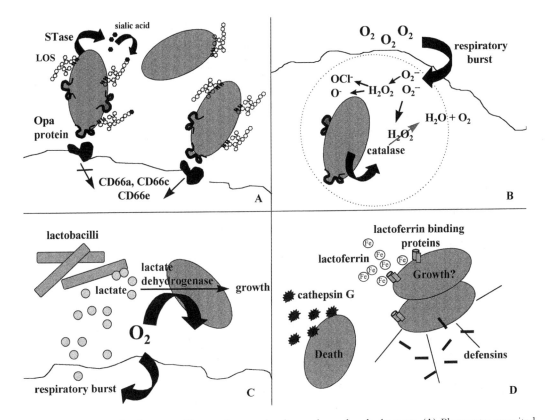

FIGURE 3 Interaction between *N. gonorrhoeae* and polymorphonuclear leukocytes. (A) Phagocytes recruited to the mucosal surface can take up *N. gonorrhoeae* in the absence of opsonins via interactions between Opa proteins and the neutrophil CD66 receptor. An Opa–negative variant that has escaped this interaction is shown; variants expressing some Opa proteins within the Opa repertoire of a strain also do not adhere to neutrophils (reviewed in reference 55). LOS sialylation catalyzed by gonococcal sialyltransferase (STase) inhibits Opa-mediated uptake by phagocytes (182). (B) Stimulation of the phagocyte respiratory burst leads to the production of toxic oxygen radicals. Unlike many other bacteria, *N. gonorrhoeae* does not make superoxide dismutase, which could neutralize the respiratory burst at an early stage in toxic radical production. *N. gonorrhoeae* does produce high levels of catalase, which is capable of cleaving H_2O_2 to oxygen and water (6). Increased production of gonococcal catalase occurs in response to sublethal concentrations of H_2O_2 (6, 250). (C) The gonococcus may effectively compete with the neutrophil for molecular O_2, which is limited on mucosal surfaces. Lactate produced by neutrophils or by commensal lactobacilli may give the gonococcus a competitive edge in that O_2 is rapidly consumed during lactose utilization by *N. gonorrhoeae* (28; reviewed in reference 203). The resultant anaerobic environment increases activity and also the expression of LOS species carrying the lactose-*N*-tetraose molecule to which sialic acid is added, which together may help prevent phagocytosis (71) (panel A). (D) Oxygen-independent killing mechanisms include the production of cathepsin G, a protease found in neutrophil lysozomes that inhibits gonococcal growth. The targets of cathepsin G are the bacterial transpeptidases used in peptidoglycan synthesis (204). *N. gonorrhoeae* is resistant to neutrophil defensins (174). Some gonococcal strains may utilize the lactoferrin released from neutrophil granules as a growth substrate (reviewed in reference 45). An additional gonococcal defense that is not shown is the capacity of *N. gonorrhoeae* to directly impair phagocyte functions, including degranulation, actin polymerization, and phagocytosis, through insertion of its major porin, P.I, into the eukaryotic cell membrane (19, 84). This direct attack on neutrophils may further promote persistence during inflammation.

of gonococci that do not undergo nonopsonic uptake by neutrophils. For example, Opa-negative variants do not adhere to neutrophils in the absence of serum in vitro and therefore are not killed. Similarly, some Opa antigenic variants do not bind to neutrophils and therefore are spared nonopsonic killing by neutrophils (12, 62, 67, 124, 155) or by stimulated monocytic and myelomonocytic cell lines (90). Posttranslational sialylation of LOS may further protect the gonococcus from Opa-mediated uptake by neutrophils. Rest and Frangipane (182) showed reduced phagocytic uptake of *N. gonorrhoeae* cultured in the presence of CMP-NANA and that preincubation of sialylated gonococci with neuraminidase reversed this effect. Consistent with these observations is the report that a gonococcal sialyltransferase mutant was highly susceptible to killing by neutrophils compared to the wild-type strain (73).

Opa-mediated uptake by phagocytes induces a respiratory burst (90, 156); no reactive oxygen intermediates are released extracellularly in vitro, however, and therefore noninternalized gonococci may thrive (156). Although most gonococci appear to succumb to neutrophil killing mechanisms following phagocytosis, there is evidence that a proportion of intracellular gonococci survive and even grow within the neutrophil (reviewed in reference 203). Gonococcal catalase may protect *N. gonorrhoeae* from H_2O_2 produced by the neutrophil during the respiratory burst (6, 89, 108). The recent cloning of the gonococcal catalase gene (109) should help elucidate the role of catalase in maintaining persistence of infection during periods of inflammation.

Evasion of Specific Immune Defenses
GENERAL OVERVIEW
Natural infection with *N. gonorrhoeae* induces the production of gonococcus-specific IgM, IgG, and IgA in serum, semen, and vaginal secretions (reviewed in reference 32). Additionally, normal human serum contains cross-reactive antibodies induced by commensal neisseriae. These antibodies primarily bind the P.I protein and LOS determinants of *N. gonor-*

rhoeae (74, 98, 192, 196) and can promote killing of *N. gonorrhoeae* by the pathways described below. Antibodies against the major porin, P.I (98), and LOS (74, 196) are bactericidal in the presence of complement, suggesting that these antibodies have a protective potential. Both cross-reactive antibodies in normal human serum (16, 181, 188) and those that are induced by natural infection (195) can opsonize gonococci, with or without complement, to promote phagocytic uptake. Gonococcus-specific secretory IgA potentially protects against colonization through direct agglutination of bacteria. Despite the many ways that the humoral response can thwart infection, *N. gonorrhoeae* appears to be capable of escaping this response, as evidenced by the fact that patients are susceptible to repeated infection with the same serovar (31, 69, 95) or strain (66) within weeks or months after treatment or are only partially protected (34, 169, 170). A variety of mechanisms by which *N. gonorrhoeae* reduces the effectiveness of the immune response have been proposed, as described below.

SERUM RESISTANCE
Gonococcal strains express one of two major porins, referred to as PorA (P.IA) or PorB (P.IB). Gonococci of the PorA (P.IA) serotype generally demonstrate stable serum resistance to complement-mediated activity of normal human serum due to structural differences inherent in the PorA molecule. In contrast, PorB (P.IB) strains are more susceptible to bactericidal killing (185). Phase variation of LOS expression may expose or block epitopes critical for this interaction, thereby increasing or reducing the degree of serum sensitivity of P.IB strains (23, 71, 82, 198). Interestingly, Bos et al. (23) showed that Opa-negative variants of a P.IB strain were more sensitive to normal human serum than were Opa-positive variants of the same LOS phenotype of this strain. This observation suggests that Opa phase variation may protect the gonococcus against bactericidal activity in hosts that were never previously infected. This finding may also explain the dramatic selection for and/or induction of

Opa protein expression that occurs in the male urethra following inoculation with a predominantly Opa-negative population of *N. gonorrhoeae* (104, 221).

Sialylation of gonococcal LOS in vivo or in vitro blocks the bactericidal activity of normal human serum (reviewed in reference 212), presumably by interfering with the deposition of complement on the bacterial surface (63). This type of serum resistance is referred to as unstable, since it is rapidly lost upon subculture in the absence of sialic acid substrate (238). LOS sialylation also increases resistance to nonopsonic phagocytosis (73, 182) and to the bactericidal activity of antibodies specific for porin (56, 63, 244) or LOS (56). Posttranslational sialylation of gonococcal LOS is well documented among urethral isolates from infected men (3), and a predominance of gonococci expressing LOS with the lactose-*N*-tetraose moiety was isolated from male volunteers inoculated with variants expressing a shorter-chain LOS (199). Collectively, these observations strongly suggest that LOS sialylation confers a survival advantage on the gonococcus. Surprisingly, however, sialylation of *N. gonorrhoeae* in vitro reduced the organism's infectivity in volunteers (200). The basis for this experimental outcome is not understood; however, the fact that gonococci are less invasive when grown in the presence of CMP-NANA (233) suggests that nonsialylated gonococci may have a functional advantage during early stages of infection.

EVASION OF HUMORAL RESPONSE THROUGH ANTIGENIC VARIATION OF SURFACE MOLECULES

Antigenic variation of gonococcal pilin, Opa proteins, and LOS in vivo theoretically could produce populations of gonococci that are not recognized by antibodies formed against variants of these molecules that were expressed earlier in infection. Antibody to gonococcal pili inhibits adherence of gonococci to cells (173), although adherence mediated by a heterologous pilin is not blocked (229). Immunization with purified pilin protects against infection with a homologous pilin variant, presumably by blocking bacterial adherence in vivo (27). The advantage that pilin antigenic variation confers on *N. gonorrhoeae* was dramatically illustrated in a large field study in which immunization with a single pilin type failed to protect volunteers from gonorrhea (24). The rapidity with which antigenic variation of pilin occurred after intraurethral inoculation of male volunteers (202, 222) suggests that immune responses formed against variants present early in infection may be easily outrun by the gonococcus; this high-level variation also ensures that the next host will most likely be immunologically naïve. The recently described pilus-associated adhesin, PilC, unfortunately also undergoes phase variation (110), and antigenic differences in PilC are found among strains (9); these characteristics are discouraging with regard to the potential of PilC as a vaccine antigen. Although the Opa repertoire expressed by a single strain of *N. gonorrhoeae* pales in comparison to that of antigenic pilin variants, antigenic variation of Opa protein expression may also facilitate immune evasion, as suggested by the demonstration that antibody to Opa proteins blocks adherence of homologous Opa variants to tissue culture cells (218). Plummer et al. (171) found an association between the titer of Opa-specific antibodies and a reduced risk of upper reproductive tract infection among commercial sex workers, suggesting that Opa-specific antibody may attenuate disease.

BLOCKING ANTIBODY

A second mechanism by which *N. gonorrhoeae* might successfully avoid antibody attack is through the expression of the conserved outer membrane protein called RmpA (reduction modifiable protein), also known as P.III. Normal human serum contains antibody to RmpA, presumably due to cross-reaction with the semihomologous *E. coli* OmpA (79). Antibody specific to RmpA blocks the bactericidal activity of antibodies against porin or LOS in vitro, thereby weakening the susceptibility of these targets to attack (184). Whether anti-P.III antibodies block bactericidal activity at appreciable levels in the genital secretions of naïve hosts is not known, however. The presence of anti-P.III antibody was associated with an increased risk of gonorrhea among commercial sex workers, suggesting that blocking antibody induced by natural infection may be advantageous to the gonococcus (171).

DIVERSION OF ANTIBODY

The tendency of *N. gonorrhoeae* to shed its outer membrane in the form of vesicles or membrane blebs also may be advantageous to the organism by providing a "sponge" of epitopes to which specific antibodies bind without effect. These blebs also contain DNA and may therefore enhance genetic exchange among different strains of *N. gonorrhoeae*, *N. meningitidis*, and commensal *Neisseria* spp. on mucosal surfaces (59).

DESTRUCTION OF ANTIBODY

The pathogenic neisseriae, like *Haemophilus* and *Bordetella*, produce a protease capable of cleaving the hinge region of IgA1, one of the two secretory subclasses of IgA found on mucosal surfaces (116). It has been proposed that this protease gives the gonococcus an advantage by destroying the protective potential of gonococcus-specific IgA1. Recently an IgA1 protease mutant was reported to retain infectivity in male volunteers (47). It is possible that IgA1 protease contributes to enhanced survival only in hosts that were previously infected; the infectivity of an IgA1 protease mutant in an artificially or naturally immunized host has not been tested. Whether cleavage of IgA1 by IgA1 protease occurs at appreciable levels during natural infection is questionable. Although IgA1 protease activity was detected in vaginal mucus of infected women (21), Hedges et al. (92) recently reported an absence of IgA1 cleavage products in cervical washes from infected women and the detection of protease inhibitors in serum and cervical mucus. Interestingly, a second way in which IgA1 protease may contribute to pathogenesis is through increasing intracellular survival of *N. gonorrhoeae* through cleavage of an endosomal membrane

protein (132). This newly described function for IgA1 protease has refreshing implications for the role of this factor in virulence.

INTRACELLULAR RETREAT

Invasion of nonprofessional phagocytes by *N. gonorrhoeae* may also serve to protect the pathogen from humoral defenses. Antigenic variation of Opa proteins may serve to provide populations of invasive gonococci that can hide from effectors of the humoral response (reviewed in reference 55). Alterations in sialylation efficiency might increase the numbers of nonsialylated gonococci in vitro, which are more invasive than sialylated gonococci through an unknown mechanism (233). There is also evidence that *N. gonorrhoeae* enters host cells via a receptor that is up-regulated in response to luteinizing hormone (77, 214). The possibility that this pathogen evolved to capitalize on hormonally regulated receptors in the female reproductive tract is intriguing.

MODELS OF PERSISTENCE

Our current understanding of how *N. gonorrhoeae* combats or evades host defenses arises from a wide variety of experimental systems, ranging from simple examination of colony morphology on solid agar plates to experimental infection of male volunteers. Insights into gonococcal resistance to isolated host factors have been derived from test tube assays designed to reproduce events that occur in vivo; similarly, mechanisms utilized by *N. gonorrhoeae* for colonization and intracellular life have been greatly elucidated by tissue culture systems. Although the development of an animal model of gonococcal genital tract infection has been slow, gonorrhea research has been fortunate in that the mildness of gonococcal urethritis in men lends itself to using human volunteers to study basic questions of gonococcal pathogenesis (reviewed in reference 44). The human model is a valuable tool for ascertaining the requirement for certain gonococcal virulence factors in causing urethritis (44, 47, 50). This model is also useful for studying the population dynamics of antigenic and phase variation of surface molecules during early urethritis (104, 199, 202, 221, 222). Insights from these studies have fostered theories regarding the functions of these molecules and the role of variable gene expression in gonococcal adaptation and transmission.

The usefulness of the human model for addressing certain questions regarding the effect of innate or acquired immune responses on gonococcal adaptation and persistence is limited by ethical restrictions against manipulating the immunological state of a volunteer or maintaining untreated experimental infection. Other more practical limitations to the human model are the restricted sample size and the fact that the expense and administration of a volunteer program are formidable for most research settings. Extrapolation of data from the male human model to infection in females is also risky, since the microenvironment of the male urethra may differ substantially from that of the female reproductive tract. We cannot directly test if events observed during experimental male infection occur during female infection due to the risk of serious complications resulting from experimental infection in women volunteers. Information concerning gonorrhea in women is currently based on the analysis of clinical specimens (42, 92, 93, 102, 166, 169), tissue culture cell systems (124, 209, 214), and cultured fallopian tube models (77, 78, 146; reviewed in reference 216). These models are limited in that they may not sufficiently mimic all the factors present in the complex microenvironment of the host, including the influence of an intact immune system on infection.

Surrogate animal models for human infection may at least partially satisfy the currently unfulfilled need for a female model of infection as well as provide intermediate steps towards eventual testing of scientific predictions in male volunteers. Research directed towards understanding gonorrhea in women lags far behind that of chlamydial research, which has been greatly accelerated by the availability of a variety of animal models. Laboratory animal models of chlamydial genital tract infection

have generated much information regarding immunopathology, tubal infertility, and hormonal influences on chlamydial infection, as well as host immune response to infection and immunization (reviewed in reference 162). Small laboratory animal models utilizing intraperitoneal injection to simulate disseminated gonococcal infection (159), implantation of subcutaneous chambers to simulate mucosal infection (127, 141), and synovial injection to simulate gonococcal arthritis (68, 75) are currently used to test gonococcal virulence. The development of animal models of gonococcal genital tract infection, however, has been severely hindered by the host specificity of *N. gonorrhoeae*. Successful genital tract infection with *N. gonorrhoeae* has only been reported in chimpanzees and mice. Male chimpanzees develop a disease that closely mimics gonococcal urethritis in humans, and sexual transmission of infection from a male to two female chimpanzees was reported. Positive cervical cultures were obtained from one of these females for 39 days postexposure, and in contrast to infected male chimpanzees, which developed an inflammatory discharge, no visible signs of infection were apparent in either of the infected females (reviewed in reference 7). Further studies designed to evaluate the similarity of infection in female chimpanzees with human infection are not feasible due to the expense and the limited availability of these animals.

Female mice are susceptible to *N. gonorrhoeae* following intrauterine (26, 217) or intravaginal (106, 117) inoculation provided they are in the proestrus stage of the estrus cycle at the time of inoculation. Colonization is short term, however, with clearance of *N. gonorrhoeae* coinciding with the transition into the metestrus and diestrus phases of the cycle. Taylor-Robinson et al. (225) successfully induced long-term gonococcal genital tract infection in germfree BALB/c mice by using 17-β estradiol treatment to increase their susceptibility to *N. gonorrhoeae*. Gonococci were associated with epithelial cells in vaginal smears, and no inflammatory response was detected. Gonococci were isolated from endometrial and ovarian tissue, suggesting that local dissemination to the upper reproductive tract occurred. My laboratory has recently devised a mouse infection protocol based on Taylor-Robinson's technique in which estradiol is delivered in a uniform fashion using a slow-release intradermal pellet and antibiotics are administered to reduce the overgrowth of inhibitory commensal flora that occurs under the influence of estradiol. Gonococci are recovered from these mice for an average of 12 to 13 days following inoculation with wild-type *N. gonorrhoeae*. Growth of *N. gonorrhoeae* occurs in vivo, suggesting that usable sources of iron may be available in murine cervical mucus. Inflammation occurs in the majority of mice, as evidenced by an influx of vaginal neutrophils that was higher than that which occurred in placebo controls, and gonococci were isolated from the endometria of 17 to 20% of the mice, suggesting that ascending infection occurred. An increase in the percentage of gonococci expressing one or more Opa proteins occurred during experimental infection of a high percentage of mice (105). This change in Opa phenotype was similar to that which occurred in male volunteers (104, 221), suggesting that some selective forces may be present in the murine genital tract that are similar to those which occur in the male urethra. The murine model may therefore allow one to address questions regarding gonococcal adaptation to the host via Opa protein phase variation.

The murine model may be a useful tool for studying other aspects of gonococcal adaptation in vivo. The genital tract of female mice shares many other features with that of humans, including similarities in oxygen tension, cervical pH, commensal flora, and hormonally driven changes in mucus and certain histological characteristics (26, 48), as well as the presence of an intact immune response. Obviously, there are certain aspects of murine infection that cannot mimic that which occurs in humans due to the absence of human-specific factors, such as the CD46 pili receptor and the CD66 Opa protein receptor. These restrictions may be overcome, however, by the use of transgenic mice that express these human receptors (61, 154). Mice that are transgenic for human transferrin, lactoferrin, and IgA1 may also be useful systems for testing questions involving these host factors.

FUTURE DIRECTIONS

N. gonorrhoeae continues to have a serious impact on public health worldwide. Women bear the greatest morbidity and mortality caused by this pathogen due to the frequency with which the gonococcus disseminates to the upper reproductive tract in females and the serious complications that can result. One might predict that the very high rate of gonorrhea among adolescent girls and young women in the United States (57) will be followed by high incidences of chronic pelvic pain, involuntary infertility, and the life-threatening condition of ectopic pregnancy. Evidence that human immunodeficiency virus transmission is increased in the presence of other sexually transmitted infections (46) further increases the seriousness of the gonorrhea epidemic. In light of the lack of an effective vaccine and the paucity of prophylactic agents against gonorrhea, public health efforts to identify and treat asymptomatically infected individuals must be maintained at a high level.

A better understanding of the mechanisms utilized by *N. gonorrhoeae* to persist in the face of host defenses is also critical in the development of strategies to curb the current epidemic of gonorrhea. Underexplored research areas include the following. First, in light of the frequency of coinfection with *N. gonorrhoeae* and *C. trachomatis*, the way in which coinfections might differ from infections with a single agent in terms of host susceptibility, symptomology, and pathology should be addressed. Models of coinfection utilizing tissue culture cells, cultured fallopian tubes, or laboratory animals might generate useful information in this area. There is also a need for a concentrated research effort to determine the combined effects of reproductive hormones, iron levels, and culture pH on gonococcal virulence to better explore adaptation of *N. gonorrhoeae* in the female host. Attempts to reproduce microenvironments in vitro that are representative of each stage of the menstrual cycle could be made using hormonally responsive tissue culture systems. The development of animal models for studying specific aspects of gonococcal infection in a female background should also be pursued, incorporating transgenic mice when possible to better mimic human infection. Such models are also greatly needed to facilitate preclinical testing of candidate vaccines and prophylactic agents, which ultimately are the only solutions for eradicating gonorrhea.

ACKNOWLEDGMENT

I thank Iris Enid Valentin-Bon for her excellent assistance in the preparation of the manuscript.

REFERENCES

1. **Anderson, J. E., P. F. Sparling, and C. N. Cornelissen.** 1994. Gonococcal transferrin-binding protein 2 facilitates but is not essential for transferrin utilization. *J. Bacteriol.* **176:**3162–3170.
2. **Apicella, M. A., K. M. Bennett, C. A. Hermerath, and D. E. Roberts.** 1981. Monoclonal antibody analysis of lipopolysaccharide from *Neisseria gonorrhoeae* and *Neisseria meningitidis*. *Infect. Immun.* **34:**751–756.
3. **Apicella, M. A., R. E. Mandrell, M. Shero, M. E. Wilson, J. M. Griffiss, G. F. Brooks, C. Lammel, J. F. Breen, and P. A. Rice.** 1990. Modification by sialic acid of *Neisseria gonorrhoeae* lipooligosaccharide epitope expression in human urethral exudates: an immunoelectron microscopic analysis. *J. Infect. Dis.* **162:**506–512.
4. **Apicella, M. A., M. Ketterer, F. K. N. Lee, D. Zhou, P. A. Rice, and M. S. Blake.** 1996. The pathogenesis of gonococcal urethritis in men: confocal and immunoelectron microscopic analysis of urethral exudates from men infected with *Neisseria gonorrhoeae*. *J. Infect. Dis.* **173:**636–646.
5. **Aral, S. O., and K. K. Holmes.** 1999. Social and behavioral determinants of the epidemiology of STDs: industrialized and developing countries, p. 39–76. *In* K. K. Holmes, P. A. Mardh, P. F. Sparling, S. M. Lemon, W. E. Stamm, P. Piot, and J. N. Wasserheit (ed.), *Sexually Transmitted Diseases*, 3rd ed. McGraw-Hill Companies, Inc., New York, N.Y.
6. **Archibald, F. S., and M. N. Duong.** 1986. Superoxide dismutase and oxygen toxicity defenses in the genus *Neisseria*. *Infect. Immun.* **51:**631–641.
7. **Arko, R. J.** 1989. Animal models for pathogenic *Neisseria* species. *Clin. Microbiol. Rev.* **2:**S56–S59.
8. **Arvidson, C. G., T. Powers, P. Walter, and M. So.** 1999. *Neisseria gonorrhoeae* PilA is an FtsY homolog. *J. Bacteriol.* **181:**731–739.
9. **Backman, M., H. Kallstrom, and A. B. Jonsson.** 1998. The phase-variable pilus-associated protein PilC is commonly expressed in clinical isolates of *Neisseria gonorrhoeae*, and shows sequence variability among strains. *Microbiology* **144:**149–156.
10. **Banerjee, A., R. Wang, S. N. Uljon, P. A. Rice, E. C. Gotschlich, and D. C. Stein.** 1998. Identification of the gene (*lgtG*) encoding the lipooligosaccharide β-chain synthesizing glucosyl transferase from *Neisseria gonorrhoeae*. *Proc. Natl. Acad. Sci. USA* **95:**10872–10877.
11. **Bartlett, J. G., and B. F. Polk.** 1984. Bacterial flora of the vagina: quantitative study. *Rev. Infect. Dis.* **6**(Suppl. 1):S67–S72.
12. **Belland, R. J., T. Chen, J. Swanson, and S. H. Fischer.** 1992. Human neutrophil response to recombinant neisserial Opa proteins. *Mol. Microbiol.* **6:**1729–1737.
13. **Berish, S. A., S. Subbarao, C. Y. Chen, D. L. Trees, and S. A. Morse.** 1993. Identification and cloning of a *fur* homolog from *Neisseria gonorrhoeae*. *Infect. Immun.* **61:**4599–4606.
14. **Bessen, D., and E. C. Gotschlich.** 1986. Interactions of gonococci with HeLa cells: attachment, detachment, replication, penetration, and the role of protein II. *Infect. Immun.* **54:**154–160.
15. **Biro, F. M., S. L. Rosenthal, and M. Kiniyalocts.** 1995. Gonococcal and chlamydial genitourinary infections in symptomatic and asymptomatic adolescent women. *Clin. Pediatr.* **34:**419–423.
16. **Bisno, A. L., I. Ofek, E. H. Beachey, R. W. Chandler, and J. W. Curran.** 1975. Human immunity to *Neisseria gonorrhoeae*: acquired serum opsonic antibodies. *J. Lab. Clin. Med.* **86:**221–229.
17. **Biswas, G. D., and P. F. Sparling.** 1995. Characterization of *lbpA*, the structural gene for a lactoferrin receptor in *Neisseria gonorrhoeae*. *Infect. Immun.* **63:**2958–2967.
18. **Biswas, G. D., J. E. Anderson, C. J. Chen, C. N. Cornelissen, and P. F. Sparling.** 1999. Identification and functional characterization of the *Neisseria gonorrhoeae lbpB* gene product. *Infect. Immun.* **67:**455–459.
19. **Bjerknes, R., H. K. Guttormsen, C. O. Solberg, and L. M. Wetzler.** 1995. Neisserial porins inhibit human neutrophil actin polymerization, degranulation, opsonin receptor expression, and phagocytosis but prime the neutrophils to increase their oxidative burst. *Infect. Immun.* **63:**160–167.
20. **Black, C. G., J. A. M. Fyfe, and J. K. Davies.** 1995. A promoter associated with the neisserial repeat can be used to transcribe the *uvrB* gene from *Neisseria gonorrhoeae*. *J. Bacteriol.* **177:**1952–1958.

21. **Blake, M. S., K. K. Holmes, and J. Swanson.** 1979. Studies on gonococcus infection. XVII. IgA1-cleaving protease in vaginal washings from women with gonorrhea. *J. Infect. Dis.* **139:**89–92.

22. **Bolan, G., A. A. Ehrhardt, and J. N. Wasserheit.** 1999. Gender perspectives and STDs, p. 117–127. *In* K. K. Holmes, P. A. Mardh, P. F. Sparling, S. M. Lemon, W. E. Stamm, P. Piot, and J. N. Wasserheit (ed.), *Sexually Transmitted Diseases,* 3rd ed. McGraw-Hill Companies, Inc., New York, N.Y.

23. **Bos, M. P., D. Hogan, and R. J. Belland.** 1997. Selection of Opa⁺ *Neisseria gonorrhoeae* by limited availability of normal human serum. *Infect. Immun.* **65:**645–650.

24. **Boslego, J. W., E. C. Tramont, R. C. Chung, D. G. McChesney, J. Ciak, J. C. Sadoff, M. V. Piziak, J. D. Brown, C. C. Brinton, and S. W. Wood.** 1991. Efficacy trial of a parenteral gonococcal pilus vaccine in men. *Vaccine* **9:** 154–162.

25. **Brandt, A. M.** 1985. Damaged goods: progressive medicine and social hygiene, p. 7–51. *In No Magic Bullet. A Social History of Venereal Disease in the United States since 1880.* Oxford University Press, New York, N.Y.

26. **Braude, A. I., L. B. Corbeil, S. Levine, J. Ito, and J. A. McCutchan.** 1978. Possible influence of cyclic menstrual changes on resistance to the gonococcus, p. 328–337. *In* G. F. Brooks, E. C. Gotschlich, K. K. Holmes, W. D. Sawyer, and F. E. Young (ed.), *Immunobiology of Neisseria gonorrhoeae.* American Society for Microbiology, Washington, D.C.

27. **Brinton, C. C., S. W. Wood, A. Brown, et al.** 1982. The development of a neisserial pilus vaccine for gonorrhea and meningococcal meningitis, p. 140–159. *In* L. Weinstein and B. N. Fields (ed.), *Seminars in Infectious Disease.* Thieme-Stratton, New York, N.Y.

28. **Britigan, B. E., D. Klapper, T. Svendsen, and M. S. Cohen.** 1988. Phagocyte derived lactate stimulates oxygen consumption by *Neisseria gonorrhoeae. J. Clin. Investig.* **81:**318–324.

29. **Britigan, B. E., M. S. Cohen, and P. F. Sparling.** 1985. Gonococcal infection: a model of molecular pathogenesis. *N. Engl. J. Med.* **312:** 1683–1694.

30. **Bro-Jorgensen, A., and T. Jensen.** 1973. Gonococcal pharyngeal infections. *Br. J. Vener. Dis.* **49:**491–499.

31. **Brooks, G. F., W. W. Darrow, and J. A. Day.** 1978. Repeated gonorrhea: an analysis of importance and risk factors. *J. Infect. Dis.* **137:**161–169.

32. **Brooks, G. F., and C. J. Lammel.** 1989. Humoral immune response to gonococcal infections. *Clin. Microbiol. Rev.* **2**(Suppl.):S5–S10.

33. **Brooks, G. F., L. Olinger, C. J. Lammel, K. S. Bhat, C. A. Calvello, M. L. Palmer, J. S. Knapp, and R. S. Stephens.** 1991. Prevalence of gene sequences coding for hypervariable regions of Opa (protein II) in *Neisseria gonorrhoeae. Mol. Microbiol.* **5:**3063–3072.

34. **Buchanan, T. M., D. A. Eschenbach, J. S. Knapp, and K. K. Holmes.** 1980. Gonococcal salpingitis is less likely to recur with *Neisseria gonorrhoeae* of the same principal outer membrane protein antigenic type. *Am. J. Obstet. Gynecol.* **138:** 978–980.

35. **Burch, C. L., R. J. Danaher, and D. C. Stein.** 1997. Antigenic variation in *Neisseria gonorrhoeae*: production of multiple lipooligosaccharides. *J. Bacteriol.* **179:**982–986.

36. **Butler, B. C., and J. W. Beakley.** 1960. Bacterial flora in vaginitis. A study before and after treatment with pure cultures of Doderlein bacillus. *Am. J. Obstet. Gynecol.* **79:**432–440.

37. **Centers for Disease Control and Prevention.** 1996. Ten leading nationally notifiable infectious diseases—United States, 1995. *Morbid. Mortal. Weekly Rep.* **45:**8834.

38. **Chen, C. J., P. F. Sparling, L. A. Lewis, D. W. Dyer, and C. Elkins.** 1996. Identification and purification of a hemoglobin binding outer protein from *Neisseria gonorrhoeae. Infect. Immun.* **64:**5008–5014.

39. **Chen, C. J., C. Elkins, and P. F. Sparling.** 1998. Phase variation of hemoglobin utilization in *Neisseria gonorrhoeae. Infect. Immun.* **66:**987–993.

40. **Chen, T., and E. C. Gotschlich.** 1996. CGM1a antigen of neutrophils, a receptor of gonococcal opacity proteins. *Proc. Natl. Acad. Sci. USA* **93:** 14851–14856.

41. **Clark, V. L., L. A. Campbell, D. A. Palermo, T. M. Evans, and K. W. Klimpel.** 1987. Induction and repression of outer membrane proteins by anaerobic growth of *Neisseria gonorrhoeae. Infect. Immun.* **55:**1359–1364.

42. **Clark, V. L., J. S. Knapp, S. Thompson, and K. W. Klimpel.** 1988. Presence of antibodies to the major anaerobically induced gonococcal outer membrane protein in sera from patients with gonococcal infections. *Microb. Pathog.* **5:**381–390.

43. **Cohen, M. S., B. E. Britigan, M. French, and K. Bean.** 1987. Preliminary observations on lactoferrin secretion in human vaginal mucus: variation during the menstrual cycle, evidence of hormonal regulation, and implications for infection with *Neisseria gonorrhoeae. Am. J. Obstet. Gynecol.* **157:**1122–1125.

44. **Cohen, M. S., J. G. Cannon, A. E. Jerse, L. M. Charniga, S. F. Isbey, and L. G. Whicker.** 1994. Human experimentation with *Neisseria gonorrhoeae*: rationale, methods, and implications for

the biology of infection and vaccine development. *J. Infect. Dis.* **169:**532–537.

45. **Cohen, M. S., and P. F. Sparling.** 1992. Mucosal infection with *Neisseria gonorrhoeae. J. Clin. Investig.* **89:**1699–1705.

46. **Cohen, M. S., and W. C. Miller.** 1998. Sexually transmitted diseases and human immunodeficiency virus infection: cause, effect or both? *Int. J. Infect. Dis.* **3:**1–4.

47. **Cohen, M. S., and J. G. Cannon.** 1999. Human experimentation with *Neisseria gonorrhoeae*: progress and goals. *J. Infect. Dis.* **179:** S375–S379.

48. **Corbeil, L. B., A. Chatterjee, L. Foresman, and J. A. Westfall.** 1985. Ultrastructure of cyclic changes in the murine uterus, cervix and vagina. *Tissue Cell.* **17:**53–68.

49. **Cornelissen, C. N., G. D. Biswas, J. Tsai, D. K. Paruchuri, S. A. Thompson, and P. F. Sparling.** 1992. Gonococcal transferrin-binding protein 1 is required for transferrin utilization and is homologous to TonB-dependent outer membrane receptors. *J. Bacteriol.* **174:**5788–5797.

50. **Cornelissen, C. N., M. Kelley, M. M. Hobbs, J. E. Anderson, J. G. Cannon, M. S. Cohen, and P. F. Sparling.** 1998. The transferrin receptor expressed by gonococcal strain FA1090 is required for the experimental infection of human male volunteers. *Mol. Microbiol.* **27:**611–616.

51. **Crawford, G., J. S. Knapp, J. Hale, and K. K. Holmes.** 1977. Asymptomatic gonorrhea in men: caused by gonococci with unique nutritional requirements. *Science* **196:**1352–1353.

52. **Cucurull, E., and L. R. Espinoza.** 1998. Gonococcal arthritis. *Rheum Dis. Clin. N. Am.* **24:**305–322.

53. **Danaher, R. J., J. C. Levin, D. Arking, C. L. Burch, R. Sandlin, and D. C. Stein.** 1995. Genetic basis of *Neisseria gonorrhoeae* lipooligosaccharide antigenic variation. *J. Bacteriol.* **177:** 7275–7279.

54. **Deheragoda, P.** 1977. Diagnosis of rectal gonorrhoea by blind anorectal swabs compared with direct vision swabs taken via a proctoscope. *Br. J. Vener. Dis.* **53:**311–313.

55. **Dehio, C., S. D. Gray-Owen, and T. F. Meyer.** 1998. The role of neisserial Opa proteins in interactions with host cells. *Trends Microbiol.* **6:** 489–495.

56. **De la Paz, H., S. J. Cooke, and J. E. Heckels.** 1995. Effect of sialylation of lipopolysaccharide of *Neisseria gonorrhoeae* on recognition and complement-mediated killing by monoclonal antibodies directed against different outer-membrane antigens. *Microbiology* **141:**913–920.

57. **Division of STD Prevention.** 1995. *Sexually Transmitted Disease Surveillance, 1994.* Centers for Disease Control and Prevention, Atlanta, Ga.

58. **Dorig, R. E., A. Marcil, and C. D. Richardson.** 1994. CD46, a primate-specific receptor for measles virus. *Trends Microbiol.* **2:**312–318.

59. **Dorwood, D. W., C. F. Garon, and R. C. Judd.** 1989. Export and intercellular transfer of DNA via membrane blebs of *Neisseria gonorrhoeae. J. Bacteriol.* **171:**2499–2505.

60. **Dyer, D. W., E. P. West, and P. F. Sparling.** 1987. Effects of serum carrier proteins on the growth of pathogenic neisseriae with heme-bound iron. *Infect. Immun.* **55:**2171–2175.

61. **Eades-Perner, A. M., H. van der Putten, A. Hirth, J. Thompson, M. Neumaier, S. von Kleist, and W. Zimmermann.** 1994. Mice transgenic for the human carcinoembryonic antigen gene maintain its spatiotemporal expression pattern. *Cancer Res.* **54:**4169–4176.

62. **Elkins, C., and R. F. Rest.** 1990. Monoclonal antibodies to outer membrane protein PII block interactions of *Neisseria gonorrhoeae* with human neutrophils. *Infect. Immun.* **58:**1078–1084.

63. **Elkins, C., N. H. Carbonetti, V. A. Varela, D. Stirewalt, D. G. Klapper, and P. F. Sparling.** 1992. Antibodies to N-terminal peptides of gonococcal porin are bactericidal when gonococcal lipopolysaccharide is not sialylated. *Mol. Microbiol.* **6:**2617–2628.

64. **Eschenbach, D. A., J. P. Harnisch, and K. K. Holmes.** 1977. Pathogenesis of acute pelvic inflammatory disease: role of contraception and other risk factors. *Am. J. Obstet. Gynecol.* **128:** 838–850.

65. **Falk, V., and G. Krook.** 1967. Do results of culture for gonococci vary with sampling phase of menstrual cycle? *Acta Derm. Venereol.* **47:** 190–193.

66. **Faruki, H., R. N. Kohmescher, W. P. McKinney, and P. F. Sparling.** 1985. A community-based outbreak of infection with penicillin-resistant *Neisseria gonorrhoeae* not producing penicillinase (chromosomally mediated resistance). *N. Engl. J. Med.* **313:**607–611.

67. **Fischer, S. H., and R. F. Rest.** 1988. Gonococci possessing only certain P.II outer membrane proteins interact with human neutrophils. *Infect. Immun.* **56:**1574–1579.

68. **Flemming, T. J., D. E. Wallsmith, and R. S. Rosenthal.** 1986. Arthropathic properties of gonococcal peptidoglycan fragments: implications for the pathogenesis of disseminated gonococcal disease. *Infect. Immun.* **52:**600–608.

69. **Fox, K. K., J. C. Thomas, D. H. Weiner, R. H. Davis, P. F. Sparling, and M. S. Cohen.** 1999. Longitudinal evaluation of serovar-specific

immunity to *Neisseria gonorrhoeae*. *Am. J. Epidemiol.* **149**:353–358.

70. **Francioli, P., H. Shio, R. B. Roberts, and M. Müller.** 1983. Phagocytosis and killing of *Neisseria gonorrhoeae* by *Trichomonas vaginalis*. *J. Infect. Dis.* **147**:87–93.

71. **Frangipane, J. V., and R. F. Rest.** 1993. Anaerobic growth and cytidine 5′-monophospho-*N*-acetylneuraminic acid act synergistically to induce high-level serum resistance in *Neisseria gonorrhoeae*. *Infect. Immun.* **61**:1657–1666.

72. **Fyfe, J. A. M., C. S. Carrick, and J. K. Davis.** 1995. The *pilE* of *Neisseria gonorrhoeae* MS11 is transcribed from a σ^{70} promoter during growth in vitro. *J. Bacteriol.* **177**:3781–3787.

73. **Gill, M. J., D. P. McQuillen, J. O. P. van Putten, L. M. Wetzler, J. Bramley, H. Crooke, N. J. Parsons, J. A. Cole, and H. Smith.** 1996. Functional characterization of a sialyltransferase-deficient mutant of *Neisseria gonorrhoeae*. *Infect. Immun.* **64**:3374–3378.

74. **Glynn, A. A., and J. E. Ward.** 1970. Nature and heterogeneity of the antigens of *Neisseria gonorrhoeae* involved in the serum bactericidal reaction. *Infect. Immun.* **2**:162–168.

75. **Goldenberg, D. L., P. L. Chisholm, and P. A. Rice.** 1983. Experimental models of bacterial arthritis: a microbiologic and histopathologic characterization of the arthritis after the intraarticular injections of *Neisseria gonorrhoeae*, *Staphylococcus aureus*, group A streptococci, and *Escherichia coli*. *J. Rheumatol.* **10**:5–11.

76. **Gorbach, S. L., K. B. Menda, H. Thadepalli, and L. Keith.** 1973. Anaerobic microflora of the cervix in healthy women. *Am. J. Obstet. Gynecol.* **8**:1053–1055.

77. **Gorby, G. L., C. M. Clemens, L. R. Barley, and Z. A. McGee.** 1991. Effect of human chorionic gonadotropin (hCG) on Neisseria gonorrhoeae invasion of and IgA secretion by human fallopian tube mucosa. *Microb. Pathog.* **10**:373–384.

78. **Gorby, G. L., and G. B. Schaefer.** 1992. Effect of attachment factors (pili plus Opa) on *Neisseria gonorrhoeae* invasion of human fallopian tube tissue in vitro: quantitation by computerized image analysis. *Microb. Pathog.* **13**:93–108.

79. **Gotschlich, E. C., M. Seiff, and M. S. Blake.** 1987. The DNA sequence of the structural gene of gonococcal protein III and the flanking region containing a repetitive sequence. Homology of protein III with enterobacterial *ompA* proteins. *J. Exp. Med.* **165**:471–482.

80. **Gotschlich, E. C.** 1994. Genetic locus for the biosynthesis of the variable portion of *Neisseria gonorrhoeae* lipooligosaccharide. *J. Exp. Med.* **180**:2181–2190.

81. **Griffiss, J. M., J. H. Schneider, R. E. Mandrell, R. Yamasaki, G. A. Jarvis, J. J. Kim, B. W. Gibson, R. Hamadeh, and M. A. Apicella.** 1988. Lipooligosaccharides: the principal glycolipids of the neisserial outer membrane. *Rev. Infect. Dis.* **10**:S287–S295.

82. **Griffiss, J. M., G. A. Jarvis, J. P. O'Brien, M. M. Eads, and H. Schneider.** 1991. Lysis of *Neisseria gonorrhoeae* initiated by binding of normal human IgM to a hexosamine-containing lipooligosaccharide epitope(s) is augmented by strain-specific, properdin-binding-dependent alternative complement pathway activation. *J. Immunol.* **147**:298–305.

83. **Haas, R., S. Veit, and T. F. Meyer.** 1992. Silent pilin genes of *Neisseria gonorrhoeae* MS11 and the occurrence of related hypervariant sequences among other gonococcal isolates. *Mol. Microbiol.* **6**:197–208.

84. **Haines, K. A., L. Yeh, M. S. Blake, P. Cristello, H. Korchak, and G. Weissmann.** 1988. Protein I, a translocatable ion channel from *Neisseria gonorrhoeae*, selectively inhibits exocytosis from human neutrophils without inhibiting O_2^- generation. *J. Biol. Chem.* **263**:945–951.

85. **Handsfield, H. H., T. O. Lipman, J. P. Harnish, E. Tronca, and K. K. Holmes.** 1974. Asymptomatic gonorrhea in men. Diagnosis, natural course, prevalence and significance. *N. Engl. J. Med.* **290**:117–123.

86. **Harkness, A. H.** 1948. The pathology of gonorrhea. *Br. J. Vener. Dis.* **24**:137–147.

87. **Harrison, W. O., R. R. Hooper, P. J. Weisner, A. F. Campbell, W. W. Karney, G. H. Reynolds, O. G. Jones, and K. K. Holmes.** 1979. A trial of minocycline given after exposure to prevent gonorrhea. *N. Engl. J. Med.* **300**:1074–1078.

88. **Harvey, H. A., M. R. Ketterer, A. Preston, D. Lubaroff, R. Williams, and M. A. Apicella.** 1997. Ultrastructural analysis of primary human urethral epithelial cell cultures infected with *Neisseria gonorrhoeae*. *Infect. Immun.* **65**:2420–2427.

89. **Hassett, D. J., L. Charniga, and M. S. Cohen.** 1990. recA and catalase in H_2O_2-mediated toxicity in *Neisseria gonorrhoeae*. *J. Bacteriol.* **172**:7293–7296.

90. **Hauck, C. R., D. Lorenzen, J. Salas, and T. F. Meyer.** 1997. An in vitro-differentiated human cell line as a model system to the interaction of *Neisseria gonorrhoeae* with phagocytic cells. *Infect. Immun.* **65**:1863–1869.

91. **Hebeler, B. H., W. W. Wong, S. A. Morse, and F. E. Young.** 1979. Cell envelope of *Neisseria gonorrhoeae* CS7: peptidoglycan-protein complex. *Infect. Immun.* **23**:353–359.

92. **Hedges, S. R., M. S. Mayo, L. Kallman, J. Mestecky, E. W. Hook, and M. W. Russell.** 1998. Evaluation of immunoglobulin A1 (IgA1) protease and IgA1 protease-inhibitory activity in human female genital infection with *Neisseria gonorrhoeae*. *Infect. Immun.* **66:**5826–5832.

93. **Hedges, S. R., D. A. Sibley, M. S. Mayo, E. W. Hook, and M. W. Russell.** 1998. Cytokine and antibody responses in women infected with *Neisseria gonorrhoeae*: effects of concomitant infections. *J. Infect. Dis.* **178:**742–751.

94. **Hipp, S. S., W. D. Lawton, N. C. Chen, and H. A. Gaafar.** 1974. Inhibition of *Neisseria gonorrhoeae* by a factor produced by *Candida albicans*. *Appl. Microbiol.* **27:**192–196.

95. **Hobbs, M. M., T. M. Alcorn, R. H. Davis, W. Fischer, J. C. Thomas, I. Martin, C. Ison, P. F. Sparling, and M. S. Cohen.** 1999. Molecular typing of *Neisseria gonorrhoeae* causing repeated infections: evolution of porin during passage within a community. *J. Infect. Dis.* **179:**371–381.

96. **Holmes, K. K., G. W. Counts, and H. N. Beaty.** 1971. Disseminated gonococcal infection. *Ann. Intern. Med.* **74:**979–993.

97. **Hook, E. W., and K. K. Holmes.** 1985. Gonococcal infections. *Ann. Intern. Med.* **102:**229–243.

98. **Hook, E. W., D. A. Olsen, and T. M. Buchanan.** 1984. Analysis of the antigen specificity of the human serum immunoglobulin G immune response to complicated gonococcal infection. *Infect. Immun.* **43:**706–709.

99. **Hook, E. W., and H. H. Handsfield.** 1999. Gonococcal infections in the adult, p. 451–472. *In* K. K. Holmes, P. A. Mardh, P. F. Sparling, S. M. Lemon, W. E. Stamm, P. Piot, and J. N. Wasserheit (ed.), *Sexually Transmitted Diseases*, 3rd ed. McGraw-Hill Companies, Inc., New York, N.Y.

100. **Householder, T. C., W. A. Belli, S. Lissenden, J. A. Cole, and V. L. Clark.** 1999. *cis*- and *trans*-acting elements involved in regulation of *aniA*, the gene encoding the major anaerobically induced outer membrane protein in *Neisseria gonorrhoeae*. *J. Bacteriol.* **181:**541–551.

101. **Ilver, D., H. Kallstrom, S. Normark, and A. B. Jonsson.** 1998. Transcellular passage of *Neisseria gonorrhoeae* involves pilus phase variation. *Infect. Immun.* **66:**469–473.

102. **James, J. F., and J. Swanson.** 1978. Color/opacity colonial variants of *Neisseria gonorrhoeae* and their relationship to the menstrual cycle, p. 338–343. *In* G. F. Brooks, E. C. Gotschlich, K. K. Holmes, W. D. Sawyer, and F. E. Young (ed.), *Immunobiology of Neisseria gonorrhoeae*. American Society for Microbiology, Washington, D.C.

103. **James, J. F., and J. Swanson.** 1978. Studies on gonococcus infection. XIII. Occurrence of color/opacity colonial variants in clinical cultures. *Infect. Immun.* **19:**332–340.

104. **Jerse, A. E., J. S. Cohen, P. M. Drown, L. G. Whicker, S. F. Isbey, H. S. Seifert, and J. G. Cannon.** 1994. Multiple gonococcal opacity proteins are expressed during experimental urethral infection in the male. *J. Exp. Med.* **179:**911–920.

105. **Jerse, A. E.** 1999. Experimental gonococcal genital tract infection and opacity protein expression in estradiol-treated mice. *Infect. Immun.* **67:**5699–5708.

106. **Johnson, A. P., M. Tuffrey, and D. Taylor-Robinson.** 1989. Resistance of mice to genital infection with *Neisseria gonorrhoeae*. *J. Med. Microbiol.* **30:**33–36.

107. **Johnson, D. W., K. K. Holmes, P. A. Kvale, C. W. Halverson, and W. P. Hirsch.** 1969. An evaluation of gonorrhea case finding in the chronically infected female. *Am. J. Epidemiol.* **90:**438–448.

108. **Johnson, S. R., B. M. Steiner, D. D. Cruce, G. H. Perkins, and R. J. Arko.** 1993. Characterization of a catalase-deficient strain of *Neisseria gonorrhoeae*: evidence for the significance of catalase in the biology of *N. gonorrhoeae*. *Infect. Immun.* **61:**1232–1238.

109. **Johnson, S. R., B. M. Steiner, and G. H. Perkins.** 1996. Cloning and characterization of the catalase gene of *Neisseria gonorrhoeae*: use of the gonococcus as a host organism for recombinant DNA. *Infect. Immun.* **64:**2627–2634.

110. **Jonsson, A. B., G. Nyberg, and S. Normark.** 1991. Phase variation of gonococcal pili by frameshift mutation in *pilC*, a novel gene for pilus assembly. *EMBO J.* **10:**477–488.

111. **Kallstrom, H., M. K. Liszewski, J. P. Atkinson, and A. B. Jonsson.** 1997. Membrane cofactor protein (MCP or CD46) is a cellular pilus receptor for pathogenic *Neisseria*. *Mol. Microbiol.* **25:**639–647.

112. **Kampmeier, R. H.** 1978. Identification of the gonococcus by Albert Neisser. *Sex. Transm. Dis.* **5:**71–72.

113. **Kellogg, D. S., Jr., I. R. Cohen, L. C. Norins, A. L. Schroeter, and G. Reising.** 1968. *Neisseria gonorrhoeae*. II. Colonial variation and pathogenicity during 35 months in vitro. *J. Bacteriol.* **96:**596–605.

114. **Kellogg, D. S., W. L. Peacock, W. E. Deacon, L. Brown, and C. I. Pirkle.** 1963. *Neisseria gonorrhoeae*. I. Virulence genetically linked to clonal variation. *J. Bacteriol.* **85:**1274–1279.

115. **Kerle, K. K., J. R. Mascola, and T. A. Miller.** 1992. Disseminated gonococcal infection. *Am. Fam. Physician* **45:**209–214.

116. **Kilian, M., J. Mestecky, and M. W. Russell.** 1988. Defense mechanisms involving Fc-dependent functions of immunoglobulin A and their subversion by bacterial immunoglobulin A proteases. *Microbiol. Rev.* **52:**296–303.

117. **Kita, E., H. Matsuura, and S. Kashiba.** 1981. A mouse model for the study of gonococcal genital infection. *J. Infect. Dis.* **143:**67–70.

118. **Kita, E., S. Takahashi, K. Yasui, and S. Kashiba.** 1985. Effect of estrogen (17β-estradiol) on the susceptibility of mice to disseminated gonococcal infection. *Infect. Immun.* **49:**238–243.

119. **Klaus, B. D., J. E. Chandler, and P. E. Dans.** 1978. Gonorrhea detection in posthysterectomy patients. *JAMA* **240:**1360–1361.

120. **Klimpel, K. W., S. A. Lesley, and V. L. Clark.** 1989. Identification of subunits of gonococcal RNA polymerase by immunoblot analysis: evidence for multiple sigma factors. *J. Bacteriol.* **171:**3713–3718.

121. **Knapp, J. S., and V. L. Clark.** 1984. Anaerobic growth of *Neisseria gonorrhoeae* coupled to nitrite reduction. *Infect. Immun.* **46:**176–181.

122. **Koch, M. L.** 1947. A study of cervical cultures taken in cases of acute gonorrhea with special reference to the phases of the menstrual cycle. *Am. J. Obstet. Gynecol.* **54:**861–866.

123. **Koch, M. L.** 1950. The bactericidal action of beta progesterone. *Am. J. Obstet. Gynecol.* **59:**168–171.

124. **Kupsch, E. M., B. Knepper, T. Kuroki, I. Heuer, and T. F. Meyer.** 1993. Variable opacity (Opa) outer membrane proteins account for the cell tropisms displayed by *Neisseria gonorrhoeae* for human leukocytes and epithelial cells. *EMBO J.* **12:**641–650.

125. **Kutteh, W. H., S. J. Prince, K. R. Hammond, C. C. Kutteh, and J. Mestecky.** 1996. Variations in immunoglobulins and IgA subclasses of human uterine cervical secretions around the time of ovulation. *Clin. Exp. Immunol.* **104:**538–542.

126. **Lambden, P. R., and J. E. Heckels.** 1979. Outer membrane protein composition and colonial morphology of *Neisseria gonorrhoeae* strain P9. *FEMS Microbiol. Lett.* **5:**263–265.

127. **Lambden, P. R., J. E. Heckels, and P. J. Watt.** 1982. Effect of anti-pilus antibodies on survival of gonococci within guinea pig subcutaneous chambers. *Infect. Immun.* **38:**27–30.

128. **Lanigan-O'Keefe, F. M.** 1974. Prepubertal gonorrhea. *Br. J. Vener. Dis.* **50:**381.

129. **Laskos, L., J. P. Dillard, H. S. Seifert, J. A. M. Fyfe, and J. K. Davies.** 1998. The pathogenic neisseriae contain an inactive *rpoN* gene and do not utilize the *pilE* σ 54 promoter. *Gene* **208:**95–102.

130. **Lebedeff, D. A., and E. B. Hochman.** 1980. Rectal gonorrhea in men: diagnosis and treatment. *Ann. Intern. Med.* **92:**463–466.

131. **Lee, B. C., and A. B. Schryvers.** 1988. Specificity of the lactoferrin and transferrin receptors in *Neisseria gonorrhoeae.* *Mol. Microbiol.* **2:**827–829.

132. **Lin, L., P. Ayala, J. Larson, M. Mulks, M. Fukuda, S. R. Carlsson, C. Enns, and M. So.** 1997. The Neisseria type 2 IgA1 protease cleaves LAMP1 and promotes survival of bacteria within epithelial cells. *Mol. Microbiol.* **24:**1083–1084.

133. **Lowe, T. L., and S. J. Kraus.** 1976. Quantitation of *Neisseria gonorrhoeae* from women with gonorrhea. *J. Infect. Dis.* **133:**621–626.

134. **Lucas, J. B., E. V. Price, J. D. Thayer, and A. Schroeter.** 1967. Diagnosis and treatment of gonorrhea in the female. *N. Engl. J. Med.* **276:**1454–1459.

135. **Magnusson, K. E., E. Kihlstrom, L. Norlander, A. Norqvist, J. Davies, and S. Normark.** 1979. Effect of colony type and pH on surface charge and hydrophobicity of *Neisseria gonorrhoeae.* *Infect. Immun.* **26:**397–401.

136. **Mandrell, R., H. Schneider, M. Apicella, W. Zollinger, P. A. Rice, and J. M. Griffiss.** 1986. Antigenic and physical diversity of *Neisseria gonorrhoeae* lipooligosaccharides. *Infect. Immun.* **54:**63–69.

137. **Mandrell, R. E., H. Smith, G. A. Jarvis, J. M. Griffiss, and J. A. Cole.** 1993. Detection and some properties of the sialyltransferase implicated in the sialylation of lipopolysaccharide of *Neisseria gonorrheae.* *Microb. Pathog.* **14:**307–313.

138. **Mandrell, R. E., and M. A. Apicella.** 1993. Lipo-oligosaccharides (LOS) of mucosal pathogens: molecular mimicry and host-modification of LOS. *Immunobiology* **187:**382–402.

139. **Mardh, P.-A., and L. Westrom.** 1976. Adherence of bacteria to vaginal epithelial cells. *Infect. Immun.* **13:**661–666.

140. **Masson, P. L., J. F. Heremans, and J. Ferin.** 1968. Presence of an iron-binding protein (lactoferrin) in the genital tract of the human female. I. Its immunohistochemical localization in the endometrium. *Fertil. Steril.* **19:**679–689.

141. **McBride, H. M., P. R. Lamden, J. E. Heckels, and P. J. Watt.** 1981. The role of outer membrane proteins in the survival of *Neisseria gonorrhoeae* P9 within guinea-pig subcutaneous chambers. *J. Gen. Microbiol.* **126:**63–67.

142. **McCormack, W. M., R. J. Stumacher, K.**

Johnson, A. Donner, and R. Rychwalski. 1977. Clinical spectrum of gonococcal infection in women. *Lancet* **2:**1182–1185.

143. **McCormack, W. M., G. H. Reynolds, and the Cooperative Study Group.** 1982. Effect of menstrual cycle and method of contraception on recovery of *Neisseria gonorrhoeae*. *JAMA* **247:**1292–1294.

144. **McCutchan, J. A., A. Wunderlich, and A. I. Braude.** 1977. Role of urinary solutes in natural immunity to gonorrhea. *Infect. Immun.* **15:**149–155.

145. **McChesney, D., E. C. Tramont, J. W. Boslego, J. Ciak, J. Sadoff, and C. C. Brinton.** 1982. Genital antibody response to a parenteral gonococcal pilus vaccine. *Infect. Immun.* **36:**1006–1012.

146. **McGee, A. A., R. L. Jensen, C. M. Clemens, D. Taylor-Robinson, A. P. Johnson, and C. R. Gregg.** 1999. Gonococcal infection of human fallopian tube mucosa in organ culture: relationship of mucosal tissue TNF-alpha concentration to sloughing of ciliated cells. *Sex. Transm. Dis.* **26:**160–165.

147. **Merz, A. J., D. B. Rifenbery, C. G. Arvidson, and M. So.** 1996. Traversal of polarized epithelium by pathogenic *Neisseriae*: facilitation by type IV pili and maintenance of epithelial barrier function. *Mol. Med.* **2:**745–754.

148. **Meyer, T. F., and J. P. M. van Putten.** 1989. Genetic mechanisms and biological implications of phase variation in pathogenic *Neisseriae*. *Clin. Microbiol. Rev.* **2:**S139–S145.

149. **Mickelsen, P. A., and P. F. Sparling.** 1981. Ability of *Neisseria gonorrhoeae, Neisseria meningitidis,* and commensal *Neisseria* species to obtain iron from transferrin and iron compounds. *Infect. Immun.* **33:**555–564.

150. **Mickelsen, P. A., E. Blackman, and P. F. Sparling.** 1982. Ability of *Neisseria gonorrhoeae, Neisseria meningitidis,* and commensal *Neisseria* species to obtain iron from lactoferrin. *Infect. Immun.* **35:**915–920.

151. **Mims, C. A.** 1997. The encounter of the microbe with the phagocytic cell, p. 60–105. *In* N. Dimmock, A. Nash, J. Stephen, and C. A. Mims (ed.), *The Pathogenesis of Infectious Disease,* 4th ed. Academic Press, Inc., San Diego, Calif.

152. **Morse, S. A., and T. J. Fitzgerald.** 1974. Effect of progesterone on *Neisseria gonorrhoeae*. *Infect. Immun.* **10:**1370–1377.

153. **Mosleh, I. M., H. J. Boxberger, M. J. Sessler, and T. F. Meyer.** 1997. Experimental infection of native human urethral tissue with *Neisseria gonorrhoeae*: adhesion, invasion, intracellular fate, exocytosis, and passage through a stratified epithelium. *Infect. Immun.* **65:**3391–3398.

154. **Mrkic, B., J. Pavlovic, T. Rulicke, P. Volpe, C. J. Buchholz, D. Hourcade, J. P. Atkinson, A. Aguzzi, and R. Cattaneo.** 1998. Measles virus spread and pathogenesis in genetically modified mice. *J. Virol.* **72:**7420–7427.

155. **Naids, F. L., B. Belisle, N. Lee, and R. F. Rest.** 1991. Interactions of *Neisseria gonorrhoeae* with human neutrophils: studies with purified PII (Opa) outer membrane proteins and synthetic opa peptides. *Infect. Immun.* **59:**4628–4635.

156. **Naids, F. L., and R. F. Rest.** 1991. Stimulation of human neutrophil oxidative metabolism by nonopsonized *Neisseria gonorrhoeae*. *Infect. Immun.* **59:**4383–4390.

157. **Naumann, M., S. Webler, C. Bartsch, B. Wieland, and T. F. Meyer.** 1997. *Neisseria gonorrhoeae* epithelial cell interaction leads to the activation of the transcription factors nuclear factor κB and activator protein 1 and the induction of inflammatory cytokines. *J. Exp. Med.* **186:**247–258.

158. **Novotny, P., E. S. Broughton, K. Cownley, M. Hughes, and W. H. Turner.** 1978. Strain related infectivity of *Neisseria gonorrhoeae* for the guinea-pig subcutaneous chamber and the variability of the immune resistance in different breeds of guinea pig. *Br. J. Vener. Dis.* **54:**88–96.

159. **Nowicki, S., M. G. Martens, and B. J. Nowicki.** 1995. Gonococcal infection in a nonhuman host is determined by human complement C1q. *Infect. Immun.* **63:**4790–4794.

160. **O'Brien, J. P., D. L. Goldenberg, and P. A. Rice.** 1983. Disseminated gonococcal infection: a prospective analysis of 49 patients and a review of pathophysiology and immune mechanisms. *Medicine* **62:**395–406.

161. **Pariser, H.** 1972. Asymptomatic gonorrhea. *Med. Clin. N. Am.* **56:**1127–1132.

162. **Patton, D. L., and R. G. Rank.** 1992. Animal models for the study of pelvic inflammatory disease, p. 85–111. *In* T. Quinn (ed.), *Advances in Host Defense Mechanisms.* Book News Inc., Portland, Oreg.

163. **Petricoin, E. F., R. J. Danaher, and D. C. Stein.** 1991. Analysis of the *lsi* region involved in lipooligosaccharide biosynthesis in *Neisseria gonorrhoeae*. *J. Bacteriol.* **173:**7896–7902.

164. **Pettit, R. K., E. S. Martin, S. M. Wagner, and V. J. Bertolino.** 1995. Phenotypic modulation of gonococcal lipooligosaccharide in acidic and alkaline culture. *Infect. Immun.* **63:**2773–2775.

165. **Pettit, R. K., M. J. Filiatrault, and E. S. Martin.** 1996. Alteration of gonococcal protein expression in acidic culture. *Infect. Immun.* **64:**1039–1042.

166. **Pettit, R. K., S. C. McAllister, and T. A. Hamer.** 1999. Response of gonococcal clinical isolates to acidic conditions. *J. Med. Microbiol.* **48:** 149–156.

167. **Phillips, R. S., P. A. Hanff, A. Wertheimer, M. D. Aronson.** 1988. Gonorrhea in women seen for routine gynecologic care: criteria for testing. *Am. J. Med.* **85:**177–182.

168. **Platt, R., P. A. Rice, and W. M. McCormack.** 1983. Risk of acquiring gonorrhea and prevalence of abnormal adnexal findings among women recently exposed to gonorrhea. *JAMA* **250:**3205–3209.

169. **Plummer, F. A., H. Chubb, J. N. N. Simonsen, M. Bosire, L. Slaney, N. J. Nagelkenke, I. MacClean, and J. O. Ndinga-Ayola.** 1994. Antibodies to opacity proteins (Opa) correlate with a reduced risk of gonococcal salpingitis. *J. Clin. Investig.* **93:**1748–1755.

170. **Plummer, F. A., J. N. Simonsen, H. Chubb, L. Sianey, J. Kimata, M. Bosire, J. O. Ndinya-Achola, and E. N. Ngugi.** 1989. Epidemiologic evidence for the development of serovar-specific immunity after gonococcal infection. *J. Clin. Investig.* **83:**1472–1476.

171. **Plummer, F. A., H. Chubb, J. N. Simonsen, M. Bosire, L. Slaney, I. Maclean, J. O. Ndinya-Achola, P. Waiyaki, and R. C. Brunham.** 1993. Antibody to Rmp (outer membrane protein 3) increases susceptibility to gonococcal infection. *J. Clin. Investig.* **91:**339–343.

172. **Porat, N., M. A. Apicella, and M. S. Blake.** 1995. *Neisseria gonorrhoeae* utilizes and enhances the biosynthesis of the asialoglycoprotein receptor expressed on the surface of the hepatic HepG2 cell line. *Infect. Immun.* **63:**1498–1506.

173. **Punsalang, A. P., and W. D. Sawyer.** 1973. Role of pili in the virulence of *Neisseria gonorrhoeae. Infect. Immun.* **8:**255–263.

174. **Qu, X. D., S. S. Harwig, A. M. Oren, W. M. Shafer, and R. I. Lehrer.** 1996. Susceptibility of *Neisseria gonorrhoeae* to protegrins. *Infect. Immun.* **64:**1240–1245.

175. **Quinn, T. C., W. E. Stamm, S. E. Goodell, E. Mkrtichian, J. Benedetti, L. Corey, M. D. Schuffler, and K. K. Holmes.** 1983. The polymicrobial origin of intestinal infections in homosexual men. *N. Engl. J. Med.* **309:**576–582.

176. **Ramsey, K. H., H. Schneider, A. S. Cross, J. W. Boslego, D. L. Hoover, T. L. Staley, R. A. Kuschner, and C. D. Deal.** 1995. Inflammatory cytokines produced in response to experimental human gonorrhea. *J. Infect. Dis.* **172:**186–191.

177. **Ravn, V., C. Stubbe, U. Mandel, and E. Dabelsteen.** 1992. The distribution of type-2 chain histo-blood group antigens in normal cycling human endometrium. *Cell Tissue Res.* **270:** 425–433.

178. **Redondo-Lopez, V., R. L. Cook, and J. D. Sobel.** 1990. Emerging role of lactobacilli in the control and maintenance of the vaginal bacterial microflora. *Rev. Infect. Dis.* **12:**856–872.

179. **Rees, E., and E. H. Annels.** 1969. Gonococcal salpingitis. *Br. J. Vener. Dis.* **45:**205–215.

180. **Reid, G., A. W. Bruce, and M. Taylor.** 1992. Influence of three-day antimicrobial therapy and lactobacillus vaginal suppositories on recurrence of urinary tract infections. *Clin. Ther.* **14:**11–16.

181. **Rest, R. F., S. H. Fischer, Z. Z. Ingham, and J. F. Jones.** 1982. Interactions of *Neisseria gonorrhoeae* with human neutrophils: effects of serum and gonococcal opacity on phagocyte killing and chemiluminescence. *Infect. Immun.* **36:** 737–744.

182. **Rest, R. F., and J. V. Frangipane.** 1992. Growth of *Neisseria gonorrhoeae* in CMP-N-acetylneuraminic acid inhibits nonopsonic (opacity-associated outer membrane protein-mediated) interactions with human neutrophils. *Infect. Immun.* **60:**989–997.

183. **Rice, P. A., and D. L. Goldenberg.** 1981. Clinical manifestations of disseminated infection caused by *Neisseria gonorrhoeae* are linked to differences in bactericidal reactivity of infecting strains. *Ann. Intern. Med.* **95:**175–178.

184. **Rice, P. A., H. E. Vayo, M. R. Tam, and M. S. Blake.** 1986. Immunoglobulin G antibodies directed against protein III block killing of serum-resistant Neisseria gonorrhoeae by immune serum. *J. Exp. Med.* **164:**1735–1748.

185. **Rice, P. A.** 1989. Molecular basis for serum resistance in *Neisseria gonorrhoeae. Clin. Microbiol. Rev.* **2:**S112–S117.

186. **Richardson, W. P., and J. C. Sadoff.** 1988. Induced engulfment of *Neisseria gonorrhoeae* by tissue culture cells. *Infect. Immun.* **56:**2512–2514.

187. **Rompalo, A. M., E. W. Hook, P. L. Roberts, M. D. Ramsey, H. Handsfield, and K. K. Holmes.** 1957. The acute arthritis-dermatitis syndrome. The changing importance of *Neisseria gonorrhoeae* and *Neisseria meningitidis. Arch. Intern. Med.* **147:**281–283.

188. **Ross, S. C., and P. Densen.** 1985. Opsonophagocytosis of *Neisseria gonorrhoeae*: interaction of local and disseminated isolates with complement and neutrophils. *J. Infect. Dis.* **151:**33–41.

189. **Rothbard, J. B., R. Fernández, L. Wang, N. H. Teng, and G. K. Schoolnik.** 1985. Antibodies to peptides corresponding to a conserved sequence of gonococcal pilins block bacterial adhesion. *Proc. Natl. Acad. Sci. USA* **82:**915–919.

190. **Saigh, J. H., C. C. Sanders, and W. E. Sanders.** 1978. Inhibition of *Neisseria gonorrhoeae* by

aerobic and facultatively anaerobic components of the endocervical flora: evidence for a protective effect against infection. *Infect. Immun.* **19:**704–710.

191. **Salit, I. E.** 1982. The differential susceptibility of gonococcal opacity variants to sex hormones. *Can. J. Biochem.* **60:**301–306.

192. **Sarafian, S. K., M. R. Tam, and S. A. Morse.** 1983. Gonococcal protein I-specific IgG in normal human serum. *J. Infect. Dis.* **148:**1025–1032.

193. **Sayeed, Z. A., U. Bhaduri, E. Howell, and H. L. Meyers.** 1972. Gonococcal meningitis. *JAMA* **219:**1730–1731.

194. **Scheuerpflug, I., T. Rudel, R. Ryll, J. Pandit, and T. F. Meyer.** 1999. Roles of PilC and PilE proteins in pilus-mediated adherence of *Neisseria gonorrhoeae* and *Neisseria meningitidis* to human erythrocytes and endothelial and epithelial cells. *Infect. Immun.* **67:**834–843.

195. **Schiller, N. L., G. L. Friedman, and R. B. Roberts.** 1979. The role of natural IgG and complement in the phagocytosis of type 4 *Neisseria gonorrhoeae* by human polymorphonuclear leucocytes. *J. Infect. Dis.* **140:**698–707.

196. **Schneider, H., J. M. Griffiss, G. D. Williams, and G. B. Pier.** 1982. Immunological basis of serum resistance of *Neisseria gonorrhoeae.* *J. Gen. Microbiol.* **128:**13–22.

197. **Schneider, H., T. L. Hale, W. D. Zollinger, R. C. Seid, C. A. Hammack, and J. M. Griffiss.** 1984. Heterogeneity of molecular size and antigenic expression within lipooligosaccharides of individual strains of *Neisseria gonorrhoeae* and *Neisseria meningitidis. Infect. Immun.* **45:**544–549.

198. **Schneider, H., J. M. Griffiss, R. E. Mandrell, and G. A. Jarvis.** 1985. Elaboration of a 3.6-kilodalton lipooligosaccharide, antibody against which is absent from human sera, is associated with serum resistance of *Neisseria gonorrhoeae. Infect. Immun.* **50:**672–677.

199. **Schneider, H., J. M. Griffiss, J. W. Boslego, P. J. Hitchcock, K. M. Zahos, and M. A. Apicella.** 1991. Expression of paragloboside-like lipooligosaccharides may be a necessary component of gonococcal pathogenesis in men. *J. Exp. Med.* **174:**1601–1605.

200. **Schneider, H., K. A. Schmidt, D. R. Skillman, L. van de Verg, R. L. Warren, H. J. Wylie, J. C. Sadoff, C. D. Deal, and A. S. Cross.** 1996. Sialylation lessens the infectivity of *Neisseria gonorrhoeae* MS11mkC. *J. Infect. Dis.* **173:**1422–1427.

201. **Seifert, H. S.** 1996. Questions about gonococcal pilus phase and antigenic variation. *Mol. Microbiol.* **21:**433–440.

202. **Seifert, H. S., C. J. Wright, A. E. Jerse, M. S. Cohen, and J. G. Cannon.** 1994. Multiple gonococcal pilin antigenic variants are produced during experimental human infections. *J. Clin. Investig.* **93:**2744–2749.

203. **Shafer, W. M., and R. F. Rest.** 1989. Interactions of gonococci with phagocytic cells. *Annu. Rev. Microbiol.* **43:**121–145.

204. **Shafer, W. M., V. C. Onunka, M. Jannoun, and L. W. Hutwaite.** 1990. Molecular mechanism for the anti-gonococcal action of lysosomal cathepsin G. *Mol. Microbiol.* **4:**1269–1277.

205. **Shapiro, R. A., C. J. Schubert, and P. A. Myers.** 1993. Vaginal discharge as an indicator of gonorrhea and Chlamydia infection in girls under 12 years old. *Pediatr. Emerg. Care* **9:**341–345.

206. **Shaw, J. H., and S. Falkow.** 1988. Model for invasion of human tissue culture cells by *Neisseria gonorrhoeae. Infect. Immun.* **56:**1625–1632.

207. **Sherrard, J., and D. Barlow.** 1996. Gonorrhea in men: clinical and diagnostic aspects. *Genitourin. Med.* **72:**422–426.

208. **Shtibel, R.** 1976. Inhibition of growth of *Neisseria gonorrhoeae* by bacterial interference. *Can. J. Microbiol.* **22:**1430–1436.

209. **Simon, D., and R. F. Rest.** 1992. *Escherichia coli* expressing a *Neisseria gonorrhoeae* opacity-associated outer membrane protein invade human cervical and endometrial epithelial cell lines. *Proc. Natl. Acad. Sci. USA* **89:**5512–5516.

210. **Singer, A.** 1975. The uterine cervix from adolescence to the menopause. *Br. J. Obstet. Gynaecol.* **82:**81–99.

211. **Skerman, J. K., and K. K. Holmes.** 1975. Disseminated gonococcal infections caused by *Neisseria gonorrhoeae. J. Infect. Dis.* **132:**204–208.

212. **Smith, H., N. J. Parson, and J. A. Cole.** 1995. Sialylation of neisserial lipopolysaccharide: a major influence on pathogenicity. *Microb. Pathog.* **19:**365–377.

213. **Sparling, P. F., J. Tsai, and C. N. Cornelissen.** 1990. Gonococci are survivors. *Scand. J. Infect. Dis.* **69:**S125–S136.

214. **Spence, J. M., C. Chen, and V. L. Clark.** 1997. A proposed role for the lutropin receptor in contact-inducible gonococcal invasion of the Hec1B cells. *Infect. Immun.* **65:**3736–3742.

215. **Spink, W. W., and C. S. Keefer.** 1937. Latent gonorrhea as a cause of acute polyarticular arthritis. *JAMA* **109:**325–328.

216. **Stephens, D. S.** 1989. Gonococcal and meningococcal pathogenesis as defined by human cell, cell culture, and organ culture assays. *Clin. Microbiol. Rev.* **2:**S104–S111.

217. **Streeter, P. R., and L. B. Corbeil.** 1981. Gonococcal infection in endotoxin-resistant and

endotoxin-susceptible mice. *Infect. Immun.* **32:** 105–110.

218. **Sugasawara, R. J., J. G. Cannon, W. J. Black, I. Nachamkin, R. L. Sweet, and G. F. Brooks.** 1983. Inhibition of *Neisseria gonorrhoeae* attachment to HeLa cells with monoclonal antibody directed against a protein II. *Infect. Immun.* **42:**980–985.

219. **Swanson, J.** 1982. Colony opacity and protein II compositions of gonococci. *Infect. Immun.* **37:** 359–368.

220. **Swanson, J.** 1972. Studies on gonococcus infection. Pili: their role in attachment of gonococci to tissue culture cells. *J. Exp. Med.* **137:**571–589.

221. **Swanson, J., O. Barrera, J. Sola, and J. Boslego.** 1988. Expression of outer membrane protein II by gonococci in experimental gonorrhea. *J. Exp. Med.* **168:**2121–2129.

222. **Swanson J., K. Robbins, O. Barrera, D. Corwin, J. Boslego, J. Ciak, M. Blake, and J. M. Koomey.** 1987. Gonococcal pilin variants in experimental gonorrhea. *J. Exp. Med.* **165:** 1344–1357.

223. **Sweet, R. L., M. Blankfort-Doyle, M. O. Robbie, and J. Schacter.** 1986. The occurrence of chlamydial and gonococcal salpingitis during the menstrual cycle. *JAMA* **255:** 2062–2064.

224. **Taha, M. K., B. Dupuy, W. Saurin, M. So, and C. Marchal.** 1991. Control of pilus expression in *Neisseria gonorrhoeae*: an original system in the family of two-component regulators. *Mol. Microbiol.* **5:**137–148.

225. **Taylor-Robinson, D., P. M. Furr, and C. M. Hetherington.** 1990. *Neisseria gonorrhoeae* colonises the genital tract of oestradiol-treated germ-free female mice. *Microb. Pathog.* **9:** 369–374.

226. **Thomas, C. E., and P. F. Sparling.** 1996. Isolation and analysis of a *fur* mutant *Neisseria gonorrhoeae*. *J. Bacteriol.* **178:**4224–4232.

227. **Tikly, M., M. Diese, N. Zannettou, and R. Essop.** 1997. Gonococcal endocarditis in a patient with systemic lupus erythematosus. *Br. J. Rheumatol.* **36:**270–272.

228. **Tonjum, T., and M. Koomey.** 1997. The pilus colonization factor of pathogenic neisserial species: organelle biogenesis and structure/ function relationship—a review. *Gene* **192:** 155–163.

229. **Tramont, E. C.** 1976. Specificity of inhibition of epithelial cell adhesion of *Neisseria gonorrhoeae*. *Infect. Immun.* **14:**593–595.

230. **Turner, C. D., and J. T. Bagnara.** 1976. Endocrinology of the ovary, p. 450–495. *In General Endocrinology*. The W. B. Saunders Company, Philadelphia, Pa.

231. **Upchurch, D. M., W. E. Brady, C. A. Reichart, and E. W. Hook III.** 1990. Behavioral contributions to acquisition of gonorrhea in patients attending an inner city sexually transmitted disease clinic. *J. Infect. Dis.* **161:**938–941.

232. **U.S. Department of Health and Human Services.** 1991. Pelvic inflammatory disease. Research directions in the 1990s. *Sex. Transm. Dis.* **18:**46–64.

233. **van Putten, J. P. M.** 1993. Phase variation of lipopolysaccharide directs interconversion of invasive and immuno-resistant phenotypes of *Neisseria gonorrhoeae*. *EMBO J.* **12:**4043–4051.

234. **Virji, M., S. M. Watt, S. Barker, K. Makepeace, and R. Doyonnas.** 1996. The N-domain of the human CD66a adhesion molecule is a target for Opa proteins of *Neisseria meningitidis* and *Neisseria gonorrhoeae*. *Mol. Microbiol.* **22:** 929–939.

235. **Virji, M., K. Makepeace, D. J. P. Ferguson, and S. M. Watt.** 1996. Carcinoembryonic antigens (CD66) on epithelial cells and neutrophils are receptors for Opa proteins of pathogenic neisseriae. *Mol. Microbiol.* **22:**941–950.

236. **Wallin, J., and M. S. Siegel.** 1979. Pharyngeal *Neisseria gonorrhoeae*: coloniser or pathogen? *Br. Med. J.* **1:**1462–1463.

237. **Wang, J., S. D. Gray-Owen, A. Knorre, T. F. Meyer, and C. Dehio.** 1998. Opa binding to cellular CD66 receptors mediates the transcellular traversal of *Neisseria gonorrhoeae* across polarized T84 epithelial cell monolayers. *Mol. Microbiol.* **30:**657–671.

238. **Ward, M. E., P. J. Watt, and A. A. Glynn.** 1970. Gonococci in urethral exudates possess a virulence factor lost on subculture. *Nature* **227:** 382–384.

239. **Ward, M. E., and P. J. Watt.** 1972. Adherence of *Neisseria gonorrhoeae* to urethral mucosal cells: electron-microscopic study of human gonorrhea. *J. Infect. Dis.* **126:**601–605.

240. **Ward, M. E., J. N. Robertson, P. M. Englefield, and P. J. Watt.** 1975. Gonococcal infection: invasion of the mucosal surfaces of the genital tract, p. 188–189. *In* D. Schlessinger (ed.), *Microbiology*. American Society for Microbiology, Washington, D.C.

241. **Washington, E., and P. Katz.** 1991. Cost of and payment source for pelvic inflammatory disease. *JAMA* **13:**2565–2569.

242. **Weinberg, E. D.** 1978. Iron and infection. *Microbiol. Rev.* **42:**45–66.

243. **Westrom, L., and D. Eschenbach.** 1999. Pelvic inflammatory disease, p. 783–809. *In* K. K. Holmes, P. A. Mardh, P. F. Sparling, S. M. Lemon, W. E. Stamm, P. Piot, and J. N. Wasserheit (ed.), *Sexually Transmitted Diseases,*

McGraw-Hill Companies, Inc., New York, N.Y.

244. **Wetzler, L. M., K. Barry, M. S. Blake, and E. C. Gotschlich.** 1992. Gonococcal lipooligosaccharide sialylation prevents complement-dependent killing by immune sera. *Infect. Immun.* **60:**39–43.

245. **Wiesner, P. J., E. Tronca, P. Bonin, A. Pedersen, and K. K. Holmes.** 1973. Clinical spectrum of pharyngeal gonococcal infection. *N. Engl. J. Med.* **288:**181–185.

246. **Wilks, M., and S. Tabaqchali.** 1987. Quantitative bacteriology of the vaginal flora during the menstrual cycle. *J. Med. Microbiol.* **24:**241–245.

247. **Wolf, D. P., J. E. Sokoloski, and M. Litt.** 1980. Composition and function of human cervical mucus. *Biochim. Biophys. Acta* **630:**545–558.

248. **Wolf, D. P., and M. Litt.** 1986. Physical and rheologic aspects of cervical mucus. *Semin. Reprod. Endocrinol.* **4:**323–332.

249. **Yang, Q. L., and E. C. Gotschlich.** 1996. Variation of gonococcal lipooligosaccharide structure is due to alterations in poly-G tracts in *lgt* genes encoding glycosyl transferases. *J. Exp. Med.* **183:**323–327.

250. **Zheng, H., D. J. Hassett, K. Bean, and M. S. Cohen.** 1992. Regulation of catalase in *Neisseria gonorrhoeae*. Effects of oxidant stress and exposure to human neutrophils. *J. Clin. Investig.* **90:**1000–1006.

251. **Zheng, H., T. M. Alcorn, and M. S. Cohen.** 1994. Effects of H_2O_2-producing lactobacilli on *Neisseria gonorrhoeae* growth and catalase activity. *J. Infect. Dis.* **170:**1209–1215.

CHLAMYDIA SPP.

Toni Darville

12

OVERVIEW OF PATHOGENESIS OF CHLAMYDIAE

The genus *Chlamydia* consists of highly specialized prokaryotic bacteria that exhibit a unique biphasic developmental cycle that ensures their survival. They exhibit morphological and structural similarities to gram-negative bacteria, including a trilaminar outer membrane, which contains lipopolysaccharide (LPS) but lacks the structurally stable peptidoglycan molecule. As a substitute for peptidoglycan, the extracellular form of chlamydiae, the elementary body (EB), exhibits extensive disulfide cross-linking both within and between outer membrane proteins, providing them with a rigid, almost spore-like structure. These tough EBs are excellent infecting forms, transiting safely between host cells. EBs attach to a susceptible host epithelial cell and induce their own phagocytosis. Once inside the cell, the EB cell wall inhibits fusion of the phagosome and lysosome and transforms into the intracellular form of chlamydiae, the delicate reticulate body (RB), which is the perfect energy parasite. The RB grows and replicates, obtaining high-energy phosphate compounds from the host cell,

all the while hidden within a protective membrane-bound vesicle called an inclusion. Once multiplication is complete, the RBs condense into EBs and the infectious progeny are released, permitting infection of new host cells.

The fact that infectious EBs can frequently be recovered from patients by cell culture and the direct observation of chlamydial inclusions containing EBs in clinical specimens indicate that productive chlamydial infection is the norm. However, RBs are relatively hidden from antibodies and cell-mediated defenses and are pampered with a rich supply of preformed nutrients in the inclusion, the perfect place to "persist" in a host. As will be discussed, different degrees of persistence seem to exist for the different species and biovars of chlamydiae. It seems that the intracellular fate of chlamydiae depends on (i) the type of host cell invaded, (ii) the infecting chlamydial species or biovar, and (iii) the state of the chlamydiae at the time of uptake. The ability to prevent fusion of lysosomes with the chlamydial inclusion is critical to intracellular survival and thus to persistence of infection. The host cell can be a hostile place, with professional phagocytic cells, such as neutrophils, monocytes, and macrophages, being better equipped than epithelial cells to kill chlamydial organisms. It seems as well that these professional phagocytes eradicate some

Toni Darville, Division of Pediatric Infectious Diseases, Department of Pediatrics and Microbiology/Immunology, University of Arkansas for Medical Sciences and Arkansas Children's Hospital, Little Rock, AR 72202.

Persistent Bacterial Infections, Edited by J. P. Nataro, M. J. Blaser, and S. Cunningham-Rundles, © 2000 ASM Press, Washington, D.C.

biovars better than others. The ability of the different chlamydial species and biovars to survive and hence to persist intracellularly in different host cell types likely determines to some extent the clinical syndromes they produce. The chlamydial biovars with greater propensities for persistence in professional phagocytes are associated with the most widespread, invasive chronic diseases. In certain instances, it is possible that monocytes and macrophages represent a mode of transport for persistent chlamydial forms to organs and tissue sites remote from the initial site of infection.

Characteristically, *Chlamydia trachomatis* infections are restricted to epithelial surfaces of the ocular or genital tract. Infection is frequently low grade or asymptomatic, and repeated infection is common, indicating that natural immunity is limited. Trachoma, due to ocular infection with *C. trachomatis* serovar A, B, Ba, or C, is currently the leading cause of infectious blindness worldwide. Below the waist, three serovars of *C. trachomatis*, L_1, L_2, and L_3, are associated with lymphogranuloma venereum (LGV), a sexually transmitted disease that is rare in the United States but is still quite prevalent in many developing countries. LGV is characterized by spread from the genital tract to the regional nodes and rectum with chronic proctitis, sometimes leading to rectal stricture. *C. trachomatis* serovars D to K are the world's most common sexually transmitted bacterial pathogens. In men, they cause urethritis and epididymitis. Women sustain a disproportionate share of the morbidity due to these *C. trachomatis* serovars through their well-known complications of pelvic inflammatory disease (PID), ectopic pregnancy, and tubal factor infertility. The annual cost of chlamydial infection is estimated to exceed $2 billion in the United States alone (22a). Babies born to infected mothers may develop pneumonia and conjunctivitis. Reactive arthritis develops in 1 to 2% of patients with *C. trachomatis* infections of the genital tract. Thus, the financial and human burden of *C. trachomatis* infection is substantial.

Another chlamydial species that causes human disease is *Chlamydia pneumoniae*. It causes pneumonia, pharyngitis, and bronchitis in humans. Epidemiological studies have revealed that *C. pneumoniae* is a fairly common cause of infection in school-aged children and young adults. Along with *Mycoplasma pneumoniae* it is probably the most common cause of community-acquired pneumonia in this age group. This agent has been implicated in the development or acceleration of atherosclerosis, asthma, and chronic obstructive pulmonary disease, and recently, it has been linked to Alzheimer's disease (AD) as well (5).

Chlamydia psittaci and *Chlamydia pecorum* are primarily agents of veterinary disease, with *C. psittaci* infecting humans only accidentally. Reports of zoonotic infections of humans with *C. psittaci* in the 1930s led to the first evidence that chlamydial infection could exist in a latent form (95). In a Grass Valley, California, outbreak, exposure to two parakeets led to the infection of several individuals. One bird had died by the time the outbreak was investigated; the other appeared to be perfectly healthy. However, Meyer and Eddie, after confirming the diagnosis in the patients and examining the recovered body of the dead bird, brought the healthy-appearing bird to the laboratory and introduced an uninfected cage mate. This sentinel bird quickly developed psittacosis and died; a series of birds were then exposed to this sentinel, leading to a similar fate for all. The judicious use of sentinel birds was instrumental in elucidating the healthy-carrier stage (95). In parakeet breeding establishments it was noted that infections would be contracted by young birds, who developed symptoms and often died. The resistance of the birds increased with age, yet when older birds were stressed by overcrowding or other conditions, they would shed increasing amounts of the organisms and would occasionally become symptomatic and die (95). A study conducted with mice in 1933 showed that a persistent carrier state could also be produced in the mouse with *C. psittaci* (96).

"Chlamydial persistence" has been described as a long-term association between chlamydiae and their host cells in which these microorganisms remain in a viable but culture-negative state (8). The term implies the absence of overt chlamydial growth, suggestive of the existence of chlamydiae in an altered state distinct from their typical intracellular morphological forms. Indeed, arrested growth of chlamydiae may correlate with a reduction in metabolic activity which restricts growth and division and delays differentiation to cultivatable EBs, thereby establishing a culture-negative "cryptic" state (100). As with viral latency, the progression of the agent through the usual developmental cycle is interrupted, and it is assumed that when conditions are more favorable for the parasite, the developmental cycle may be resumed, resulting once again in a "productive" infection. Distinct from viral latency, chlamydial DNA does not integrate into the host genome, and nonreplicating persistent forms of chlamydiae remain in the host cell cytoplasm. As described in detail later in this chapter, although "reactivation" of such persistent forms has been shown to occur in vitro, it has not been demonstrated conclusively in animals or humans.

There are numerous reports describing the detection of chlamydial antigen, DNA, and even rRNA transcripts in the tissues of patients with chronic disease ascribed to chlamydial infection, in the absence of detectable replicating organisms. In addition, more recent studies using transmission electron microscopy reveal morphologically atypical chlamydial forms in sites of chronic tissue pathology in vivo, concurrent with reverse transcription (RT)-PCR detection of chlamydial rRNA and mRNA transcripts. These studies suggest that potentially viable chlamydiae persist in the host in a nonreplicative and thus nonculturable state, but documentation of such a cryptic state in natural infections remains to be verified and established conclusively. A key question is whether such persistent chlamydial forms play a role in the immunopathology of disease.

Chlamydial infections are prevalent in most societies, and host immunity to chlamydia is transient. Thus, repeated reinfection is well documented, making it essentially impossible to prove persistence of chlamydial infection in humans. Clarification of whether persistent infection occurs is significant, since persistently infected persons may be particularly at risk for chlamydia-induced immunopathology and may be more resistant to treatment with certain antibiotic regimens. In addition, reactivation of a persistent infection allows for ongoing transmission of the infection to others.

CONSIDERATION OF RELEVANT CLINICAL CHARACTERISTICS OF *CHLAMYDIA* SPP.

Evidence for Persistence of *C. trachomatis* In Vivo

Although productive chlamydial infection is the norm, multiple studies suggest the presence of nonculturable persistent chlamydial organisms in host tissues. More importantly, these persistent forms are often found in sites of chronic disease.

TRACHOMA

Strong evidence for the continued presence of trachoma-causing organisms in a culture-negative state comes from studies of patients with trachoma and a primate model for ocular disease in which chlamydial rRNA was detected in conjunctival swabs long after antigen detection was negative (25, 60, 62). Because RNA molecules are very labile, these data indicate the chlamydia were nonreplicating but viable. The presence of such quiescent chlamydial forms is further suggested by studies of individuals who left areas where trachoma was endemic and developed acute trachoma several decades later (127). Furthermore, studies of trachoma in older individuals with chronic conjunctival scarring from whom it is rare to isolate viable chlamydiae reveal a significant association of chronic antigen carriage (88) or antigen and DNA carriage (59) with conjunctival scarring. Progressive-scarring disease occurs with these culture-negative infections, indicating that individuals may harbor a cryptic form of chlamydiae in their eye tissue and that these cryptic forms may induce inflammation beyond the time when standard techniques can detect the organism.

Several studies report the delayed appearance and prolonged carriage of genital tract *C. trachomatis* strains acquired perinatally. These strains have been isolated from the rectovaginal areas and pharynxes of perinatally exposed infants for up to 3 years (10, 127). One study reported reisolation of *C. trachomatis* from the eyes or nasopharynxes of 7 of 22 babies treated for 2 weeks with both topical ocular tetracycline and oral erythromycin, although compliance with medication was not monitored (10).

GENITAL TRACT DISEASE
Epidemiologically, high antibody titers against *C. trachomatis* correlate with increased incidence of infertility, severe tubal disease, and ectopic pregnancy. Are these increased antibody titers due to repeated infection (recurrences) or to a persistently low level of intermittent antigen stimulation (relapse of a persistent infection)? Of course, high antibody titers are also seen in patients with recent acute infection with no previous history of sexually transmitted disease. Whether chlamydiae persist subclinically in the upper genital tracts of women with resulting infertility remains unclear.

A study by Patton et al. (109) demonstrated *C. trachomatis* DNA or antigens in 19 of 24 tubal-biopsy specimens from women with postinfectious tubal infertility, 17 of whom had received antichlamydial antibiotics during the previous year. Serological tests showed that all were chronically infected except one woman with immunoglobulin M (IgM) antibody. Only 3 of 25 were positive by culture from the tubal biopsy (109). This is just one example among multiple studies describing the detection of chlamydial DNA or antigen in women with tubal infertility, the majority of whom are culture negative (21, 75, 141, 152). The presence of chlamydial antigen and nucleic acids is suggestive but does not prove the presence of persistent viable organisms in the tissues. It is possible that tissue culture procedures may not be sensitive enough to detect low but poten-

tially immunologically significant levels of replicating chlamydiae. Alternatively, these individuals may harbor aberrant nonreplicating (and therefore nonculturable) but viable forms of chlamydiae with the capacity to stimulate immunopathologic changes. Unfortunately, there is as yet a lack of longitudinal evidence for a long-term culture-negative persistent state of chlamydia infection in patients with *C. trachomatis* genital tract infections.

Evidence against persistence after antimicrobial treatment comes from a study performed with women from Seattle (159). Twenty women were followed for up to 5 months after completion of doxycycline therapy; 384 cervical, rectal, and urethral specimens were examined by culture and PCR for chlamydial DNA. All specimens were negative except for those from one woman with apparent reinfection with a different serotype (F) than the original infecting strain (E). Thus, this study found no evidence to indicate that doxycycline failed to eradicate lower genital tract infections and found no evidence of persistent chlamydial infection after therapy. The authors mentioned some caveats with their study. First, 60% of their patients had serological evidence of acute infection, and it is possible that chronic infection, in which organisms may be less metabolically active, would be more difficult to eradicate. Second, they did not sample the upper genital tract for persistent infection. Lastly, they used a very active drug regimen against chlamydial infection, and it is possible that diminished compliance or a drug with less activity would not be as successful.

This last caveat was supported in a study by Hooton et al. (61) that examined the effectiveness of ciprofloxacin for nongonococcal urethritis in 178 men. Among patients who initially had cultures positive for chlamydia, *C. trachomatis* was isolated again within 4 weeks after treatment in 11 (52%) of 21 patients treated with 750 mg of ciprofloxacin twice daily and in 6 (38%) of 16 patients treated with 1,000 mg of ciprofloxacin twice daily, compared to none of 10 doxycycline-treated patients. Each of the recurrent strains was identical in serotype to the original infecting strain. Thus, this study indicated that *C. trachomatis* persists for at least 1 month in males if treatment is inadequate.

These studies suggest that when patients are compliant with an active drug regimen, relapse of infection after cessation of adequate therapy is not a common cause of persistent or chronic infection. Rather, chronic infection may more often arise from failure to identify infections because of lack of adequate screening programs. These conclusions are supported by a study by Scholes et al. (131) in which screening and treatment of cervical chlamydial infection led to a dramatic 56% decrease in the incidence of PID. However, a recent study suggests that although persistent infections may not be common after accepted treatment regimens are administered, they may indeed occur (33). Dean and colleagues studied seven women attending the Seattle King County Health Department sexually transmitted disease clinic and found that each had multiple relapses of chlamydial infection with their originally infecting genotype strain over 2 to 5 years (33). After each positive culture, the patients were treated with either doxycycline or azithromycin and had sex partner follow-up. Cultures became negative after the receipt of antibiotics, but the same genotype returned weeks to months later. Genotyping of the outer membrane protein 1 (Omp1) gene that encodes the major outer membrane protein (MOMP) of *C. trachomatis* revealed that in three of the patients nucleotide mutations occurred in the original genotype after several rounds of chemotherapy. Although only seven isolates were identified in the course of ongoing studies over 8 years, these data suggest that certain *C. trachomatis* genotypes may persist in the genital tract despite appropriate antimicrobial treatment. These latent organisms may then develop mutations as a result of selective antimicrobial or immune pressure. A comparison of these results with those of Workowski et al. (159) suggests that certain serovars (notably the C complex) may be more prone to persistence.

A disturbing study of adolescent females was reported recently by Katz et al. (71). These investigators followed 106 female subjects (mean age, 16.9 years) with chlamydial infection who returned for a 1- or 3-month examination including a urine-based chlamydia PCR. All subjects received azithromycin treatment at the time chlamydial infection was diagnosed. The incidence of persistent or recurrent infection was 16% (17 of 106) at 1 month and 19% (15 of 79) at 3 months. At 1 month, 31 adolescents who reported no interval sex had a 9.7% infection rate. At 3 months, 15 adolescents who reported no interval sex had a 13.3% infection rate. A similar, although slightly higher, rate was observed for those who claimed to use a condom for each coital event. The high infection rates observed in those who reported abstinence or 100% condom use are particularly disconcerting, suggesting a persistence rate in adolescent females of about 10% despite what should have been adequate therapy. Although cultures were not done on follow-up, it seems extremely unlikely that intact DNA would remain for up to 3 months in the absence of productive infection.

It is well known that many men and most women infected with *C. trachomatis* in the genital tract are either asymptomatic or minimally symptomatic, and presentation for diagnosis is often a result of screening or a contact being symptomatic. Screening studies show that approximately 10% of sexually active asymptomatic men are infected, and among sexually active women, the proportion infected ranges from 8 to 40%, with a median of about 15%. Unrecognized infection can progress in the female and result in PID and subsequent tubal infertility. Because so many infections are asymptomatic, they may go undiagnosed and therefore untreated. Resolution of infection is thus often left to the immune response, but the high rates of unrecognized infection suggest an ability of the organism to evade the host immune response. The study by Katz et al. suggests that even when the infection is diagnosed and treated, chlamydial organisms can persist for up to 3 months in adolescent females (71).

More studies need to be done with larger sample sizes to confirm these results.

Although chlamydiacidal antibiotics may kill the parasite, chlamydial antigens may persist for prolonged periods, and there is evidence that these nonviable forms may lead to continued inflammation. This has recently been shown in an elegant in vitro study by Wyrick et al. (162). These investigators found that azithromycin-loaded-neutrophil exposure of *C. trachomatis* serovar E-infected human endometrial epithelial (HEC-1B) cells results in the formation of pronounced outer membrane blebbing of metabolically active RBs as well as several juxtaposed vacuoles external to the inclusions. The vacuoles are filled with outer membrane blebs, which react specifically with gold-conjugated anti-chlamydial LPS monoclonal antibody and with anti-chlamydial MOMP antibody. These chlamydial antigens were also detected on the surfaces of the infected cells as well as extracellularly (162). The timing of the appearance of chlamydial antigens on the host cell surfaces, approximately 36 h postinfection, coincided with polymorphonuclear neutrophil (PMN) chemotaxis. mRNA for two chemokines, ENA-78 and GCP-2, was detected in infected cultures. Furthermore, in cultures monitored for 1 month after azithromycin exposure, residual chlamydial envelopes and MOMP and LPS antigens were detected, and these 1-month-old cultures continued to stimulate PMN chemotaxis. These data provide one plausible explanation for the theory that a prolonged inflammatory response to persistent chlamydial antigens may be responsible for the damage and sequelae in chlamydial infections.

Macaques with experimentally induced chronic salpingitis and PID (110) were given doxycycline, doxycycline plus ibuprofen, doxycycline plus triamcinolone, or placebo to assess the effects of antimicrobial and anti-inflammatory drugs on oviductal pathology. Despite negative posttreatment cervical cultures, persistence of chlamydial MOMP and chlamydial plasmid DNA was found in multiple tissues in the majority of treated animals when they were examined at 4 to 6 weeks posttreatment. Although antibiotic treatment resulted in negative cultures, there was no evidence that it had any effect on gross or histological pathology. Thus, when doxycycline is given after a chronic chlamydial infection of the upper genital tract is established, irreversible damage may already have been done.

REACTIVE ARTHRITIS

Alan P. Hudson, together with multiple collaborators, has published some of the most convincing evidence for the existence of persistent viable *C. trachomatis* forms in the joints of the human host. His studies have shown that biopsy material from the synovial membranes of patients with chlamydia-induced arthritis often contain both atypical chlamydiae and intact chlamydial DNA and RNA, even as late as 12 years after the onset of disease (105). He and others showed via Northern blot analysis that apparently intact chlamydial RNA is present in synovial tissues from patients with Reiter's syndrome but not in similar preparations from most patients with other forms of arthritis (55, 115). Synovial tissue is the source of choice for PCR screening for chlamydial DNA (14), as synovial fluid may be negative due to the fact that the chlamydiae often reside in discrete cell layers well beneath the synovial lining (12, 13). By immunoelectron microscopy, Nanagara et al. (105) showed atypical aberrant forms of RBs in fibroblasts and macrophages in five of six synovial membrane samples from patients who had either early or chronic arthritis. Four of the patients had received antichlamydial antibiotics. Gold-conjugated antibodies to chlamydial LPS and MOMP produced weak but specific signals on the RBs compared to very strong signals in infected HeLa cell controls. In addition, atypical EBs were found extracellularly among fibrinous substances or within vacuoles of macrophages or fibroblasts. As with the RBs, staining was weak but specific. Of special note, intact chlamydial particles were not found in monocytes of the synovial fluid; rather, only chlamydial debris was seen in monocyte phagolysosomes (105). The authors suggested that decreased surface membrane protein expression is a means by which chlamydiae persist in synovial tissues. A lowered level of antigen expression may prevent immune eradication, as well as failure of organism detection and isolation from synovial membranes by conventional techniques.

Detection of intact nucleic acids and identification of aberrant chlamydial forms by electron microscopy indicate that chlamydial forms are indeed present in synovial tissues. But are the organisms viable, and if so, are they metabolically active? The rate of transcriptional initiation at promoters of rRNA operons is directly related to the cellular growth rate; thus, Gerard et al. reasoned that the observation of such transcripts in patient samples would be evidence for viable, metabolically active chlamydial cells in those samples (44). They detected rRNA transcripts in samples from 14 of 16 arthritic patients that were PCR positive for chlamydial DNA. These same 14 samples were also RT-PCR positive for mRNA of the chlamydial glycyl tRNA synthetase enzyme and the chlamydial genes encoding the ribosomal proteins S5 and L5, as well as for mRNA from the chlamydial heat shock protein 60 (Hsp60) gene. Patients PCR negative for chlamydial DNA, and those who were PCR positive without primary rRNA transcripts, were negative for genes required for chlamydial protein synthesis and for Hsp60. Interestingly, none of the 14 samples from PCR-positive patients whose RNA preparations included chlamydial rRNA and protein synthesis-related transcripts, as well as Hsp60 mRNA, contained detectable messenger for the *omp1* gene, encoding the MOMP. Thus, while synovial chlamydiae are viable and metabolically active, they produce at best extremely low levels of transcripts from *omp1*, a gene normally expressed at high levels during chlamydial replication (44). However, preliminary data from this same group reveal that the expression of all outer membrane proteins is not attenuated, as several of the 14 PCR- and mRNA-positive patient RNA samples have tested positive for transcripts of the

omp2 gene, which encodes a 60,000-M_r cysteine-rich envelope protein (44).

The MOMP is abundant in both EBs and RBs, where it provides structural integrity to the cell. One can hypothesize that the low level of mRNA for MOMP detected by RT-PCR in synovial samples (44) would lead to a low level of MOMP protein, thus making MOMP unavailable for maintenance of a strong chlamydial cell wall. This may explain the atypical morphology of RBs and EBs seen in patients' synovial tissues (105). On the other hand, the weak but persistent expression of chlamydial LPS by these aberrant forms could induce chronic inflammation. Interleukin 1 and tumor necrosis factor alpha (TNF-α) are released by monocytes in response to chlamydial LPS (65, 123). Thus, chlamydial LPS is an attractive candidate for stimulation of chronic inflammation in chlamydia-induced reactive arthritis, which is reported in 1 to 3% of patients after genital infection with *C. trachomatis*.

The above-mentioned studies raise two questions. First, how do these chlamydiae reach the synovial tissues in the first place? And second, why do these forms manifest an irregular pattern of gene expression? One potential method of transport of the chlamydiae from the genital epithelium to the joint is via peripheral blood monocytes. Using *C. trachomatis* serovar K, investigators demonstrated persistence of chlamydial DNA, RNA, MOMP, and LPS in human monocytes in vitro over a culture period of 14 days (130); no replication of the organism was observed in these experiments. Transmission electron microscopy of serovar K-infected human peripheral blood monocytes revealed morphologically atypical chlamydiae within monocyte vesicles that were immunoreactive for MOMP and LPS at the chlamydial plasma membrane. Chlamydial LPS was also detected at the membranes of the monocyte vesicles and in the monocyte cytoplasm, but chlamydial MOMP was not. To investigate the metabolic state of these aberrant forms, RT-PCR analysis was performed to detect primary transcripts from chlamydial rRNA operons. Functional processed 16S rRNA molecules were detected in monocytes throughout 10 days of infection. Despite the organism's non-replicative state, the presence of several apparently intact chlamydial macromolecules clearly suggests that potentially viable bacteria persist in monocytes for at least a few days following infection. However, Nanagara et al. did not find intact chlamydial particles in monocytes from the synovial fluid of patients with reactive arthritis; rather, only chlamydial debris was seen in monocyte phagolysosomes (105). It is likely that over time, the monocytes render the chlamydiae nonviable, but possibly not until some viable forms have been deposited in fibroblasts and macrophages of the synovial tissues.

An answer to the second question regarding aberrant gene expression has been proposed by Gerard et al. (44). Increased levels of gamma interferon (IFN-γ) transcripts have been found in RNA preparations from synovial tissues of chlamydia-infected patients with reactive arthritis (78). Gerard and colleagues proposed that IFN-γ may lead to the irregular gene expression of chlamydial forms found in affected joints (44). Indeed, as will be discussed in detail later in the chapter, data of Beatty et al. (7, 8) reveal that serovar A-infected cells treated with IFN-γ in vitro show low levels of MOMP and develop large, aberrant noninfectious but viable forms of chlamydiae.

Evidence for Persistence of C. pneumoniae In Vivo

RESPIRATORY TRACT INFECTION

Since the description of C. pneumoniae as a pathogen in 1986 (49), it has become recognized as a common infectious agent found worldwide. It is now known to cause about 10% of cases of community-acquired pneumonia. Primary infections are documented most often in school children and young adults and lead to only partial immunity, with reinfection prominent among the elderly. The illness can be quite mild, as only 10% of primary infections in young Scandinavian military recruits led to clinical manifestations of pneumonia (11, 36). As with C. trachomatis, it is likely that many

C. pneumoniae infections go undiagnosed and untreated, with resolution of infection being left to the immune response. Also, as with C. trachomatis, proving the existence of persistent in vivo infection is difficult, as only temporary resistance to reinfection is induced in the host, making it difficult to distinguish persistent infection from repeated reinfection.

One of the first efforts to pursue the detection of chronic respiratory tract infection with C. pneumoniae was reported by Hammerschlag et al. (56). They were able to obtain follow-up nasopharyngeal cultures from 9 of 14 patients who had had symptomatic culture-proven C. pneumoniae infections. Five of the nine (56%) were documented to have persistently positive cultures. The patients were felt to have had acute infection at enrollment based on serological tests. Four of the patients with persistently positive cultures had a flulike illness with pharyngitis, and one had bronchitis. One subject remained culture positive for 2 months and one for 3 months. Three remained positive for 11 months despite 10- to 21-day courses of tetracycline or doxycycline. Four of the five patients had a moderate to good clinical response to therapy despite persistently positive cultures. One female patient appeared to have a clinical relapse 3 months after an initial course of 10 days of tetracycline but clinically improved after a course of doxycycline. Eleven months after her acute episode, she was feeling well, but cultures of nasopharyngeal swab specimens were still positive for C. pneumoniae (56). In addition to this study, a case report by Yamazaki et al. (163) describes a 5-year-old girl with pneumonia who had positive cultures from her nasopharynx 2 weeks after completion of 18 days of rokitamycin (a macrolide antibiotic) despite clinical improvement on the antibiotic.

These observations suggest that persistent respiratory infection with C. pneumoniae may frequently (more than half of the time) follow acute infection and that individuals may remain infected or colonized for many months. Indeed, such individuals may serve as reservoirs for spread of the organism. C. pneumoniae may not be eradicated from the patient's respiratory tract by use of currently available antibiotics even if there is a clinical response to therapy. This is similar to reports of patients with pneumonia due to *M. pneumoniae* for whom tetracycline or erythromycin treatment resulted in clinical improvement despite continued shedding of *M. pneumoniae* from the respiratory tract (139).

Asymptomatic carriage of *C. pneumoniae* has been investigated in several recent studies. A prevalence of 4.7% was detected from oropharyngeal specimens of healthy adults attending a Swedish travel clinic (45), and nasopharyngeal carriage was detected in 2 of 103 healthy hospital workers in New York: one was culture positive, and one was PCR and enzyme immunoassay positive (64). Interestingly, the New York study noted that 19 of these 103 healthy subjects with negative nasopharyngeal specimens met serological criteria for acute infection (49), and the overall seroprevalence was 82%. The fact that positive serology could be obtained from asymptomatic apparently healthy people with negative nasopharyngeal specimens raises some questions. First, how specific is the microimmunofluorescence (MIF) test for acute *C. pneumoniae* infection? Some researchers have claimed that the MIF test lacks both sensitivity (63) and specificity (46, 47); others insist that when the test is performed properly with paired sera, it is more sensitive than culture or even PCR for throat specimens (47, 50). If the MIF test is specific, and the serological results from these 19 subjects were true positives, it indicates they had recently been infected with *C. pneumoniae*. But, if persistent nasopharyngeal infection or colonization is frequent after acute infection, why were all of these subjects culture negative? Perhaps persistent infection or colonization occurs more often after symptomatic disease. These studies suggest that caution should be exercised when interpreting the meaning of a single serological assay for *C. pneumoniae*, and studies that rely solely on serum antibody titers to link *C. pneumoniae* infection to chronic disease should be regarded with caution.

In an investigation by von Hertzen and colleagues (155) of a link between chronic *C. pneumoniae* infection and chronic obstructive pulmonary disease (COPD), IgG titers were no different in elderly patients with or without chronic lung disease. However, *C. pneumoniae*-specific IgA antibodies were found more frequently and in higher concentrations in patients with COPD than in disease-free controls. Because of the short half-life of IgA antibodies, these investigators proposed that stable elevated IgA antibody titers are a useful marker for chronic *C. pneumoniae* infection. Indeed, they found elevated IgA in patients during exacerbations of COPD and suggested these were due to a continuous or intermittently activated inflammatory process induced by *C. pneumoniae* in the bronchi (155). A similar study has linked asthma exacerbations to recrudescence of a persistent *C. pneumoniae* infection (53).

CHRONIC CARDIOVASCULAR DISEASE
An excellent recent review summarizes the studies associating *C. pneumoniae* infection with atherosclerosis, in addition to discussing preliminary in vitro and in vivo studies suggesting the plausibility of a causative role (20). An association of *C. pneumoniae* with atherosclerosis has been documented seroepidemiologically in over 20 studies; most have an odds ratio of 2.0 or greater (29). The actual presence of *C. pneumoniae* in atherosclerotic lesions has been documented by PCR, immunocytochemical staining, and electron microscopy by various laboratories (48, 80–82, 138), with over 50% of the examined tissues being positive at the site of lesions and only 5% of the tissues being positive when they appeared normal (29). One study, however, which examined 58 atheroma specimens from patients in Brooklyn by culture and PCR found all of them negative, except one that was positive by PCR. Twenty-two of the specimens were examined with electron microscopy by two different investigators, and all were negative. Antibody titers to *C. pneumoniae* were higher in controls than in patients (157). The organism has been cultured from

atherosclerotic lesions of patients (87, 116), albeit rarely, which is not surprising, as isolation from infected tissues in chronic chlamydial infection is extremely difficult.

Multiple in vitro studies suggest that *C. pneumoniae* has the potential to persistently infect vascular cells and to promote atherogenic responses. Vascular cells are susceptible to persistent infection with the organism, and *C. pneumoniae* produces productive infection in human macrophages, endothelial cells, and arterial smooth muscle cells (43, 46), all key cellular components in atherosclerosis. It has been proposed that the ability of the organism to multiply in cells of monocyte/macrophage lineage allows it to disseminate from the respiratory tract via the bloodstream (76). Several laboratories have demonstrated the ability of the organism to induce release of adhesins, cytokines, and proteases by human vascular endothelial cells and by monocytes and macrophages (41, 57, 72, 98), all of which could lead to endothelial injury or activation, resulting in monocyte/macrophage adherence and migration to the subendothelium. In addition, exposure of human monocyte-derived macrophages to *C. pneumoniae* followed by the addition of low-density lipoprotein results in foam cell formation and the accumulation of cholesteryl esters (69). Ultrastructural studies have demonstrated *C. pneumoniae* in human foam cells and smooth muscle cells that take up lipids, and it has been found by immunocytochemical staining to be present in macrophages within aortic atheromatous lesions (81).

Several questions need to be answered regarding the link between *C. pneumoniae* and atherosclerosis. First, although *C. pneumoniae* antigen and DNA are often found in atheromas, isolation-positive lesions are rare. Thus, do PCR and immunocytochemistry (ICC) positivity reflect persistent infection with viable chlamydiae or just partially degraded organisms and pieces of chlamydial DNA? Second, there are difficulties in interpretation of the MIF test, especially with reinfection in which IgM is absent and interpretations of IgG titer vary between laboratories. Thus, it is difficult

to know if a subject has an elevated IgG titer because of reactivation of a persistent chlamydial infection or because of recent reinfection. If the antigens and DNA detected in atheromas represent viable chlamydial organisms, are they from a persistent infection of the involved host cells or have they recently been deposited there from activated mononuclear phagocytes that gobbled them up after an acute reinfection of the lung, or even after recent reactivation of a persistent infection in the lung? Of course, as proposed with *C. trachomatis* in the genital tract, the presence of persistent *C. pneumoniae* antigen alone may contribute to atherogenesis through prolonged stimulation of inflammation, e.g., chlamydial LPS induction of cytokine release (65, 123).

Murine studies with the lung model of *C. pneumoniae* infection support the possibility that detection of DNA and antigen may represent persistent viable organisms from a chronic infection (84). Two separate studies with *C. pneumoniae*-infected mice support the possibility of reactivation of a persistent lung infection due to suppression of the immune system by steroids (84, 89). Laitinen and colleagues found that 60% of cortisone-treated mice turned culture positive for chlamydiae when steroid treatment was started as late as 30 days after primary infection, but not with saline treatment (84). Malinverni used PCR to demonstrate a similar response (89). Although these studies cannot distinguish between reactivation of a persistent infection and enhancement of a low-grade infection, they provide direct evidence of the persistent nature of *C. pneumoniae*. A third study looked at mice infected with live versus UV-inactivated organisms (97). Alveolar macrophages were examined for organisms by culture and PCR at various time points after infection. When live organisms were used, the organism could be cultured and detected by PCR for up to 7 days, but when UV-inactivated organisms were used, they could only be detected by PCR immediately after inoculation (97). These experiments demonstrated that DNA from dead organisms is rapidly degraded. Thus, DNA is unlikely to be detected at a site remote from that of inoculation unless it is produced by a productive infection at the remote site.

A study of New Zealand White rabbits suggests not only that *C. pneumoniae* appears to exacerbate atherosclerosis but that the organism may persist despite treatment with antibiotics (102). The rabbits were fed a diet with 0.25% cholesterol and were inoculated intranasally three times with *C. pneumoniae*. The infected rabbits and controls were treated for 7 weeks with azithromycin. Three months after the final inoculation, the maximal intimal thickness of the thoracic aortas increased in infected rabbits but not in controls. The maximal intimal thicknesses of azithromycin-treated rabbits were less than those of untreated infected rabbits and similar to those of controls. However, organisms were detected by immunofluorescence with a genus-specific anti-lipoprotein antibody in the aortas of treated rabbits as frequently as in untreated rabbits.

A prospective human study of atherosclerosis suggests that a chronic *C. pneumoniae* infection may best be indicated by the detection of elevated IgA antibody titers that persist for 3 to 6 months and by persistent detection of chlamydial-LPS-containing immune complexes (125). In 103 patients with myocardial infarction and 103 controls followed prospectively in the Helsinki heart study with serum collected every 3 months, there was no difference in the seroprevalence of positive IgG ($\geq$16) or IgA ($\geq$8) titers to *C. pneumoniae*. However, when persistence of elevated IgA antibody titers ($\geq$64 at baseline and at 3 to 6 months before the cardiac event) was examined for cases and controls, the odds ratio for the development of a cardiac event was 2.5 (confidence interval, 0.9 to 6.5). When persistently positive immune complexes were combined with persistently elevated IgA titers, the odds ratio increased to 2.9 (confidence interval, 1.5 to 5.4). Although baseline seroprevalence was high in cases and controls, persistent elevations in IgA and IgG and the presence of immune complexes were clearly more common among case patients than controls, thus supporting an association between chronic *C. pneumoniae* infection and the risk for coronary heart disease (125).

ALZHEIMER'S DISEASE

Perhaps one of the most exciting and controversial recent reports is that infection with *C. pneumoniae* may be a risk factor for late-onset AD. A group of investigators, including Alan Hudson and Herve Gerard, who have previously identified *C. pneumoniae* in synovial tissues from patients with reactive arthritis, recently reported the identification and localization of *C. pneumoniae* in the AD-affected brain (5). These investigators used multiple techniques to demonstrate that *C. pneumoniae* is present, viable, and transcriptionally active in areas of neuropathology in the AD-affected brain. PCR assay for DNA revealed that brain areas with typical neuropathology were positive in 17 of 19 patients and negative in 18 of 19 controls. Chlamydial DNA was uncommon in unaffected or less AD-affected areas of brain tissues. Electron and immunoelectron microscopy identified chlamydial EBs and RBs in neuropathologic tissues of AD-affected brains but not in controls. RT-PCR assays for the gene required for chlamydial LPS synthesis and for a gene specifying a protein containing an epitope specific for *C. pneumoniae* revealed transcripts in affected areas of patients' brains but not in those of controls. Immunohistochemical staining identified *C. pneumoniae* within pericytes, microglia, and astroglia of affected areas in AD-affected brain but not in those of controls. Significantly, homogenates of AD-affected brain tissues, but not those from controls, productively infected a monocytic cell line in culture. Available clinical data for the patients studied did not identify any who were suspected to have chlamydial pneumonia, and as many controls as patients died of pulmonary-related causes. No serology was done.

While these data do not establish a causal relationship between central nervous system infection with *C. pneumoniae* and development of late-onset AD, they suggest that further investigations are needed. The nonneuronal cell types found to be infected are directly involved in inflammatory responses in the brain. It is possible that chronic infection of glial cells with *C. pneumoniae* may result in alteration of mechanisms that regulate production and deposition of β-amyloid peptide that composes the neuritic senile plaques seen in AD.

MEANS BY WHICH *CHLAMYDIA* SPP. ESTABLISH PERSISTENCE

Avoidance of Phagosome-Lysosome Fusion

When intracellular parasites enter host cells, they must avoid destruction by whatever antiparasitic activities the host cells are able to mobilize. One such capability shared by both professional and nonprofessional phagocytes is fusion of their lysosomes with parasite-containing phagosomes and release of acid hydrolases into the resulting phagolysosomes. Chlamydiae may evade lysosomal killing by not provoking the fusion of lysosomes with parasite-laden phagosomes. However, not every chlamydia-containing phagosome escapes fusion with lysosomes. Whether or not there is phagosome-lysosome fusion depends on the kind of host cell, the condition of the chlamydiae, and the conditions under which the chlamydiae are ingested. The relative ability of the different chlamydial species and serovars to inhibit phagosome-lysosome fusion likely determines to some extent the clinical syndromes they produce. Those species with the greatest ability to survive within professional phagocytes are associated with more-disseminated disease, suggesting that monocytes and macrophages may serve to transport these hardy chlamydial species to sites remote from the epithelium that served as the initial site of infection.

Persistent *C. psittaci* infections were noted in birds and nonhuman mammals soon after the organism was first isolated (94, 137). The 6BC strain of *C. psittaci* was isolated from a parrot in 1941 by Meyer and Eddie, and the Cal 10 meningopneumonitis strain (MN/Cal 10) was isolated in 1936 from ferrets inoculated with throat washings from a human with a suspected case of influenza (39). The results of early in vitro studies performed with these *C. psittaci* agents revealed some important information regarding the ability of chlamydial species to evade phagosome-lysosome fusion (100).

EVASION OF PHAGOSOME-LYSOSOME FUSION IN HOST CELLS

Twelve to 20 h after mouse fibroblasts (L cells) have ingested infectious EBs of *C. psittaci* 6BC and MN/Cal 10, the cytoplasm of the L cells contains inclusions in which the EBs have differentiated into RBs and started to divide. There is no morphological evidence of fusion with lysosomes, and the inclusions do not stain for acid phosphatase (40, 77). Failure to provoke fusion with L-cell lysosomes depends on preservation of as-yet-undefined structures in the EB cell wall and not on maintenance of infectivity. UV-inactivated *C. psittaci* does not trigger phagosome-lysosome fusion in L cells, although it does not multiply (35). The fact that inhibitory structures reside in the cell wall was demonstrated by the observation that cell walls purified from *C. psittaci* MN/Cal 10 EBs and labeled with a tritiated reagent released label in trichloroacetic acid-soluble form almost as slowly as similarly labeled intact infectious EBs (35, 90). These proposed structures may be inactivated by heating, because heated EBs enter L cells in phagosomes that quickly fuse with lysosomes (40). After 24 h of infection with *C. psittaci*, RBs have multiplied extensively, many have differentiated into EBs, and the developmental cycle draws to a close. Lysosomes are then released into the cytoplasm of the host cells, which begin to disintegrate and lyse (77, 154). The fact that all species and strains of chlamydiae produce productive infection of appropriate host cells is evidence of their ability to evade phagosome-lysosome fusion.

EVASION OF PHAGOSOME-LYSOSOME FUSION IN PROFESSIONAL PHAGOCYTIC CELLS

The developmental cycle of *C. psittaci* in mouse peritoneal macrophages is identical in all respects to the cycle observed in cell lines when the multiplicity of infection is not greater than 1 (161). Infectious EBs are ingested in phagosomes that do not fuse with ferritin-labeled lysosomes, whereas heat-inactivated EBs are promptly destroyed in ferritin-marked phagolysosomes (161). Thus, at low multiplicities of infection, the relation between *C. psittaci* and lysosomes is much the same in mouse macrophages and L cells. At higher multiplicities of infection, many of the macrophages are rapidly destroyed and are thus unable to support a productive infection.

Macrophages, unlike L cells, will ingest RBs. When radioactively labeled RBs of *C. psittaci* MN/Cal 10 are taken up by macrophages, their label is rapidly released in trichloroacetic acid-soluble form, indicating that they are being destroyed (161). Thus, the elements in the EB wall required for evasion of phagosome-lysosome fusion are either absent from the RB wall or present in an inactive state. However, the constant presence of the EB wall is not required. By 8 to 12 h after infection, there are no longer any EBs in the *C. psittaci* inclusions and yet these inclusions do not provoke lysosomal fusion for many hours thereafter (77, 154). Chlamydia-induced inhibition of fusion is not generalized but is strictly limited to the phagosomes containing intact EBs. When mouse macrophages simultaneously ingest infectious EBs of *C. psittaci* MN/Cal 10 and whole cells of either *Saccharomyces cerevisiae* or *Escherichia coli*, the yeast- and bacterium-laden phagosomes fuse with lysosomes and their contents are degraded to the same extent as in macrophages that phagocytized *S. cerevisiae* or *E. coli* alone (34). Small differences in membrane proteins may account for the occurrence or nonoccurrence of lysosomal fusion. When phagosomes were taken from mouse peritoneal macrophages 1 h after inoculation with either infectious or heat-inactivated *C. psittaci* EBs, the phagosome membranes surrounding the two kinds of chlamydial cells shared several proteins, as determined by polyacrylamide gel electrophoresis, but a small number of proteins were unique to each kind of phagosome (166).

Experiments done more recently have further elucidated the protective function of the chlamydial inclusion by monitoring the trafficking of 6-[*N*-(7-nitrobenzo-2-oxa-1,3-diazol-4-yl)aminocaproyl sphingosine] (C6-NBD-ceramide), a fluorescent analog of ceramide, through the chlamydial developmental cycle (Fig. 1) (51, 52, 58). This probe is a vital stain for the Golgi apparatus and has been used in conjunction with either fluorescence or electron microscopy to study sphingolipid trafficking in viable cells. Like endogenous ceramide, C6-NBD-ceramide is enzymatically converted to sphingomyelin at the *cis*- or medial-Golgi compartment before transport to the plasma membrane. When cells infected with *C. trachomatis* are labeled with C6-NBD-ceramide, a substantial proportion of the sphingomyelin endogenously synthesized from the added fluorescent ceramide analog is diverted to the chlamydial inclusion, where it is subsequently incorporated into the cell walls of the chlamydiae. Immediately after being labeled with C6-NBD-ceramide, the fluorescent analog is observed only in the Golgi apparatus, which is typically adjacent to the chlamydial inclusion. With time, increasing amounts of the fluorescent probe are acquired by the intracellular chlamydiae (52). Quantitative estimates made by using thin-layer chromatography of extracted fluorescent lipids (151) suggest that up to 40 to 50% of the sphingomyelin endogenously synthesized from C6-NBD-ceramide is retained by chlamydiae. Once exposed on the inner surface of the inclusion membrane, sphingomyelin appears to be acquired rapidly by chlamydiae within the inclusion by what probably represents preferential lipid solubility in a membrane of appropriate composition. C6-NBD-sphingomyelin introduced directly into the plasma membrane is not delivered in significant amounts to the chlamydial inclusion (51), indicating that the primary route of sphingomyelin delivery to the inclusion is direct from the Golgi apparatus rather than from the plasma membrane as a result of fusion with endocytic vesicles.

Although the chlamydial inclusion starts at

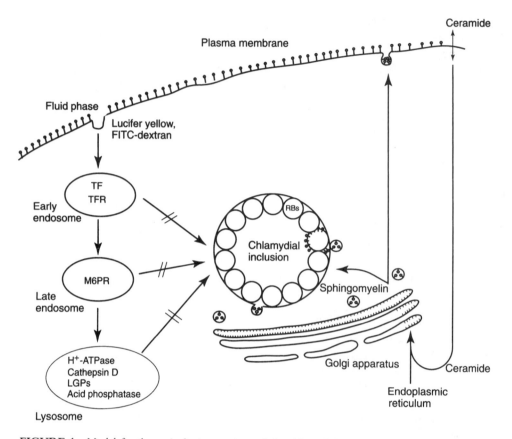

FIGURE 1 Model for the vesicular interactions of the chlamydial inclusion. By 2 h postinfection, in a process that requires early protein synthesis, endocytosed *C. trachomatis* EBs transform the properties of the endocytic vesicles such that they no longer interact with endocytic pathways but begin to intercept sphingolipids from an exocytic pathway. Fluid phase markers or markers for early and later endosomes or lysosomes are not associated with the chlamydial inclusion. Instead, the chlamydial inclusion fuses with a subset of sphingomyelin-containing vesicles in transit to the plasma membrane. Fusion of these vesicles exposes the sphingomyelin on the luminal surface of the inclusion membrane, from which it is adsorbed by the chlamydial RBs and incorporated into their cell walls. (Reprinted from reference 51 with permission.)

the plasma membrane, it might best be described as an aberrant Golgi-derived vesicle situated distal to the *trans*-Golgi apparatus such that it receives host-derived lipids from an exocytic pathway (Fig. 1) (51). The acquisition of host sphingolipids by bacteria is distinctly unusual. In this model, the chlamydial inclusion represents an exocytic vesicle which is delayed somehow in its transport to and fusion with the plasma membrane. This proposal is consistent with the observation that certain serovars of *C. trachomatis* do not lyse the host cell at the

completion of replication but are released through fusion of the inclusion membrane with the plasma membrane.

This model suggests a novel mechanism by which chlamydiae may evade lysosomal fusion. Although the majority of intracellular parasites are believed to block the maturation of endosomes to lysosomes at an appropriate stage and then remain within those vesicles, chlamydiae appear to dissociate themselves entirely from this pathway. By appearing as a secretory vesicle, the chlamydial inclusion is apparently not perceived by the host cell as a vesicle destined to fuse with lysosomes. This interpretation is consistent with observations indicating that suppression of lysosomal fusion is limited to the inclusion and is not a general inhibition of lysosomal function in chlamydia-infected cells (34, 58).

Both transport to the Golgi region and acquisition of fluorescent sphingomyelin are dependent on early chlamydial protein synthesis, suggesting that chlamydiae actively modify the inclusion membrane in order to establish interactions with the exocytic pathway (133). When early chlamydial protein synthesis is inhibited, the endocytosed EBs are eventually degraded within lysosomes (133). This suggests that chlamydiae actively modify the response of the host cell to infection by a process that requires de novo chlamydial protein synthesis. Insertion of chlamydial polypeptides into the inclusion membrane is a likely means to modify the early chlamydial vacuole such that it is targeted to an exocytic pathway. It is known that routing of transport vesicles throughout a cell is mediated by proteins present on the transport vesicle membrane (124). Bannantine et al. and Rockey et al. have identified three *C. psittaci* proteins, termed IncA, -B, and -C, that are localized to the inclusion membranes of infected cells (122; J. P. Banantine, D. D. Rockey, and T. Hackstadt, *Abstr. 97th Gen. Meet. Am. Soc. Microbiol.*, abstr. D-004, 1997). IncA is exposed on the cytoplasmic face of the inclusion membrane and is phosphorylated by the host cell (121, 122), suggesting that these proteins may mediate some type of interaction or communication with the infected cell. Scidmore-Carlson and colleagues have described a protein, IncD, that is associated with the inclusion membrane in *C. trachomatis* (serovar L2)-infected cells and is a distant homolog of IncA (134). IncD is transcribed within the first 2 h following chlamydial uptake, making IncD an ideal candidate for an early communication device between the inclusion and the host cell. Identification of the signals used by the chlamydiae to govern vesicular trafficking to the inclusion remains a significant challenge in understanding the interaction of chlamydiae with the host cell.

One hypothesis in which the inclusion does not fuse with lysosomes is based on the retention of Na^+,K^+-ATPases within the parasite-containing vesicular membrane. Upon entering the host cell, the EB endosome pH only drops to 6.2 before stabilizing at 6.6, possibly due to retention of the endosomal Na^+,K^+-ATPase (132). The ion pumps Na^+,K^+-ATPase and the vacuolar proton ATPase (H^+-ATPase) are involved in regulating the pH of endocytic compartments and controlling their acidification (19, 42). The action of the Na^+,K^+-ATPase, internalized with ligands during endocytosis, creates an interior-positive membrane potential in the endosome, which limits acidification by the H^+-ATPase. Thus, the pH of early endosomes does not fall below 6.0 until the Na^+,K^+-ATPase is removed from the vesicle, permitting acidification to lysosomal levels. It is thought that *C. trachomatis* L2 may reside within vesicles originating from the host cell plasma membrane which retain the characteristics of early endosomes by avoiding fusion with H^+-ATPase-containing vesicles. If so, these serovar L2-containing vesicles are guaranteed to avoid fusion with lysosomes because early endosomes are unable to fuse with lysosomes (103) while late endosomes readily do so (104). If chlamydia-containing vesicles retain Na^+,K^+-ATPases, any H^+-ATPases incorporated into these vesicles will remain inactive until the NA^+,K^+-ATPases are removed or inactivated. This is a novel method for the inhibition of vesicle acidification by intracellular parasites and warrants further investigation. It first needs to be determined if Na^+,K^+-ATPases and H^+-ATPases exist in the inclusion membrane.

Avoidance of lysosomal destruction is an obvious necessity for prolonged chlamydial survival in a host cell, and thus prolonged existence in a host. Chlamydia RBs replicate within an inclusion membrane which takes up host sphingomyelin, as well as other eukaryotic glycerophospholipids, such as phosphatidyl choline; phosphatidylinositol, normally made within the endoplasmic reticulum; cardiolipin, normally contained in mitochondria; and cholesterol (160). Thus, the RBs are enclosed within a membrane that mimics the membranes of host cellular organelles, and there is no evidence that chlamydia-specific molecules are exchanged for cellular sphingolipids intercepted from the exocytic pathway.

All chlamydial species can survive and multiply in host epithelial cells, but their abilities to survive and reproduce in professional phagocytes vary. The guinea pig inclusion conjunctivitis (GPIC) strain of *C. psittaci* does not grow in macrophages, yet the 6BC and MN/Cal 10 strains do. The LGV strains of *C. trachomatis* grow poorly in human macrophages, but human macrophages support little or no growth of the oculogenital strains of *C. trachomatis* (91, 164). Fresh human monocytes are potently chlamydiacidal against both LGV and oculogenital trachoma biovars. Monocyte lysosomes fuse with phagosomes of both LGV and trachoma biovars. However, when monocytes are cultured for 8 days to yield monocyte-derived macrophages, they support the growth of LGV, with LGV phagosomes avoiding lysosome fusion, but continue to kill oculogenital strains through the successful fusion of lysosomes with oculogenital phagosomes (164). The demise of trachoma organisms in monocyte-derived macrophages implies sensitivity of the organisms to nonoxidative systems, because oxidative metabolism is low in these phagocytes. These findings may reflect differences in disease syndromes, with organisms from the trachoma biovar preferentially infecting mucosal epithelial cells, causing a more peripheral infection, and organisms from the LGV biovar primarily infecting lymph nodes and causing systemic infection.

C. pneumoniae has also been shown to produce a productive infection in macrophages, but in monocytes, no infectious progeny have been found (73). However, *C. pneumoniae* organisms remain metabolically active for at least 3 days after monocyte infection. *C. trachomatis* serovar K has also been shown to remain viable in human monocytic cells for 10 days, although

in noncultivatable form (76). Monocytes may thus offer a hiding place for the parasite with the potential for reactivation under favorable conditions. Infected human blood monocytes may act as transporters of these nonreplicating but viable chlamydiae. Proposed theories include monocyte dissemination of *C. pneumoniae* from respiratory epithelial cells to blood vessel cells, where they induce or accelerate atherosclerosis, or to phagocytic cells of the brain, where they augment AD. For *C. trachomatis*, monocytes may carry the organisms from the genital tract to peripheral joints, where they induce reactive arthritis, or monocytes may leave the genital tract and recirculate to induce relapsing disease. Further work is needed to explain the different responses to chlamydial infection in human monocytes and human monocyte-derived macrophages.

Work by Rasmussen and colleagues suggests that the presence or absence of replication in persistent infection may be of significance (118). Their in vitro data revealed that cervical epithelial cells and primary endocervical cells release interleukin 1α after chlamydial infection and that this response requires productive infection, as chlamydia-infected cells treated with chloramphenicol did not release this proinflammatory cytokine. Chlamydial LPS was not sufficient to elicit epithelial cell cytokine production. Of course, in the in vivo situation persistent antigen (LPS) alone likely stimulates continued release of proinflammatory mediators from infiltrating inflammatory cells.

PMNs are the only myeloid cells whose lysosomes readily fuse with phagosomes containing intact EBs of either *C. trachomatis* (trachoma or LGV strains) or *C. psittaci*. EBs of both the LGV and trachoma biovars activate complement in the absence of antibody and exert a strong chemotactic effect on human PMNs (93). Both oxygen-dependent and oxygen-independent mechanisms are active in the killing of chlamydiae by PMNs (140, 164, 168). Although chlamydiae are killed by PMNs, as discussed earlier, in human endometrial epithelial cell cultures monitored for more than 1 month after exposure to azithromycin (a chlamydiacidal antibiotic)-loaded PMNs, residual chla-mydial envelopes and MOMP and LPS anti-gens were detected and continued to stimulate PMN chemotaxis (162). In addition, Wyrick has shown that exposure of penicillin-induced persistent forms to azithromycin-loaded PMNs did not result in eradication of the persistent forms of chlamydiae (P. B. Wyrick, personal communication). Thus, even though chlamyd-iae may not be able to reproduce in PMNs, their antigens may persist for some time after the organisms are killed, inducing continued inflammation and tissue damage in the host.

Dendritic cells (DC) have also recently been shown to readily kill *C. trachomatis* and *C. psit-taci*. The chlamydiae are internalized by the DC in a nonspecific manner through macropino-cytosis, and the macropinosomes subsequently fuse with DC lysosomes expressing major his-tocompatibility complex class II molecules. The interaction induces maturation of the DC, and the DC stimulate antigen-specific CD4$^+$ T cells (106). These professional antigen-pre-senting cells must be programmed in such a way that they do not allow the chlamydiae time to do whatever is required to prevent phago-some-lysosome fusion. One mechanism by which chlamydiae may cause repeated reinfec-tion in the host is by stimulation of short-lived CD4-dependent immunity. The enhanced an-tigen-presenting capacity of DC for chlamyd-iae has been capitalized on recently in a vaccine study in which chlamydia-fed DC were used for immunization and were found to be quite protective (146).

Methods of Attachment and Entry of Chlamydiae into the Host Cell

Chlamydial infection begins by contact of in-fectious EB with the epithelial apical surface. Attachment of chlamydiae may involve multi-ple different adhesins or specific adhesins. The following EB envelope components have been proposed as adhesins: (i) the MOMP, whose role in adherence is based on the inhibitory properties of trypsin and of monoclonal anti-bodies which target surface-exposed domains of MOMP (147, 148); (ii) a 38-kDa cytadhesin

shown to bind specifically to glutaraldehyde-fixed HeLa cells (67, 68); (iii) an unidentified glycosaminoglycan-like molecule implicated in a trimolecular mechanism involving uniden-tified glycosaminoglycan receptors on EBs and host cells (26, 167); (iv) an unidentified glycan presumed to be covalently linked to MOMP (149); (v) the heat shock protein Hsp70 or a genetically linked gene product, whose role in attachment and invasion was suggested by the use of recombinant methods (120, 129); and (vi) the developmentally regulated cysteine-rich envelope protein, outer membrane pro-tein 2 (Omp2), that is present only in the infec-tious EB form (153).

There is evidence that the first and last ad-hesins mentioned above may be somewhat hidden from immune surveillance and thus may allow continued propagation of chlamyd-iae in the host. Data from Su et al. (147) suggest that negatively charged divergent sequences in exposed MOMP variable domains (VDs) func-tion in the binding of chlamydiae to host cells via electrostatic interactions, followed by a more specific hydrophobic interaction involv-ing an invariant nonapeptide sequence located in VD IV. This nonapeptide, which is normally inaccessible to antibody on native EBs, be-comes immunoaccessible in heat-treated or-ganisms. The hydrophobic nonapeptide is flanked at both its N- and C-termini by hyper-variable domains containing hydrophilic and charged residues, suggesting that the invariant sequence may form a hydrophobic depression or cleft. On the basis of these properties, this invariant region of VD IV may be a cryptic binding site that functions in the attachment of chlamydiae to host cells (147). In this model, all chlamydiae utilize a common binding domain that is protected from immune surveillance. The protruding sequences of VD IV flanking this region would be expected to exhibit se-quence variation, as they indeed do, since they are surface-exposed charged sites and therefore primary targets for immunological attack.

The last-mentioned proposed adhesin, Omp2, is susceptible to trypsin activity even at low concentrations of the protease, suggesting its presence on the EB surface, and yet only a small portion of Omp2 seems to be immunoaccessible, as some studies using Omp2-specific antibodies have failed to detect it (28, 156). This would partially protect this potential adhesin from antibody binding and thus from interference with cellular attachment.

These multiple options for attachment provide flexibility for chlamydiae in different mucosal environments to attach to and enter epithelial cells with vastly different physiological functions, which may be reflected by an array of different surface receptors. They may also explain mechanisms for differential growth of chlamydia species in professional phagocytes. For example, attachment of LGV serovars to the host cell involves heparan sulfate-like glycosaminoglycans as a critical ligand (167). Perhaps heparan sulfate-like glycosaminoglycans are endocytosed with the LGV EBs and inhibit lysosomal fusion in a manner similar to sulfatides, which have been proposed to prevent lysosomal fusion with *Mycobacterium tuberculosis*-containing vesicles (3).

THE DEVELOPMENT OF CRYPTIC BODIES: MOULDER'S HYPOTHESIS

Do chlamydiae persist in a quiescent, nonproductive form in the mammalian host, waiting for the right moment to revive and proliferate? Perhaps the first step in developing an answer to this question is to examine the data suggesting that chlamydiae can persist in such a form in vitro in cell culture. Support for such a cryptic chlamydial form was first provided by Moulder and colleagues in 1980 (101) with monolayer cultures of mouse fibroblasts (L cells) infected with strain 6BC of *C. psittaci*. When L cells were infected in suspension with 0.01 to 10 50% infectious doses of *C. psittaci* per host cell and then plated out in 25-cm^2 plastic cell culture flasks, the resulting monolayers appeared to be totally destroyed by infection in 4 to 14 days, depending on the multiplicity of infection. However, if these monolayers were washed to remove detached cells, covered with fresh medium, and incubated for another 2 to 3 weeks, a few colonies of L cells appeared in

some of the flasks. Microscopic examination of Giemsa-stained monolayers revealed that some of the L cells contained chlamydial inclusions in their cytoplasm while others showed no sign of chlamydial infection. However, on continued propagation of these inclusion-negative colonies, all eventually produced inclusion-bearing cells.

Moulder et al. (101) suggested that chlamydiae persisted in these cells as cryptic bodies and that some factor periodically initiated the conversion of cryptic bodies into reproductive RB. Conversion of the RBs into infectious EBs completes the chlamydial developmental cycle, and most of the host cells are destroyed by overt chlamydial multiplication. However, a few cryptically infected L cells do not convert to overt infection, and these cells survive to initiate a new cycle of host cell regrowth.

Virtually all of the microscopically inclusion-free L cells were immune to infection with exogenous chlamydiae but gave rise to infected clones. Thus, one must assume that all of the cells in a persistent infection are either overtly or cryptically infected and that in some as yet unexplained way cryptic infection confers immunity to superinfection. The resistance seemed to be due to a defect in entry, as ^{14}C-labeled *C. psittaci* cells failed to attach and resistance to superinfection could be circumvented by centrifuging the inoculum onto the host cells. Interestingly, the inclusion-positive and inclusion-negative L cells from persistently infected cultures had a pattern of surface-exposed proteins different from the patterns of uninfected and acutely infected wild-type L cells. Superinfection refractoriness and abnormal surface protein patterns disappeared simultaneously when L cells were cured of persistent infection, either spontaneously or with tetracycline or rifampin. The fact that rifampin and tetracycline were effective in curing the L cells of cryptic infection suggests that reproduction of the cryptic body required transcription and translation of chlamydial genes (101).

Moulder's cryptic body hypothesis raises many questions. What kind of a host-parasite interaction is it that yields a cryptically infected cell? What is the physical nature of the cryptic body? What initiates the development of the cryptic body, and what eventually stimulates its conversion into a replicating RB? What is the mechanism of host cell resistance to super-infection? Finally, can these data be extrapolated to the in vivo situation? Do cryptic bodies exist in vivo? Long-term persistent chlamydial infection, whether in cell culture or in natural hosts, must be based on establishment of a mutually acceptable balance between multiplication of chlamydiae and their host cells. The host cell cycle is not disrupted at low multiplicities of infection, and some infected cells continue to divide. Chlamydiae depend on the host cell for both synthetic intermediates and energy in the form of ATP. Multiplying RBs must compete with their host cells because metabolic pools of the host are the feedstock for both host and chlamydial biosynthesis. Thus, perhaps one mechanism of induction of cryptic-body formation in vivo may be the fact that in certain circumstances, the host cell is at a relative advantage in competing for nutrients and the RB is deprived. Any situation that prevents RB multiplication and continuation of the chlamydial developmental cycle may prompt the conversion of RBs into cryptic forms. In vitro correlates of such situations have been demonstrated with the use of medium formulations lacking specific nutrients and with drugs that inhibit chlamydial multiplication. Such situations may induce development of aberrant persistent forms of chlamydiae.

INDUCTION OF PERSISTENCE BY NUTRIENT DEPLETION

Allan and Pearce found that the availability of certain amino acids in the growth medium determined whether dormant or productive infection was expressed in McCoy cells infected with the *C. psittaci* strain GPIC (2). Depletion of an essential nutrient may block multiplication not only of chlamydiae but of host cells as well. For a limited time, both host and parasite survive in nonmultiplying states from which they may be revived when the nutrient is supplied (145). Interestingly, different strains of *C. trachomatis* and *C. psittaci* exhibit differential re-

quirements for specific amino acids in their growth media. Differences in requirements for the *C. trachomatis* strains correlate with the associated clinical syndrome, with trachoma serotypes A, B, and C exhibiting a requirement for the addition of tryptophan while six strains of oculogenital origin, representing serotypes D to I, exhibited no requirement for tryptophan. Of four *C. psittaci* strains from different hosts, three showed distinct patterns of amino acid requirements. Thus, *C. psittaci* amino acid requirements may reflect the nutritional environments in which the various strains have evolved (1).

INDUCTION OF PERSISTENCE BY ANTIBIOTICS

Previous studies of chlamydial development in the presence of antibiotics showed that these agents cause interruptions in the normal developmental cycle of chlamydiae, and several studies implicate the generation of abnormal developmental forms (27, 79, 92, 126). Examples include the following. (i) The addition of aminopterin and thymidine 20 h after infection of McCoy cells with *C. psittaci* results in no visible inclusions and no infectivity for fresh McCoy cells for as long as 4 weeks, although chlamydial multiplication may be restored at any time by the addition of folinic acid. Aminopterine inhibits dihydrofolate reductase, which prevents reorganization of RBs to EBs. A rare RB must survive passage to await removal of the aminopterin block (114). (ii) Penicillin blocks the conversion of RBs into EBs, and abnormal "penicillin forms" accumulate for at least 40 h. The effect of penicillin, which is possibly due to its inhibition of synthesis of the cysteine-rich 60-kDa envelope protein (23), is reversible after contact with infected cells for as long as 48 h (66).

The fact that multiple mechanisms may result in alterations in chlamydial growth and differentiation implies that there may be multiple mechanisms by which persistence is generated. In fact, it is remarkable how many different ways to produce persistent chlamydial infections in cell culture have been described and how differently these persistent in vitro infections behave. It seems unlikely that chlamydiae, with one of the smallest of all eubacterial genomes, would have evolved such a variety of ways of interacting with host cells without at least some of them being of adaptive value.

INDUCTION OF PERSISTENCE BY CYTOKINES

Production of persistently infected cell cultures by adding an inhibitor of chlamydial multiplication or by withholding a nutrient essential to growth may be a laboratory curiosity, but the demonstration that IFN-γ reversibly blocks growth of chlamydiae by inducing an enzyme that breaks down tryptophan, an essential amino acid for chlamydiae (18), suggests that this in vitro mechanism may well have an in vivo counterpart.

IFN-γ is known to be an important immune effector molecule for intracellular parasitic and bacterial pathogens. This immune-regulated cytokine has been shown in vivo and in cell culture models to protect against infection by *C. trachomatis* and *C. psittaci* (18, 22, 117). The suggested mechanism of protection is not a result of the direct effect of the cytokine on chlamydiae but rather is a result of alterations in the host cell that interfere with normal chlamydial growth. IFN-γ affects human host cells by inducing indoleamine 2,3-dioxygenase, a nonconstitutive enzyme that catalyzes the initial step in the degradation of tryptophan to N-formylkynurenine and kynurenine. Depletion of exogenous tryptophan correlates with growth inhibition of chlamydiae in a wide spectrum of human host cells, including monocyte-derived macrophages, fibroblasts, epithelial cells, and primary conjunctival cells (17, 18, 22, 117).

Uptake of chlamydiae and differentiation of EBs into RBs are not affected by IFN-γ treatment; instead, the cytokine adversely affects

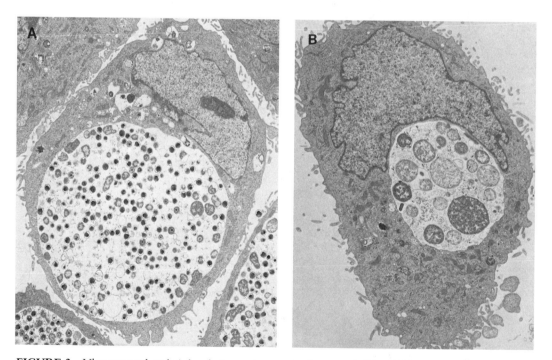

FIGURE 2 Ultrastructural analysis by electron microscopy of untreated (A) and IFN-γ-treated (B) cells 48 h after infection. Note the typical RB and EB forms in inclusions of untreated cells. The IFN-γ-treated cells do not contain typical chlamydial forms; instead, large atypical RB forms characterize the inclusions. (Photomicrographs provided by Gerald I. Byrne.)

normal growth and division of RBs and interrupts their redifferentiation into infectious EBs (135). IFN-γ-mediated tryptophan catabolism results in an alteration of growth characterized by a decrease in the structural components of chlamydiae, including MOMP, the 60-kDa OMP, and LPS (7), major components of the outer membrane complex that are required for proper division of RBs and differentiation into EBs (Fig. 2). The amino acid sequence of *C. trachomatis* serovar A MOMP reveals seven tryptophan residues (4), and these are conserved for all *C. trachomatis* MOMP sequences reported to date, including the genital serovars H (54), E (112), and F (168) and the LGV serovars L1 (113) and L2 (168). Sequence analysis of the 60-kDa chlamydial OMP reveals four tryptophan molecules (30). Under conditions of IFN-γ-mediated deprivation of tryptophan, a decrease in MOMP and 60-kDa OMP expression may be the result of the inability to synthesize these structural constituents effi-

ciently, leading to aberrant chlamydial growth. The synthesis of the chlamydial 60-kDa heat shock protein (Hsp60), a proposed immunopathological antigen, is maintained under these conditions. The chlamydial Hsp60 contains no tryptophan residues, as deduced from the nucleotide sequence (99). Another possibility is that under conditions of stress, mRNA for stress response proteins continues to be transcribed, whereas that for structural proteins is downregulated.

Transmission electron microscopic studies of IFN-γ-induced persistence revealed the morphological development of infectious chlamydiae from aberrant forms following IFN-γ removal (9). Aberrant chlamydial forms demonstrating budding from RBs were observed early in the recovery process (Fig. 3A). In addition, single aberrant organisms displaying multiple nucleoid-like regions of condensation were observed late in the recovery process (Fig. 3B), indicating that the reorganization of ge-

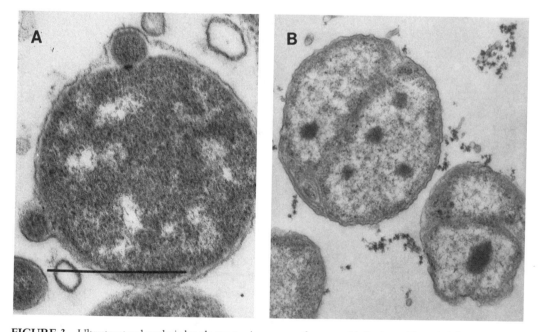

FIGURE 3 Ultrastructural analysis by electron microscopy of rescue of infectious chlamydial forms from cells treated with IFN-γ for 48 h after infection and subsequently cultured in the absence of IFN-γ. At 12 h following the removal of IFN-γ, budding from enlarged RBs (A) was observed. By 24 h following the removal of IFN-γ, nucleoid-like structures were observed within aberrant forms (B). Bar, 1 μm. (Reprinted from reference 9 with permission.)

netic material occurred during the recovery process. This was confirmed by labeling with the thymidine analog BrdU, which was used to detect the presence of DNA. Immuno-electron microscopy with anti-BrdU specific antibodies was done to identify and localize DNA. Specific labeling was associated with dense nucleoid structures by 24 h after IFN-γ removal (Fig. 4). The localization of chlamydial DNA to nucleoid-like masses suggested that multiple genomes were present in persistent forms and underwent reorganization to produce multiple infectious EBs from a single aberrant form of the organism.

Thus, Beatty et al. showed that treatment of *C. trachomatis* serovar A-infected HeLa cells with low levels of IFN-γ resulted in the development of large, aberrant noninfectious forms of chlamydiae (7) and that upon removal of IFN-γ from the culture or by addition of exogenous tryptophan the atypical forms revert to morphologically typical infectious EBs (9). These studies substantiated the notion that cryptic bodies can be induced and viability can be maintained during this persistent state. The fact that IFN-γ has been shown to induce cryptic chlamydial forms through degradation of tryptophan may provide a link between cell culture descriptions of persistence via nutrient deprivation and the actual process of chlamydial persistence in natural infections.

A potential problem proposed with the IFN-γ model is that not all chlamydia strains require exogenous tryptophan for in vitro growth (1), and thus the model may not be applicable to all strains. Byrne et al. have published data using serovar A of *C. trachomatis*, but this group has induced many other serovars (including many of the genital strains) into a persistent state with IFN-γ treatment (G. I. Byrne, personal communication). Serovars that grow more rapidly in vitro are more difficult to induce into a persistent state, and it may be that the more rapidly growing serovars are better at competing with the host cell for essential nutrients (Byrne, personal communication). A recent study from Byrne's laboratory indicated that the in vitro culture system used can also affect induction of persistence. In polarized cells, intracellular soluble tryptophan pools are larger than those in nonpolarized cells, explaining the fact that substantially larger quantities of IFN-γ are required to induce persistent forms of chlamydiae in polarized cell cultures (70).

A recent study by Wyrick examined the ability of azithromycin to kill penicillin-induced persistent forms of serovar E in HEC-1B cells (P. B. Wyrick, personal communication). Aberrant large persistent forms of *C. trachomatis* serovar E were successfully induced in polarized HEC-1B cells by exposure to penicillin. At 72 h postinfection, azithromycin was added in addition to penicillin. At 144 h postinfection, the antibiotics were removed and the cul-

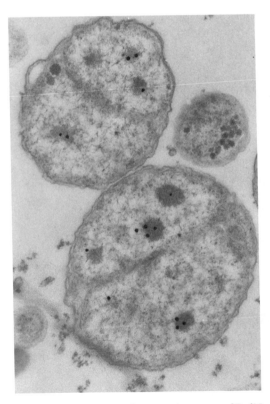

FIGURE 4 Immuno-electron microscopy of BrdU incorporation during the recovery process. At 24 h after removal of IFN-γ, anti-BrdU antibodies localized DNA synthesis to dense nucleoid masses. (Reprinted from reference 9 with permission.)

tures were incubated for an additional 72 h to allow for recovery. The number of inclusions recovered was large and no different from the recovered penicillin control (Wyrick, personal communication). A study by Kutlin and Hammerschlag with *C. pneumoniae* in a continuous-infection model in HEp-2 cells revealed that treatment of cells that had been persistently infected with chlamydiae for over 2 years with azithromycin or ofloxacin reduced but did not completely eliminate the organism (83). This was in contrast to primarily infected cells, where antibiotic treatment completely killed the chlamydiae. These data indicate that slowly metabolizing chlamydiae are apparently refractory to the bactericidal effects of antibiotics. Therefore, one explanation for treatment failure may be that if these cryptic aberrant forms of chlamydiae are present in vivo, they are less susceptible to the bactericidal effects of standard antimicrobial regimens.

TNF-α, another cytokine that has been implicated in host defense against chlamydiae (158), has also been shown to induce irregular developmental forms in vitro. Electron microscopic analysis of HEp-2 cells infected with *C. trachomatis* L2 48 h after treatment with TNF-α revealed small inclusion bodies containing a high proportion of irregular developmental forms and enlarged RBs (136). Thus, cytokines that are released by the host in order to kill chlamydiae may induce the development of persistent forms.

It has been suggested that when chlamydiae exist in an aberrant form, as seen with IFN-γ treatment (9), penicillin treatment (23, 150), or amino acid depletion (6, 27), they are able to evade immune clearance because persistence within the cell protects the organisms from antibody-mediated neutralization. However, both CD4+ and CD8+ cells are activated in a primary response to chlamydial infection (142), with the primary function of CD8+ cells being to lyse infected target cells. One group of investigators has suggested that if these in vitro aberrant forms are a satisfactory model for in vivo persistence, then the aberrant forms should not only evade the humoral immune response but also be resistant to cell-mediated killing. When the ability of *Chlamydia*-specific cytotoxic T lymphocytes to kill IFN-γ- and penicillin-treated serovar L2- or serovar A-infected cells was tested in vitro, these cultures were killed as efficiently as the untreated controls (119). Regardless of whether the chlamydial forms were typical or aberrant, they were efficiently killed by specific CD8+ cells. Thus, there is no direct evidence that such aberrant forms are capable of completely evading the immune response. One could envision a scenario in which the majority of chlamydial organisms were successfully neutralized by antibody and all infected cells, whether or not aberrant or persistent forms were present, would be killed by cytotoxic T lymphocytes. Although this would lead to the resolution of infection, it might also contribute to disease pathogenesis. Of course, these in vitro studies do not take into account the need for the CD8+ cells to home to the site of persistent infection. Nevertheless, the existence of cryptic forms of chlamydiae in vivo remains to be proven.

Effects on Apoptosis

Chlamydiae have been shown to protect infected cells from apoptosis due to other ligands, including TNF-α, Fas antibody, and granzyme B or perforin, and that protection is evident within 4 h of infection (38). Thus, the antiapoptotic activity may protect infected cells during the initial stages of chlamydial invasion, allowing time for mechanisms which, at least in epithelial cells, ensure avoidance of phagosome-lysosome fusion to play out. The antiapoptotic activity of chlamydia infection is due to inhibition of caspase 3 activation (38), which is required for apoptosis following the TNF-α and Fas pathways. Interestingly, *C. psittaci* has been shown to induce apoptosis in epithelial cells and macrophages, a phenomenon that is measurable within 1 day of infection and requires productive infection by the bacteria (107). Inhibition of either of two proapoptotic enzymes, caspase-1 or caspase-3, did not significantly affect chlamydia-induced apoptosis, suggesting that chlamydial infection triggers an apoptotic pathway that is independent of known caspases (107). Hence, there may be a fine balance struck between the anti- and proapoptotic activities of chlamydiae during the course of infection. Antiapoptotic activity may protect infected cells from lysis by cells and effector molecules of the immune system, while proapoptotic activity may contribute to the continued release of infectious progeny. The exact contribution of each of these activities to the propagation of chlamydiae and to the pathology of the infection remains to be determined.

Antigenic Variation
Antigenic variation by microbial pathogens represents a fundamental virulence capability that promotes persistence by evasion of the host immune response. Four factors support the conclusion that the antibody response to the only known variant surface antigen, MOMP, is an important mediator of immunity to *C. trachomatis* infection: the presence of a polymorphic MOMP surface antigen, the serovar specificity of resistance to challenge, the demonstration that antibodies specific for serovariant-specific surface antigens can neutralize infection experimentally in vivo (169), and the selection of MOMP allelic variants in human populations with a high prevalence of chlamydial infection (15, 32). The MOMP quantitatively dominates the surface architecture of the chlamydial EB and defines serovar specificity; however, its physical and antigenic structures are complex and not understood beyond the level of primary sequence (16, 143). Using chlamydial MOMP expressed in *E. coli* for absorption of mouse immune sera, Fan and Stephens recently showed that neutralization of infectivity was highly serovar specific and dependent upon thermolabile antigens of MOMP (37). Monoclonal antibody studies using a variety of serovars have shown that antibody reactivities to individual MOMP VD peptides played a minor role in neutralization compared with those of conformational antigens defined by the authentic structure of the entire protein. Antigenic determinants of *C.*

pneumoniae may be similar, as studies have shown that antisera elicited by EBs neutralize infectivity but antisera elicited by MOMP peptides could not (111). The antigen conformation dependence of chlamydial neutralization and the sequence-variant character of MOMP suggest that minor changes in MOMP primary sequence, found even among strains of the same serovar designation (32), may affect the efficacy of conformation-dependent neutralization sufficiently to initially facilitate escape from neutralization.

Analysis of major genotypic variants suggests that recombination may be a substantial mechanism by which genetic diversity of the *omp1* gene, and thus antigenic diversity of MOMP, is generated in *C. trachomatis* (15, 85).

Recombination depends on coinfection of the host with multiple *C. trachomatis* serovars, which has been reported as 6% in a group of sex workers (15) and more recently as high as 48% in men and 57% in their female sex partners, identified as infected at a sexually transmitted disease clinic in Boston (86). Consistent with this hypothesis is recent analysis of the sequenced *C. trachomatis* genome, which reveals extensive representation of genes for DNA repair and recombination systems, indicating that chlamydiae have considerable recombination capabilities (144).

Two recent genotyping studies by Deborah Dean and colleagues suggest that antigenic variation arises in response to antimicrobial and/or immune pressure; one was conducted with women with *C. trachomatis* infections of the genital tract, and one was done with patients with *C. pneumoniae* infections of the respiratory tract. As discussed earlier in this chapter, seven women had repeatedly positive endocervical cultures that revealed nucleotide mutations in the original genotype after several rounds of chemotherapy. These organisms produced relapsing infection over 2 to 5 years (33). In a study of two patients who were intermittently symptomatic and culture positive with *C. pneumoniae* infection for up to 7 years, it was found that both patients had initial infections with prototype genotypes and, following their first course of treatment, developed an infection with a new genotype, CP1. This genotype appeared repeatedly in these two patients despite treatment with appropriate antibiotics and lack of contact between them (31). Although preliminary, these studies suggest that newly identified genotypes may emerge under antimicrobial and/or immune pressure and may play a role in persistence and disease pathogenesis.

CONCLUSIONS

Although significánt circumstantial evidence exists, a latent form of chlamydiae has not been clearly documented in the human host. Unfortunately, there is not currently a "marker" for persistent chlamydial infection, and so multiple methods are utilized in attempts to prove its existence and its relationship to the pathology of chlamydial disease.

Perhaps the efforts of Alan Hudson and colleagues have come the closest to proving the persistence of chlamydial infection in patients with reactive arthritis (12, 13, 44, 105, 115). These studies suggest that the chlamydiae are viable but not actively replicating; hence, they are in a latent form. The problem with these studies is the difficulty inherent in proving the presence of chronic chlamydial infection as opposed to recent reinfection. Despite the fact that many patients had symptoms for years, serology was frequently not done, and even if it had been, the accuracy of serological tests for the diagnosis of acute versus chronic infection with *C. trachomatis* is debatable.

The same problem exists with *C. pneumoniae*. Population surveys have shown that *C. pneumoniae* is ubiquitous and that specific IgG antibodies may persist for years, which diminishes the value of IgG as a marker of persistent infection. The persistence of chlamydia-specific IgA antibodies has been proposed as a better marker of chronic *C. pneumoniae* infections (125), and of chronic *C. trachomatis* infections as well (24). Perhaps studies that look at IgA levels in patients with chronic disease in conjunction with immuno-electron microscopy and molecular biological investigations of the patients' tissues would help to confirm both methodologies.

The problem with studying persistent chlamydial infection in the human host is the logistical difficulty of examining individual patients over time. Studies that have best conquered this dilemma have perhaps come from collaborations between chlamydiologists working in different laboratories. As an example, the genotyping study reported in 1998 by Dean et al. (31) was performed on *C. pneumoniae* isolates obtained over 7 years from patients who were initially in a study conducted by Hammerschlag et al. in 1992 (56).

The unique characteristics of persistent chlamydiae described by Beatty et al. (decreased MOMP expression in the presence of normal levels of Hsp60) have been proposed as potentially important attributes of these organisms that may facilitate in vivo identification (8), and yet, since actively replicating chlamydiae make Hsp60, these altered levels of protein expression are far from a perfect marker of persistent latent infection. What is needed for the future is documentation of expression of a protein or other cellular product that is produced by persistent chlamydial forms and is not produced by actively replicating forms of chlamydiae. Such a marker of chlamydial persistence would not only allow proof of persistence in vivo but could also help explain chlamydial disease pathogenesis if the marker was found associated with actual chlamydial disease.

ACKNOWLEDGMENTS

I thank David M. Ojcius for his ideas and Priscilla B. Wyrick for her ideas and the personal communication of pertinent data. I am indebted to Roger G. Rank, Kathleen A. Kelly, and Gerald I. Byrne for their critical review of this work. I am particularly indebted to Gerald I. Byrne for his insightful discussions and for contributing photomicrographs of persistent chlamydial forms for this chapter.

REFERENCES

1. **Allan, I., and J. H. Pearce.** 1983. Amino acid requirements of strains of *Chlamydia trachomatis* and *Chlamydia psittaci* growing in McCoy cells:

relationship with clinical syndrome and host origin. *J. Gen. Microbiol.* **129:**2001–2007.

2. **Allan, I., and J. H. Pearce.** 1983. Differential amino acid utilization by *Chlamydia psittaci* (strain guinea pig conjunctivitis) and its regulatory effect on chlamydial growth. *J. Gen. Microbiol.* **129:** 1991–2000.

3. **Armstrong, J. A.** 1975. Phagosome-lysosome interactions in cultured macrophages infected with virulent tubercle bacilli. Reversal of the usual nonfusion pattern and observations on bacterial survival. *J. Exp. Med.* **142:**1–16.

4. **Baehr, W., Y. X. Zhang, T. Joseph, H. Su, F. E. Nano, K. D. E. Everett, and H. D. Caldwell.** 1988. Mapping antigenic domains expressed by Chlamydia trachomatis major outer membrane protein genes. *Proc. Natl. Acad. Sci. USA* **85:** 4000–4004.

5. **Balin, B. J., H. C. Gerard, E. J. Arking, D. M. Appelt, P. J. Branigan, J. T. Abrams, J. A. Whittum-Hudson, and A. P. Hudson.** 1998. Identification and localization of *Chlamydia pneumoniae* in the Alzheimer's brain. *Med. Microbiol. Immunol.* **187:**23–42.

6. **Beatty, W. L., T. A. Belanger, A. A. Desai, R. P. Morrison, and G. I. Byrne.** 1994. Tryptophan depletion as a mechanism of gamma interferon-mediated chlamydial persistence. *Infect. Immun.* **62:**3705–3711.

7. **Beatty, W. L., G. I. Byrne, and R. P. Morrison.** 1993. Morphologic and antigenic characterization of interferon-γ-mediated persistent *Chlamydia trachomatis* infection in vitro. *Proc. Natl. Acad. Sci. USA* **90:**3998–4002.

8. **Beatty, W. L., R. P. Morrison, and G. I. Byrne.** 1994. Persistent chlamydiae: from cell culture to a paradigm for chlamydial pathogenesis. *Microbiol. Rev.* **58:**686–699.

9. **Beatty, W. L., R. P. Morrison, and G. I. Byrne.** 1995. Reactivation of persistent *Chlamydia trachomatis* infection in cell culture. *Infect. Immun.* **63:**199–205.

10. **Bell, T. A., W. E. Stamm, C. C. Kuo, S. P. Wang, K. K. Holmes, and J. T. Grayston.** 1987. Delayed appearance of *Chlamydia trachomatis* infections acquired at birth. *Pediatr. Infect. Dis. J.* **6:**928–931.

11. **Berdal, B. P., O. Scheel, A. R. Ogaard, T. Hoel, T. J. Gutteberg, and G. Anestad.** 1992. Spread of subclinical *Chlamydia pneumoniae* infection in a closed community. *Scand. J. Infect. Dis.* **24:**431–436.

12. **Beutler, A. M., H. R. Schumacher, J. A. Whittum-Hudson, W. A. Salameh, and A. P. Hudson.** 1995. *In situ* hybridization for detection of inapparent infection with *Chlamydia trachomatis* in synovial tissue of a patient with Reiter's syndrome. *Am. J. Med. Sci.* **310:**206–213.

13. **Beutler, A. M., J. A. Whittum-Hudson, R. Nanagara, H. R. Schumacher, and A. P. Hudson.** 1994. Intracellular location of inapparently infecting chlamydia in synovial tissue from patients with Reiter's syndrome. *Immunol. Res.* **13:**163–171.

14. **Branigan, P. J., H. C. Gerard, A. P. Hudson, and H. R. Schumacher.** 1996. Comparison of synovial tissue and synovial fluid as the source of nucleic acids for detection of *Chlamydia trachomatis* by polymerase chain reaction. *Arthritis Rheum.* **39:** 1740–1746.

15. **Brunham, R., C. Yang, I. Maclean, J. Kimani, G. Maitha, and F. Plummer.** 1994. *Chlamydia trachomatis* from individuals in a sexually transmitted disease core group exhibit frequent sequence variation in the major outer membrane protein (ompl) gene. *J. Clin. Investig.* **94:**458–463.

16. **Brunham, R. C., and R. W. Peeling.** 1994. *Chlamydia trachomatis* antigens: role in immunity and pathogenesis. *Infect. Agents Dis.* **3:**218–233.

17. **Byrne, G. I., and D. A. Krueger.** 1983. Lymphokine-mediated inhibition of *Chlamydia* replication in mouse fibroblasts is neutralized by anti-gamma interferon immunoglobulin. *Infect. Immun.* **42:**1152–1158.

18. **Byrne, G. I., L. K. Lehmann, and G. J. Landry.** 1986. Induction of tryptophan catabolism is the mechanism for gamma-interferon-mediated inhibition of intracellular *Chlamydia psittaci* replication in T24 cells. *Infect. Immun.* **53:** 347–351.

19. **Cain, C. C., D. M. Sipe, and R. F. Murphy.** 1989. Regulation of endocytic pH by Na, K-ATPase in living cells. *Proc. Natl. Acad. Sci. USA* **86:**544–548.

20. **Campbell, L. A., C. C. Kuo, and J. T. Grayston.** 1998. *Chlamydia pneumoniae* and cardiovascular disease. *Emerg. Infect. Dis.* **4:**571–579.

21. **Campbell, L. A., D. L. Patton, D. E. Moore, A. L. Cappuccio, B. A. Mueller, and S. P. Wang.** 1993. Detection of *Chlamydia trachomatis* deoxyribonucleic acid in women with tubal infertility. *Fertil. Steril.* **59:**45–50.

22. **Carlin, J. M., E. C. Borden, and G. I. Byrne.** 1989. Interferon-induced indoleamine 2,3-dioxygenase activity inhibits *Chlamydia psittaci* replication in human macrophages. *J. Interferon Res.* **9:** 329–337.

22a.**Cates, W., Jr., and J. N. Wasserheit.** 1991. Genital chlamydial infections: epidemiology and reproductive sequelae. *Am. J. Obstet. Gynecol.* **164:**1771–1781.

23. **Cevenini, R., M. Donati, and M. La Placa.** 1988. Effects of penicillin on the synthesis of

membrane proteins of *Chlamydia trachomatis* LGV2 serotype. *FEMS Microbiol. Lett.* **56**:41–46.

24. **Chaim, W., B. Sarov, I. Sarov, B. Piura, A. Cohen, and V. Insler.** 1989. Serum IgG and IgA antibodies to chlamydia in ectopic pregnancies. *Contraception* **40**:59–71.

25. **Cheema, M. A., H. R. Schumacher, and A. P. Hudson.** 1991. RNA-directed molecular hybridization screening: evidence for inapparent chlamydial infection. *Am. J. Med. Sci.* **302**:261–268.

26. **Chen, J. C., and R. S. Stephen.** 1994. Trachoma and LGV biovars of *Chlamydia trachomatis* share the same glycosaminoglycan-dependent mechanism for infection of eukaryotic cells. *Mol. Microbiol.* **11**:501–507.

27. **Coles, A. M., D. J. Reynolds, A. Harper, A. Devitt, and J. H. Pearce.** 1993. Low-nutrient induction of abnormal chlamydial development: a novel component of chlamydial pathogenesis? *FEMS Microbiol. Lett.* **106**:193–200.

28. **Collett, B. A., W. J. Newhall, R. A. Jersild, and R. B. Jones.** 1989. Detection of surface-exposed epitopes on *Chlamydia trachomatis* by immune electron microscopy. *J. Gen. Microbiol.* **135**:85–94.

29. **Danesh, J., R. Collins, and R. Peto.** 1997. Chronic infections and coronary heart disease: is there a link? *Lancet* **350**:430–436.

30. **de la Maza, L. M., T. J. Fielder, E. J. Carlson, B. A. Markoff, and E. M. Peterson.** 1991. Sequence diversity of the 60-kilodalton protein and of a putative 15-kilodalton protein between the trachoma and lymphogranuloma venereum biovars of *Chlamydia trachomatis*. *Infect. Immun.* **59**:1196–1201.

31. **Dean, D., P. Roblin, L. Mandel, J. Schachter, and M. Hammerschlag.** 1998. Molecular evaluation of serial isolates from patients with persistent *Chlamydia pneumoniae* infections, p. 219–222. *In* R. S. Stephens, G. I. Byrne, G. Christiansen, I. N. Clarke, J. T. Grayston, R. G. Rank, G. L. Ridgway, P. Saikku, J. Schachter, and W. E. Stamm (ed.), *Chlamydial Infections. Proceedings of the Ninth International Symposium on Human Chlamydial Infection.* Napa, Calif.

32. **Dean, D., J. Schachter, C. R. Dawxon, and R. S. Stephens.** 1992. Comparison of the major outer membrane protein variant sequence regions of B/Ba isolates: a molecular epidemiologic approach to *Chlamydia trachomatis* infections. *J. Infect. Dis.* **166**:383–392.

33. **Dean, D., R. J. Suchland, and W. E. Stamm.** 1998. Apparent long-term persistence of *Chlamydia trachomatis* cervical infections—analysis of *Ompl* genotyping, p. 31–34. *In* R. S. Stephens, G. I. Byrne, G. Christiansen, I. N. Clarke, J. T. Grayston, R. G. Rank, G. L. Ridgway, P. Saikku, J. Schachter, and W. E. Stamm (ed.), *Chlamydial Infections. Proceedings of the Ninth International Symposium on Human Chlamydial Infection.* Napa, Calif.

34. **Eissenberg, L. G., and P. B. Wyrick.** 1981. Inhibition of phagolysosome fusion is localized to *Chlamydia psittaci*-laden vacuoles. *Infect. Immun.* **32**:880–896.

35. **Eissenberg, L. G., P. B. Wyrick, C. H. Davis, and J. W. Rumpp.** 1983. *Chlamydia psittaci* elementary body envelopes: ingestion and inhibition of phagolysosome fusion. *Infect. Immun.* **40**:741–751.

36. **Ekman, M. R., J. T. Grayston, R. Visakorpi, M. Kleemola, C. C. Kuo, and P. Saikku.** 1993. An epidemic of infections due to *Chlamydia pneumoniae* in military conscripts. *Clin. Infect. Dis.* **17**:420–425.

37. **Fan, J., and R. S. Stephens.** 1997. Antigen conformation dependence of *Chlamydia trachomatis* infectivity neutralization. *J. Infect. Dis.* **176**:713–721.

38. **Fan, T., H. Lu, L. Lu, L. Shi, G. A. McClarty, D. M. Nance, A. H. Greenberg, and G. Zhong.** 1998. Inhibition of apoptosis in *Chlamydia*-infected cells: blockage of mitochondrial cytochrome c release and caspase activation. *J. Exp. Med.* **187P**:487–497.

39. **Francis, T. F., and T. P. Magill.** 1938. An unidentified virus producing acute meningitis and pneumonitis in experimental animals. *J. Exp. Med.* **68**:147–160.

40. **Friis, R. R.** 1972. Interaction of L cells and *Chlamydia psittaci*: entry of the parasite and host responses to its development. *J. Bacteriol.* **110**:706–721.

41. **Fryer, R. H., E. P. Schwobe, M. L. Woods, and G. M. Rodgers.** 1997. Chlamydia species infect human vascular endothelial cells and induce procoagulant activity. *J. Investig. Med.* **45**:168–174.

42. **Fuchs, R., S. Schmidt, and I. Mellman.** 1989. A possible role for Na+, K+-ATPase in regulating ATP-dependent endosome acidification. *Proc. Natl. Acad. Sci. USA* **86**:539–543.

43. **Gaydos, C. A., J. T. Summersgill, N. N. Sahney, J. A. Ramirez, and T. C. Quinn.** 1996. Replication of *Chlamydia pneumoniae* in vitro in human macrophages, endothelial cells, and aortic artery smooth muscle cells. *Infect. Immun.* **64**:1614–1620.

44. **Gerard, H. C., P. J. Branigan, H. R. Schumacherz, Jr., and A. P. Hudson.** 1998. Synovial *Chlamydia trachomatis* in patients with reactive arthritis/Reiter's syndrome are viable but show aberrant gene expression. *J. Rheumatol.* **25**:734–742.

45. **Gnarpe, J., H. Gnarpe, and B. Sundelof.**

1991. Endemic prevalence of *Chlamydia pneumoniae* in subjectively healthy persons. *Scand. J. Infect. Dis.* **23**:387–388.

46. **Godzik, K., E. R. O'Brien, S. W. Wang, and C. C. Kuo.** 1995. In vitro susceptibility of human vascular wall cells to infection with *Chlamydia pneumoniae. J. Clin. Microbiol.* **33**:2411–2414.

47. **Grayston, J. T., M. B. Aldous, and A. Easton.** 1993. Evidence that *Chlamydia pneumoniae* causes pneumonia and bronchitis. *J. Infect. Dis.* **168**:1231–1235.

48. **Grayston, J. T., C. C. Kuo, A. S. Coulson, L. A. Campbell, R. D. Lawrence, and L. Ming-Jong.** 1995. *Chlamydia pneumoniae* (TWAR) in atherosclerosis of the carotid artery. *Circulation* **93**:3397–3400.

49. **Grayston, J. T., C. C. Kuo, S. P. Wang, and J. Altman.** 1986. A new *Chlamydia psittaci* strain, TWAR, isolated in acute respiratory tract infections. *N. Engl. J. Med.* **315**:161–168.

50. **Grayston, J. T., S. P. Wang, L. J. Yeh, and C. C. Kuo.** 1985. Importance of re-infection in the pathogenesis of trachoma. *Rev. Infect. Dis.* **7**:717–725.

51. **Hackstadt, T., D. D. Rockey, R. A. Heinzen, and M. A. Scidmore.** 1996. Chlamydia trachomatis interrupts an exocytic pathway to acquire endogenously synthesized sphingomyelin in transit from the Golgi apparatus to the plasma membrane. *EMBO J.* **15**:964–977.

52. **Hackstadt, T., M. A. Scidmore, and D. D. Rockey.** 1995. Lipid metabolism in Chlamydia trachomatis-infected cells: directed trafficking of Golgi-derived sphingolipids to the chlamydial inclusion. *Proc. Natl. Acad. Sci. USA* **92**:4877–4881.

53. **Hahn, D. L., T. Anttila, and P. Saikku.** 1996. Association of *Chlamydia pneumoniae* IgA antibodies with recently symptomatic asthma. *Epidemiol. Infect.* **117**:513–517.

54. **Hamilton, P. T., and D. P. Malinowski.** 1989. Nucleotide sequence of the major outer membrane protein gene from *Chlamydia trachomatis* serovar H. *Nucleic Acids Res.* **17**:8366.

55. **Hammer, M., E. Nettelnbreker, S. Hopf, E. Schmitz, K. Porschke, and H. Zeidler.** 1992. Chlamydial RNA in the joints of patients with *Chlamydia*-induced arthritis and undifferentiated arthritis. *Clin. Exp. Rheumatol.* **10**:63–66.

56. **Hammerschlag, M. R., K. Chirgwin, P. M. Roblin, M. Gelling, W. Dumornay, L. Mandel, P. Smith, and J. Schachter.** 1992. Persistent infection with *Chlamydia pneumoniae* following acute respiratory illness. *Clin. Infect. Dis.* **14**:178–182.

57. **Heinemann, M., M. Susa, U. Simnacher, R. Marre, and A. Essig.** 1996. Growth of *Chlamydia pneumoniae* induces cytokine production and

expression of CD14 in a human monocytic cell line. *Infect. Immun.* **64**:4872–4887.

58. **Heinzen, R. A., M. A. Scidmore, D. D. Rockey, and T. Hackstadt.** 1996. Differential interaction with endocytic and exocytic pathways distinguish [sic] parasitophorous vacuoles of *Coxiella burnetii* and *Chlamydia trachomatis. Infect. Immun.* **64**:796–809.

59. **Holland, M. J., R. L. Bailey, L. J. Hayes, H. C. Whittle, and D. C. Mabey.** 1993. Conjunctival scarring in trachoma is associated with depressed cell-mediated immune responses to chlamydial antigens. *J. Infect. Dis.* **168**:1528–1531.

60. **Holland, S. M., A. P. Hudson, L. Bobo, J. A. Whittum-Hudson, R. P. Viscidi, T. C. Quinn, and H. R. Taylor.** 1992. Demonstration of chlamydial RNA and DNA during a culture-negative state. *Infect. Immun.* **60**:2040–2047.

61. **Hooton, T. M., E. Rogers, T. G. Medina, L. E. Kuwamura, C. Ewers, P. L. Roberts, and W. E. Stamm.** 1990. Ciprofloxacin compared with doxycycline for nongonococcal urethritis. Ineffectiveness against *Chlamydia trachomatis* due to relapsing infection. *JAMA* **264**:1418–1421.

62. **Hudson, A. P., C. M. McEntee, M. Reacher, J. A. Whittum-Hudson, and H. R. Taylor.** 1992. Inapparent ocular infection by *Chlamydia trachomatis* in experimental and human trachoma. *Curr. Eye Res.* **11**:279–283.

63. **Hyman, C. L., M. H. Augenbraun, P. M. Roblin, J. Schachter, and M. R. Hammerschlag.** 1991. Asymptomatic respiratory tract infection with *Chlamydia pneumoniae* TWAR. *J. Clin. Microbiol.* **29**:2082–2083.

64. **Hyman, C. L., P. M. Roblin, C. A. Gaydos, T. C. Quinn, J. Schachter, and M. R. Hammerschlag.** 1995. Prevalence of asymptomatic nasopharyngeal carriage of *Chlamydia pneumoniae* in subjectively healthy adults: assessment by polymerase chain reaction-enzyme immunoassay and culture. *Clin. Infect. Dis.* **20**:1174–1178.

65. **Ingalls, R. R., P. A. Rice, N. Qureshi, K. Takayama, J. Shin Lin, and D. T. Golenbock.** 1995. The inflammatory cytokine response to *Chlamydia trachomatis* infection is endotoxin mediated. *Infect. Immun.* **63**:3125–3130.

66. **Johnson, F. W. A., and D. Hobson.** 1977. The effect of penicillin on genital strains of *Chlamydia trachomatis* in tissue culture. *J. Antimicrob. Chemother.* **3**:49–56.

67. **Joseph, T. D., and S. K. Bose.** 1991. A heat-labile protein of Chlamydia trachomatis binds to HeLa cells and inhibits the adherence of chlamydiae. *Proc. Natl. Acad. Sci. USA* **88**:4054–4058.

68. **Joseph, T. D., and S. K. Bose.** 1991. Further characterization of an outer membrane protein of

Chlamydia trachomatis with cytadherence properties. *FEMS Microbiol. Lett.* **68:**167–171.

69. **Kalayoglu, M. V., and G. I. Byrne.** 1998. Induction of macrophage foam cell formation by *Chlamydia pneumoniae. J. Infect. Dis.* **177:**725–729.

70. **Kane, C. D., R. M. Vena, S. P. Ouelette, and G. I. Byrne.** 1999. Intracellular tryptophan pool sizes may account for differences in gamma interferon-mediated inhibition and persistence of chlamydial growth in polarized and nonpolarized cells. *Infect. Immun.* **67:**1666–1671.

71. **Katz, B. P., D. Fortenberry, and D. Orr.** 1998. Factors affecting chlamydial persistence or recurrence one and three months after treatment, p. 35–38. *In* R. S. Stephens, G. I. Byrne, G. Christiansen, I. N. Clarke, J. T. Grayston, R. G. Rank, G. L. Ridgway, P. Saikku, J. Schachter, and W. E. Stamm (ed.), *Chlamydial Infections. Proceedings of the Ninth International Symposium on Human Chlamydial Infection.* Napa, Calif.

72. **Kaukoranta-Tolvanen, S. S., T. Ronni, M. Leinonen, P. Saikku, and K. Laitinen.** 1996. Expression of adhesion molecules on endothelial cells stimulated by *Chlamydia pneumoniae. Microb. Pathog.* **21:**407–411.

73. **Kaukoranta-Tolvanen, S. S., A. M. Teppo, K. Laitinen, P. Saikku, K. Linnavuori, and M. Leinonen.** 1996. Growth of *Chlamydia pneumoniae* in cultured peripheral blood mononuclear cells and induction of a cytokine response. *Microb. Pathog.* **21:**215–221.

74. **Kern, D. G., M. A. Neill, and J. Schachter.** 1993. A seroepidemiologic study of *Chlamydia pneumoniae* in Rhode Island. Evidence of serologic cross-reactivity. *Chest* **104:**208–213.

75. **Kiviat, N. B., P. Wolner-Hanssen, M. Peterson, J. Wasserheit, W. E. Stamm, D. A. Eschenbach, J. Paavonen, J. Lingenfelter, T. Bell, V. Zabriskie, B. Kirby, and K. K. Holmes.** 1986. Localization of *Chlamydia trachomatis* infection by direct immunofluorescence and culture in pelvic inflammatory disease. *Am. J. Obstet. Gynecol.* **154:**865–873.

76. **Koehler, L., E. Nettelnbreker, A. P. Hudson, N. Ott, H. C. Cerard, P. J. Branigan, H. R. Schumacher, W. Drommer, and H. Zeidler.** 1997. Ultrastructural and molecular analyses of the persistence of *Chlamydia trachomatis* (serovar K) in human monocytes. *Microb. Pathog.* **22:**133–142.

77. **Kordova, N., J. C. Wilt, and M. Sadiq.** 1971. Lysosomes in L cells infected with *Chlamydia psittaci* strain 6BC. *Can. J. Microbiol.* **17:**955–959.

78. **Kotake, S., H. R. Schumacher, and R. L. Wilder.** 1996. A simple nested RT-PCR method for quantitation of the relative amounts of multiple cytokine mRNAs in small tissue samples. *J. Immunol. Methods* **199:**193–203.

79. **Kramer, M. J., and F. B. Gordon.** 1971. Ultrastructural analysis of the effects of penicillin and chlortetracycline on the development of a genital tract. *Chlamydia. Infect. Immun.* **3:**333–341.

80. **Kuo, C. C., A. S. Coulson, L. A. Campbell, A. L. Cappuccio, R. D. Lawrence, and S. P. Wang.** 1997. Detection of *Chlamydia pneumoniae* in atherosclerotic plaques in the walls of arteries of lower extremities from patients undergoing bypass operation for arterial obstruction. *J. Vasc. Surg.* **26:**29–31.

81. **Kuo, C. C., A. M. Gown, E. P. Benditt, and J. T. Grayston.** 1992. Detection of *Chlamydia pneumoniae* in aortic lesions of atherosclerosis by immunocytochemical stain. *Arterioscler. Thromb.* **13:**1501–1504.

82. **Kuo, C. C., A. Shor, L. A. Campbell, H. Fukushi, D. L. Patton, and J. T. Grayston.** 1993. Demonstration of *Chlamydia pneumoniae* in atherosclerotic lesions of coronary arteries. *J. Infect. Dis.* **167:**841–849.

83. **Kutlin, A., P. M. Roblin, and M. R. Hammerschlag.** 1999. In vitro activities of azithromycin and ofloxacin against *Chlamydia pneumoniae* in a continuous-infection model. *Antimicrob. Agents Chemother.* **43:**2268–2272.

84. **Laitinen, K., A. L. Laurila, M. Leinonen, and P. Saikku.** 1996. Reactivation of *Chlamydia pneumoniae* infection in mice by cortisone treatment. *Infect. Immun.* **64:**1488–1490.

85. **Lampe, M. F., R. J. Suchland, and W. E. Stamm.** 1993. Nucleotide sequence of the variable domains within the major outer membrane protein gene from serovariants of *Chlamydia trachomatis. Infect. Immun.* **61:**213–219.

86. **Lin, J.-S. L., P. Donegan, T. C. Heeren, M. Greenberg, E. E. Flaherty, R. Haivanis, X.-H. Su, D. Dean, W. J. Newhall, J. S. Knapp, S. K. Sarafian, R. J. Rice, S. A. Morse, and P. A. Rice.** 1998. Transmission of *Chlamydia trachomatis* and *Neisseria gonorrhoeae* among men with urethritis and their female sex partners. *J. Infect. Dis.* **178:**1707–1712.

87. **Maass, M., C. Bartels, P. M. Engel, U. Mamat, and H. H. Sievers.** 1998. Endovascular presence of viable *Chlamydia pneumoniae* is a common phenomenon in coronary artery disease. *J. Am. Coll. Cardiol.* **31:**827–832.

88. **Mabey, D. C. W., M. E. Ward, and J. N. Robertson.** 1987. Detection of *Chlamydia trachomatis* by enzyme immunoassay in patients with trachoma. *Lancet* **2:**1491–1492.

89. **Malinverni, R., C. C. Kuo, L. A. Campbell, and J. T. Grayston.** 1995. Reactivation of *Chlamydia pneumoniae* infection in mice by cortisone treatment. *J. Infect. Dis.* **172:**593–594.

90. **Manire, G. P., and A. Tamura.** 1967. Preparation and chemical composition of the cell walls of mature infectious dense forms of meningopneumonitis organisms. *J. Bacteriol.* **94:** 1178–1183.

91. **Manor, E., and I. Sarov.** 1986. Fate of *Chlamydia trachomatis* in human monocytes and monocyte-derived macrophages. *Infect. Immun.* **54:**90–95.

92. **Matsumoto, A., and G. P. Manire.** 1970. Electron microscopic observations on the effects of penicillin on the morphology of *Chlamydia psittaci.* *J. Bacteriol.* 101:278–285.

93. **Megram, D. W., H. G. Stiver, and W. R. Bowie.** 1985. Complement activation and stimulation of chemotoxin by *Chlamydia trachomatis.* *Infect. Immun.* **49:**670–673.

94. **Meyer, K. F.** 1967. The host spectrum of psittacosis-lymphogranuloma venereum (PL) agents. *Am. J. Ophthalmol.* 63:1225–1246.

95. **Meyer, K. F., and B. Eddie.** 1933. Latent psittacosis infections in shell parakeets. *Proc. Exp. Biol. Med.* **30:**484–488.

96. **Meyer, K. F., and B. Eddie.** 1933. Latent psittacosis infections in mice. *Proc. Soc. Exp. Biol. Med.* 30:483–484.

97. **Moazed, T. C., C. C. Kuo, J. T. Grayston, and L. A. Campbell.** 1998. Systemic dissemination of *Chlamydia pneumoniae* infection via macrophages. *J. Infect. Dis.* **177:**132–135.

98. **Molestina, R. E., D. Dean, J. A. Ramirez, and J. T. Summersgill.** 1998. Characterization of a strain of *Chlamydia pneumoniae* isolated from a coronary atheroma by analysis of the *omp1* gene and biological activity in human endothelial cells. *Infect. Immun.* **66:**1360–1376.

99. **Morrison, R. P., H. Su, K. Lyng, and Y. Yuan.** 1990. The *Chlamydia trachomatis hyp* operon is homologous to the *groEL* stress response of *Escherichia coli.* *Infect. Immun.* **58:**2701–2705.

100. **Moulder, J. W.** 1991. Interaction of chlamydiae and host cells in vitro. *Microbiol. Rev.* **55:** 143–190.

101. **Moulder, J. W., N. J. Levy, and L. P. Schulman.** 1980. Persistent infection of mouse fibroblasts (L cells) with *Chlamydia psittaci:* evidence for a cryptic chlamydial form. *Infect. Immun.* **30:** 874–883.

102. **Muhlestein, J. B., J. L. Anderson, E. H. Hammond, L. Zhao, S. Trehan, E. P. Schwobe, and J. F. Carlquist.** 1998. Infection with *Chlamydia pneumoniae* accelerates the development of atherosclerosis and treatment with azithromycin prevents it in a rabbit model. *Circulation* **97:**633–636.

103. **Mullock, B. M., W. J. Branch, M. van Schaik, L. K. Gilbert, and J. P. Luzio.** 1989. Reconstitution of an endosome-lysosome interaction in a cell-free system. *J. Cell Biol.* **108:** 2093–2099.

104. **Mullock, B. M., J. H. Perez, T. Kuwana, S. R. Gray, and J. P. Luzio.** 1994. Lysosomes can fuse with a late endosomal compartment in a cell-free system from rat liver. *J. Cell Biol.* **126:** 1173–1182.

105. **Nanagara, R., L. Feng, A. Beutler, A. P. Hudson, and H. R. Schumacher.** 1995. Alteration of *Chlamydia trachomatis* biologic behavior in synovial membranes. *Arthritis Rheum.* **38:** 1410–1417.

106. **Ojcius, D. M., Y. Bravo de Alba, J. M. Kanellopoulos, R. A. Hawkins, K. A. Kelly, R. G. Rank, and A. Dautry-Vaarsat.** 1998. Internalization of *Chlamydia* by dendritic cells and stimulation of *Chlamydia*-specific T cells. *J. Immunol.* **160:**1297–1303.

107. **Ojcius, D. M., P. Souque, J.-L. Perfettini, and A. Dautry-Varsat.** 1998. Apoptosis of epithelial cells and macrophages due to infection with the obligate intracellular pathogen *Chlamydia psittaci.* *J. Immunol.* **161:**4220–4226.

108. **Ozanne, G., and J. Lefebvre.** 1992. Specificity of the microimmunofluorescence assay for the serodiagnosis of *Chlamydia pneumoniae* infections. *Can. J. Microbiol.* **38:**1185–1189.

109. **Patton, D. L., M. Askienazy-Elbhar, J. Henry-Suchet, L. A. Campbell, A. Cappuccio, W. Tannous, S. P. Wang, and C. C. Kuo.** 1994. Detection of *Chlamydia trachomatis* in fallopian tube tissue in women with postinfectious tubal infertility. *Am. J. Obstet. Gynecol.* **171:** 95–101.

110. **Patton, D. L., Y. C. Sweeney, N. J. Bohannon, A. M. Clark, J. P. Hughes, A. Cappuccio, L. A. Campbell, and W. E. Stamm.** 1997. Effects of doxycycline and antiinflammatory agents on experimentally induced chlamydial upper genital tract infection in female macaques. *J. Infect. Dis.* **175:**648–654.

111. **Peterson, E. M., X. Cheng, Z. Qu, and L. M. de la Maza.** 1996. Characterization of the murine antibody response to peptides representing the variable domains of the major outer membrane protein of *Chlamydia pneumoniae.* *Infect. Immun.* **64:**3354–3359.

112. **Peterson, E. M., B. A. Markoff, and L. M. de la Maza.** 1990. The major outer membrane protein nucleotide sequence of *Chlamydia trachomatis,* serovar E. *Nucleic Acids Res.* **18:**3414.

113. **Picket, M. A., M. E. Ward, and I. N. Clarke.** 1987. Complete nucleotide sequence of the major outer membrane protein gene from *Chlamydia trachomatis* serovar L₁. *FEMS Microbiol. Lett.* **42:**185–190.

114. **Pollard, M., and N. Sharon.** 1963. Induction of prolonged latency in psittacosis infected cells by aminopterin. *Proc. Soc. Exp. Biol. Med.* **112:** 51–54.

115. **Rahman, M. U., M. A., Cheema, H. R. Schumacher, and A. P. Hudson.** 1992. Molecular evidence for the presence of chlamydia in the synovium of patients with Reiter's syndrome. *Arthritis Rheum.* **35:**521–529.

116. **Ramirez, J. A.** 1996. Isolation of *Chlamydia pneumoniae* from the coronary artery of a patient with coronary atherosclerosis. The *Chlamydia pneumoniae*/atherosclerosis Study Group. *Ann. Intern. Med.* **125:**979–982.

117. **Rapoza, P. A., S. G. Tahija, J. M. Carlin, S. L. Miller, M. L. Padilla, and G. I. Byrne.** 1991. Effect of interferon on a primary conjunctival epithelial cell model of trachoma. *Investig. Ophthalmol. Vis. Sci.* **32:**2919–2923.

118. **Rasmussen, S. J., L. Eckmann, A. J. Quayle, L. Shen, Y.-X. Zhang, D. J. Anderson, J. Fierer, R. S. Stephens, and M. F. Kagnoff.** 1997. Secretion of proinflammatory cytokines by epithelial cells in response to chlamydia infection suggests a central role for epithelial cells in chlamydial pathogenesis. *J. Clin. Investig.* **99:**77–87.

119. **Rasmussen, S. J., P. Timms, P. R. Beatty, and R. S. Stephens.** 1996. Cytotoxic-T-lymphocyte-mediated cytolysis of L cells persistently infected with *Chlamydia* spp. *Infect Immun.* **64:** 1944–1949.

120. **Raulston, J. E., C. H. Davis, D. H. Schmiel, M. W. Morgan, and P. B. Wyrick.** 1993. Molecular characterization and outer membrane association of a *Chlamydia trachomatis* protein related to the hsp70 family of proteins. *J. Biol. Chem.* **268:**23139–23147.

121. **Rockey, D. D., D. Grosenbach, D. E. Hruby, M. G. Peacock, R. A. Heinzen, and T. Hackstadt.** 1997. *Chlamydia psittaci* IncA is phosphorylated by the host cell and is exposed on the cytoplasmic face of the developing inclusion. *Mol. Microbiol.* **24:**217–228.

122. **Rockey, D. D., R. A. Heinzen, and T. Hackstadt.** 1995. Cloning and characterization of a *Chlamydia psittaci* gene coding for a protein localized in the inclusion membrane of infected cells. *Mol. Microbiol.* **15:**617–626.

123. **Rothermel, C. D., J. Schachter, P. Lavrich, E. C. Lipsitz, and T. Francus.** 1989. *Chlamydia trachomatis* induced production of interleukin-1 by human monocytes. *Infect. Immun.* **57:** 2705–2711.

124. **Rothman, J. E., and F. T. Wieland.** 1996. Protein sorting by transport vesicles. *Science* **272:** 227–234.

125. **Saikku, P., M. Leinonen, L. Tenkanen, E.** Linnanmaki, M. R. Ekman, V. Manninen, M. Manttari, M. H. Frick, and J. K. Huttunen. 1992. Chronic *Chlamydia pneumoniae* infection as a risk factor for coronary heart disease in the Helsinki Heart Study. *Ann. Intern. Med.* **116:** 273–278.

126. **Sardinia, L. M., E. Segal, and D. Ganem.** 1988. Developmental regulation of the cysteine-rich outer membrane proteins of murine *Chlamydia trachomatis*. *J. Gen. Microbiol.* **134:** 997–1004.

127. **Schachter, J.** 1978. Chlamydial infections. *N. Engl. J. Med.* **298:**428–435.

128. **Schachter, J., M. Grossman, R. T. Sweet, J. Halt, C. Jordan, and E. Bishop.** 1986. Prospective study of perinatal transmission of *Chlamydia trachomatis*. *JAMA* **225:**3374–3377.

129. **Schmiel, D. H., S. T. Knight, J. E. Raulston, J. Choong, C. H. Davis, and P. B. Wyrick.** 1991. Recombinant *Escherichia coli* clones expressing *Chlamydia trachomatis* gene products attach to human endometrial epithelial cells. *Infect. Immun.* **59:**4001–4012.

130. **Schmitz, E., E. Nettelnbreker, H. Zeidler, M. Hammer, E. Manor, and J. Wollenhaupt.** 1993. Intracellular persistence of chlamydial major outer membrane protein, lipopolysaccharide and rRNA after non-productive infection of human monocytes with *Chlamydia trachomatis* serovar K. *J. Med. Microbiol.* **38:** 278–285.

131. **Scholes, D., A. Stergachis, F. E. Heidrich, H. Andrilla, K. K. Holmes, and W. E. Stamm.** 1996. Prevention of pelvic inflammatory disease by screening for cervical chlamydial infection. *N. Engl. J. Med.* **334:**1362–1366.

132. **Schramm, N., C. R. Bagnell, and P. B. Wyrick.** 1996. Vesicles containing *Chlamydia trachomatis* serovar L2 remain above pH 6 within HEC-1B cells. *Infect. Immun.* **64:**1208–1214.

133. **Scidmore, M. A., D. D. Rockey, E. R. Fischer, R. A. Heinzen, and T. Hackstadt.** 1996. Vesicular interactions of the *Chlamydia trachomatis* inclusion are determined by chlamydial early protein synthesis rather than route of entry. *Infect. Immun.* **64:**5366–5372.

134. **Scidmore-Carlson, M., E. I. Shaw, C. A. Dooley, and T. Hackstadt.** 1997. Identification and characterization of putative *Chlamydia trachomatis* inclusion membrane proteins, p. 103–106. *In* R. S. Stephens, G. I. Byrne, G. Christiansen, I. N. Clarke, J. T. Grayston, R. G. Rank, G. L. Ridgway, P. Saikku, J. Schachter, and W. E. Stamm (ed.), *Chlamydial Infections*. Laboratory of Intracellular Parasites, Rocky Mountain Laboratories, National Institute of Al-

lergy and Infectious Diseases, National Institutes of Health, Hamilton, Mont.

135. **Shemer, Y., and I. Sarov.** 1985. Inhibition of growth of *Chlamydia trachomatis* by human gamma interferon. *Infect. Immun.* **48:**592–596.

136. **Shemer-Avni, Y., D. Wallach, and I. Sarov.** 1988. Inhibition of *Chlamydia trachomatis* growth by recombinant tumor necrosis factor. *Infect. Immun.* **56:**2503–2506.

137. **Shewen, P. E.** 1980. Chlamydial infection in animals: a review. *Can. Vet. J.* **21:**2–11.

138. **Shor, A., C. C. Kuo, and D. L. Patton.** 1992. Detection of *Chlamydia pneumoniae* in coronary arterial fatty streaks and atheromatous plaques. *S. Afr. Med. J.* **82:**158–161.

139. **Smith, C. B., W. J. Friedewald, and R. M. Chanock.** 1967. Shedding of *Mycoplasma pneumoniae* after tetracycline and erythromycin therapy. *N. Engl. J. Med.* **276:**1172–1175.

140. **Soderlund, G., C. Dahlgren, and E. Kihlstrom.** 1984. Interaction between polymorphonuclear leukocytes and *Chlamydia trachomatis*. *FEMS Microbiol. Lett.* **22:**21–25.

141. **Soong, Y. K., S. M. Kao, C. J. Lee, P. S. Lee, and C. C. Pao.** 1990. Endocervical chlamydial deoxyribonucleic acid in infertile women. *Fertil. Steril.* **54:**815–818.

142. **Stagg, A. J., W. A. Elsley, M. A. Pickett, M. E. Ward, and S. C. Knight.** 1993. Primary human T-cell responses to the major outer membrane protein of *Chlamydia trachomatis*. *Immunology* **79:**1–9.

143. **Stephens, R. S.** 1992. Challenge of chlamydia research. *Infect. Agents Dis.* **1:**279–293.

144. **Stephens, R. S., S. Kalman, C. Lammel, J. Fan, R. Marathe, L. Aravind, W. Mitchell, L. Olinger, R. L. Tatusov, J. Qixun, E. V. Koonin, and R. W. Davis.** 1998. Genome sequence of an obligate intracellular pathogen of humans: *Chlamydia trachomatis*. *Science* **282:**754–759.

145. **Stirling, P., I. Allan, and J. H. Pearce.** 1983. Interference with transformation of chlamydiae from reproductive to infected body forms by deprivation of cysteine. *FEMS Microbiol. Lett.* **19:**133–136.

146. **Su, H., R. Messer, W. Whitmore, E. Fischer, J. C. Portis, and H. D. Caldwell.** 1998. Vaccination against chlamydial genital tract infection after immunization with dendritic cells pulsed ex vivo with nonviable chlamydiae. *J. Exp. Med.* **188:**809–818.

147. **Su, H., N. G. Watkins, Y. X. Zhang, and H. D. Caldwell.** 1990. *Chlamydia trachomatis*-host cell interactions: role of the chlamydial major outer membrane protein as an adhesin. *Infect. Immun.* **58:**1017–1025.

148. **Su, H., Y. X. Zhang, O. Barrera, N. G. Watkins, and H. D. Caldwell.** 1988. Differential effect of trypsin on infectivity of *Chlamydia trachomatis*: loss of infectivity requires cleavage of major outer membrane protein variable domains II and IV. *Infect. Immun.* **56:**2094–2100.

149. **Swanson, A. F., and C. C. Kuo.** 1994. Binding of the glycan of the major outer membrane protein of *Chlamydia trachomatis* to HeLa cells. *Infect. Immun.* **62:**24–28.

150. **Tamura, A., and G. P. Manire.** 1968. Effect of penicillin on the multiplication of meningopneumonitis organisms (*Chlamydia psittaci*). *J. Bacteriol.* **96:**875–880.

151. **Taraska, T., D. M. Ward, R. S. Ajioka, P. B. Wyrick, S. R. Davis-Kaplan, C. H. Davis, and J. Kaplan.** 1996. The late chlamydial inclusion membrane is not derived from the endocytic pathway and is relatively deficient in host proteins. *Infect. Immun.* **64:**3713–3727.

152. **Thejis, H., J. Gnarpe, O. Lundkvist, G. Heimer, G. Larsson, and A. Victor.** 1991. Diagnosis and prevalence of persistent chlamydia infection in infertile women: tissue culture, direct antigen detection, and serology. *Fertil. Steril.* **55:**304–310.

153. **Ting, L.-M., R.-C. Hsia, C. G. Haidaris, and P. M. Bavoil.** 1995. Interaction of outer envelope proteins of *Chlamydia psittaci* GPIC with the HeLa cell surface. *Infect. Immun.* **63:**3600–3608.

154. **Todd, W. J., and J. Storz.** 1975. Ultrastructural cytochemical evidence for the activation of lysosomes in the cytocidal effect of *Chlamydia psittaci*. *Infect. Immun.* **12:**638–646.

155. **von Hertzen, L., R. Isoaho, M. Leinonen, R. Koskinen, P. Laippala, M. Toyryla, S. L. Kivela, and P. Saikku.** 1996. *Chlamydia pneumoniae* antibodies in chronic obstructive pulmonary disease. *Int. J. Epidemiol.* **25:**658–664.

156. **Watson, M. W., P. R. Lambden, J. S. Everson, and J. N. Clarke.** 1994. Immunoreactivity of the 60 kDa cysteine-rich proteins of Chlamydia trachomatis, Chlamydia psittaci, and Chlamydia pneumoniae expressed in Escherichia coli. *Microbiology* **140:**2003–2011.

157. **Weiss, S. M., P. M. Roblin, C. A. Gaydos, P. Cummings, D. L. Patton, N. Schulhoff, J. Shani, R. Frankel, K. Penney, T. C. Quinn, M. R. Hammerschlag, and J. Schachter.** 1996. Failure to detect Chlamydia pneumoniae in coronary atheromas of patients undergoing atherectomy. *J. Infect. Dis.* **173:**957–962.

158. **Williams, D. M., D. M. Magee, L. F. Bonewald, J. G. Smith, C. A. Bleicker, G. I. Byrne, and J. Schachter.** 1990. A role in vivo

for tumor necrosis factor alpha in host defense against *Chlamydia trachomatis*. *Infect. Immun.* **58:** 1572–1576.

159. **Workowski, K. A., M. F. Lampe, K. G. Wong, M. B. Watts, and W. E. Stamm.** 1993. Long-term eradication of *Chlamydia trachomatis* genital infection after antimicrobial therapy. Evidence against persistent infection. *JAMA* **270:**2071–2075. (Erratum, **271:**348, 1994).

160. **Wylie, J. L., G. M. Hatch, and G. McClarty.** 1997. Host cell phospholipids are trafficked to and then modified by *Chlamydia trachomatis*. *J. Bacteriol.* **179:**7233–7242.

161. **Wyrick, P. B., and E. A. Brownridge.** 1978. Growth of *Chlamydia psittaci* in macrophages. *Infect. Immun.* **19:**1054–1060.

162. **Wyrick, P. B., S. T. Knight, T. R. Paul, R. G. Rank, and C. S. Barbier.** 1999. Persistent chlamydial envelope antigens in antibiotic-exposed infected cells trigger neutrophil chemotaxis. *J. Infect. Dis.* **179:**954–966.

163. **Yamazaki, T., H. Nakada, N. Sakurai, C. C. Kuo, S. P. Wang, and J. T. Grayston.** 1990. Transmission of *Chlamydia pneumoniae* in young children in a Japanese family. *J. Infect. Dis.* **162:**1390–1392.

164. **Yong, E. C., E. Y. Chi, and C. C. Kuo.** 1987. Differential antimicrobial activity of human mononuclear phagocytes against the human bio-vars of *Chlamydia trachomatis*. *J. Immunol.* **139:** 1297–1302.

165. **Yong, E. C., S. J. Klebanoff, and C. C. Kuo.** 1982. Toxic effect of human polymorphonuclear leukocytes and *Chlamydia trachomatis*. *Infect. Immun.* **57:**422–426.

166. **Zeichner, S. L.** 1983. Isolation and characterization of macrophage phagosomes containing infectious and heat-inactivated *Chlamydia psittaci*: two phagosomes with different intracellular behavior. *Infect. Immun.* **40:**956–966.

167. **Zhang, J. P., and R. S. Stephens.** 1992. Mechanism of *Chlamydia trachomatis* attachment to eukaryotic host cells. *Cell* **69:**861–869.

168. **Zhang, Y. X., S. G. Morrison, and H. D. Caldwell.** 1990. The nucleotide sequence of the major outer membrane protein gene of *Chlamydia trachomatis* serovar F. *Nucleic Acids Res.* **18:** 1061.

169. **Zhang, Y. X., S. Stewart, T. Joseph, H. R. Taylor, and H. D. Caldwell.** 1987. Protective monoclonal antibodies recognize epitopes located on the major outer membrane protein of *Chlamydia trachomatis*. *J. Immunol.* **138:**575–581.

170. **Zvillich, M., and I. Sarov.** 1985. Interaction between human polymorphonuclear leukocytes and *Chlamydia trachomatis* elementary bodies: electron microscopy and chemiluminescent response. *J. Gen. Microbiol.* **131:**2627–2635.

HELICOBACTER PYLORI

Andre Dubois, Anthony Welch, Douglas E. Berg,
and Martin J. Blaser

13

Helicobacter pylori is extraordinary among bacteria in its ability to colonize the stomachs of more than half of all people worldwide and often to persist for years or decades once it has become established (100). This persistence entails bacterial growth on the surfaces of gastric epithelial cells, in the overlying mucin, and perhaps within certain epithelial cells as well. The gastric mucosa, like other mucosal tissues, is constantly turning over, with a half-life typically of only a few days. Thus, *H. pylori* cannot simply elude the host in a quiescent state, as is the case with persistent infections by certain pathogens, such as *Mycobacterium tuberculosis* (see chapter 16). This active *H. pylori* growth, which we postulate is essential for its persistence, occurs despite important host defenses, including gastric acidity, peristalsis, epithelial cell turnover, and immune and inflammatory responses. In fact, persistence might even depend on a moderate inflammatory response, because the collateral host cell injury such responses also elicit releases cellular macromolecules and metabolites that *H. pylori* may utilize as nutrients for growth. In contrast, excessive inflammation may well eradicate *H. pylori*, either by direct killing of the bacterium or by destruction of the normal gastric epithelial tissue milieu upon which it depends for survival. Thus, success in persistent colonization may depend on a proper balance between inciting and downregulating host responses (13).

No other bacterial species except the closely related *Helicobacter heilmannii* and *Helicobacter bizzozeronii* colonizes healthy human gastric mucosa. Only when the capacity for gastric acid secretion is impaired (which can occur transiently or permanently in some *H. pylori*-colonized persons) will other bacteria colonize the stomach. Conversely, *H. pylori* is thought not to colonize other sites in the human body, except when developmental changes (some of which it may help trigger) result in gastric-type epithelial cells in the esophagus or duodenum. There is evidence from PCR that *H. pylori* strains may also colonize certain microaerobic sites in the mouth, although to our knowledge attempts to culture the bacterium from these sites have not been successful. *H. pylori* appears

Andre Dubois, Laboratory of Gastrointestinal and Liver Studies, Digestive Diseases Division, Department of Medicine, Uniformed Services University of the Health Sciences, Bethesda, Md. *Anthony Welch*, Laboratory of Gastrointestinal and Liver Studies, Digestive Diseases Division, Department of Medicine, Uniformed Services University of the Health Sciences, Bethesda, and Bioqual Inc., Rockville, Md. *Douglas E. Berg*, Departments of Molecular Microbiology and of Genetics, Washington University Medical School, St. Louis, Mo. *Martin J. Blaser*, Departments of Medicine and Microbiology, New York University School of Medicine, and New York Harbor VA Medical Center, New York, N.Y.

Persistent Bacterial Infections, Edited by J. P. Nataro, M. J. Blaser, and
S. Cunningham-Rundles, © 2000 ASM Press, Washington, D.C.

to be quite specific for humans, nonhuman primates (36), and cats (53), although certain strains that can colonize a few other mammalian species have been found in the search for convenient animal infection models. Other gastric *Helicobacter* species also have been found, each in a number of different mammalian species. Thus, persistent gastric colonization by members of this genus seems to be widespread, although the human-*H. pylori* association has received by far the most attention.

Much of the research on *H. pylori*, with the issue of persistence as a major focus, is driven by the importance of the bacterium as a human pathogen: persistent (decades-long) colonization by this microbe is an important risk factor for gastric and duodenal ulcers; an early risk factor for gastric adenocarcinoma, one of the most frequently lethal malignancies worldwide; and also a risk factor for the less common and developmentally different MALT lymphomas. Yet a majority of *H. pylori*-positive persons are completely asymptomatic, and it has been proposed that its colonization of the stomach may actually be beneficial (11). Just which bacterial, host, and environmental factors collectively determine these varied clinical outcomes is beginning to be understood.

Not all *H. pylori* colonizations persist for decades, however, and some are actually quite transient, lasting for only 1 or 2 weeks at most (see below). In interpreting this phenomenon, we believe it is important to note at the outset that *H. pylori* is an extremely diverse species genetically and that we humans may be equivalently diverse in traits that could be important to individual strains: a reflection of our own genetics and physiology, the specificity and potency of our immune and inflammatory responses, and the environments in which we live. It is our thesis that some of the phenotypic diversity of *H. pylori* has been selected for by our human diversity and that only a subset of *H. pylori* strains may be able to colonize any given human host. All clinical isolates, however, represent relatively successful end products of many years (perhaps millions) of bacterium-host evolution, and those strains that would not be successful in colonizing one individual host should be relatively well adapted to others in the same community. Exactly how various *H. pylori* strains cope with, and indeed probably exploit, distinctive features and responses of different hosts for long and balanced life in the potentially hostile gastric mucosa is most intriguing. No less important is an understanding of events or factors that underlie those cases in which *H. pylori* fails to achieve or maintain colonization. Understanding these issues should be beneficial to medicine, in terms of development of drugs and vaccines that will more efficiently eradicate *H. pylori* when warranted, and possibly also in mimicking some of the potentially or putatively beneficial effects of certain colonizations (in terms of suppression of gastroesophageal reflux disease or lowered risk of esophageal cancer) when appropriate.

EPIDEMIOLOGY

There is a pressing need to better understand how *H. pylori* is transmitted and maintained within at-risk populations and what the risk factors for colonization are. This is complicated by the fact that most colonizations are not immediately clinically apparent or even sufficient for investigation. Typically only after decades of chronic carriage are patients likely to develop symptoms sufficient to warrant tests for *H. pylori* carriage. *H. pylori* can be detected and analyzed by a variety of different methods, as described under "Diagnostic Methods" below.

Seroepidemiological studies performed in the United States and abroad have demonstrated the worldwide presence of *H. pylori* in a large majority of individuals from low socioeconomic groups and also in many people of higher socioeconomic status (100). There is a high frequency of seropositivity in many developing countries, including those of Eastern Europe (up to 100% in some age groups). The acquisition of the organisms during infancy is characteristic of groups living in crowded or poor hygienic conditions, and it appears to be independent of gender and ethnic origin. In adults of higher socioeconomic groups, the rate of seroconversion is estimated to be about

0.5%/year, and the prevalence of seropositivity increases with age to eventually reach 40% or more. The increase in frequency of positivity with age might be due to years of low but cumulative risk of acquisition and/or to a higher rate of *H. pylori* acquisition in Western countries in past years than during recent years, representing a cohort effect (25).

Although the exact route of transmission of *H. pylori* is not known, it appears to be preferentially intrafamilial in industrialized countries (31). In addition, direct contact and/or consumption of food or water (64) contaminated by saliva (48), gastric contents, or feces (101) may be a major factor. The recent observation that *H. pylori* can be isolated from cats (53) and that cats can be colonized by *H. pylori* following inoculation (94) suggests that transmission from pets to humans (or humans to pets) is also possible.

PATHOGENICITY AND CLINICAL ASSOCIATIONS

H. pylori has generally been considered a pathogen because (i) its presence is always associated with chronic active gastritis and (ii) eradication of the bacterium is always followed by resolution of the gastritis. However, the vast majority of persons carrying *H. pylori* do not report any related clinical symptoms, and it has been argued that inflammation of the stomach mucosa is a "normal" event (10), by analogy with the bacterial colonization and the associated tissue infiltration by inflammatory cells of the small intestine and colon. Nonetheless, the fact that nearly all patients with duodenal ulcer disease have *H. pylori* gastritis and that ulcer relapse after *H. pylori* eradication is exceptional indicates that *H. pylori* plays a permissive role, although other factors must also be involved (68). Therefore, when disease occurs, it is probably because of colonization by particularly virulent strains and/or because yet undefined host or environmental (e.g., dietary) cofactors exacerbate normally benign conditions.

Persons carrying *H. pylori* also have an increased risk of developing both intestinal-type and diffuse-type noncardia gastric adenocarci-

noma (3, 85, 88). In addition, the association of *H. pylori* with either gastric ulcer or gastric cancer may be underestimated in these studies. The atrophic gastritis that may follow long-term carriage makes the gastric niche less hospitable for *H. pylori*, which may cause its elimination or suppression. Nevertheless, atrophic gastritis per se is believed to be a precancerous lesion that may lead to carcinogenesis without the need for the continued presence of *H. pylori*. In total, it has become clear that the carriage of *H. pylori* increases the risk for gastric and duodenal ulcers, noncardia gastric adenocarcinoma, and non-Hodgkin's gastric lymphoma compared to that for noncarriers. Conversely, epidemiological evidence is emerging that carriage of *H. pylori* decreases the risk for gastroesophageal reflux disease, Barrett's esophagus, and adenocarcinoma of the distal esophagus and proximal stomach (cardia) (11). Thus, the overall assessment of whether *H. pylori* is chiefly a pathogen or a symbiont may depend on the particular context.

DIAGNOSTIC METHODS

The presence of *H. pylori* can be diagnosed from gastric-biopsy specimens harvested at endoscopy. Histology can demonstrate the presence of *H. pylori* in close proximity to surface epithelial cells, especially if Gram or silver (Warthin-Starry) stains are used. The combination of hematoxylin and eosin, silver, and Alcian blue stains (Genta-Robason stain) on the same histologic section is also very useful, as it allows the concurrent visualization of *H. pylori* (silver stained), mono- and polynuclear infiltration (hematoxylin and eosin) and, if present, intestinal metaplasia (Alcian blue positive) (51). In *H. pylori*-positive subjects, culture of biopsies under microaerobic conditions (90% N_2, 5% O_2, and 5% CO_2) for up to 7 days can produce "water spray" colonies that are urease, catalase, and oxidase positive, and 3- to 6-μm-long gram-negative spiral or curved bacteria should be visualized by light microscopy. One advantage of this approach is that it is highly specific and it provides information on the genotype of the strain(s) that has colonized a particular individual. The PCR technique also provides such information. However, because *H. pylori* colonization is focal, negative biopsies do not exclude the possibility of colonization in areas that were not sampled.

H. pylori colonization can be diagnosed most easily and cost-effectively by determining plasma or salivary immunoglobulin G (IgG) and/or A levels using enzyme-linked immunosorbent assays (31, 90). The technique is noninvasive, specific, and sensitive and is believed to reflect the mucosal and systemic immune responses induced by *H. pylori*.

The urea breath test (UBT) also represents a noninvasive test of *H. pylori* colonization (5). It is based on the fact that *H. pylori* produces urease in sufficient amounts to digest urea introduced into the stomach. ^{14}C- or ^{13}C-urea introduced into an *H. pylori*-colonized stomach is broken down by urease, and $^{14}CO_2$ or $^{13}CO_2$ diffuses through the gastric mucosa into the bloodstream and is exhaled from the lungs within 20 min. It should be noted that the UBT is not specific for *H. pylori*, since other *Helicobacter* spp., in particular *H. heilmannii*, also synthesize urease and therefore will give a positive reaction. However, *H. heilmannii* is much less (<1%) frequent than *H. pylori* in humans (33), and the only other gastric *Helicobacter* sp. shown to colonize the human stomach (*H. bizzozeronii*) is also rare.

MECHANISM OF COLONIZATION AND PERSISTENCE

Once established, *H. pylori* may persist for decades in the stomach in a majority of the world's population (13). Following acquisition, lifelong colonization is believed to be the rule based on extrapolations from humans with well-established, long-term colonization. Those subjects often are identified during population screens or because of persistent gastroduodenal disease symptoms. However, some adults can become transiently colonized, even in the absence of antimicrobial therapy (73, 77, 78, 106). Further evidence for spontaneous clearance comes from seroepidemiological and UBT studies of children that demonstrated dramatic fluctuations over time in gastric urease levels among many children in the study group (52, 63; J. E. Thomas, personal communication). These results support the hypothesis that transient colonization is common in humans when first exposed to *H. pylori*. If persistence is not inevitable, then a better understanding of the mechanisms leading to transience would be gained by closer examination of the early stages of colonization. Unfortunately, such studies are difficult because experimental inoculation of humans with *H. pylori* is rarely done and because natural colonization by *H. pylori* is often asymptomatic, at least initially. Studies of animals could help resolve this question, although the relevance of observations in many models is limited by differences in the physiology and immune response of the host. It is possible that only studies of nonhuman primates would be immediately relevant (34).

Although the mechanisms allowing persistence of *H. pylori* are unknown, it is likely that multiple bacterial, host, and environmental factors play a role.

Bacterial Factors

When *H. pylori* enters the stomach, it must survive until it reaches its mucosal niche, despite low intragastric pH, proteolytic enzymes, and powerful peristaltic waves that grind and mix food with saliva and gastric secretions. Production of NH_4OH by *H. pylori* urease is essential for initial survival in the acidic luminal contents of the stomach, as suggested by observations that urease-negative mutants cannot colonize the stomachs of experimentally inoculated gnotobiotic pigs (38). That urease function may also be important for persistence is suggested by the observation that *Helicobacter* spp. can be eradicated from mice and ferrets following immunization of colonized animals with urease (24, 87). However, urease may not be essential for persistence in humans, since urease-negative mutants have been isolated occasionally (80, 91) and immunization with urease did not cure colonized human volunteers (75).

By the to-and-fro motion that grinds and mixes food within the stomach prior to gastric

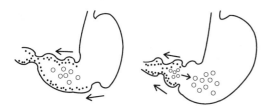

FIGURE 1 Schematic representation of the flow of particles within the stomach lumen (arrows indicate direction of peristaltic waves or flow).

emptying, small particles (among which *H. pylori* cells are presumably located) tend to accumulate near the antral mucosa (32), thereby placing *H. pylori* in close proximity to the unstirred mucus layer (Fig. 1). The bacteria can then enter the mucus layer, presumably by their flagellar movements, interact with microvilli that cover superficial epithelial cells, and attach to pedestals induced by their interaction. Extensive genetic control of flagellar synthesis and function has been described (2, 70, 102).

Epithelial cell adherence is considered important in bacterial colonization and persistence (9). In addition, oligosaccharides linked to glycoproteins and glycolipids on epithelial cell membranes are specifically recognized by bacterial adhesins. Furthermore, free oligosaccharides found in secretions, including human breast milk, have been shown to inhibit bacterial attachment to epithelial cells that line the mucous membranes (112). *H. pylori* isolates differ in the ability to adhere to gastric epithelial cells from various mammals (14, 44) or to various cell lines, such as HeLa, Hep2, and Kato cells (47, 55, 83). These various adherence properties are believed to reflect specific adhesin proteins expressed by different *H. pylori* strains under culture conditions. The three main *H. pylori* adhesins described to date are the sialyllactose adhesin *hpaA* (42), the BabA (histo-blood group antigen-binding activity) (56), and the predicted porin-like outer membrane protein encoded by the recently described *alpAB* genes (86). Host structures recognized by these adhesins include the oligosaccharide 3′-sialyllactose, NeuAcα2-3Galβ1-

4Glc (3′SL) (43), and the fucosylated histo-blood group antigens (blood group antigens H and Lewis b) of the gastric epithelial cells (14). The importance of adherence in the persistence of *H. pylori* is suggested by both mathematical modeling (12) and in vitro tests showing that the oligosaccharide 3′SL inhibited binding of *H. pylori* to various gastrointestinal epithelial cells and that *H. pylori* could be detached from these cells by 3′SL (99). In addition, 3′SL given orally to rhesus monkeys persistently colonized by *H. pylori* was able to permanently eradicate the bacterium in two of six animals (82). In this context, it is noteworthy that the major ganglioside detected by chemical analysis of human gastric mucosa is NeuAcα2-3Galβ1-4Glc-ceramide, a glycolipid that contains the same sugar structure as 3′SL (61, 96). More complex polyglycosylceramides isolated from human erythrocytes and other cells also have been identified as potent adherence receptors whose activity likewise depends upon the presence of sialic acid α2-3 linked to galactose (76).

H. pylori strains also differ in the ability to hemagglutinate reticulocytes from different sources, which probably reflects bacterial specificity for different receptors (69). Finally, *H. pylori* cells differ in length, shape, and the stage at which they convert from comma shaped to spherical, which may affect mobility in the gastric mucus and survival outside the human host (J. Lewala-Guruge and T. Wadstrom, personal communication).

Soon after *H. pylori* has become established in the unstirred mucus layer or is attached to mucosal cells, it induces immune responses that eventually could eradicate it, unless the bacterium is able to develop a protective strategy. Antigen mimicry, which utilizes the autotolerance that the host needs to survive its own immune responses, is believed to be extensively used by *H. pylori*. Lewis (Le) expression on bacterial lipopolysaccharide (LPS) is believed to represent such a mimicry. Le antigen expression by *H. pylori* isolates appears to be related to the Le phenotype of the human host from which it was isolated. Specifically, the strains isolated from Le[a] subjects predominantly express Le^x (both monofucosylated glycoconjugates), whereas Le^b subjects are colonized by strains that predominantly express Le^y (both difucosylated glycoconjugates) (110). This suggests that selection of host-adapted bacterial populations is occurring. Whether the host Le phenotype selects for particular bacterial Le phenotypes was examined prospectively following experimental *H. pylori* infection of rhesus monkeys (109). Four rhesus monkeys from whom natural *H. pylori* colonization had been eradicated 6 months earlier were inoculated with a mixture of seven human *H. pylori* isolates (35). Gastric biopsy specimens were harvested at endoscopy at regular intervals up to 10 months after inoculation and cultured. Single-colony isolates were fingerprinted by random amplified polymorphic DNA-PCR, and their Le expression was examined by enzyme-linked immunosorbent assay. Hemagglutination inhibition of Le antigens in saliva and gastric juice and immunohistochemistry of gastric biopsy specimens demonstrated that two monkeys were of the Le(a + b −) phenotype and that the two other monkeys were of the Le(a − b +) phenotype. After experimental inoculation, all four monkeys remained colonized for up to 10 months. At 1 week, the four animals harbored two to four of the seven inoculated strains (J166, J170, J238, and J258); at 14 weeks, just three strains (J166, J238, and J170) could be isolated. At 10 months, three monkeys carried a single strain (J166) whereas the fourth animal still had two strains (75% J166 and 25% J238), as determined by random amplified polymorphic DNA-PCR (35). The single strain (J166) that was dominant among the four animals at 10 months mostly expressed the Le^y phenotype at the time of inoculation, and yet it equally colonized animals that were of the Le^a or Le^b phenotype. However, the pattern of bacterial Le expression clearly became different in monkeys of different Le phenotype. *H. pylori* isolates from monkeys with an Le(a + b −) phenotype at 10 months had high Le^x-Le^y expression, whereas those from Le(a − b +)-phenotype monkeys had low Le^x-Le^y expression. These data indicate that a single strain of

H. pylori can change Le phenotype over time. The mechanism of this switching may be related to the presence of redundant fucosyltransferase genes in the *H. pylori* genome (102) as well as phase shifts due to slipped-strand DNA replication (107). In addition, it provides an example of how a clinically relevant animal model permits a prospective analysis of clinical observations.

The LPSs of gram-negative bacteria are among the dominant surface features in terms of their abilities to induce host response; this is primarily a function of their lipid A components. However, the LPS of *H. pylori* has far lower biological activity than those of *Escherichia coli* or *Salmonella* (62, 81, 92), for example. From 3,000 to 30,000 times more *H. pylori* LPS is required to induce macrophage activation or to produce tumor necrosis factor alpha (TNF-α), superoxide, or proinflammatory eicosanoids than is needed for equivalent activation by LPS from enteric organisms (92). A parallel, but less defined, phenomenon has been observed for the LPS of *Bacteroides* species, other persistent colonizers of the human gut.

Those bacteria that are now found to colonize and persist in the human stomach represent the culmination of many years (perhaps millions) of evolution. They must be exquisitely specialized to persist in the stomach for the lives of most, but not all, exposed humans. In addition, the bacteria further specialize for specific human subtypes, and in an ongoing manner, as demonstrated by the variable Le expression discussed above. Interestingly, some genetic traits of *H. pylori* are polymorphic in the population and appear to be associated with overt disease, such as peptic ulcer or cancer. These include the vacuolating cytotoxin (*vacA s1*) (4, 16), the cytotoxin-associated gene (*cag*) pathogenicity island (1, 15, 104), and the gene induced by contact with gastric epithelial cells (*iceA*) (89, 105). Why these determinants of virulence have appeared and persisted worldwide even though they might potentially shorten the ultimate duration of colonization is unknown. Perhaps these genes provide advantages to the bacteria that are not directly related to disease induction, and the cost to *H. pylori* of disease (and premature mortality of the host) is compensated for by benefits to the bacteria, such as colonization ability and transmission to new hosts. Alternatively, these traits might cause severe damage to hosts only because of cofactors that appeared relatively recently, such as modern dietary habits, environmental factors, or stress (68), and to which *H. pylori* has not yet had time to adapt. The recent sequencing of the entire genomes of two *H. pylori* strains (2, 102) has opened new avenues to research on which genetic factors are important for colonization, persistence, and pathogenicity of the bacterium; new developments can be expected in the coming years.

The extensive genetic diversity among *H. pylori* strains may be adaptive, but which of such bacterial traits are important is at present unknown. This diversity probably reflects continuous selection for variants that are increasingly fit for a given colonized host phenotype, even as the host may change over time. A strain with such a history might often be imperfectly suited to the next host to ingest it, and in the extreme, either fail to colonize that host or result in only transient colonization. Therefore, it is also important to consider the role of host factors.

Host Factors

IMMUNE RESPONSE

Long-term gastric colonization is associated with intense humoral and cellular immune responses. However, these responses are usually unable to eradicate *H. pylori* and they may, in fact, play a role in the persistence of the bacterium and/or in the production of disease. Therefore, a better understanding of the host's responses to *H. pylori* is critical in the development of new treatments and vaccines.

The humoral response is primarily of the IgA and IgG subclasses (79, 90). Analysis of the antigen specificity of plasma from humans colonized by *H. pylori* has identified a number of immunogenic proteins. These include urease (33), the Hsp60 heat shock protein homolog (HspB) (50, 93), the CagA protein (21), the

vacuolating cytotoxin (VacA) (17, 18), catalase (84), surface-exposed outer membrane antigens, and flagellar antigens (30).

In addition, an intense T-cell response is the hallmark of the host's cellular response. Two subsets of CD4$^+$ T-helper (Th) cells (Th1 cells and Th2 cells) have been described in mice. Th1 cells express the cytokines gamma interferon (IFN-γ) and interleukin 2 (IL-2), whereas Th-2 cells express IL-4, IL-5, IL-6, and IL-10. Whether equivalent subtypes of Th cells are present in humans is controversial at present, and we therefore prefer to refer to these as Th1-like or Th2-like when discussing studies of humans or monkeys.

Studies of humans persistently colonized by *H. pylori* have led to two different hypotheses as to the role of Th1- and Th2-like cellular immune responses in persistence. Each suggests that an "inappropriate" balance in Th1-like versus Th2-like responses results in persistent colonization as opposed to natural clearance. One hypothesis proposes that an excessive Th1-like response and a weak or absent Th2-like response to *H. pylori* are responsible for the chronic inflammation and subsequent pathology (40, 41). This implies that a protective immunity that would prevent persistence would require a more intense Th2-like response to give a better Th1- and Th2-like balance. This hypothesis is supported by the observation that patients with persistent *H. pylori* express IFN-γ, IL-12, and TNF-α in gastric biopsies (8, 28, 29, 54). An alternative hypothesis invokes a suppressed Th-1-like response (45). This implies that protective immunity would require a switch from Th2- to Th1-like response. This model is supported by observations that expression of IFN-γ, the levels of IFN-γ-secreting cells, and T-cell activation as determined by thymidine incorporation were all decreased in *H. pylori*-positive patients compared to *H. pylori*-negative patients (46, 57). The two hypotheses are not mutually exclusive, since either "imbalance" might occur in different subsets of individuals in the heterogeneous human population.

In addition to specific B- and T-cell responses to *H. pylori*, phagocytic cells, such as macrophages and neutrophils, infiltrate gastric submucosa, leading to increased permeability of the vascular endothelium to support further cellular infiltration and fluid drainage to lymph nodes. Macrophages are activated by the LPSs of gram-negative bacteria to secrete the cytokines TNF-α, IL-1β, IL-6, IL-8, and IL-12. IL-8, a potent chemotactic factor for neutrophils, is secreted by epithelial cells incubated with *H. pylori* (especially of the more virulent *cag*+ type), and this may be an important inducer of neutrophil infiltration into the site of colonization (20, 22, 23, 98). This is probably indirect, via activation of transcription of the gene for NF-κB in gastric epithelial cells (59, 97). NF-κB is an important transcriptional regulator of many inflammatory response genes, including those for chemokines such as IL-8, cytokines such as TNF-α, and immunoglobulin superfamily members such as major histocompatibility complex (MHC) class II molecules and the cellular adhesion molecule ICAM-1. Thus, activation of NF-κB during *H. pylori* initial colonization may be an important defense response by gastrointestinal epithelial cells. In addition, *cag*+ strains induce NF-κB to a greater extent than do *cag*− cells (1, 15, 19, 71). Mutational tests have begun to identify genes in the 40-kb *cag* pathogenicity island that are important in the induction of IL-8 (or NF-κB) secretion and its regulation, but much remains to be learned concerning how or if the host responses affect the persistence or transience of colonization.

Importantly, the majority of the data discussed above were obtained by comparing *H. pylori*-positive patients to *H. pylori*-negative patients, and the *H. pylori*-positive patients had been colonized for an undefined period of time (years to decades). We suggest that the response observed in persistently colonized hosts might have prevented initial colonization if it had been present immediately upon *H. pylori* entry into the stomach. This hypothesis is based on our finding that rhesus monkeys that became only transiently colonized after experimental inoculation had rapid cellular (108) and humoral immune responses (Fig. 2) (34), whereas

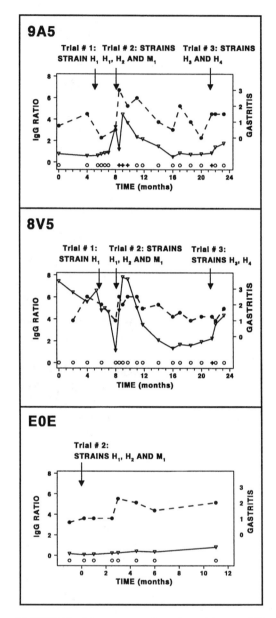

FIGURE 2   Time course of antral gastritis score (●) and plasma IgG (▽) before and after transient or unsuccessful colonization. Absence of the organism is indicated by ○, and positivity for *H. pylori* by culture and/or histology is indicated by +. Animal 9A5 was not colonized in trial 1 but developed transient colonization during trials 2 and 3. Animal 8V5 was not colonized during trials 1 and 2 but developed transient colonization during trial 3. Animal E0E was included only in trial 2 and did not become colonized with *H. pylori* (34).

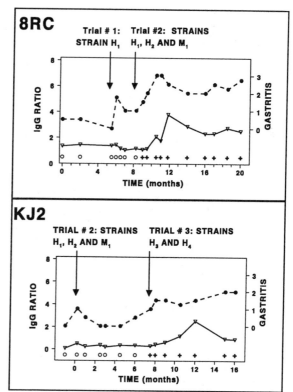

FIGURE 3 Time course of antral gastritis score (●) and plasma IgG (▽) before and after successful colonization. Absence of the organism is indicated by ○, and positivity for *H. pylori* by culture and/or histology is indicated by +. Animal 8RC became persistently colonized in trial 2, and the plasma IgG and gastritis scores increased after a 3-month delay. Animal KJ2 did not become colonized in trial 2 but was colonized by one of the human strains from a patient with gastric ulcer used in trial 3 (34).

the animals that became persistently infected did not develop intense gastritis and peak IgG levels until 3 to 4 months after inoculation (Fig. 3) (34). A similar delay in antibody response was observed in the only long-term study of persistent *H. pylori* colonization after experimental challenge of a human (79). Thus, rapid immune response may reflect protective immunity, although the serum antibodies measured in the patient and in the monkeys only approximated the more relevant gastric mucosal immune responses. That maternal antibodies can protect infants against colonization by *H. pylori* is suggested by the following anecdotal observation in rhesus monkeys: a weanling from an *H. pylori*-positive mother was seronegative at 1 year, whereas a weanling from an *H. pylori*-negative mother was seropositive at the same age (A. Dubois, unpublished data). Thus, a strong early tissue and/or humoral immune response might help the host eliminate newly acquired *H. pylori*.

To understand why the immune response observed in persistently colonized hosts does not eliminate *H. pylori*, it may be useful to examine the mechanism of the protection produced by immunization. The classical view is that mucosal defense is principally mediated by secretory IgA (65). Studies using the mouse model have supported this view. Protection against experimental infection was achieved by intragastric administration of anti-*Helicobacter felis* monoclonal IgA at the time of the challenge. In addition, oral immunization with bacterial antigens resulted in both protection against infection and elevated anti-*H. felis* IgA, and also IgG, titers (26). Similarly, production of secretory IgA against urease was correlated with successful protection against challenge of mice with *H. felis* following administration of recombinant urease (rUre) vaccine (66, 87). In contrast, other studies have shown a lack of relation between protection of mice following immunization using rUre and levels of specific

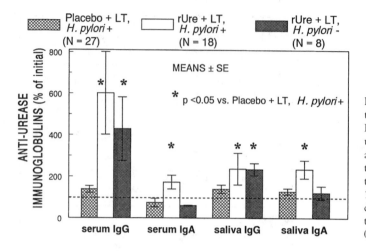

FIGURE 4 Effect of administration of rUre plus LT or placebo plus LT on conversion in specific anti-urease serum and saliva IgG and IgA at 1 week after the fourth immunization. The *H. pylori* + or − designation reflects the status at endoscopy 11.5 months after immunization. The dotted line represents 100% of the initial immunoglobulin level. *, P < 0.05 (36). SE, standard error.

IgA in gastric mucosa, blood, feces (60), and/or intestinal secretions (74). A similar observation was recently reported in rhesus monkeys immunized against natural colonization by *H. pylori* with rUre plus *E. coli* heat-labile enterotoxin (LT) compared to those immunized with LT alone (Fig. 4 and 5) (36). Thus, neither serum nor secretory IgA appears to play a protective role, which is consistent with the observation of persistent colonization in humans despite increased production of anti-*H. pylori* IgA. This apparent paradox may be explained by findings that only a fraction of *H. pylori* cells present in the gastric lumen are coated with IgA, that the bacteria located deep in gastric pits are not (58, 116), and that no IgA-coated *H. pylori* cells have been observed in gastric brushings of *H. pylori*-positive patients (27). Therefore, it is possible that even mucosal IgA may not have access to the *H. pylori* cells most critically involved in persistence of colonization.

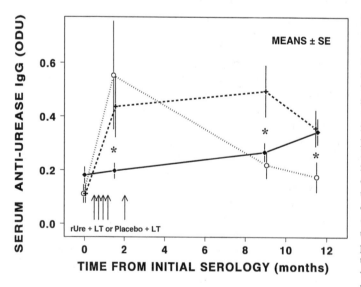

FIGURE 5 Time course of serum anti-urease IgG. Following administration of rUre plus LT, mean IgG initially increased (○ and +). IgG subsequently decreased in animals that were *H. pylori*-negative at the endoscopy performed at 11.5 months (○; n = 8), whereas it did not change significantly in those who were *H. pylori* positive at 11.5 months (+; n = 18). In animals given placebo plus LT, IgG initially did not change and then increased progressively in the animals that were *H. pylori* positive at the endoscopy performed at 11.5 months (◆; n = 27). IgG remained low in the two animals that had received placebo plus LT and remained *H. pylori* negative (data not illustrated). *, P < 0.05 versus placebo plus LT and *H. pylori* positive at 11.5 months. SE, standard error. (Adapted from reference 36.)

If IgA is not involved in the protection conferred by immunization, then it is worth considering the possible role of IgG, which is generally neglected when mucosal immunity is discussed (95). Parenteral or oral administration of IgG is sufficient to confer passive protection against most infections, including gastrointestinal infections (95), and it can opsonize *H. pylori* for destruction by mononuclear cells (103). Further support of a role for IgG in *Helicobacter* clearance is provided by the observation that immunization against *H. felis* induces proliferation of IgG-secreting cells in the protected animals but no gastric anti-*H. pylori* IgA response, whereas colonization is associated with recruitment of IgA-producing plasma cells (49). In rhesus monkeys, a rapid rise in specific anti-urease IgG was observed immediately following administration of rUre plus LT but not in those receiving placebo plus LT (Fig. 4 and 5). Although the levels of immunoglobulin in gastric secretion were not determined, the observed rise in serum anti-*H. pylori* IgG is probably associated with a concurrent rise in IgG in the stomach mucosa and in the gastrointestinal fluids (95). The possible role of IgG in immunity is also supported by the observation that administration of the GroES homolog of *H. pylori* (HspB), alone or in association with urease, increased the production of specific anti-*H. pylori* IgG1 in mice and concurrently protected against experimental infection by *H. felis* (50). However, the situation appears to be complex, since a long-term study of rhesus monkeys showed that serum anti-urease IgG decreased in immunized animals that remained protected against *H. pylori* infection despite their continuous exposure to hyperenzootic transmission conditions (Fig. 5) (36). Continued antigenic stimulation may explain why serum anti-urease IgG increased over time in sham-immunized animals that became *H. pylori* positive (by histology and/or culture of gastric biopsy specimens) and the fact that levels remained elevated in the vaccinated animals that were not protected against *H. pylori* challenge (Fig. 5) (36). Similar to the conclusions drawn for the role of IgA, this observation suggests

that the efficacy of immunization does not depend solely on elevated serum anti-urease IgG.

Recently, the basis of protective immunity in two mouse models was demonstrated to be independent of a humoral immune response (39; A. Akhian, M. Kjerrulf, R. Redline, J. Nedrud, S. J. Czinn, and N. Lycke. *Proc. 3rd Int. Workshop Pathog. Host Response Helicobacter Infect.*, abstr C1, 1999). Both studies used knockout mice to study the efficacy of protection by immunization with either the urease B subunit (39) or an *H. felis* lysate (Akhian et al., *Proc. 3rd Int. Workshop Pathog. Host Response Helicobacter Infect.*, 1999). In the first study, wild-type mice and mice that were deficient in B-cell ($\mu MT^{-/-}$), MHC-class I (β_2-microglobulin$^{-/-}$), or MHC-class II (I-A$^{b-/-}$) immune response were immunized orally with urease plus *E. coli* LT (39). In these experiments, only the MHC-class II knockout (I-A$^{b-/-}$) mice were not protected against a subsequent challenge with *H. pylori*. These results indicate that neither antibody- nor MHC class I-mediated immune responses contributed to the observed protection in this model. In a study addressing the roles of IgA and CD4$^+$ Th1- and Th2-directed responses in protective immunity, wild-type, IgA$^{-/-}$, IFN-$\gamma^{-/-}$ (Th1-deficient), and IL-4$^{-/-}$ (Th2-deficient) animals were orally immunized with *H. felis* lysate plus cholera toxin (Akhian et al., *Proc. 3rd Int. Workshop Pathog. Host Response Helicobacter Infect.*, 1999). Upon challenge with *H. felis*, protection was observed in both wild-type and IgA$^{-/-}$ mice, but no protection was observed in either the IFN-$\gamma^{-/-}$ or IL-4$^{-/-}$ mice. These studies indicate that both IFN-γ- and IL-4-directed responses are critical to protection in this model. Taken together, these data indicate a specific requirement for a CD4$^+$-mediated T-cell response to generate the observed protective immunity.

Thus, data from vaccine studies of animals are consistent with the hypothesis that the humoral immune response is not essential for protection. Instead, protective immunity may depend on specific cellular immune responses that are absent or unsuccessful during persistent colonization by *H. pylori*. Interestingly, vaccination can reduce the severity of antral gastritis in mice (87), ferrets (24), and monkeys (36). However, immunization can eliminate colonization by *H. pylori* in mice (87) and ferrets (24) but not in monkeys (36) or humans (75). Thus, a better dissection of the differences in colonization and/or cellular immune responses among these bacterial and host species may help us understand the mechanism of persistence versus transience of *H. pylori* colonization in humans and open new strategies for the eradication of this bacterium.

HOST GENOTYPE

Genetically determined host traits (72) in combination with age of acquisition and environmental or dietary cofactors may play an important role in determining the outcome of initial contact of particular *H. pylori* strains with the gastric mucosa.

Particular HLA alleles may be important in strain-specific responses because of the pivotal role they play in cellular immunity. Having observed that the accidental inoculation of a gastroenterologist with *H. pylori* was followed by only transient colonization, a group of investigators attributed this anecdotal finding to his carrying the DQA1*0102 allele of the HLA-DQ class II gene (77). In turn, this gene would result in an aSHyet-undefined immune defense. The same group subsequently expanded the basis for this theory by demonstrating that the frequency of the DQA1*0102 genotype was higher in *H. pylori*-negative than in *H. pylori*-positive Japanese patients with duodenal ulcer, whereas the opposite applied to the DQA1*0301 genotype (7). Similarly, the DQA1*0301 allele was less frequent, and the DQA1*0102 allele was more frequent, in *H. pylori*-positive subjects with atrophic gastritis or intestinal type adenocarcinoma than in *H. pylori*-negative controls. Interestingly, a group of *H. pylori*-positive subjects with superficial gastritis were also preferentially of the DQA1*0102 allele genotype (6). These results suggest that there are genetic differences between *H. pylori*-positive and *H. pylori*-negative

patients with duodenal ulcer or intestinal-type adenocarcinoma and also between *H. pylori*-positive subjects with or without atrophic gastritis in Japan. These genetic differences in turn could be responsible for differences in susceptibility to colonization by *H. pylori* and/or in inflammatory responses to the bacterium.

In contrast, a U.S. group did not find an increased frequency of DQA1*0301 in Caucasian patients with gastric adenocarcinoma; however, they observed that the DQB1*0301 allele was more frequent in gastric adenocarcinoma but not pancreatic or colorectal adenocarcinoma (67). This study also showed that *H. pylori* was less frequent in patients with gastric adenocarcinoma if they carried the DQB1*0301 allele than if they did not. These discrepancies could be related to the reported clearance of *H. pylori* in gastric cancer attributed to proliferation of other bacteria, to the fact that the authors did not separate intestinal-type adenocarcinoma from undifferentiated adenocarcinoma, or to genetic differences between Caucasian and Japanese subjects. Nonetheless, these observations suggest that host immunogenetic factors could be important in susceptibility or resistance to *H. pylori* and/or formation of precancerous and cancerous lesions.

HOST RESPONSE AND PATHOGENESIS

H. pylori colonization is always associated with the host tissue response termed gastritis, but the intensity of the cellular response varies markedly among colonized subjects. In some hosts, the tissue response is mild and acid output is not modified (although it is important to remember that only a minority of patients with peptic ulcer disease [PUD] have increased gastric acidity). In other individuals, the development of atrophy with resulting suppression of acid output and intestinal metaplasia facilitates the growth of other bacteria that may in turn compete with *H. pylori* and eliminate it. Although this outcome might appear advantageous to the host, it is not without risk, since these alterations of the gastric mucosa appear to be irreversible, and they substantially increase the risk for carcinogenesis.

The full set of factors determining the varied final outcomes of *H. pylori* colonization in humans (i.e., asymptomatic, PUD, or gastric cancer) is at present unknown, although PUD and gastric cancer are more frequently observed in subjects colonized by strains possessing virulence genes (the *cagA* pathogenicity island [1], *vacA s1* [4], and/or *iceA1* [89]) than in those colonized by *H. pylori* with the more benign genotype. The immune response to colonization by *H. pylori* has been proposed as being responsible in part for the production of these diseases. Thus, ulceration of the gastroduodenal mucosa may be caused by antibodies directed against host antigens or by the production of proinflammatory cytokines that may contribute to persistent inflammation, tissue injury, or changes in gastric acid secretory physiology. In addition, persistent *H. pylori* infection may induce precancerous lesions, but the final steps of carcinogenesis may evolve in its absence.

CONCLUSIONS AND FUTURE RESEARCH

Since the first isolation of *H. pylori* and the demonstration of its role in PUD about 16 years ago, our knowledge of the bacterium has expanded enormously. This organism has brought together gastroenterologists, infectious-disease specialists, pathologists, microbiologists, molecular biologists, immunologists, geneticists, and pharmacologists in collaborative teams to explore its biological and clinical significance. The results have been substantial, and our understanding of the illnesses associated with *H. pylori* has markedly improved. However, many questions remain unanswered, and ongoing studies using genetic, molecular, biochemical, and cell biology techniques certainly will provide much information. However, it is likely that only studies of humans and appropriate animal models will be able to provide definitive answers to the following three important questions: (i) what are the exact mechanisms that permit persistence of the bacterium in the stomachs of a large proportion of humankind, (ii) why do some subjects develop gastric ulcer, duodenal ulcer, or gastric cancer, whereas a majority of colonized individuals remain free of clinical disease; and (iii) what is the impact of *H. pylori* on the production of extragastric diseases?

ACKNOWLEDGMENTS

Support was provided by grants NIH RO1 AI38166, DK53727, and DK53707 and by the Medical Research Service of the Department of Veterans Affairs.

REFERENCES

1. **Akopyants, N. S., S. W. Clifton, D. Kersulyte, J. E. Crabtree, B. E. Youree, C. A. Reece, B. A. Roe, N. O. Bukanov, E. S. Drazek, and D. E. Berg.** 1998. The *cag* pathogenicity island of *Helicobacter pylori*. *Mol. Microbiol.* **28:** 37–54.
2. **Alm, R. A., L. S. Ling, D. T. Moir, B. L. King, E. D. Brown, P. C. Doig, D. R. Smith, B. Noonan, B. C. Guild, B. L. de Jonge, G. Carmel, P. J. Tummino, A. Caruso, M. Uria-Nickelsen, D. M. Mills, C. Ives, R. Gibson, D. Merberg, S. D. Mills, Q. Jiang, D. E. Taylor, G. F. Vovis, and T. J. Trust.** 1999. Genomic-sequence comparison of two unrelated isolates of the human gastric pathogen *Helicobacter pylori*. *Nature* **397:**176–180.
3. **Anonymous.** 1994. Helicobacter pylori in peptic ulcer disease. NIH Consensus Conference. *JAMA* **272:**65–69.
4. **Atherton, J. C., R. M. Peek, Jr., K. T. Tham, T. L. Cover, and M. J. Blaser.** 1997. Clinical and pathological importance of heterogeneity in *vacA*, the vacuolating cytotoxin gene of *Helicobacter pylori*. *Gastroenterology* **112:**92–99.
5. **Atherton, J. C., and R. C. Spiller.** 1999. The urea breath test for *Helicobacter pylori*. *Gut* **35:** 723–725.
6. **Azuma, T., S. Ito, F. Sato, Y. Yamazaki, H. Miyaji, Y. Ito, H. Suto, M. Kuriyama, T. Kato, and Y. Kohli.** 1998. The role of the HLADQA1 gene in resistance to atrophic gastritis and gastric adenocarcinoma induced by *Helicobacter pylori* infection. *Cancer* **82:**1013–1018.
7. **Azuma, T., J. Konishi, Y. Ito, M. Hirai, Y. Tanaka, S. Ito, T. Kato, and Y. Kohli.** 1995. Genetic differences between duodenal ulcer patients who were positive or negative for *Helicobacter pylori*. *J. Clin. Gastroenterol.* **21:**S1514.
8. **Bamford, K. B., X. Fan, S. E. Crowe, J. F. Leary, W. K. Gourley, G. K. Luthra, E. G.**

Brooks, D. Y. Graham, V. E. Reyes, and P. B. Ernst. 1998. Lymphocytes in the human gastric mucosa during *Helicobacter pylori* have a T helper cell 1 phenotype. *Gastroenterology* **114:** 482–492.

9. Beachey, E. H. 1981. Bacterial adherence: adhesin-receptor interactions mediating the attachment of bacteria to mucosal surfaces. *J. Infect. Dis.* **143:**325–345.

10. Blaser, M. J. 1998. Helicobacters are indigenous to the human stomach: duodenal ulceration is due to changes in gastric microecology in the modern era. *Gut* **43:**721–727.

11. Blaser, M. J. 1999. The changing relationship of *Helicobacter pylori* and humans: implications for health and disease. *J. Infect. Dis.* **179:**1523–1530.

12. Blaser, M. J., and D. Kirschner. 1999. Dynamics of *Helicobacter pylori* colonization in relation to the host response. *Proc. Natl. Acad. Sci. USA* **96:** 8359–8364.

13. Blaser, M. J., and J. Parsonnet. 1994. Parasitism by the "slow" bacterium *Helicobacter pylori* leads to altered gastric homeostasis and neoplasia. *J. Clin. Investig.* **94:**4–8.

14. Boren, T., P. Falk, K. A. Roth, G. Larson, and S. Normark. 1993. Attachment of *Helicobacter pylori* to human gastric epithelium mediated by blood group antigens. *Science* **262:**1892–1895.

15. Censini, S., C. Lange, Z. Xiang, J. E. Crabtree, P. Ghiara, M. Borodovsky, R. Rappuoli, and A. Covacci. 1996. *cag*, a pathogenicity island of *Helicobacter pylori*, encodes type I-specific and disease-associated virulence factors. *Proc. Natl. Acad. Sci. USA* **93:**14648–14653.

16. Cover, T. L. 1996. The vacuolating cytotoxin of *Helicobacter pylori*. *Mol. Microbiol.* **20:**241–246.

17. Cover, T. L., P. Cao, U. K. Murth, M. S. Sipple, and M. J. Blaser. 1992. Serum neutralizing antibody response to the vacuolating cytotoxin of *Helicobacter pylori*. *J. Clin. Investig.* **90:**913–918.

18. Cover, T. L., C. P. Dooley, and M. J. Blaser. 1990. Characterization of a human serologic response to proteins in *Helicobacter pylori* broth culture supernatant with vacuolizing cytotoxin activity. *Infect. Immun.* **58:**603–610.

19. Crabtree, J. E., D. Kersulyte, S. D. Li, I. J. D. Lindley, and D. E. Berg. 1999. Modulation of *Helicobacter pylori*-induced IL-8 synthesis in gastric epithelial cells mediated by *cag* PAI-encoded VirD4 homologue. *J. Clin. Pathol.* **52:**653–657.

20. Crabtree, J. E., P. Peichl, J. I. Wyatt, U. Stachl, and I. J. Lindley. 1993. Gastric interleukin-8 and IgA Il-8 autoantibodies in *Helicobacter pylori* infection. *Scand. J. Immunol.* **37:**65–70.

21. Crabtree, J. E., J. D. Taylor, J. I. Wyatt, R. V. Heatley, T. M. Shalicross, D. S. Tompkins, and B. J. Rathbone. 1991. Mucosal IgA

recognition of *Helicobacter pylori* 120 kDa protein, peptic ulceration, and gastric pathology. *Lancet* **338:**335.

22. Crabtree, J. E., J. I. Wyatt, L. K. Trejdosiewicz, P. Peichl, P. H. Nichols, N. Ramsay, J. N. Primrose, and I. J. D. Lindley. 1994. Interleukin-8 expression in *Helicobacter pylori*-infected, normal, and neoplastic gastroduodenal mucosa. *J. Clin. Pathol.* **47:**61–66.

23. Crowe, S. E., L. Alvarez, P. M. Sherman, Y. Jin, M. Dytoc, R. H. Hunt, H. Patel, M. J. Muller, and P. B. Ernst. 1995. Expression of interleukin 8 and CD54 by human gastric epithelium after *H. pylori* infection in vitro. *Gastroenterology* **108:**65–74.

24. Cuenca, R., T. G. Blanchard, S. J. Czinn, J. G. Nedrud, T. P. Monath, C. K. Lee, and R. W. Redline. 1996. Therapeutic immunization against *Helicobacter mustelae* in naturally infected ferrets. *Gastroenterology* **110:**1170–1175.

25. Cullen, D. J., B. J. Collins, B. J. Christiansen, J. R. Warren, R. Surveyor, and K. J. Cullen. 1993. When is *Helicobacter pylori* infection acquired? *Gut* **34:**1681–1682.

26. Czinn, S. J., A. Cai, and J. G. Nedrud. 1993. Protection of germ-free mice from infection by *Helicobacter felis* after active oral or passive IgA immunization. *Vaccine* **11:**637–642.

27. Darwin, P. E., M. B. Sztein, Q. X. Zheng, S. P. James, and G. T. Fantry. 1996. Immune evasion by *Helicobacter pylori*: gastric spiral bacteria lack surface immunoglobulin deposition and reactivity with homologous antibodies. *Helicobacter* **1:** 20–27.

28. D'Elios, M. M., M. Manghetti, F. Almerigogn, E. Arnedel, F. Costa, D. Burroni, C. T. Baldari, S. Romagnani, J. L. Telford, and G. Del Prete. 1997. Different cytokine profile and antigens specificity repertoire in *Helicobacter pylori* specific T cell clones from the antrum of chronic gastritis patients with or without peptic ulcer. *Eur. J. Immunol.* **27:**1751–1755.

29. D'Elios, M. M., M. Manghetti, M. De Carli, F. Costa, C. T. Baldari, D. Burroni, J. L. Telford, S. Romagnani, and G. Del Prete. 1997. T helper 1 effector cells specific for *Helicobacter pylori* in the gastric antrum of patients with peptic ulcer disease. *J. Immunol.* **158:**962–967.

30. Doig, P. C., and T. J. Trust. 1994. Identification of surface exposed outer membrane antigens of *Helicobacter pylori*. *Infect. Immun.* **62:**4526–4533.

31. Drumm, B., G. I. Perez-Perez, M. J. Blaser, and P. M. Sherman. 1990. Intrafamilial clustering of *Helicobacter pylori* infection. *N. Engl. J. Med.* **322:**359–363.

32. Dubois, A. 1989. Functional causes of disturbed gastric function, p. 143–170. *In* W. P. Snape (ed.),

Pathogenesis of Functional Bowel Disease. Plenum Medical Book Company, New York, N.Y.

33. **Dubois, A.** 1995. Spiral bacteria in the human stomach: the gastric helicobacters. *Emerg. Infect. Dis.* **1:**79–85.

34. **Dubois, A., D. E. Berg, E. T. Incecik, N. Fiala, L. M. Heman-Ackah, G. I. Perez-Perez, and M. J. Blaser.** 1996. Transient and persistent experimental infection of nonhuman primates with *Helicobacter pylori*: implications for human disease. *Infect. Immun.* **64:**2885–2891.

35. **Dubois, A., D. E. Berg, E. T. Incecik, N. Fiala, L. M. Heman-Ackah, M. Yang, H. P. Wirth, G. I. Perez-Perez, and M. J. Blaser.** 1999. Host specificity of *Helicobacter pylori* strains and host responses in experimentally challenged nonhuman primates. *Gastroenterology* **116:**90–96.

36. **Dubois, A., C. P. Lee, P. T. Mehlman, N. Fiala, H. Kleanthous, and T. Monath.** 1998. Immunization against natural *Helicobacter pylori* infection in rhesus monkeys. *Infect. Immun.* **66:**4340–4346.

37. **Dunn, B. E., C. C. Sung, N. S. Taylor, and J. G. Fox.** 1991. Purification and characterization of *Helicobacter mustelae* urease. *Infect. Immun.* **59:**3343–3345.

38. **Eaton, K., D. R. Morgan, C. L. Brooks, and S. Krakowka.** 1991. Essential role of urease in pathogenesis of gastritis induced by *Helicobacter pylori* in gnotobiotic piglets. *Infect. Immun.* **59:**2470–2475.

39. **Ermak, T. H., P. J. Giannasca, R. Nichols, G. A. Myers, J. Nedrud, R. Weltzin, C. K. Lee, H. Kleanthous, and T. P. Monath.** 1998. Immunization of mice with urease vaccine affords protection against *Helicobacter pylori* infection in the absence of antibodies and is mediated by MHC class II-restricted responses. *J. Exp. Med.* **188:**2277–2288.

40. **Ernst, P. B., S. E. Crowe, and V. E. Reyes.** 1995. The immunopathogenesis of gastroduodenal disease associated with *Helicobacter pylori* infection. *Curr. Opin. Gastroenterol.* **11:**512–518.

41. **Ernst, P. B., S. E. Crowe, and V. E. Reyes.** 1997. How does *Helicobacter pylori* cause mucosal damage? The inflammatory response. *Gastroenterology* **113:**S35–S42.

42. **Evans, D. G., D. J. Evans, H. C. Lampert, and D. Y. Graham.** 1995. Restriction fragment length polymorphism in the adhesin gene hpaA of Helicobacter pylori. *Am. J. Gastroenterol.* **90:**1282–1288.

43. **Evans, D. G., D. J. Evans, J. J. Moulds, and D. Y. Graham.** 1988. *N*-acetylneuraminyllactose-binding fibrillar hemagglutinin of *Campylobacter pylori*: a putative colonization factor antigen. *Infect. Immun.* **56:**2896–2906.

44. **Falk, P., K. A. Roth, T. Boren, T. U. Westblom, J. I. Gordon, and S. Normark.** 1993. An in vitro adherence assay reveals that *Helicobacter pylori* exhibits cell lineage-specific tropism in the human gastric epithelium. *Proc. Natl. Acad. Sci. USA* **90:**2035–2039.

45. **Fan, X. G., J. Yakoob, X. J. Fan, and P. W. N. Keeling.** 1996. Enhanced T helper 2 lymphocyte responses: immune mechanism of *Helicobacter pylori* infection. *Ir. J. Med. Sci.* **165:**37–39.

46. **Fan, X. J., A. Chua, C. N. Shahi, J. McDevitt, P. W. N. Keeling, and D. Kelleher.** 1994. Gastric T lymphocyte responses to *Helicobacter pylori* in patients with *H. pylori* colonization. *Gut* **35:**1379–1384.

47. **Fauchere, J., and M. J. Blaser.** 1990. Adherence of *Helicobacter pylori* cells and their surface components to HeLa cell membranes. *Microb. Pathog.* **9:**427–439.

48. **Ferguson, D. A., C. Li, N. R. Patel, W. R. Mayberry, D. S. Chi, and E. Thomas.** 1993. Isolation of *Helicobacter pylori* from saliva. *J. Clin. Microbiol.* **31:**2802–2804.

49. **Ferrero, R. L., J.-M. Thiberge, and A. Labigne.** 1997. Local immunoglobulin G antibodies in the stomach may contribute to immunity against *Helicobacter* infection in mice. *Gastroenterology* **113:**185–194.

50. **Ferrero, R. L., J. M. Thiberge, I. Kansau, N. Wuscher, M. Huerre, and A. Labigne.** 1995. The GroES homolog of *Helicobacter pylori* confers protective immunity against mucosal infection in mice. *Proc. Natl. Acad. Sci. USA* **92:**6499–6503.

51. **Genta, R. M., G. O. Robason, and D. Y. Graham.** 1994. Simultaneous visualization of *Helicobacter pylori* and gastric morphology: a new stain. *Hum. Pathol.* **25:**221–226.

52. **Granstrom, M., Y. Tindberg, and M. Blennow.** 1997. Seroepidemiology of *Helicobacter pylori* infection in a cohort of children monitored from 6 months to 11 years of age. *J. Clin. Microbiol.* **35:**468–470.

53. **Handt, L. K., J. G. Fox, F. E. Dewhirst, G. J. Fraser, B. J. Paster, L. L. Yan, H. Rozmiarek, R. Rufo, and I. H. Stalis.** 1994. *Helicobacter pylori* isolated from the domestic cat: public health implications. *Infect. Immun.* **62:**2367–2374.

54. **Handt, L. K., M. Kubin, K. B. Bamford, R. Carofalo, D. Y. Graham, F. El-Zaatari, S. E. Kartunen, S. E. Crowe, V. E. Reyes, and P. B. Ernst.** 1997. Differential stimulation of interleukin 12 (IL-12) and IL-10 by live and killed *Helicobacter pylori* in vitro and association of IL-12 production with gamma interferon-producing T cells in the human gastric mucosa. *Infect. Immun.* **65:**4229–4235.

55. **Hemalatha, S. G., B. Drumm, and P. J. Sher-**

man. 1991. Adherence of *Helicobacter pylori* to human gastric epithelial cells in vitro. *Med. Microbiol.* **35**:197–202.

56. **Ilver, D., A. Arnqvist, J. Ogren, I. M. Frick, D. Kersulyte, E. T. Incecik, D. E. Berg, A. Covacci, L. Engstrand, and T. Boren.** 1998. *Helicobacter pylori* adhesin binding fucosylated histo-blood group antigens revealed by retagging. *Science* **279**:373–377.

57. **Karttunen, R., T. Karttunen, H.-P. T. Ekre, and T. T. MacDonald.** 1995. Interferon gamma and interleukin 4 secreting cells in the gastric antrum in *Helicobacter pylori* positive and negative gastritis. *Gut* **36**:341–345.

58. **Kazi, J. L., R. Sinniah, N. A. Jaffrey, S. M. Alam, V. Zman, S. J. Zuberi, and A. M. Kazi.** 1989. Cellular and humoral immune responses in *Campylobacter pylori*-associated chronic gastritis. *J. Pathol.* **159**:231–237.

59. **Keates, S., Y. S. Hitti, M. Upton, and C. P. Kelly.** 1997. *Helicobacter pylori* infection activates NF-κB in gastric epithelial cells. *Gastroenterology* **113**:1099–1109.

60. **Kelly, S. M., M. C. Pitcher, S. M. Farmery, and G. R. Gibson.** 1994. Isolation of *Helicobacter pylori* from feces of patients with dyspepsia in the United Kingdom. *Gastroenterology* **107**:1671–1674.

61. **Keranen, A.** 1975. Gangliosides of the human gastrointestinal mucosa. *Biochim. Biophys. Acta* **409**:320–328.

62. **Kirkland, T., S. Viriyakosol, G. I. Perez-Perez, and M. J. Blaser.** 1997. *Helicobacter pylori* lipopolysaccharide can activate 70Z/3 cells via CD14. *Infect. Immun.* **65**:604–608.

63. **Klein, P. D., R. H. Gilman, R. Leon-Barua, F. Diaz, E. O. Smith, and D. Y. Graham.** 1994. The epidemiology of *Helicobacter pylori* in Peruvian children between 6 and 30 months of age. *Am. J. Gastroenterol.* **89**:2196–2200.

64. **Klein, P. D., D. Y. Graham, A. Gaillour, A. R. Opekun, and E. O. Smith.** 1991. Gastrointestinal Physiology Working Group. Water source as risk factor for *Helicobacter pylori* infection in Peruvian children. *Lancet* **337**:1503–1506.

65. **Lee, A.** 1996. Therapeutic immunization against *Helicobacter* infection. *Gastroenterology* **110**:2003–2006.

66. **Lee, C. K., R. Weltzin, W. D. Thomas, Jr., H. Kleanthous, T. H. Ermak, G. Soman, J. E. Hill, S. K. Ackerman, and T. P. Monath.** 1995. Oral immunization with recombinant *Helicobacter pylori* urease induces secretory IgA antibodies and protects mice from challenge with *Helicobacter felis*. *J. Infect. Dis.* **172**:161–172.

67. **Lee, J. E., A. M. Lowy, W. A. Thompson, M. Lu, P. T. Loflin, J. M. Skibber, D. B.**

Evans, S. A. Curley, P. F. Mansfield, and J. D. Reveille. 1996. Association of gastric adenocarcinoma with the HLA class II gene DQB10301. *Gastroenterology* **111**:426–432.

68. **Levenstein, S., S. Ackerman, J. K. Kiecolt-Glaser, and A. Dubois.** 1999. Stress and peptic ulcer disease. *JAMA* **281**:10–11.

69. **Lewala-Guruge, J., A. Ljungh, and T. Wadstrom.** 1992. Haemagglutination patterns of *Helicobacter pylori*. Frequency of sialic acid-specific and nonsialic acid-specific haemagglutinins. *APMIS* **100**:908–913.

70. **Leying, H., S. Suerbaum, G. Geis, and R. Haas.** 1992. Cloning and genetic characterization of a *Helicobacter pylori* flagellin gene. *Mol. Microbiol.* **6**:2863–2874.

71. **Li, S. D., D. Kersulyte, I. J. Lindley, B. Neelam, D. E. Berg, and J. E. Crabtree.** 1999. Multiple genes in the left half of the *cag* pathogenicity island of *Helicobacter pylori* are required for tyrosine kinase-dependent transcription of interleukin-8 in gastric epithelial cells. *Infect. Immun.* **67**:3893–3899.

72. **Malaty, H. M., L. Engstrand, N. L. Pedersen, and D. Y. Graham.** 1994. *Helicobacter pylori* infection: genetic and environmental influences. *Ann. Intern. Med.* **120**:982–986.

73. **Marshall, B. J., J. A. Armstrong, D. B. McGechie, and R. J. Glancy.** 1985. Attempt to fulfill Koch's postulate for pyloric *Campylobacter*. *Med. J. Aust.* **142**:436–439.

74. **Michetti, P., I. E. Corthesy-Theulaz, C. Davin, R. Haas, A.-C. Vaney, M. Heitz, J. Bille, J.-P. Krahenbuhl, E. Saraga, and A. L. Blum.** 1994. Immunization of BALB/c mice against *Helicobacter felis* infection with *Helicobacter pylori* urease. *Gastroenterology* **107**:1002–1011.

75. **Michetti, P., C. Kreiss, K. L. Kotloff, N. Porta, J.-L. Blanco, D. Bachmann, M. Herranz, P. F. Saldinger, I. E. Corthesy-Theulaz, G. Lozonsky, R. Nichols, M. Stolte, S. Ackerman, T. P. Monath, and A. L. Blum.** 1999. Oral immunization with urease and *Escherichia coli* heat-labile enterotoxin is safe and immunogenic in *Helicobacter pylori*-infected adults. *Gastroenterology* **116**:804–812.

76. **Miller-Podraza, H., M. A. Mihl, S. Teneberg, and K. A. Karlsson.** 1997. Binding of *Helicobacter pylori* to sialic acid-containing glycolipids of various origins separated by thin-layer chromatograms. *Infect. Immun.* **65**:2480–2482.

77. **Miyaji, H., Y. Kohli, T. Azuma, Y. Ito, M. Hirai, T. Kato, M. Kuriyama, and Y. Abe.** 1995. Endoscopic cross-infection with *Helicobacter pylori*. *Lancet* **345**:464.

78. **Moriai, T., and N. Hirahara.** 1999. Clinical course of acute gastric mucosal lesions caused by

acute infection with *Helicobacter pylori*. *N. Engl. J. Med.* **341:**456–458.

79. **Morris, A. J., M. R. Ali, G. I. Nicholson, G. I. Perez-Perez, and M. J. Blaser.** 1991. Long term follow-up of voluntary ingestion of *Helicobacter pylori*. *Ann. Intern. Med.* **114:**662–663.

80. **Muraoka, H., I. Kobayashi, M. Hasegawa, T. Saika, H. Toda, M. Nishida, J. Suzuki, T. Mine, and T. Fujita.** 1997. Urease-negative Helicobacter pylori isolates from gastrointestinal mucosa of patients with peptic ulcer. *Kansenshogaku Zasshi* **71:**1216–1220.

81. **Mutiola, A., I. M. Helander, L. Pyhala, T. U. Kosunen, and A. P. Moran.** 1992. Low biological activity of *Helicobacter pylori* lipopolysaccharide. *Infect. Immun.* **60:**1714–1716.

82. **Mysore, J. V., P. M. Simon, D. Zopf, L. M. Heman-Ackah, and A. Dubois.** 1999. Treatment of *Helicobacter pylori* infection in rhesus monkeys using a novel antiadhesive compound. *Gastroenterology* **117:**1316–1325.

83. **Neman-Simba, V., and F. Megraud.** 1988. In vitro model for *Campylobacter pylori* adherence properties. *Infect. Immun.* **56:**3329–3333.

84. **Newell, D. G., and A. R. Staccy.** 1994. B cell responses in *H. pylori* infection, p. 309–320. *In* R. H. Hunt and G. N. Tytgat (ed.), *H. pylori: Basic Mechanisms to Clinical Cure.* Kluwer Academic Publishers, Amsterdam, The Netherlands.

85. **Nomura, A., G. N. Stemmermann, P. H. Chyou, I. Kato, G. I. Perez-Perez, and M. J. Blaser.** 1994. *Helicobacter pylori* infection and gastric carcinoma among Japanese Americans in Hawaii. *Ann. Intern. Med.* **120:**977–981.

86. **Odenbreit, S., M. Till, D. Hofreuter, G. Faller, and R. Haas.** 1999. Genetic and functional characterization of the *alpAB* locus essential for the adhesion of *Helicobacter pylori* to human gastric tissue. *Mol. Microbiol.* **31:**1537–1548.

87. **Pappo, J., W. D. J. Thomas, Z. Kabok, N. S. Taylor, J. C. Murphy, and J. G. Fox.** 1995. Effect of oral immunization with recombinant urease on murine *Helicobacter felis* gastritis. *Infect. Immun.* **63:**1246–1252.

88. **Parsonnet, J., S. Hansen, L. Rodriguez, A. B. Gelb, R. A. Warnke, E. Jellum, N. Orentreich, J. H. Vogelman, and G. D. Friedman.** 1994. *Helicobacter pylori* infection and gastric lymphoma. *N. Engl. J. Med.* **330:**1267–1271.

89. **Peek, R. M., S. Thompson, J. P. Donahue, K. T. Tham, J. C. Atherton, M. J. Blaser, and G. G. Miller.** 1998. Adherence to epithelial cells induces expression of a *Helicobacter pylori* gene, *iceA*, that is associated with clinical outcome. *Proc. Am. Assoc. Physicians* **110:**531–544.

90. **Perez-Perez, G. I., B. M. Dworkin, J. E. Chodos, and M. J. Blaser.** 1988. Campylobacter

pylori antibodies in humans. *Ann. Intern. Med.* **109:**11–17.

91. **Perez-Perez, G. I., A. Z. Olivares, T. L. Cover, and M. J. Blaser.** 1992. Characteristics of *Helicobacter pylori* variants selected for urease deficiency. *Infect. Immun.* **60:**3658–3663.

92. **Perez-Perez, G. I., V. L. Shepherd, J. D. Morrow, and M. J. Blaser.** 1999. Activation of human THP-1 cells and rat bone marrow-derived macrophages by *Helicobacter pylori* lipopolysaccharide. *Infect. Immun.* **63:**1183–1187.

93. **Perez-Perez, G. I., S. M. Thiberge, A. Labigne, and M. J. Blaser.** 1996. Relationship of immune response to heatshock protein A and characteristics of *Helicobacter pylori* infected patients. *J. Infect. Dis.* **174:**1050.

94. **Perkins, S. E., J. G. Fox, R. P. Marini, Z. Shen, C. A. Dangler, and Z. Ge.** 1998. Experimental infection in cats with a *cagA*[+] human isolate of *Helicobacter pylori*. *Helicobacter* **3:**225–235.

95. **Robbins, J. B., R. Schneerson, and S. C. Szu.** 1995. Perspective: hypothesis: Serum IgG antibody is sufficient to confer protection against infectious diseases by inactivating inoculum. *J. Infect. Dis.* **171:**1387–1398.

96. **Saitoh, T., H. Natomi, W. Zhao, K. Okuzumi, K. Sugano, M. Iwamori, and Y. Nagai.** 1991. Identification of glycolipid receptors for *Helicobacter pylori* by TLC-immunostaining. *FEBS Lett.* **282:**385–387.

97. **Sharma, S. A., M. K. Tummuru, M. J. Blaser, and L. D. Kerr.** 1998. Activation of IL8 gene expression by *Helicobacter pylori* is regulated by transcription factor nuclear factor κB in gastric epithelial cells. *J. Immunol.* **160:**2401–2407.

98. **Sharma, S. A., M. K. Tummuru, G. G. Miller, and M. J. Blaser.** 1995. Interleukin-8 response of gastric epithelial cell lines to *Helicobacter pylori* stimulation in vitro. *Infect. Immun.* **63:**1681–1687.

99. **Simon, P. M., P. L. Goode, A. Mobasseri, and D. Zopf.** 1997. Inhibition of *Helicobacter pylori* binding to gastrointestinal epithelial cells by sialic acid-containing oligosaccharides. *Infect. Immun.* **65:**750–757.

100. **Taylor, D. N., and M. J. Blaser.** 1991. The epidemiology of *Helicobacter pylori* infection. *Epidemiol. Rev.* **13:**42–59.

101. **Thomas, J. E., G. R. Gibson, M. K. Darboe, A. Dale, and L. T. Weaver.** 1992. Isolation of *H. pylori* from human faeces. *Lancet* **340:**1194–1195.

102. **Tomb, J. F., O. White, A. R. Kerlavage, R. A. Clayton, G. G. Sutton, R. D. Fleischmann, K. A. Ketchum, H. P. Klenk, S. Gill,**

B. A. Dougherty, K. Nelson, J. Quackenbush, L. Zhou, E. F. Kirkness, S. Peterson, B. Loftus, D. Richardson, R. Dodson, H. G. Khalak, A. Glodek, K. McKenney, L. M. Fitzgerald, N. Lee, M. D. Adams, E. K. Hickey, D. E. Berg, J. D. Gocayne, T. R. Utterback, J. D. Peterson, J. M. Kelley, M. D. Cotton, J. M. Weidman, C. Fujii, C. Bowman, L. Watthey, E. Wallin, W. S. Hayes, M. Borodovsky, P. D. Karp, H. O. Smith, C. M. Fraser, and J. C. Venter. 1997. The complete genome sequence of the gastric pathogen *Helicobacter pylori*. *Nature* **388**:539–547.

103. **Tosi, M. F., and S. J. Czinn.** 1990. Opsonic activity of specific human IgG against *Helicobacter pylori*. *J. Infect. Dis.* **162**:156–162.

104. **Tummuru, M. K., S. A. Sharma, and M. J. Blaser.** 1995. *Helicobacter pylori* picB, a homologue of the *Bordetella pertussis* toxin secretion protein, is required for induction of IL-8 in gastric epithelial cells. *Mol. Microbiol.* **18**:867–876.

105. **Van Doorn, L. J., C. Figueiredo, R. Sanna, A. Plaisier, P. Schneeberger, W. De Boer, and W. Quint.** 1998. Clinical relevance of the *cagA, vacA,* and *iceA* status of *Helicobacter pylori*. *Gastroenterology* **115**:58–66.

106. **Veldhuyzen van Zanten, S., D. Malatjalian, R. Tanton, D. Leddin, R. H. Hunt, and W. Blanchard.** 1995. The effect of eradication of *Helicobacter pylori* (HP) on symptoms of non-ulcer dyspepia (NUD): randomized double-blind placebo controlled trial. *Gastroenterology* **108**: A2050.

107. **Wang, G., D. A. Rasko, R. Sherbourne, and D. E. Taylor.** 1999. Molecular genetic basis for the variable expression of Lewis Y antigen in *Helicobacter pylori*: analysis of the alpha(1,2) fucosyltransferase gene. *Mol. Microbiol.* **31**: 1265–1274.

108. **Welch, A., L. Jones, T. Wigginton, R. Kampen, A. Kirk, and A. Dubois.** 1999. Cytokine mRNA expression during experimental *H. pylori* infection in rhesus monkeys. *Gut* **45**: A36.

109. **Wirth, H. P., M. Yang, A. Dubois, D. E. Berg, and M. J. Blaser.** 1999. Host Lewis phenotype-dependent selection of *H. pylori* Lewis expression in rhesus monkeys. *Gut* **43**(Suppl. 2): A26.

110. **Wirth, H. P., M. Yang, R. M. Peek, K. T. Tham, and M. J. Blaser.** 1997. *Helicobacter pylori* Lewis expression is related to the host Lewis phenotype. *Gastroenterology* **113**:1091–1098.

111. **Wyatt, J. I., B. J. Rathbone, and R. V. Heatley.** 1986. Local immune response to gastric *Campylobacter* in non-ulcer dyspepsia. *J. Clin. Pathol.* 863–870.

112. **Zopf, D., and S. Roth.** 1996. Oligosaccharide anti-infective agents. *Lancet* **347**:1017–1021.

LYME BORRELIOSIS

Stephen W. Barthold

14

Lyme borreliosis (Lyme disease) is unequivo-cally a persistent infectious disease. *Borrelia burg-dorferi*, the agent of Lyme disease, persists in both humans and animals, despite a vigorous and effective immune response by the infected host. Persistence is the norm, in fact, the rule, in a wide variety of experimental animal spe-cies, including mice (17), rats (115), hamsters (81), dogs (168), and monkeys (125, 142). Al-though natural infections are less well con-trolled and defined, there is convincing, albeit circumstantial, evidence that persistence also occurs in naturally infected humans (98, 119, 134, 151).

Considering that the vector (*Ixodes persulca-tus* complex) has a long and somewhat ineffi-cient life cycle (2 to 6 years, depending upon geographic latitude) and that *B. burgdorferi* is not significantly transmitted transovarially in ticks (3), it is not surprising that *B. burgdorferi* spirochetes have evolved a strategy to persis-tently infect their reservoir hosts. The agent of Lyme disease also owes its survival to its pro-pensity to infect a wide variety of mammalian and avian hosts (3), thereby allowing geo-graphic spread and adaptation to new niches.

Finally, it has evolved to cause relatively mild or no disease in its hosts (although patients with Lyme disease would rightfully challenge that statement).

B. BURGDORFERI

The agent of Lyme borreliosis belongs to a ge-nospecies complex, *B. burgdorferi* sensu lato, based upon gene sequence data. Several mem-bers of the complex have been validated as sep-arate species, whereas others have been vali-dated as DNA groups. The three major species are *B. burgdorferi* sensu stricto, *Borrelia afzelii*, and *Borrelia garinii*. *B. burgdorferi* sensu stricto is the dominant species in North America and also occurs in Europe but not in Asia. Other species in North America include *Borrelia ander-soni* and the DN127 DNA group, which can also be found in Europe. *B. afzelii* and *B. garinii* predominate in Europe and Asia but are absent in America. Europe also hosts *Borrelia lusitaniae*, and *Borrelia valaisiana* occurs in Europe and Asia. Additional Asian species include *Borrelia japonica*, *Borrelia tanukii*, and *Borrelia turdi*. The *B. burgdorferi* sensu lato complex is related to the relapsing fever borrelia, and newly identified species with relationships to both groups in-clude *Borrelia lonestari* and *Borrelia miyamotoi* (101, 177).

B. burgdorferi sensu lato evolved millions of

Stephen W. Barthold, Center for Comparative Medicine, Schools of Medicine and Veterinary Medicine, University of California, One Shields Ave., Davis, CA 95616.

Persistent Bacterial Infections, Edited by J. P. Nataro, M. J. Blaser, and S. Cunningham-Rundles, © 2000 ASM Press, Washington, D.C.

years ago and further evolved within geographically isolated niches circumpolarly in palearctic regions of the receding ice age. Each original niche was associated with different related members of the relict tick species *I. persulcatus* (11), which continued to evolve in Eurasia (*I. persulcatus*), Europe (*Ixodes ricinus*), and North America (*Ixodes scapularis* in the Northeast and Midwest and *Ixodes pacificus* in the Northwest), among many other areas. Geographic, environmental, and wildlife factors have merged and mixed these genetically distinct but closely related *Borrelia* species. It has recently been proposed that the North American *B. burgdorferi* sensu stricto, which is highly diverse genetically, has been introduced to Europe, where *B. burgdorferi* sensu stricto isolates are more homogeneous, via post-Columbian human migrations. In turn, *B. burgdorferi* sensu stricto in North America possibly evolved from *B. garinii*, of European origin, introduced via migratory seabirds millions of years ago (110). In Europe, *B. burgdorferi* sensu stricto shares reservoirs and vectors with *B. garinii*, which was probably original to the area, and *B. afzelii*, which spread from Eurasia after the recession of the last ice age (11, 14). Furthermore, wherever *B. burgdorferi* sensu lato evolved within its specific niches, including within *Ixodes* vectors and reservoir hosts, it commonly coevolved with a guild of unrelated tick-borne agents, including ehrlichia, babesia, and tick-borne encephalitis virus, which share reservoir hosts and vectors. The pattern is similar around the world (172).

B. burgdorferi sensu lato infects a wide variety of reservoir hosts, allowing maintenance within its niches, as well as allowing spread via migratory birds. Although not thoroughly examined, it appears that most *B. burgdorferi* sensu lato isolates are relatively nonpathogenic in their hosts. Clinical disease in humans is associated with only a few of these *Borrelia* species, including *B. burgdorferi* sensu stricto, *B. afzelii*, *B. garinii*, and, to a limited degree, *B. japonica*. Mixed infections of single patients with different *B. burgdorferi* sensu lato species have been documented (50, 123). Other members of the group overlap geographically with these major species and infect the same vectors and reservoir hosts but have not been isolated from humans with Lyme disease. Mixed infections of single ticks with different *B. burgdorferi* sensu lato species have been documented in Europe (83, 141). It has not been determined to what extent different species or isolates of *B. burgdorferi* influence disease, but there does seem to be an association between infecting species and disease syndromes (8, 175). In rodent models, *B. burgdorferi* sensu stricto, *B. afzelii*, *B. garinii*, 25015 (13), and *B. japonica* (92) all induce similar patterns of disease with different degrees of severity, and different degrees of disease severity occur among different isolates of a single *B. burgdorferi* sensu stricto species (13).

CLINICAL CHARACTERISTICS OF LYME DISEASE

Lyme disease in humans is the result of multisystemic infection following local and hematogenous spread of *B. burgdorferi* from the site of a tick bite. The majority (60 to 80%) of patients with Lyme disease develop an expanding annular skin lesion (erythema migrans) at the site of the tick bite. Erythema migrans, like most Lyme disease manifestations, is ephemeral, disappearing naturally without benefit of antibiotic treatment. Other ephemeral manifestations follow, including general symptoms of flu-like illness; migratory pain in joints, tendons, muscle, and bone; secondary erythema migrans; meningitis; cranial neuritis; encephalitis; lymphadenopathy; splenomegaly; atrioventricular nodal block; and myopericarditis. Attempts have been made to "stage" these events, but they are highly variable in onset and prevalence and should simply be considered manifestations of disseminated infection. Oligoarticular arthritis occurs in about 50% of untreated patients, with recurrent episodes becoming longer in duration in the late stages of infection (161). Notably, there is correlation between positive PCR for *B. burgdorferi* gene targets in synovial fluid and active arthritis during these recurrent bouts (119). Experimental studies of rodents suggest close correlation between the presence of active infection and

PCR reactivity (108). In Europe, a common variation is acrodermatitis chronica atrophicans (ACA), often at the site of earlier erythema migrans. ACA lesions remain PCR and culture positive for years (6). These observations underscore the fact that humans, like animals, become persistently infected with *B. burgdorferi*.

LYME DISEASE IN EXPERIMENTAL ANIMAL MODELS

Because *B. burgdorferi* readily infects a broad array of species, Lyme disease can be investigated in a number of experimental animal models. However, much of our understanding of *B. burgdorferi* pathogenesis is based upon studies with *B. burgdorferi* sensu stricto in mice, with extrapolation to larger species, such as dogs and monkeys (which preclude intensive experimental investigation), and with other *B. burgdorferi* sensu lato species. Because of similar patterns of disease, disease course, and persistence induced by different *B. burgdorferi* sensu lato species in rodents (13), it can be safely assumed that mechanisms of persistence are similar for each of the major subspecies of the *B. burgdorferi* sensu lato complex.

The most thoroughly investigated model system has been the laboratory mouse infected with *B. burgdorferi* sensu stricto. Not surprisingly, different inbred strains of mice vary in susceptibility to disease following infection with *B. burgdorferi* (17, 22), but all strains of mice are equally susceptible to infection (12). The disease-susceptible C3H mouse has been used to define the kinetics of *B. burgdorferi* infection, disease pathogenesis, and mechanisms of persistence. Mice can be infected by syringe with cultured spirochetes, by transplantation of infected tissue (skin) from other mice, and by tick-borne transmission. These different forms of spirochetes represent organisms that have adapted to significantly different environmental conditions, with profound impact upon our understanding of the biology of this pathogen. Regardless of the infecting form of the spirochete, *B. burgdorferi* organisms disseminate following dermal inoculation, with evidence of distant tissue invasion within 4 to 5 days. Silver stains reveal that spirochetes penetrate the walls of small arteries and enter surrounding tissue, with a universal predilection for connective tissue, particularly the attachment sites of ligaments and tendons to bone, skin, and the great vessels at the base of the heart. Based upon silver staining, PCR, immunohistochemistry, in situ DNA hybridization, and culture, the onset of inflammation in joint and heart tissue is concomitant with the presence of invading spirochetes. Remarkably, spirochetes can invade other tissues, such as the skin, nervous system, and spleen, with minimal inflammation (21). These observations suggest that unique events are occurring in certain target tissues, thereby eliciting inflammation, whereas other tissues, which also contain visible spirochetes, may not have inflammation.

In the immunocompetent mouse, arthritis and carditis progress over the next 2 to 3 weeks and then undergo immune-mediated resolution. In the ensuing months, the mice remain persistently infected, with spirochetes readily detectable in their tissues but without active inflammation. At a year or more after infection, the skin is the most consistent site of infection (a logical outcome for a vector-borne agent). During the course of persistent infection, arthritis, carditis, and spirochetemia undergo periodic bouts of exacerbation and remission, reminiscent of relapsing fever (17). Unlike relapsing fever, however, where myriads of spirochetes appear in peripheral blood during relapses, there are only small numbers of spirochetes in peripheral blood in Lyme disease (152).

In the absence of acquired immunity, severe combined immunodeficient (SCID) mice develop progressively severe arthritis. In addition, carditis remains active (but does not become progressively severe) (22, 148). Thus, disease evolution is not mediated by acquired immune responses, but disease resolution is immune mediated. In both immunodeficient and immunocompetent mice, there is a predilection of spirochetes for specific tissues and a universal predilection for connective tissue, with particular tropism for the dermis at all stages of infection (17, 21).

HOST IMMUNITY DURING PERSISTENT INFECTION

Despite the fact that *B. burgdorferi* establishes persistent infection, the infected host develops demonstrably strong immune responses to infection. When serum from persistently infected, immunocompetent mice (immune serum) is transferred to naïve mice, remarkably small amounts of immune serum will provide protection against challenge with high doses of cultured spirochetes. Indeed, passive transfer of immune serum for up to 4 to 5 days after challenge inoculation with cultured spirochetes will actually eliminate early infection, but higher doses of immune sera fail to eliminate infection beyond that point (10, 16, 18). Similar protective activity can be demonstrated in sera of humans and dogs with natural Lyme disease, by passive immunization of mice (20, 67). When immune serum is transferred from persistently infected, immunocompetent mice into SCID mice with established infection and progressive disease, there is resolution of arthritis, but the tissues of the mice continue to be culture positive, the mice continue to be spirochetemic, and carditis remains active (16, 18).

Thus, immune serum from actively infected mice contains antibody directed against *B. burgdorferi* antigenic targets that effectively generates protective and disease-resolving immunity. In contrast to the potent passive protective and arthritis-resolving activity in immune serum from actively infected mice, hyperimmune serum, generated against killed, cultured spirochetes, is passively protective, but only if given prior to or at the time of challenge inoculation (but not after), requires much higher doses for protection, and does not resolve arthritis (16, 18). Furthermore, when immune serum is used to probe infected tissue, via indirect immunohistochemistry, spirochetes can be labeled in tissues of the joints and heart but apparently not other tissue (including

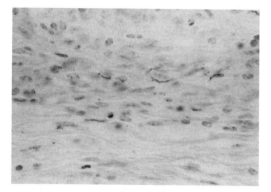

FIGURE 1 Indirect immunohistochemistry of joint tissue from an infected SCID mouse probed with immune serum from a *B. burgdorferi*-infected immunocompetent mouse. Immune serum contains antibodies that are reactive to spirochetes in joint tissue, but the target antigen(s) has not been implicated.

adjacent skin) (Fig. 1). When hyperimmune sera against cultured, heat-killed *B. burgdorferi* are used to probe tissues, spirochetes are not labeled (16).

These observations suggest that *B. burgdorferi* spirochetes express undefined antigens during infection and possibly express antigens within the specific context of selected tissues, such as the joints and heart. Because of the proinflammatory nature of lipoproteins (120), with which the spirochete is abundantly endowed, the antigens that are expressed in selected tissues during infection of the mammalian host may very well be eliciting the inflammation in the context of specific tissues and may very well be the targets that allow immune-mediated disease resolution but not cure of infection.

CLUES TO MECHANISMS OF PERSISTENCE IN THE BORRELIA GENOME

The genome of *B. burgdorferi* sensu stricto B31 has recently been sequenced as a prototype species. *B. burgdorferi* is unique among the eubacteria in that its genome is organized into a linear chromosome of approximately 910,000 bp and numerous (up to 20) linear and circular plasmids with a combined size of 530,000 bp (72). The presence of linear extrachromosomal elements ("minichromosomes") is similar to other borreliae but differs from other spirochetes, such as treponemae, which have no linear DNA (23). Borrelia plasmids are fundamentally different from plasmids of other bacteria in that they contain essential, rather than nonessential, extrachromosomal elements of the genome. This is true for both linear and circular plasmids of *B. burgdorferi* (167). The rather small genome size of *B. burgdorferi* can be attributed to the apparent absence of cellular biosynthetic pathways, with no genes for synthesis of amino acids, fatty acids, enzyme cofactors, or nucleotides, similar to Myoplasma. Many of its genes encode transport and binding proteins, allowing the organism to live within the mammalian or avian host. More than 6% of the chromosomal genes are involved in motility and chemotaxis. Nearly 40% of plasmid genes represent paralogs that form 47 gene families of unknown function. The uncommon degree of gene redundancy within extrachromosomal elements of the *B. burgdorferi* genome is puzzling. It is a paradox that 32-kb circular plasmids contain repetitive genetic material equivalent to nearly a fourth of the chromosome. These paralog families represent good candidates for a role in antigenic variation and immune evasion. Furthermore, the *B. burgdorferi* genome encodes approximately 150 outer surface (lipo)proteins (Osp), likely to be expressed on the cell membrane and to serve as the interface between the bacterium and host immunity. Most of the genes encoding Osp proteins are localized to linear or circular plasmids, underscoring the importance of extrachromosomal elements as key determinants for the biology of this organism. Clearly, attributing functions to the genes of *B. burgdorferi* is critical to understanding persistence.

EVIDENCE FOR GENE REARRANGEMENTS: MECHANISM FOR ANTIGENIC VARIATION?

Antigenic variation implies changes in structure or expression of antigens during persistent infection at a frequency greater than the spontaneous mutation rate (156). Antigenic variation through orderly gene rearrangement is a well-established phenomenon with *Borrelia hermsii*, a relapsing fever agent. *B. hermsii* relies upon a complex and sophisticated antigenic-variation mechanism. Surface-exposed lipoproteins, termed variable major proteins (Vmp), are encoded by homologous genes located in linear plasmids with covalently closed telomeres. These relapsing fever spirochetes contain at least 26 *vmp* genes, most of which remain unexpressed in "storage plasmids." Only one *vmp* gene, located near one of the telomeres of a different plasmid (the expression plasmid), is expressed at any given time. Antigenic variation occurs when the expressed *vmp* is replaced completely or partially by one of the silent *vmp* genes through interplasmid recombination and post-switch rearrangement (95, 183). These events occur spontaneously, allowing relapsing fever spirochetes to develop a selective advantage in an immunologically hostile environment (154).

Early studies with *B. burgdorferi* demonstrated changes in plasmid profiles and protein profiles among spirochetes isolated from persistently infected rodents (17, 153, 180). However, it is now known that *B. burgdorferi* isolates, particularly those derived from ticks, are mixed populations. Mixed infections have been documented in both ticks (30, 83) and mammals, including humans (85, 103, 111, 117). Natural tick-borne infection results in infections with mixed populations of *B. burgdorferi*, with variation in dominant subpopulations during persistent infection (85). However, when mice were experimentally infected with clonal populations of spirochetes, persistent infection resulted in subsequent isolation of organisms that had no overt genetic differences, based upon genomic macrorestriction analysis and fine sequence analysis of *ospA*, *ospB*, and *ospC* (127, 162).

These findings have not discouraged pursuit of the antigenic-variation hypothesis as an explanation for immune evasion and persistence. Notable in this regard is *ospC*, in that it is a highly heterogeneous gene among various isolates and species, and it shows evidence of having undergone extensive recombination (104, 110, 173, 174, 181). The 33-kDa Vmp of *B. hermsii* has more amino acid similarity to OspC than to other Vmp proteins of *B. hermsii*, and OspC has more similarity to Vmp33 than to other *B. burgdorferi* Osp proteins (OspA, OspB, and OspD). In addition, serological cross-reactivity exists between Vmp-33 and OspC (35). As noted above, *B. burgdorferi* causes somewhat similar relapsing features, so an analogy would be logical. However, *ospC* does not seem to undergo any genetic change during persistent infection. Analysis of spirochetes isolated from persistently infected mice, following original injection with a clonal inoculant of *B. burgdorferi* sensu stricto, revealed virtually no *ospC* gene variation (162). Although there is genetic evidence of recombination among *ospC* genes to explain the genetic diversity of *ospC* among *B. burgdorferi* isolates, it has been concluded that it is likely to be due to lateral transfer between spirochetes rather than to exchange of genetic material within a single organism (89, 104). Lateral transfer requires mixed infection in the tick or host, both of which have been well documented. Evidence for lateral gene exchange has also been found with *ospD*, but this gene is not required for infectivity or virulence (109, 122). There is also genetic evidence for recombination between *ospA* and *ospB* genes, with resulting deletions and chimeric fusions of gene segments (145), which may account for the diversity in decorin binding protein A (DbpA) (143). The phenomenon of lateral gene transfer and recombination may have selective advantages in mixed populations of spirochetes but does not provide an explanation for the immune evasion of clonal populations of spirochetes during persistent infection.

Simpson et al. (160) first described repeated DNA sequences that were associated with circular plasmids of *B. burgdorferi*, and they hypothesized that these gene families encoded functionally similar but antigenically distinct proteins. Other gene paralog families were noted with P39, or BmpA, a lipoprotein that is the product of one of four closely related tandomly arranged chromosomal genes of unknown function (5, 139, 159).

Genetic rearrangements among a diverse and repetitive family of genes have been described for the genes encoding the Erp (OspEF-related) proteins of *B. burgdorferi* and have also been suggested as a means for persistence and evasion of the immune response (165). The genes for OspE and OspF represent a bicistronic operon on the 45-kb linear plasmid (100). Investigation of OspE and OspF led to the discovery of additional loci that contain nonallelic paralogous genes related to *ospE* and *ospF*, which represent a closely related gene family designated *erp*. Two loci, *erpAB* and *erpCD*, are each bicistronic operons like *ospEF* but located on separate 32-kb circular plasmids. The *ospE*, *erpA*, and *erpC* genes are similar to one another, while the *ospF*, *erpB*, and *erpC* genes are divergent. Another locus, within a separate 32-kb circular plasmid, contains a single gene termed *erpG*, with a downstream *bapA* gene which lacks similarity to any of the *erp* genes (167). Examination of other "B31" isolates has revealed additional 32-kb circular plasmid genes that encode Erp proteins: *erpH*, *erpIJ*, *erpK*, and *erpL*. Similar multiple circular 32-kb plasmids containing *erp* genes are present among a variety of *B. burgdorferi* sensu stricto and sensu lato isolates (37). In studies utilizing *B. burgdorferi* sensu stricto B31, recombinants among these plasmids have not been found in bacteria maintained either in culture or through a tick-mouse cycle (37), but evidence for recombination involving both individual genes and entire *erp* loci has been found (165). These genes share a conserved upstream control sequence element that may represent an environmentally cued regulon (170). It has been postulated that the sizes, gene orders, and transcription patterns of the 32-kb circular plasmids resemble those of prophages, with precedent for lysogenic bacteriophage-carried genes playing a role in the interaction of pathogenic bacteria with their hosts (36, 40).

Another genetic locus (2.9 locus) has at least seven copies within circular plasmids of *B. burgdorferi* sensu stricto 297 (133). Each locus contains an operon of four genes (*ABCD*) and open reading frames, designated *rep*⁺ and *rep*⁻, which encode multiple repeat motifs. Downstream from the *rep*⁺ genes are two distinct (genetic and antigenic) classes of lipoprotein genes possessing similar signal sequences but variable mature polypeptides. The *ABCD* operon has a single upstream promoter, but a number of promoters appear to regulate the lipoprotein genes. Elements of this complex gene family appear to be separately transcribed, suggesting that they are functionally unrelated, despite their conserved genetic organization. The repetitiveness, diversity, and complexity of the 2.9 gene locus family, for reasons yet to be determined, must play a role in the survival and adaptability of this spirochete.

Recently, a homologous genetic locus, termed *vmp*-like sequence (*vls*), has been identified in *B. burgdorferi* because of its similarity to the *vmp* genes of *B. hermsii*. A *vls* expression site (*vlsE*) and 15 additional silent *vls* cassettes were found on a 28-kb linear plasmid (lp28-1). During infection of mice with *B. burgdorferi* sensu stricto B31, it was revealed that portions of several of the silent *vls* cassette regions recombined into the central *vlsE* cassette region, resulting in antigenic variation of the expressed lipoprotein (183). Although this is intriguing, it remains to be determined whether this gene complex is involved in biologically relevant antigenic variation that has significance for immune evasion in a manner equivalent to that manifested by relapsing fever borrelia. There is evidence that isolates lacking this plasmid have lost their infectivity, suggesting, at the very least, that this complex may be needed in some way for invasion and dissemination within the host (183). The *vlsE* gene has been shown to undergo extensive genetic (and antigenic) variation within 28 days of infection of mice. Sequence changes were apparent within 4 days of infection and occurred in both SCID and immunocompetent mice, but no sequence changes were detected in spirochetes cultured in vitro for up to 84 days (184). These studies suggest that *vlsE* changes are prompted by infection of the host but are not induced by adaptive immune responses. The significance of the *vlsE* complex for persistence remains to be elucidated.

PERSISTENCE VIA ANTIGENIC VARIATION

Based upon the above discussion, it appears incontrovertible that *B. burgdorferi* undergoes genetic variation, but it is unclear whether this variation is a means to avoid immune clearance, analogous to that of *B. hermsii*. The most likely candidate gene products for this activity, OspC, Erp proteins, the 2.9 locus, and Vls, all show evidence that these proteins are expressed in the mammalian host and stimulate serum antibody responses during infection (2, 38, 48, 77, 126, 169, 176, 183, 184). OspC does not appear to undergo any genetic change during infection (162). Erp proteins are more intriguing. Experimentally infected mice seroconvert to OspE during early infection and to OspF during later stages of infection (100). Other, but not all, members of the Erp family appear to be expressed preferentially in vivo (2, 38, 164, 169, 176). In one study, seroconversion and reverse transcription (RT)-PCR data suggested that ErpG (P21, or PG) was not expressed during the first few weeks of infection in laboratory mice but was upregulated during later stages of infection (48). The Rev protein of the 2.9 gene locus family also stimulates antibody responses following tick-borne infection (77), but the relevance to antigenic variation has not been determined. Notably, the Vls proteins also elicit antibody responses during infection (77), and the rate of genetic change among Vls variants is higher in the immunologically intact mouse than in immunodeficient SCID mice (184).

The proof of the pudding for antigenic variation is whether antigenic changes in spirochetes provide selective advantages for the variant subpopulation in evading immune clearance. No evidence for this phenomenon has been observed with *B. burgdorferi*. Indeed, there is strong evidence to negate a role for antigenic variation as a significant means of immune evasion by *B. burgdorferi*. Mice that had immunizing infections with a clonal population of *B. burgdorferi*, followed by antibiotic sterilization, were completely resistant to reinfection by inoculation with the original clonal inoculant or by *B. burgdorferi* isolated from ear biopsies 90 days after infection (prior to antibiotic treatment), including autologous *B. burgdorferi* isolates. By necessity, that experiment required growth of the original and "late" isolates of *B. burgdorferi* in vitro, which could have obscured any antigenic change in vivo. Therefore, using the same approach, additional mice were immunized by infection, treated with antibiotics, and then challenged by subcutaneous autografts of ear skin pieces that had been biopsied and frozen prior to antibiotic treatment. The mice were infected for 15, 90, or 180 days before biopsy and antibiotic treatment. Control (nonimmune) mice were susceptible to infection with skin transplants, whereas immune mice were resistant to infection following autograft challenge, regardless of the interval of biopsy (10). In addition, immune sera from mice that were persistently infected for 1 year, when passively transferred to naïve mice, had equal titers of protective activity against either the original clonal inoculant or *B. burgdorferi* isolates obtained from mice infected for 1 year (15). These studies suggest no discernible antigenic advantage for *B. burgdorferi* isolates obtained from persistently infected, immunocompetent hosts.

PERSISTENCE VIA ANTIGENIC MODULATION

In contrast to the lack of firm evidence for antigenic variation as a significant means of evading immune clearance, there is much stronger evidence for antigenic modulation by *B. burgdorferi*. Antigenic modulation refers to variation in the expression of antigens as a means of evading immune clearance. In the case of *B. burgdorferi*, there is also a strong case for antigenic modulation as a means of adapting to different environments. *B. burgdorferi* must adapt to vastly different environments within the resting (unfed or flat) tick, the feeding tick, and the mammalian host. Part of this adaptation must incorporate a mechanism by which immunologically vulnerable antigen targets on the outer membrane of the organism do not preclude the critical acts of transmission or persistence. Indeed, the *B. burgdorferi* genome potentially encodes over 150 lipoproteins (72) that could be expressed in the lipidated outer membrane of the spirochete and are likely to be highly immunogenic. It is the lipidated moieties of *B. burgdorferi* Osp proteins that elicit a variety of proinflammatory responses (56, 62, 76, 106, 116, 120, 121, 137, 171, 178, 182) and that act as adjuvants to the appended protein (63). This abundance of proinflammatory and immunogenic lipoproteins must be important to the spirochete, but their presence is counter to the spirochete's best interests for surviving immune-mediated attack.

OspA has been singularly critical in unraveling the mysteries of *B. burgdorferi* biology in the tick and the mammalian host. OspA has been estimated to represent nearly 30% of the total protein of *B. burgdorferi* when cultured in vitro (43). On protein gels, OspA is a major component of the spirochete, and it is obvious why this protein drew early attention as a possible vaccine candidate. When OspA was initially described, it was shown to be on the outer surfaces of the spirochetes in culture and on spirochetes in the midguts of flat (unfed, or resting) ticks (9). Paradoxically, human patients (and dogs) with naturally acquired Lyme disease do not seroconvert to OspA or may seroconvert only after months of infection (1, 20, 61, 91). The lack of OspA antibody during naturally acquired infection was confirmed in a variety of experimental-animal species, including monkeys, dogs, mice, and hamsters, following tick-borne infection (75, 79, 129, 144).

Despite this evidence, efforts to develop OspA as a potential vaccine were not deterred. Active immunization with recombinant OspA, or passive immunization with OspA hyperimmune serum or OspA monoclonal antibodies, protected laboratory mice against challenge infection with cultured *B. burgdorferi* (65, 147). This immediately led to debate that tick-borne spirochetes might be different (partially based upon the argument that tick-borne infection did not elicit an OspA antibody response in humans) and therefore the vaccine might fail against tick-borne challenge. Experiments with mice confirmed that OspA vaccination was protective against tick-borne challenge, leading to the long road of clinical trials in humans; confirmatory studies showed that OspA vaccination protected against tick-borne challenge in a range of species, including hamsters, dogs, and monkeys, and against a broad range of *B. burgdorferi* isolates (39, 46, 65, 70, 74, 90, 105, 130, 136).

The immunogenicity of OspA following vaccination (proof of its protective effect against tick-borne challenge) but the lack of seroconversion to OspA following natural infection prompted examination of spirochetes within ticks and the mammalian host. These studies confirmed original observations (9) that OspA was abundantly expressed by spirochetes in the midguts of flat ticks (53) (Fig. 2). When the midguts of ticks were examined following their feeding on OspA-vaccinated mice, direct killing of spirochetes was seen within the ticks (Fig. 3), with apparent "cure" of the ticks following the subsequent molt (53, 69). This prompted further investigation of OspA expression by spirochetes in the tick. Spirochetes in the flat tick are located principally

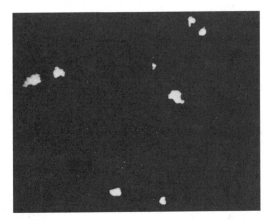

FIGURE 3 Indirect immunofluorescence of the midgut of a tick that has fed upon a mouse immunized with OspA. Ingestion of OspA antibody has killed *B. burgdorferi* organisms, with no viable spirochetes remaining in the midgut. (Reprinted from reference 69.)

within the midgut, where they aggregate along the microvillar brush border and between gut epithelial cells, with only small numbers of spirochetes infecting other tick tissues (31, 33). Within hours of tick attachment and commencement of feeding, spirochetes penetrate the gut wall and disseminate to the salivary glands (51, 140, 186). Using different approaches, other laboratories showed that OspA was rapidly shed (downregulated?) during tick feeding, with most spirochetes in the gut and salivary glands of the feeding tick being OspA-negative within 24 h of attachment (Fig. 4) (34, 54, 71, 155). Thus, spirochetes entering the mammalian host during tick feeding do not express significant amounts of OspA, and spirochetes that invade and disseminate within the mammalian host also do not express significant amounts of OspA, thereby explaining why naturally infected humans (and dogs) do not seroconvert to this protein.

To confirm the hypothesis that host-adapted spirochetes do not express OspA during infection, mice were hyperimmunized against OspA, and then challenged with equivalent doses of cultured spirochetes or with spirochetes within transplants of infected skin from donor mice, with the hypothesis that spi-

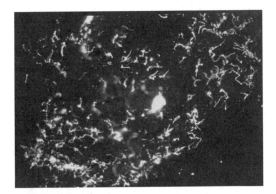

FIGURE 2 Indirect immunofluorescence of the midgut of a flat (resting) tick labeled with antiserum to *B. burgdorferi* OspA. Spirochetes within the midgut of the tick are strongly reactive with OspA antibody. (Reprinted from reference 69.)

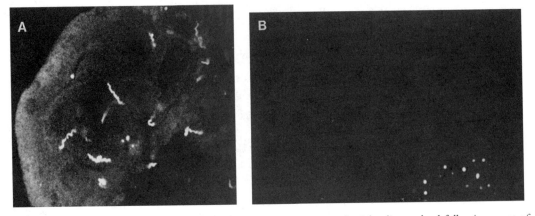

FIGURE 4 Indirect immunofluorescence and confocal microscopy of a tick salivary gland following onset of feeding, demonstrating loss of OspA following migration to salivary glands during feeding. Spirochetes are labeled with antiserum to *B. burgdorferi* (A) but are not labeled with antiserum to OspA (B). (With permission from E. Fikrig.)

rochetes that had adapted to the host (transplant origin) had downregulated OspA. Mice immunized against OspA were resistant to challenge with cultured spirochetes (which express OspA) but were fully susceptible to challenge with transplants of tissue containing host-adapted spirochetes (which do not express OspA). Spirochetes introduced by transplantation disseminated and caused disease, unfettered by OspA immunity (19). Subsequent passive-immunization studies in which OspA hyperimmune sera were administered to mice at intervals relative to tick attachment and feeding showed that OspA antibody protection was effective against tick-borne challenge for up to 24 h after tick attachment but was ineffective against tick challenge at 48 or more hours. The OspA-mediated protection directly correlated with the presence of OspA on spirochetes while they remained in the midguts of the ticks (52, 53). Notably, OspA immunity in the host also precludes successful acquisition of infection by the feeding tick by killing incoming spirochetes as they upregulate OspA in the process of adapting to the new environment of the tick midgut (55). In the final analysis, therefore, OspA antibody is indeed antithetical to the welfare of *B. burgdorferi*.

The OspA story awakened the scientific community to the fact that *B. burgdorferi* is a very dynamic organism that must rapidly adapt to vastly different environments (resting tick, feeding tick, and mammalian host). It was simultaneously discovered that other proteins, such as OspC, are upregulated during feeding in ticks and within the mammalian host (53, 71, 155). The cues that stimulate these dramatic changes in Osp expression by spirochetes remain undefined, but the onset of feeding by ticks and increased temperature are two factors known to upregulate OspC (155, 166). Increased temperature-related differential expression of other Osp proteins has also been documented in vitro, including upregulation of OspE, OspF, and other Erp proteins (164, 166). Growth phase and cell density in culture also influence protein expression in *B. burgdorferi*. Lipoprotein P35 and a 7.5-kDa lipoprotein (whose open reading frame is downstream from *p35*) are upregulated at the onset of stationary phase in vitro (88). Further studies have shown that at least 13 additional genes, including *ospC*, *bmpD*, and *groEL*, were upregulated, a gene encoding a 28-kDa protein was downregulated, and *ospA*, *ospB*, *p72*, *flagellin*, and *bmpA* remained unchanged during the transition from logarithmic to stationary phase in culture (138). These observations represent a small window on the complex biology of differential gene expression by *B. burgdorferi* in the flat and feeding tick.

Other than OspA and OspC, differential expression of other *B. burgdorferi* proteins within the flat and feeding tick have not been extensively evaluated. Immunization of mice against OspE and OspF resulted in partial destruction of spirochetes within feeding ticks and partial protection of some mice against tick-borne infection (118). Based upon immunolabeling, it has been shown that P21, a member of the Erp family, is expressed by spirochetes in mice but not in flat or feeding ticks, whereas OspE is expressed by spirochetes in flat and feeding ticks (48).

BIOLOGICALLY RELEVANT ANTIGENS

The phenomena of antibody-mediated protective immunity, and probably antibody-mediated arthritis resolution, are universal among the members of the *B. burgdorferi* sensu lato complex but are species specific, so immunity in mice infected with one *B. burgdorferi* species does not cross protect against challenge with an unrelated species (13). Because of these antibody-mediated events that evolve in response to active infection, immune serum can be used as a mirror to reflect what the host encounters antigenically during infection with *B. burgdorferi*. It would seem intuitive that probing *B. burgdorferi* lysates with immune serum would identify the antigens that seem to be eliciting these biologically relevant antibodies. When laboratory mice were infected for as little as 2 weeks with *B. burgdorferi* sensu stricto N40, their sera contained protective and arthritis-resolving activities. When these early sera, with demonstrable biological activity, were reacted against *B. burgdorferi* lysates on single-dimension immunoblots, a limited repertoire of antigens was labeled, including BmpA (P39), OspC, and flagellin (18). However, none of these antigens, at least in recombinant form, elicit antibody that possesses protective or arthritis-resolving activity against *B. burgdorferi* sensu stricto N40 (18). An exception to this

statement is OspC, which can induce protective immunity against a homologous strain of *B. burgdorferi* but is not cross protective (25, 136). In addition, OspC protection against a homologous *B. burgdorferi* sensu stricto isolate is variable and does not protect against some homologous strains, such as *B. burgdorferi* sensu stricto N40 (18, 25). In a single study, passive immunization of SCID mice with OspC hyperimmune sera revealed cure of infection and disease (*B. burgdorferi* sensu stricto ZS7) (185), but this has not been repeated with other strains of *B. burgdorferi*. With the exception of that single study, the very strong protective and arthritis-resolving activities in immune serum cannot be attributed to OspC and most certainly cannot be attributed to OspC with *B. burgdorferi* sensu stricto N40.

Thus, the protective and disease-modulating antibodies that are present in immune sera are directed against unidentified antigens that are not apparent on single-dimension immunoblots for which cultured spirochetes were used as the antigen substrate. This could be explained by a number of possibilities, including comigration (and thus masking) of target proteins by flagellin, BmpA, or OspC; differential expression of target proteins in vivo (thus not being expressed by cultured spirochetes, which serve as the antigen substrate in vitro); or the fact that the target antigens are not proteins, or that protective epitopes are conformational, so that denaturation and processing of native antigens may preclude detection.

All of these possibilities may be valid. OspC, with a molecular mass of approximately 22 to 24 kDa, comigrates with, and thus obscures, a number of other similarly sized proteins of *B. burgdorferi* that are known to elicit antibody during infection (reviewed in reference 64). Decorin binding proteins (Dbp) A and B are illustrative. They comigrate with OspC but are highly immunogenic and elicit early antibody responses during infection. Indeed, much of the seroreactivity attributed to OspC on Western blots may be due to reactivity to DbpA (64, 84). Immunization with DbpA, and to a lesser extent DbpB, elicits protective immunity against syringe-borne challenge, and immunization studies suggest that passive immunization with antibody to DbpA will eliminate infection up to 4 days after syringe challenge inoculation (84). This fits the pattern of protective activity of immune serum (15). Studies to examine tick-borne challenge of DbpA-immunized mice and expression of DbpA in flat or feeding ticks are needed. DbpA does not elicit immunity that can induce arthritis resolution in either passive- or active-immunization experiments (64). These DbpA data provide evidence that protective immunity and arthritis-resolving immunity may be mediated by different antigenic targets.

There is also growing evidence that *B. burgdorferi* expresses antigens exclusively in vivo and that these antigens have therefore gone undetected on immunoblots that utilize cultured spirochetes as the antigen substrate. Immune sera from infected mice (and humans) have been used to probe *B. burgdorferi* sensu stricto genomic expression libraries, revealing a number of clones with genes expressing immunoreactive proteins that are upregulated during mammalian infection (169, 176). Alternate approaches have likewise revealed in vivo-expressed antigens (2, 38). Notably, most of these in vivo-expressed antigens are paralogs of the Erp family. Alternatively, as with OspA, other proteins appear to be downregulated in vivo (99).

Investigation of the temporal sequence of OspE and P21 (an Erp) expression in infected mouse tissue by RT-PCR and by seroconversion has found that OspE is expressed during early infection whereas P21 is expressed at later intervals (48). Serological evidence also suggests a temporal difference in expression of OspE and OspF, with seroconversion to OspE occurring earlier than that to OspF (even though these antigens are expressed in vitro and in the tick) (100, 118). A recently discovered protein, ErpT, has been shown not to be expressed (based upon RT-PCR) by cultured spirochetes, to be expressed in flat ticks, but not to be expressed in engorged ticks. Analysis of mouse tissues during infection suggested that

ErpT expression did not occur in the skin during early infection but became upregulated in other tissues, but not the skin, during later stages of infection. ErpT elicited an antibody response during infection but did not elicit protective or disease-resolving immunity. These studies demonstrated the possibility that *B. burgdorferi* genes are differentially expressed in a temporal as well as tissue-specific fashion within the infected host (68).

Two unrelated gene products, P35 and P37, have also been shown to be expressed in vivo. Their genes are located on different plasmids, and one (p37) encodes a lipoprotein. Both antigens stimulate early antibody responses in infected mice. RT-PCR of infected mouse tissue suggested that neither gene was expressed at the site of inoculation at 48 h, but at 7 days and beyond, tissues at the site of inoculation as well as distant sites (infected with disseminated spirochetes) became p37 positive. Active and passive immunization of mice against P35 and P37 induced partial protective immunity against syringe challenge, and protective immunity was enhanced by immunization against both antigens (66).

Differential expression of *B. burgdorferi* proteins in vivo is now well established, but the dogma of strict in vivo expression is not likely to be absolute. As noted earlier, different culture and environmental conditions could very well stimulate differential gene expression by these organisms. It is apparent, however, that *B. burgdorferi* preferentially expresses certain gene products in vivo. OspC and BmpA are notable in this regard, but their functions have not been determined. Other gene products have been ascribed a function, such as DbpA, which binds decorin on collagen, a logical function given the organism's propensity for collagenous connective tissue and dermis. Immunization against DbpA appears to prevent dissemination from the site of inoculation (64; unpublished observations). *B. burgdorferi* proteins bind a number of host ligands with logical hypothetical functions for invasion, dissemination, and tissue tropism, including plasminogen (44, 86), fibronectin (82), glycosaminoglycans (heparan sulfate and dermatan sulfate) (102), integrins (42), and glycosphingolipids (7).

Regardless of function, many of these activities are mediated by surface-exposed lipoproteins that in turn are likely to stimulate host immune responses that are deleterious to the spirochete. DbpA and DbpB, its bicistronic partner, stimulate early and very strong antibody responses following syringe and tick-borne infection, and both passive and active immunization with these proteins stimulates a protective immune response against syringe challenge (64, 84). OspC, which is upregulated during early infection, can likewise stimulate protective immune responses (at least with some *B. burgdorferi* isolates or strains) (25, 136). Thus, it appears as if *B. burgdorferi* must express immunologically vulnerable antigens upon its surface in order to successfully invade and disseminate within the host. It therefore must accomplish this before immune clearance and then cease expression of these antigens or develop other means of evasion.

Titration of the protective antibody response in immune serum from actively infected mice reveals a rapid rise in titer during early infection, peak titers within 2 to 4 weeks, and then progressive decline in titer over the course of persistent infection (15). These kinetics suggest that the inciting antigen(s) is expressed during early infection and then becomes occult to the immune system once the persistent phase of infection is established. This is not true for overall antibody responses to *B. burgdorferi* lysates, which rise during early infection and persist (64). Thus, the immune response continues to recognize *B. burgdorferi* antigens, but the most immunologically vulnerable antigens (yet to be determined), which stimulate strong protective immunity, may be downregulated or masked following the essential function of dissemination in the preimmune phase of infection.

AN IMMUNOLOGICAL SHELL GAME

Elicitation of strong protective immunity, induced by active infection of the mammalian host, would seem to be deleterious to successful transmission of spirochetes from the host to the vector and from the vector to the host. However, spirochetes readily infect ticks following their feeding upon persistently infected mice, although the rate of transmission may be somewhat lower during late infection than during early infection. There is no adverse effect on spirochetal infectivity to ticks which feed on mice with high levels of spirochetal antibody (157). As noted above, immune serum from actively infected mice contains potent protective antibody if that serum is passively transferred to mice that are challenged by syringe with cultured spirochetes. However, when immune serum with a high titer of protective activity (against cultured spirochetes) is passively transferred to mice prior to challenge by tick-borne infection or challenge with host-adapted spirochetes, the mice become infected. Host-adapted spirochetes can be introduced by transplantation of skin containing infectious organisms from an infected donor mouse or by syringe inoculation with spirochetes that were grown within 0.1-μm-pore-size filter chambers implanted in the peritoneal cavities of uninfected donor mice (52). Chamber-derived spirochetes undergo antigenic modulation, with loss of OspA (S. Nazario and F. Kantor, personal communication). Passive transfer of immune serum to mice at 4 days after challenge inoculation eliminates infection following syringe inoculation with cultured spirochetes but has no effect on spirochetes introduced by transplantation. The resistance of tick- and host-adapted spirochetes to the protective activity of immune serum cannot be overcome with high doses of immune serum, but OspA antiserum prevents tick-borne infection. In these experiments, although mice became infected when challenged by tick-, transplant-, or chamber-derived spirochetes, the presence of immune serum did not prevent dissemination of spirochetes within the mouse but did abrogate arthritis (52).

These results highlight the importance of the quality of the immune serum. Immune sera generated by the infection of mice by transplant, tick, or syringe inoculation with cultured spirochetes all contain protective activity against syringe-borne cultured-spirochete challenge (13). It is the process of active infection, not the nature of the inoculum, that determines the protective activity in immune sera from actively infected mice, but the protective activity is effective only against challenge with cultured organisms. This suggests that the target antigens for protective immunity are present on cultured spirochetes (rather than expressed exclusively in vivo), but host-adapted spirochetes, or spirochetes entering the host via the tick, have devised a means by which they are no longer vulnerable to the effects of immune serum.

The OspA story tells us that the spirochetes within the midgut of the feeding tick are vulnerable to the effects of appropriately targeted (OspA) antibody, but OspA is not expressed in the host, so antibody deleterious to the spirochete is usually not generated. On the other hand, spirochetes departing the tick via the salivary glands seem to have achieved a status of invulnerability to the potent effects of immune serum. This is evolutionary intelligence at its best.

Not all of the host's defenses reside in antibody. In studies utilizing SCID mice and adoptive lymphocyte transfer, T cells did not provide protection but transfer of T and B cells, or B cells alone, did (57, 149). Nevertheless, actively immunized, immunocompetent mice that have had an immunizing infection and are then treated with antibiotic are resistant to challenge by syringe, by transplantation of infected tissue, or by tick-borne challenge (13, 132). This bodes well for developing strategies against tick-borne spirochetes.

The search for biologically relevant antigens that drive protective and disease-resolving immunity continues, but the antigens have not been defined, despite extensive efforts to implicate them by probing genomic expression libraries with immune serum. It may be a matter of time and luck to identify these antigens among the "haystack" of immunoreactive antigens. On the other hand, the inability to identify relevant antigens may be due to a lack of appropriate conformational epitopes on recombinant proteins, or it may be that the target antigens are not proteins. Nonprotein *B. burgdorferi* antigens, including lipooligosaccharides, have been shown to react with sera from patients with Lyme disease. These antigens, which are in nonaqueous fractions of the organism, are not likely to be present in aqueous whole-cell lysate antigens used for enzyme-linked immunosorbent assay or immunoblotting, thereby also escaping detection by antibody screening (41, 179).

ALTERNATIVE THEORIES FOR IMMUNE EVASION

A popular explanation for *B. burgdorferi* persistence and immune evasion has been intracellular localization, or sequestration in an immunologically privileged site. Proof of this assertion has been largely based upon in vitro studies, which have little relevance to life in a host. Nevertheless, spirochetes have been shown to enter a variety of cultured cell types, including endothelial cells, synovial cells, macrophages, and fibroblasts (28, 45, 78, 97, 114). Most spirochetes that encounter macrophages in vitro are killed, whether they are opsonized or not (112, 113), which is in keeping with immunohistochemical localization of spirochetes in the hearts of infected mice, where intracellular forms are particulate and degrading (4). More convincing evidence of intracellular localization is the observation by electron microscopy of spirochetes within cardiac endothelial cells and myocytes of infected mice (124). Although this could explain persistence in the presence of host immunity, a more intriguing observation is the consistent finding of fully elongated, extracellular spirochetes in the dermis of mice infected for 1 year. Indeed, every mouse examined had discernible organisms in the collagen of the dermis after 1 year of persistent infection (17). Others (49) have likewise found no evidence of intracellular localization of spirochetes in tissues of immunodeficient mice, whereas extracellular forms were abundant. Clearly, *B. burgdorferi*, although capable of intracellular life (probably due to its invasive propensity), typically lives in the extracellular milieu.

The dermatotropism of spirochetes during persistent infection makes evolutionary sense for the pathogen, since skin is the host–vector interface. In studies with persistently infected mice, skin was the most consistently infected tissue, based upon culture, PCR, and silver staining (17). The predilection of spirochetes for collagenous connective tissue (including the dermis) may provide a novel mechanism for persistence. It has been proposed that the paucity of spirochetes in fluids relative to their abundance in viscous tissue may be explained by the physical properties of collagenous tissue ground substance. In studies that examined the motility of *B. burgdorferi* in fluids of varying viscosity, spirochetes were found to migrate most rapidly through viscous matrices (94). It was proposed that the ability of spirochetes to migrate rapidly through viscous substances, such as skin, may assist their escape from host inflammatory and immune responses. Indeed, phagocytes are not as motile within viscous tissues and may be incapable of "catching up with" their prey. It is difficult to directly discern the motility of spirochetes within tissues. Morphological elements of silver-stained *B. burgdorferi* in the skin of mice indicate elongated rather than spiral forms and the presence of bulbous ends on the organism (17, 21). This pattern is in keeping with a "forward-and-reverse" motility of spirochetes, as illustrated in published figures (80) and more readily demonstrated on videotapes of motile *B. burgdorferi* organisms (N. Charon, personal communication).

An unexplained behavior of *B. burgdorferi* is the phenomenon of "blebbing." Blebs, or extracellular membrane-bound vesicles, are structures that are shed from the surface of the spirochete. The protein content of these structures is related to the membrane protein content of intact organisms, and the blebs contain plasmid but not chromosomal DNA (73, 158). A possibly related phenomenon is "target imbalance." When PCR is utilized to detect *B. burgdorferi* in tissues or exudates, plasmid-encoded DNA targets are far more sensitive than chromosomally encoded DNA targets. This has been noted in synovial fluid from patients with Lyme disease (128), as well as experimentally infected mice (108). Blebs, which contain plasmid but not chromosomal DNA, may explain this phenomenon. The physiological role of blebbing and how it relates to immune evasion and persistence have yet to be determined. It may be a mechanism by which the spirochete sheds potentially harmful host factors, such as antibody, or a mechanism by which the spirochete can rapidly eliminate surface elements as it adapts to different environments (tick-, host-, and host tissue-specific antigen modulation).

B. burgdorferi is also capable of incorporating a number of host proteins (and other substances) into its outer membrane. This is well illustrated by its plasminogen binding activity (44, 96). Nonspecific immunoglobulin M binding to the outer surface of *B. burgdorferi* has been reported (60), and *B. burgdorferi* spirochetes also bind lymphocyte antigens (58). A striking but not yet fully explained phenomenon is invasion of both T and B lymphocytes by spirochetes. This may cause transient or sustained immunosuppression via lymphocyte killing (59) and could explain the transient immunosuppression that has been demonstrated in the early phase of infection of laboratory mice (57).

OBSCURED IMMUNOGENICITY: THE STEALTH BOMBER HYPOTHESIS

It is becoming increasingly apparent that *B. burgdorferi* does not necessarily express significant amounts of immunogenic lipoproteins on its surface during persistent infection of the host. Cryosection immuno-electron microscopy and cell fractionation studies have suggested that only minor amounts of lipoproteins are exposed on the outer membrane. Analysis of the outer and inner membranes of spirochetes indicates that the majority of protein is associated with the inner membrane (24) and that proteins associated with the outer membrane, including OspC, may have only limited surface exposure (47). *B. burgdorferi* spirochetes have significantly lower protein-to-lipid ratios in their outer membranes than gram-negative bacteria, and membrane lipoproteins are immunogenic but are membrane anchored by N-terminal lipids and may be predominantly tethered to the inner leaflet of the outer membrane, thereby being less accessible to antibody. One hypothesis is that spirochetes may possess a secretory apparatus for translocating lipoproteins across the outer membrane for surface exposure when needed. In addition, those polypeptides that are membrane spanning are less abundant and are poorly immunogenic (47).

There are also a number of publications that document B. burgdorferi L-form variants, spheroplasts, or cystic forms (26, 29, 87, 135). These forms have defective cell walls and are beta-lactam antibiotic resistant (150). They do not expose several known surface antigens (87), making them potentially antigenically inert. They can be induced in vitro by antibiotics in the medium (93, 150), the presence of antibody (146), the absence of serum (27), changes in pH, metabolites, and aging (32). These are all in vitro phenomena, but cystic forms have been documented in tissues from infected humans (87, 107). When spirochetes are inoculated into spinal fluid, they convert to cyst forms within 24 h and can be converted back to motile forms following placement in BSK-H medium (26). Recently, a method for culturing cell wall-deficient B. burgdorferi from the blood of patients with chronic Lyme disease was described and revealed an astonishingly high rate of infection (131). This study demonstrated that B. burgdorferi may be maintained in the blood in an altered state which cannot be cultured on routine media. Could antigenically inert L forms, which periodically revert to motile, invasive forms that express proinflammatory antigens, explain the relapsing course of B. burgdorferi infection?

CONCLUSION

This review has documented evidence for B. burgdorferi persistence and has discussed a number of potential mechanisms by which the Lyme disease spirochete can evade host immunity. Hopefully, this review also reinforces the fact that the scientific community has a long way to go before mechanisms of host-agent interactions during persistent infection with B. burgdorferi are fully understood. The Lyme disease story has not ended with the advent of a recombinant OspA vaccine, which can only prevent, but not abrogate, infection or disease. Persistent infection and chronic Lyme disease remain crucial but difficult issues for biomedical research. B. burgdorferi offers very well-defined model systems and techniques for incisive investigation of these issues. The major roadblock in understanding B. burgdorferi pathogenesis is the current inability to genetically manipulate the pathogen, but inroads are being made in this regard (163).

REFERENCES

1. Aguero-Rosenfeld, M. E., J. Nowakowski, D. F. McKenna, C. A. Carbonaro, and G. P. Wormser. 1993. Serodiagnosis in early Lyme disease. J. Clin. Microbiol. 31:3090–3095.
2. Akins, D. R., S. F. Porcella, T. G. Popova, D. Shevchenko, S. I. Baker, M. Li, M. V. Norgard, and J. D. Radolf. 1995. Evidence for in vivo but not in vitro expression of a Borrelia burgdorferi outer surface protein F (OspF) homologue. Mol. Microbiol. 18:507–520.
3. Anderson, J. F., and L. A. Magnarelli. 1993. Epizootiology of Lyme disease-causing borreliae. Clin. Dermatol. 11:339–351.
4. Armstrong, A. L., S. W. Barthold, D. H. Persing, and D. S. Beck. 1992. Carditis in Lyme disease susceptible and resistant strains of laboratory mice infected with Borrelia burgdorferi. Am. J. Trop. Med. Hyg. 47:249–258.
5. Aron, L., M. Alekshun, L. Perlee, I. Schwartz, H. Godfrey, and F. Cabello. 1994. Cloning and DNA sequence analysis of bmpC, a gene encoding a potential membrane lipoprotein of Borrelia burgdorferi. FEMS Microbiol. Lett. 123:75–82.
6. Asbrink, E., and A. Hovmark. 1985. Successful cultivation of spirochetes from skin lesions of patients with erythema chronica migrans afzelius and acrodermatitis chonica atrophicans. Acta Pathol. Microbiol. Immunol. Scand. 93:161–163.
7. Backenson, P. B., J. L. Coleman, and J. L. Benach. 1995. Borrelia burgdorferi shows specificity of binding to glycosphingolipids. Infect. Immun. 63:2811–2817.
8. Balmelli, T., and J. C. Piffaretti. 1995. Association between different clinical manifestations of

Lyme disease and different species of *Borrelia burgdorferi* sensu lato. *Res. Microbiol.* **146:**329–340.

9. **Barbour, A. G., S. L. Tessier, and W. J. Todd.** 1983. Lyme disease spirochetes and Ixodid tick spirochetes share a common surface antigenic determinant defined by monoclonal antibody. *Infect. Immun.* **41:**795–804.

10. **Barthold, S. W.** 1993. Antigenic stability of *Borrelia burgdorferi* during chronic infections of immunocompetent mice. *Infect. Immun.* **61:**4955–4961.

11. **Barthold, S. W.** 1996. The globilisation of Lyme borreliosis. *Lancet* **348:**1603–1604.

12. **Barthold, S. W.** 1991. Infectivity of *Borrelia burgdorferi* relative to route of inoculation and genotype in laboratory mice. *J. Infect. Dis.* **163:**419–420.

13. **Barthold, S. W.** 1999. Specificity of infection-induced immunity among *Borrelia burgdorferi* sensu lato species. *Infect. Immun.* **67:**36–42.

14. **Barthold, S. W.** 1998. Spirochetes, ticks, and DNA. *Parasitol. Today* **14:**444.

15. **Barthold, S. W., and L. K. Bockenstedt.** 1993. Passive immunizing activity of sera from mice infected with *Borrelia burgdorferi*. *Infect. Immun.* **61:**4696–4702.

16. **Barthold, S. W., M. deSouza, and S. Feng.** 1996. Serum-mediated resolution of Lyme arthritis in mice. *Lab. Investig.* **74:**57–67.

17. **Barthold, S. W., M. S. deSouza, J. L. Janotka, A. L. Smith, and D. H. Persing.** 1993. Chronic Lyme borreliosis in the laboratory mouse. *Am. J. Pathol.* **143:**951–971.

18. **Barthold, S. W., S. Feng, L. K. Bockenstedt, E. Fikrig, and K. Feen.** 1997. Protective and arthritis-resolving activity in serum from mice infected with *Borrelia burgdorferi*. *Clin. Infect. Dis.* **25:**S9–S17.

19. **Barthold, S. W., E. Fikrig, L. K. Bockenstedt, and D. H. Persing.** 1995. Circumvention of outer surface protein A immunity by host-adapted *Borrelia burgdorferi*. *Infect. Immun.* **63:**2255–2261.

20. **Barthold, S. W., S. A. Levy, E. Fikrig, L. K. Bockenstedt, and A. L. Smith.** 1995. Serologic response of naturally exposed or vaccinated dogs to *Borrelia burgdorferi*, the agent of Lyme borreliosis. *J. Am. Vet. Med. Assoc.* **207:**1435–1440.

21. **Barthold, S. W., D. H. Persing, A. L. Armstrong, and R. A. Peeples.** 1991. Kinetics of *Borrelia burgdorferi* dissemination and evolution of disease following intradermal inoculation of mice. *Am. J. Pathol.* **139:**263–273.

22. **Barthold, S. W., C. L. Sidman, and A. L. Smith.** 1992. Lyme borreliosis in genetically resistant and susceptible mice with severe combined immunodeficiency. *Am. J. Trop. Med. Hyg.* **47:**605–613.

23. **Bergstrom, S., C. F. Garon, and A. G. Barbour.** 1992. Extrachromosomal elements of spirochetes. *Res. Microbiol.* **143:**623–628.

24. **Bledsoe, H. A., J. A. Carroll, T. R. Whelchel, M. A. Farmer, D. W. Dorward, and F. C. Gherardini.** 1994. Isolation and partial characterization of *Borrelia burgdorferi* inner and outer membranes by using isopycnic centrifugation. *J. Bacteriol.* **176:**7447–7455.

25. **Bockenstedt, L. K., E. Hodzic, S. Feng, K. W. Bourell, A. deSilva, R. Montgomery, J. D. Radolf, and S. W. Barthold.** 1997. *Borrelia burgdorferi* strain-specific OspC-mediated immunity in mice. *Infect. Immun.* **65:**4661–4667.

26. **Brorson, O., and S. H. Brorson.** 1998. In vitro conversion of *Borrelia burgdorferi* to cystic forms in spinal fluid, and transformation to mobile spirochetes by incubation in BSK-H medium. *Infection* **26:**144–150.

27. **Brorson, O., and S. H. Brorson.** 1997. Transformation of cystic forms of Borrelia burgdorferi to normal, mobile spirochetes. *Infection* **25:**240–246.

28. **Brouqui, P., S. Badiaga, and D. Raoult.** 1996. Eukaryotic cells protect *Borrelia burgdorferi* from the action of penicillin and ceftriaxone but not from the action of doxycline and erythromycin. *Antimicrob. Agents Chemother.* **40:**1552–1554.

29. **Bruck, D. K., M. L. Talbor, R. G. Cluss, and J. T. Boothby.** 1995. Ultrastructural characterization of the stages of spheroplast preparation of *Borrelia burgdorferi*. *J. Microbiol. Methods* **23:**219.

30. **Brunet, L. R., A. Spielman, E. Fikrig, and S. R. Telford III.** 1997. Heterogeneity of Lyme disease spirochaetes within individual vector ticks. *Res. Microbiol.* **148:**437–445.

31. **Burgdorfer, W., S. Hayes, and J. Benach.** 1988. Development of *Borrelia burgdorferi* in ixodid tick vectors. *Ann. N. Y. Acad. Sci.* **539:**172–179.

32. **Burgdorfer, W., and S. F. Hayes.** 1989. Vector-spirochete relationships in louse-borne and tick-borne borreliosis with emphasis on Lyme disease. *Adv. Dis. Vector Res.* **6:**127–150.

33. **Burgdorfer, W., S. F. Hayes, and D. Corwin.** 1989. The pathophysiology of the Lyme disease spirochete, *Borrelia burgdorferi*, in ixodid ticks. *Rev. Infect. Dis.* **110:**S1442–S1450.

34. **Burkot, T. R., J. Piesman, and R. A. Wirtz.** 1994. Kinetics of the *Borrelia burgdorferi* outer surface protein A (OspA) in the tick, *Ixodes scapularis*, p. 224–227. *In* R. Cevinini, V. Sambri, and M. LaPlaca (ed.), *Advances in Lyme Borreliosis Research. Proceedings of the VIth International Conference on Lyme Borreliosis.* University of Bologna, Bologna, Italy.

35. **Carter, C. J., S. Bergstrom, S. J. Norris, and A. G. Barbour.** 1994. A family of surface-ex-

posed proteins of 20 kilodaltons in the genus *Borrelia*. *Infect. Immun.* **62:**2792–2799.

36. **Casjens, S., G. Hatfull, and R. Hendrix.** 1992. Evolution of dsDNA tailed-bacteriophage genomes. *Semin. Virol.* **3:**383–397.

37. **Casjens, S., R. van Vugt, K. Tilly, P. A. Rosa, and B. Stevenson.** 1997. Homology throughout the multiple 32-kilobase circular plasmids present in Lyme disease spirochetes. *J. Bacteriol.* **179:**217–227.

38. **Champion, C. I., D. R. Blanco, J. T. Skare, D. A. Haake, M. Giladi, D. Foley, J. N. Miller, and M. A. Lovett.** 1994. A 9.0 kilobase-pair circular plasmid of *Borrelia burgdorferi* encodes an exported protein: evidence for expression only during infection. *Infect. Immun.* **62:**2653–2661.

39. **Chang, Y. F., M. J. G. Appel, R. H. Jacobson, S. J. Shin, P. Harpending, R. Straubinger, L. A. Patrician, H. Mohammed, and B. A. Summers.** 1995. Recombinant OspA protects dogs against infection and disease caused by *Borrelia burgdorferi*. *Infect. Immun.* **63:**3543–3549.

40. **Cheetham, B., and M. Katz.** 1995. A role for bacteriophages in the evolution and transfer of bacterial virulence determinants. *Mol. Microbiol.* **18:**201–208.

41. **Cinco, M., E. Banfi, D. Balanzin, C. Godeas, and E. Panfili.** 1991. Evidence for (lipo) oligosaccharides in *Borrelia burgdorferi* and their surrounding serological specificity. *FEMS Microbiol. Lett.* **76:**33–38.

42. **Coburn, J., L. Magoun, S. C. Bodary, and J. M. Leong.** 1998. Integrins alpha(v)beta and alpha5beta1 mediate attachment of Lyme disease spirochetes to human cells. *Infect. Immun.* **66:**1946–1952.

43. **Coleman, J. L., and J. L. Benach.** 1987. Isolation of antigenic components from the Lyme disease spirochete: their role in early diagnosis. *J. Infect. Dis.* **155:**756–765.

44. **Coleman, J. L., J. A. Gebbia, J. Piesman, J. L. Degen, T. H. Bugge, and J. L. Benach.** 1997. Plasminogen is required for efficient dissemination of *Borrelia burgdorferi* in ticks and for enhancement of spirochetemia in mice. *Cell* **89:**1111–1119.

45. **Comstock, L. E., and D. D. Thomas.** 1991. Characterization of *Borrelia burgdorferi* invasion of cultured endothelial cells. *Microb. Pathog.* **10:**137–148.

46. **Coughlin, R. T., D. Fish, T. N. Mather, J. N. Ma, C. Pavia, and P. Bulger.** 1995. Protection of dogs from Lyme disease with a vaccine containing outer surface protein (Osp) A, OspB and the saponin adjuvant QS21. *J. Infect. Dis.* **171:**1049–1052.

47. **Cox, C. L., D. R. Akins, K. W. Bourell, P.** Lahdenne, M. V. Norgard, and J. D. Radolf. 1996. Limited surface exposure of *Borrelia burgdorferi* outer surface lipoproteins. *Proc. Natl. Acad. Sci. USA* **93:**7973–7978.

48. **Das, S., S. W. Barthold, S. S. Giles, R. R. Montgomery, S. R. Telford III, and E. Fikrig.** 1997. Temporal pattern of *Borrelia burgdorferi* p21 gene expression in ticks and the mammalian host. *J. Clin. Investig.* **99:**987–995.

49. **Defosse, D. L., P. H. Duray, and R. C. Johnson.** 1992. The NIH-3 immunodeficient mouse is a model for Lyme borreliosis myositis and carditis. *Am. J. Pathol.* **141:**3–10.

50. **Demaerschalck, I., A. BenMessaoud, M. DeKesel, B. Hyois, Y. Lobet, P. Hoet, G. Bigaignon, A. Bollen, and E. Godfroid.** 1995. Simultaneous presence of different *Borrelia burgdorferi* genospecies in biological fluids of Lyme disease patients. *J. Clin. Microbiol.* **33:**602–608.

51. **deSilva, A., and E. Fikrig.** 1995. Growth and migration of *Borrelia burgdorferi* in *Ixodes* ticks during blood feeding. *Am. J. Trop. Med. Hyg.* **53:**397–404.

52. **deSilva, A., E. Fikrig, E. Hodzic, S. R. Telford III, and S. W. Barthold.** 1998. Immune evasion by tick-borne and host-adapted *Borrelia burgdorferi*. *J. Infect. Dis.* **177:**395–400.

53. **deSilva, A., S. R. Telford, L. R. Brunet, S. W. Barthold, and E. Fikrig.** 1996. *Borrelia burgdorferi* OspA arthropod-specific transmission-blocking Lyme disease vaccine. *J. Exp. Med.* **183:**271–275.

54. **deSilva, A. M., and E. Fikrig.** 1997. Arthropod- and host-specific gene expression by *Borrelia burgdorferi*. *J. Clin. Investig.* **99:**377–379.

55. **deSilva, A. M., D. Fish, T. R. Burkot, Y. Zhang, and E. Fikrig.** 1997. OspA antibodies inhibit the acquisition of *Borrelia burgdorferi* by Ixodes ticks. *Infect. Immun.* **65:**3146–3150.

56. **deSouza, M. S., E. Fikrig, A. L. Smith, R. A. Flavell, and S. W. Barthold.** 1992. Nonspecific proliferative responses of murine lymphocytes to *Borrelia burgdorferi* antigens. *J. Infect. Dis.* **165:**471–478.

57. **deSouza, M. S., A. L. Smith, D. S. Beck, G. A. Terwilliger, E. Fikrig, and S. W. Barthold.** 1993. Long-term study of cell-mediated responses to *Borrelia burgdorferi* in the laboratory mouse. *Infect. Immun.* **61:**1814–1822.

58. **Dorward, D. W.** 1998. Immune ultrastructural evidence of lymphocytic antigen binding by Lyme disease spirochetes. *Scanning* **20:**197–199.

59. **Dorward, D. W., E. R. Fischer, and D. M. Brooks.** 1997. Invasion and cytopathic killing of human lymphocytes by spirochetes causing Lyme disease. *Clin. Infect. Dis.* **25:**S22–S8.

60. **Dorward, D. W., E. D. Huegenel, G. Davis,**

and C. F. Garon. 1992. Interactions between extracellular *Borrelia burgdorferi* proteins and non-*Borrelia*-directed immunoglobulin M antibodies. *Infect. Immun.* **60**:838–844.

61. Dressler, F., J. A. Whalen, B. N. Reinhardt, and A. C. Steere. 1993. Western blotting in the serodiagnosis of Lyme disease. *J. Infect. Dis.* **167**: 392–400.

62. Ebnet, K., K. D. Brown, U. K. Siebenlist, M. M. Simon, and S. Shaw. 1997. *Borrelia burgdorferi* activates nuclear factor-KB and is a potent inducer of chemokine and adhesion molecule gene expression in endothelial cells and fibroblasts. *J. Immunol.* **158**:3285–3292.

63. Erdile, L. F., M. A. Brandt, D. J. Warakomski, G. J. Westrack, A. Sadziene, A. G. Barbour, and J. P. Mays. 1993. Role of attached lipid in immunogenicity of *Borrelia burgdorferi* OspA. *Infect. Immun.* **61**:81–90.

64. Feng, S., E. Hodzic, B. Stevenson, and S. W. Barthold. 1998. Humoral Immunity to *Borrelia burgdorferi* N40 decorin binding proteins during infection of laboratory mice. *Infect. Immun.* **66**: 2827–2835.

65. Fikrig, E., S. W. Barthold, F. S. Kantor, and R. A. Flavell. 1990. Protection of mice against the Lyme disease agent by immunizing with recombinant OspA. *Science* **250**:553–556.

66. Fikrig, E., S. W. Barthold, W. Sun, W. Feng, S. R. I. Telford, and R. A. Flavell. 1997. *Borrelia burgdorferi* P35 and P37 proteins, expressed in vivo, elicit protective immunity. *Immunity* **6**: 531–539.

67. Fikrig, E., L. K. Bockenstedt, S. W. Barthold, M. Chen, H. Tao, P. Ali-Salaam, S. R. Telford, and R. A. Flavell. 1994. Sera from patients with chronic Lyme disease protect mice from Lyme borreliosis. *J. Infect. Dis.* **169**:568–574.

68. Fikrig, E., M. Chen, S. W. Barthold, J. Anguita, W. Feng, S. R. Telford III, and R. A. Flavell. 1999. *Borrelia burgdorferi* erpT expression in the arthropod vector and murine host. *Mol. Microbiol.* **31**:281–290.

69. Fikrig, E., S. R. Telford III, S. W. Barthold, F. S. Kantor, A. Spielman, and R. A. Flavell. 1992. Elimination of *Borrelia burgdorferi* from vector ticks feeding on OspA-immunized mice. *Proc. Natl. Acad. Sci. USA* **89**:5418–5421.

70. Fikrig, E., S. R. Telford III, R. Wallich, M. Chen, Y. Lobet, F. R. Matuschka, R. B. Kimsey, F. S. Kantor, S. W. Barthold, A. Spielman, and R. A. Flavell. 1995. Vaccination against Lyme disease caused by diverse *Borrelia burgdorferi*. *J. Exp. Med.* **181**:215–221.

71. Fingerle, V., U. Hauser, G. Liegl, B. Petko, V. Preac-Mursic, and B. Wilske. 1995. Expression of outer surface proteins A and C of

Borrelia burgdorferi in *Ixodes ricinus*. *J. Clin. Microbiol.* **33**:1867–1869.

72. Fraser, C. M., S. Casjens, W. M. Huang, G. G. Sutton, R. Clayton, R. Lathigra, O. White, K. A. Ketchum, R. Dodson, E. K. Hickey, M. Gwinn, B. Dougherty, J. F. Tomb, R. D. Fleischmann, D. Richardson, J. Peterson, A. R. Kerlavage, J. Quackenbush, S. Salzberg, M. Hanson, R. van Vugt, N. Palmer, M. D. Adams, J. Gocayne, J. Weidman, T. Utterback, L. Watthey, L. McDonald, P. Artiach, C. Bowman, S. Garland, C. Fujii, M. D. Cotton, K. Horst, K. Roberts, B. Hatch, H. O. Smith, and J. C. Venter. 1997. Genomic sequence of a Lyme disease spirochaete, *Borrelia burgdorferi*. *Nature* **390**:580–586.

73. Garon, C. F., D. W. Dorward, and M. D. Corwin. 1989. Structural features of *Borrelia burgdorferi*—the Lyme disease spirochete: silver staining for nucleic acids. *Scanning Microsc.* **3**:109–115.

74. Gern, L., O. Rais, C. Capiau, P. Hauser, Y. Lobet, E. Simoen, P. Voet, and J. Petre. 1994. Immunization of mice by recombinant OspA preparations and protection against *Borrelia burgdorferi* infection induced by *Ixodes ricinus* ticks. *Immunol. Lett.* **39**:249–258.

75. Gern, L., U. E. Schaible, and M. M. Simon. 1993. Mode of inoculation of the Lyme disease agent *Borrelia burgdorferi* influences infection and immune responses in inbred strains of mice. *J. Infect. Dis.* **167**:971–975.

76. Giambartolomei, G. H., V. A. Dennis, B. L. Lasater, and M. T. Philipp. 1999. Induction of pro- and anti-inflammatory cytokines by *Borrelia burgdorferi* lipoproteins in monocytes is mediated by CD14. *Infect. Immun.* **67**:140–147.

77. Gilmore, R. D., Jr., and M. L. Mbow. 1998. A monoclonal antibody generated by antigen inoculation via tick bite is reactive to *Borrelia burgdorferi* Rev protein, a member of the 2.9 gene family locus. *Infect. Immun.* **66**:980–986.

78. Girschick, H. J., H. I. Huppertz, H. Russmann, V. Krenn, and H. Karch. 1996. Intracellular persistence of *Borrelia burgdorferi* in human synovial cells. *Rheumatol. Int.* **16**:125–132.

79. Golde, W. T., K. J. Kappel, G. Dequesne, C. Feron, D. Plainchamp, C. Capiau, and Y. Lobet. 1994. Tick transmission of *Borrelia burgdorferi* to inbred strains of mice induces an antibody response to P39 but not to outer surface protein A. *Infect. Immun.* **62**:2625–2627.

80. Goldstein, S. F., N. W. Charon, and J. A. Kreiling. 1994. *Borrelia burgdorferi* swims with a planar waveform similar to that of eukaryotic flagella. *Proc. Natl. Acad. Sci. USA* **91**:3433–3437.

81. Goodman, J. L., P. Jurkovich, C. Kodner, and R. C. Johnson. 1991. Persistent cardiac and

urinary tract infections with *Borrelia burgdorferi* in experimentally infected Syrian hamsters. *J. Clin. Microbiol.* **29**:894–896.

82. **Grab, D. J., C. Givens, and R. Kennedy.** 1998. Fibronectin-binding activity in *Borrelia burgdorferi*. *Biochim. Biophys. Acta* **1407**:135–145.

83. **Guttman, D. S., P. W. Wang, I. N. Wang, E. M. Bosler, B. J. Luft, and D. E. Dykhuizen.** 1996. Multiple infections of *Ixodes scapularis* ticks by *Borrelia burgdorferi* as revealed by single-strand conformation polymorphism analysis. *J. Clin. Microbiol.* **34**:652–656.

84. **Hanson, M. S., D. R. Cassatt, B. P. Guo, N. K. Patel, M. P. McCarthy, D. W. Dorward, and M. Hook.** 1998. Active and passive immunity against *Borrelia burgdorferi* decorin binding protein A (DbpA) protects against infection. *Infect. Immun.* **66**:2143–2153.

85. **Hofmeister, E. K., and J. E. Childs.** 1995. Analysis of *Borrelia burgdorferi* sequentially isolated from *Peromyscus leucopus* captured at a Lyme disease enzootic site. *J. Infect. Dis.* **172**:462–469.

86. **Hu, L. T., S. D. Pratt, G. Perides, L. Katz, R. A. Rogers, and M. S. Klempner.** 1997. Isolation, cloning, and expression of a 70-kilodalton plasminogen binding protein of *Borrelia burgdorferi*. *Infect. Immun.* **65**:4989–4995.

87. **Hulinska, D., P. Bartak, J. Hercogova, J. Hancil, J. Basta, and J. Schramlova.** 1994. Electron microscopy of Langerhans cells and *Borrelia burgdorferi* in Lyme disease patients. *Zentbl. Bakteriol.* **280**:348–359.

88. **Indest, K. J., R. Ramamoorthy, M. Sole, R. D. Gilmore, B. J. B. Johnson, and M. T. Philipp.** 1997. Cell-density-dependent expression of *Borrelia burgdorferi* lipoproteins in vitro. *Infect. Immun.* **65**:1165–1171.

89. **Jauris-Heipke, S., G. Liegl, V. Preac-Mursic, D. Rossler, E. Schwab, E. Spitscjel, G. Will, and B. Wilske.** 1995. Molecular analysis of genes encoding outer surface protein C (OspC) of *Borrelia burgdorferi* sensu lato: relationship to OspA genotype and evidence of lateral gene exchange of OspC. *J. Clin. Microbiol.* **33**:1860–1866.

90. **Johnson, B. J. B., S. L. Sviat, C. M. Happ, J. J. Dunn, J. C. Frantz, L. W. Mayer, and J. Piesman.** 1995. Incomplete protection of hamsters vaccinated with unlipidated OspA from *Borrelia burgdorferi* infection is associated with low levels of antibody to an epitope defined by mAb La-2. *Vaccine* **13**:1086–1094.

91. **Kalish, R. A., J. M. Leong, and A. C. Steere.** 1995. Early and late antibody responses to full-length and truncated constructs of outer surface protein A of *Borrelia burgdorferi* in Lyme disease. *Infect. Immun.* **63**:2228–2235.

92. **Kaneda, K., T. Masuzawa, M. M. Simon,** E. Isogai, H. Isogai, K. Yasugami, T. Suzuki, Y. Suzuki, and Y. Yanagihara. 1998. Infectivity and arthritis induction of *Borrelia japonica* on SCID mice and immune competent mice: possible role of galactosylceramide binding activity on initiation of infection. *Microbiol. Immunol.* **42**:171–175.

93. **Kersten, A., C. Poitschek, S. Rauch, and E. Aberer.** 1995. Effects of penicillin, ceftriaxone, and doxycycline on morphology of *Borrelia burgdorferi*. *Antimicrob. Agents Chemother.* **39**:1127–1133.

94. **Kimsey, R. B., and A. Spielman.** 1990. Motility of Lyme disease spirochetes in fluid as viscous as the extracellular matrix. *J. Infect. Dis.* **162**:1205–1208.

95. **Kitten, T., and A. Barbour.** 1990. Juxtaposition of expressed variable antigen genes with a conserved telomere in the bacterium *Borrelia hermsii*. *Proc. Natl. Acad. Sci. USA* **87**:6077–6081.

96. **Klempner, M. S., R. Noring, M. P. Epstein, B. McCloud, and R. A. Rogers.** 1996. Binding of human urokinase type plasminogen activator and plasminogen to Borrelia species. *J. Infect. Dis.* **174**:97104.

97. **Klempner, M. S., R. Noring, and R. A. Rogers.** 1993. Invasion of human skin fibroblasts by the Lyme disease spirochete, *Borrelia burgdorferi*. *J. Infect. Dis.* **167**:1074–1081.

98. **Kuiper, H., A. P. van Dam, L. Spanjaard, B. M. de Jongh, A. Widjojokusumo, T. C. P. Ramselaar, I. Cairo, K. Vos, and J. Dankert.** 1994. Isolation of *Borrelia burgdorferi* from biopsy specimens taken from healthy-looking skin of patients with Lyme borreliosis. *J. Clin. Microbiol.* **32**:715–720.

99. **Lahdenne, P., S. F. Porcella, K. E. Hagman, D. R. Akins, T. G. Popova, D. D. Cox, L. I. Katona, J. D. Radolf, and M. V. Norgard.** 1997. Molecular characterization of 6.6-kilodalton *Borrelia burgdorferi* outer membrane-associated lipoprotein (lp6.6) which appears to be downregulated during mammalian infection. *Infect. Immun.* **65**:412–421.

100. **Lam, T. T., T. K. Nguyen, R. R. Montgomery, F. S. Kantor, E. Fikrig, and R. A. Flavell.** 1994. Outer surface proteins E and F of *Borrelia burgdorferi*, the agent of Lyme disease. *Infect. Immun.* **62**:290–298.

101. **LeFleche, A., D. Postic, K. Girardet, O. Peter, and G. Baranton.** 1997. Characterization of *Borrelia lusitaniae* sp. nov. by 16S ribosomal DNA sequence analysis. *Int. J. Syst. Bacteriol.* **47**:921–925.

102. **Leong, J. M., H. Wang, L. Magoun, J. A. Field, P. E. Morrissey, D. Robbins, J. B. Tatro, J. Coburn, and N. Parveen.** 1998. Dif-

ferent classes of proteoglycan contribute to the attachment of *Borrelia burgdorferi* to cultured endothelial and brain cells. *Infect. Immun.* **66:** 994–999.

103. **Liveris, D., G. P. Wormser, J. Nowakowski, R. Nadelman, S. Bittker, D. Cooper, S. Varde, F. H. Moy, G. Forsetter, C. S. Pavia, and I. Schwartz.** 1996. Molecular typing of *Borrelia burgdorferi* from Lyme disease patients by PCR-restriction fragment length polymorphism analysis. *J. Clin. Microbiol.* **34:**1306–1309.

104. **Livey, I., C. P. Gibbs, R. Schuster, and F. Dormer.** 1995. The role of lateral transfer and recombination in OspC variation in Lyme disease Borrelia. *Mol. Microbiol.* **18:**257–269.

105. **Lovrich, S. D., S. M. Callister, B. K. DuChateau, L. C. L. Lim, J. Winfrey, S. P. Day, and R. F. Schell.** 1995. Abilities of OspA proteins from different seroprotective groups of *Borrelia burgdorferi* to protect hamsters from infection. *Infect. Immun.* **63:**2113–2119.

106. **Ma, Y., K. P. Seiler, K.-F. Tai, L. Yang, M. Woods, and J. J. Weis.** 1994. Outer surface lipoproteins of *Borrelia burgdorferi* stimulate nitric oxide production by the cytokine-inducible pathway. *Infect. Immun.* **62:**3663–3671.

107. **MacDonald, A. B.** 1998. Concurrent neocortical borreliosis and Alzheimer's disease. *Ann. N. Y. Acad. Sci.* **539:**468–470.

108. **Malawista, S. M., S. W. Barthold, and D. H. Persing.** 1994. Fate of *Borrelia burgdorferi* DNA in tissues of infected mice after antibiotic treatment. *J. Infect. Dis.* **170:**1312–1316.

109. **Marconi, R. T., D. S. Samuels, R. K. Landry, and C. F. Garon.** 1994. Analysis of the distribution and molecular heterogeneity of the *ospD* gene among the Lyme disease spirochetes: evidence for lateral gene exchange. *J. Bacteriol.* **176:**4572–4582.

110. **Marti Ras, N., D. Postic, M. Foretz, and G. Baranton.** 1997. *Borrelia burgdorferi* sensu stricto, a bacterial species "made in the U.S.A."? *Int. J. Syst. Bacteriol.* **47:**1112–1117.

111. **Mitchell, P. D., K. D. Reed, and J. M. Hofkes.** 1996. Immunoserologic evidence of coinfection with *Borrelia burgdorferi*, *Babesia microti*, and human granulocytic *Ehrlichia* species in residents of Wisconsin and Minnesota. *J. Clin. Microbiol.* **34:**724–727.

112. **Modolell, M., U. E. Schaible, M. Rittig, and M. M. Simon.** 1994. Killing of *Borrelia burgdorferi* by macrophages is dependent on oxygen radicals and nitric oxide and can be enhanced by antibodies to outer surface proteins of the spirochete. *Immunol. Lett.* **40:**139–146.

113. **Montgomery, R. R., and S. E. Malawista.** 1996. Entry of *Borrelia burgdorferi* into macro-

phages is end-on and leads to degradation in lysosomes. *Infect. Immun.* **64:**2867–2872.

114. **Montgomery, R. R., M. H. Nathanson, and S. E. Malawista.** 1993. The fate of *Borrelia burgdorferi*, the agent for Lyme disease, in mouse macrophages: destruction, survival, recovery. *J. Immunol.* **150:**909–915.

115. **Moody, K. D., S. W. Barthold, G. A. Terwilliger, D. S. Beck, G. M. Hansen, and R. O. Jacoby.** 1990. Experimental chronic Lyme borreliosis in Lewis rats. *Am. J. Trop. Med. Hyg.* **42:**65–74.

116. **Morrison, T. B., J. H. Weis, and J. J. Weis.** 1997. *Borrelia burgdorferi* outer surface protein A (OspA) activates and primes human neutrophils. *J. Immunol.* **158:**4838–4845.

117. **Nakao, M., and K. Miyamoto.** 1995. Mixed infection of different *Borrelia* species among *Apodemus speciosus* mice in Hokkaido, Japan. *J. Clin. Microbiol.* **33:**490–492.

118. **Nguyen, T. K., T. T. Lam, S. W. Barthold, S. R. Telford III, R. A. Flavell, and E. Fikrig.** 1994. Partial destruction of *Borrelia burgdorferi* within ticks engorged on OspE- or OspF-immunized mice. *Infect. Immun.* **62:**2079–2084.

119. **Nocton, J. J., F. Dressler, R. J. Rutledge, P. N. Rys, D. H. Persing, and A. C. Steere.** 1994. Detection of *Borrelia burgdorferi* DNA by polymerase chain reaction in synovial fluid from patients with Lyme arthritis. *N. Engl. J. Med.* **330:**229–234.

120. **Norgard, M., B. Riley, J. Richardson, and J. Radolf.** 1995. Dermal inflammation elicited by synthetic analogs of *Treponema pallidum* and *Borrelia burgdorferi* lipoproteins. *Infect. Immun.* **63:** 1507–1515.

121. **Norgard, M. V., L. L. Arndt, D. R. Akins, L. L. Curetty, D. A. Harrich, and J. D. Radolf.** 1996. Activation of human monocytic cells by *Treponema pallidum* and *Borrelia burgdorferi* lipoproteins and synthetic lipopeptides via a pathway distinct from that of lipopolysaccharide involves the transcriptional activator of NF-κB. *Infect. Immun.* **64:**3845–3852.

122. **Norris, S. J., C. J. Carter, J. K. Howell, and A. G. Barbour.** 1992. Low-passage associated proteins of *Borrelia burgdorferi* B31: characterization and molecular cloning of OspD, a surface-exposed, plasmid-encoded lipoprotein. *Infect. Immun.* **60:**4662–4672.

123. **Oksi, J., M. Marjamaki, K. Koski, J. Nikoskelainen, and M. Viljanen.** 1995. Bilateral facial palsy and meningitis caused by borrelia double infection. *Lancet* **345:**1583–1584.

124. **Pachner, A. R., J. Basta, E. Delaney, and D. Hulinska.** 1995. Localization of *Borrelia burg-*

dorferi in murine Lyme borreliosis by electron microscopy. *Am. J. Trop. Med. Hyg.* **52**:128–133.

125. **Pachner, A. R., E. Delaney, and T. ONeill.** 1995. Neuroborreliosis in the nonhuman primate: *Borrelia burgdorferi* persists in the central nervous system. *Ann. Neurol.* **38**:667–669.

126. **Padula, S. J., F. Dias, A. Sampieri, R. B. Craven, and R. W. Ryan.** 1994. Use of recombinant OspC from *Borrelia burgdorferi* for serodiagnosis of early Lyme disease. *J. Clin. Microbiol.* **32**:1733–1738.

127. **Persing, D. H., D. Mathiesen, D. Podzorski, and S. W. Barthold.** 1994. Genetic stability of *Borrelia burgdorferi* recovered from chronically infected immunocompetent mice. *Infect. Immun.* **62**:3521–3527.

128. **Persing, D. H., B. J. Rutledge, P. N. Rys, D. S. Podzorski, P. D. Mitchell, K. D. Reed, B. Liu, E. Fikrig, and S. E. Malawista.** 1994. Target imbalance: disparity of *Borrelia burgdorferi* genetic material in synovial fluid from Lyme arthritis patients. *J. Infect. Dis.* **169**:668–672.

129. **Philipp, M. T., M. K. Aydintug, R. P. Bohm, Jr., F. B. Cogswell, V. A. Dennis, H. N. Lanners, R. C. Lowrie, Jr., E. D. Roberts, M. D. Conway, M. Karacorlu, G. A. Peyman, D. J. Gubler, B. J. B. Johnson, J. Piesman, and Y. Gu.** 1993. Early and early disseminated phases of Lyme disease in the rhesus monkey: a model for infection in humans. *Infect. Immun.* **61**:3047–3059.

130. **Philipp, M. T., Y. Lobet, R. P. Bohm, Jr., E. D. Roberts, V. A. Dennis, Y. Gu, R. C. Lowrie, Jr., P. Desmons, P. H. Duray, J. D. Englands, P. Hauser, J. Piesman, and K. Xu.** 1997. The outer surface protein A (OspA) vaccine against Lyme disease: efficacy in the rhesus monkey. *Vaccine* **15**:1872–1887.

131. **Phillips, S. E., L. H. Mattman, D. Hulinska, and H. Moayad.** 1998. A proposal for the reliable culture of *Borrelia burgdorferi* from patients with chronic Lyme disease, even from those previously aggressively treated. *Infection* **26**:364–367.

132. **Piesman, J., M. C. Dolan, C. M. Happ, B. J. Luft, S. E. Rooney, T. N. Mather, and W. T. Golde.** 1997. Duration of immunity to reinfection with tick-transmitted *Borrelia burgdorferi* in naturally infected mice. *Infect. Immun.* **65**:4043–4047.

133. **Porcella, S. F., T. G. Popova, D. R. Akins, M. Y. Li, J. D. Radolf, and M. V. Norgard.** 1996. *Borrelia burgdorferi* supercoiled plasmids encode multicopy tandem open reading frames and a lipoprotein gene family. *J. Bacteriol.* **178**:3293–3307.

134. **Preac-Mursic, V., H. W. Pfister, B. Wilske, B. Gross, A. Baumann, and J. Prokop.** 1989. Survival of *Borrelia burgdorferi* in antibiotically treated patients with Lyme borreliosis. *Infection* **17**:355–359.

135. **Preac-Mursic, V., G. Wanner, S. Reinhardt, B. Wilske, U. Busch, and W. Marget.** 1996. Formation and cultivation of *Borrelia burgdorferi* spheroplast-L-form variants. *Infection* **24**:218–226.

136. **Probert, W. S., M. Crawford, R. B. Cadiz, and R. B. LeFebvre.** 1997. Immunization with outer surface protein (Osp) A, but not OspC, provides cross-protection of mice challenged with North American isolates of *Borrelia burgdorferi*. *J Infect. Dis.* **175**:400–405.

137. **Radolf, J. D., L. L. Arndt, D. R. Akins, L. L. Curetty, M. E. Levi, Y. N. Shen, L. S. Davis, and M. V. Norgard.** 1995. *Treponema pallidum* and *Borrelia burgdorferi* lipoproteins and synthetic lipopeptides activate monocytes/macrophages. *J. Immunol.* **154**:2866–2877.

138. **Ramamoorthy, R., and M. T. Philipp.** 1998. Differential expression of *Borrelia burgdorferi* proteins during growth in vitro. *Infect. Immun.* **66**:5119–5124.

139. **Ramamoorthy, R., L. Povinelli, and M. T. Philipp.** 1996. Molecular characterization, genomic arrangement, and expression of *bmpD*, a new member of the *bmp* class of genes encoding membrane proteins of *Borrelia burgdorferi*. *Infect. Immun.* **64**:1259–1264.

140. **Ribeiro, J. M. C., T. N. Mather, J. Piesman, and A. Spielman.** 1987. Dissemination and salivary delivery of Lyme disease spirochetes in vector ticks (Acari: Ixodidae). *J. Med. Entomol.* **24**:201–205.

141. **Rijpkema, S. G. T., M. J. C. H. Molkenboer, L. M. Schouls, F. Jongejan, and J. F. P. Schellekens.** 1995. Simultaneous detection and genotyping of three genomic groups of *Borrelia burgdorferi* sensu lato in Dutch *Ixodes ricinus* ticks by characterization of the amplified intergenic spacer region between 5S and 23S rRNA genes. *J. Clin. Microbiol.* **33**:3091–3095.

142. **Roberts, E. D., R. F. Bohm, F. B. Cogswell, H. Norbert-Lanners, R. C. Lowrie, L. Povinelli, J. Piesman, and M. T. Philipp.** 1995. Chronic Lyme disease in the rhesus monkey. *Lab. Investig.* **72**:146–160.

143. **Roberts, W. C., B. A. Mullikin, R. Lathigra, and M. S. Hanson.** 1998. Molecular analysis of sequence heterogeneity among genes encoding decorin binding proteins A and B of *Borrelia burgdorferi* sensu lato. *Infect. Immun.* **66**:5275–5285.

144. **Roehrig, J. T., J. Piesman, A. R. Hunt, M. G. Keen, C. M. Happ, and B. J. B. Johnson.**

1992. The hamster immune response to tick transmitted *Borrelia burgdorferi* differs from the response to needle-inoculated, cultured organisms. *J. Immunol.* **149:**3648–3653.

145. **Rosa, P. A., T. Schwan, and D. Hogan.** 1992. Recombination between genes encoding major outer surface proteins A and B of *Borrelia burgdorferi. Mol. Microbiol.* **6:**3031–3040.

146. **Sadziene, A., P. Rosa, D. Hogan, and A. Barbour.** 1992. Antibody-resistant mutants of *Borrelia burgdorferi*: in vitro selection and characterization. *J. Exp. Med.* **176:**799–809.

147. **Schaible, U. E., M. D. Kramer, K. Eichmann, M. Modolell, C. Museteanu, and M. M. Simon.** 1990. Monoclonal antibodies specific for the outer surface protein A (OspA) of *Borrelia burgdorferi* prevent Lyme borreliosis in severe combined immunodeficiency (scid) mice. *Proc. Natl. Acad. Sci. USA* **87:**3768–3772.

148. **Schaible, U. E., M. D. Kramer, C. Museteanu, G. Zimmer, H. Mossmann, and M. Simon.** 1990. Lyme borreliosis in the severe combined immunodeficiency (scid) mouse manifests predominantly in the joints, heart and liver. *Am. J. Pathol.* **137:**811–820.

149. **Schaible, U. E., R. Wallich, M. D. Kramer, G. Nerz, T. Stehle, C. Museteanu, and M. M. Simon.** 1994. Protection against *Borrelia burgdorferi* infection in SCID mice is conferred by presensitized spleen cells and partially by B- but not T-cells alone. *Intern. Immun.* **6:**671–681.

150. **Schaller, M., and U. Neubert.** 1994. Ultrastructure of *Borrelia burgdorferi* after exposure to benzylpenicillin. *Infection* **22:**401–406.

151. **Schmidli, J., T. Hunziker, P. Moesli, and U. B. Schaad.** 1988. Cultivation of *Borrelia burgdorferi* from joint fluid three months after treatment of facial palsy due to Lyme borreliosis. *J. Infect. Dis.* **158:**905–906.

152. **Schwan, T. G.** 1996. Ticks and Borrelia: Model systems for investigating pathogen-arthropod interactions. *Infect. Agents Dis.* **5:**167–181.

153. **Schwan, T. G., W. Burgdorfer, and C. F. Garon.** 1988. Changes in infectivity and plasmid profile of the Lyme disease spirochete, *Borrelia burgdorferi*, as a result of in vitro cultivation. *Infect. Immun.* **56:**1831–1836.

154. **Schwan, T. G., and B. J. Hinnebusch.** 1998. Bloodstream- versus tick-associated variants of a relapsing fever bacterium. *Science* **280:**1938–1940.

155. **Schwan, T. G., J. Piesman, W. T. Golde, M. C. Dolan, and P. A. Rosa.** 1995. Induction of outer surface protein on *Borrelia burgdorferi* during tick-feeding. *Proc. Natl. Acad. Sci. USA* **92:**2909–2913.

156. **Seifert, H. S., and M. So.** 1988. Genetic mechanisms of bacterial antigenic variation. *Microbiol. Rev.* **52:**327–336.

157. **Shih, C.-M., L.-P. Liu, and A. Spielman.** 1995. Differential spirochetal infectivities to vector ticks of mice chronically infected by the agent of Lyme disease. *J. Clin. Microbiol.* **33:** 3164–3168.

158. **Shoberg, R. J., and D. D. Thomas.** 1995. *Borrelia burgdorferi* vesicle production occurs via a mechanism independent of immunoglobulin M. *Infect. Immun.* **63:**4857–4861.

159. **Simpson, W. J., W. Cieplak, M. E. Schrumpf, A. G. Barbour, and T. G. Schwan.** 1994. Nucleotide sequence and analysis of the gene in *Borrelia burgdorferi* encoding the immunogenic P39 antigen. *FEMS Microbiol. Lett.* **119:**381–388.

160. **Simpson, W. J., C. R. Garon, and T. G. Schwan.** 1990. *Borrelia burgdorferi* contains repeated DNA sequences that are species specific and plasmid associated. *Infect. Immun.* **58:** 847–853.

161. **Steere, A. C.** 1989. Lyme disease. *N. Engl. J. Med.* **321:**586–596.

162. **Stevenson, B., L. K. Bockenstedt, and S. W. Barthold.** 1994. Expression and gene sequence of outer surface protein C of *Borrelia burgdorferi* reisolated from chronically infected mice. *Infect. Immun.* **62:**3568–3571.

163. **Stevenson, B., J. L. Bono, A. Elias, K. Tilly, and P. Rosa.** 1998. Transformation of the Lyme disease spirochete *Borrelia burgdorferi* with heterologous DNA. *J. Bacteriol.* **180:**4850–4855.

164. **Stevenson, B., J. L. Bono, T. G. Schwan, and P. Rosa.** 1998. *Borrelia burgdorferi* Erp proteins are immunogenic in mammals infected by tick bite, and their synthesis is inducible in cultured bacteria. *Infect. Immun.* **66:**2648–2654.

165. **Stevenson, B., S. Casjens, and P. Rosa.** 1998. Evidence of past recombination events among the genes encoding the Erp antigens of *Borrelia burgdorferi. Microbiology* **144:**1869–1879.

166. **Stevenson, B., T. G. Schwan, and P. A. Rosa.** 1995. Temperature-related differential expression of antigens in the Lyme disease spirochete, *Borrelia burgdorferi. Infect. Immun.* **63:** 4535–4539.

167. **Stevenson, B., K. Tilly, and P. A. Rosa.** 1996. A family of genes located on four separate 32-kilobase circular plasmids in *Borrelia burgdorferi* B31. *J. Bacteriol.* **178:**3508–3516.

168. **Straubinger, R. K., B. A. Summers, Y. F. Chang, and M. J. G. Appel.** 1997. Persistence of *Borrelia burgdorferi* in experimentally infected dogs after antibiotic treatment. *J. Clin. Microbiol.* **35:**111–116.

169. Suk, K., S. Das, W. Sun, B. Jwang, S. W. Barthold, R. A. Flavell, and E. Fikrig. 1995. *Borrelia burgdorferi* genes selectively expressed in the infected host. *Proc. Natl. Acad. Sci. USA* **92:** 4269–4273.

170. Sung, S.-Y., C. L. Lavoie, J. A. Carlyon, and R. T. Marconi. 1998. Genetic divergence and evolutionary instability of *ospE*-related members of the upstream homology box gene family in *Borrelia burgdorferi* sensu lato complex isolates. *Infect. Immun.* **66:**4656–4668.

171. Tai, K. F., Y. Ma, and J. J. Weis. 1994. Normal human B lymphocytes and mononuclear cells respond to the mitogenic and cytokine-stimulatory activities of *Borrelia burgdorferi* and its lipoprotein OspA. *Infect. Immun.* **62:**520–528.

172. Telford, S. R., III, P. M. Armstrong, P. Katavolos, I. Foppa, A. S. Olmeda-Garcia, M. L. Wilson, and A. Spielman. 1997. A new tick-borne encephalitis-like virus infecting New England deer ticks, *Ixodes dammini*. *Emerg. Infect. Dis.* **3:**165–170.

173. Theisen, M., B. Frederiksen, A.-M. Lebech, J. Vuust, and K. Hansen. 1993. Polymorphism in the *ospC* gene of *Borrelia burgdorferi* and immunoreactivity of OspC protein: implications for taxonomy and for use of OspC protein as a diagnostic antigen. *J. Clin. Microbiol.* **31:**2570–2576.

174. Theisen, M., M. Borre, M. J. Mathiesen, B. Mikkelsen, A. M. Lebech, and K. Hansen. 1995. Evolution of the *Borrelia burgdorferi* outer surface protein C. *J. Bacteriol.* **177:**3036–3044.

175. van Dam, A. P., H. Kuiper, K. Vos, A. Widojojokusumo, L. Spanjaard, B. M. de Jongh, A. C. P. Bamselaar, M. D. Kramer, and J. Dankert. 1993. Different genospecies of *Borrelia burgdorferi* are associated with distinct clinical manifestations of Lyme borreliosis. *Clin. Infect. Dis.* **17:**708–717.

176. Wallich, R., C. Brenner, M. D. Kramer, and M. M. Simon. 1995. Molecular cloning and immunological characterization of a novel linear-plasmid-encoded gene, *pG*, of *Borrelia burgdorferi* expressed only in vivo. *Infect. Immun.* **63:** 3327–3335.

177. Wang, G., A. P. van Dam, A. LeFleche, D. Postic, O. Peter, G. Baranton, R. deBoer, L. Spanjaard, and J. Dankert. 1997. Genetic and phenotypic analysis of *Borrelia valaisiana* sp.

178. Weis, J. J., Y. Ma, and L. F. Erdile. 1994. Biological activities of native and recombinant *Borrelia burgdorferi* outer surface protein A: dependence on lipid modification. *Infect. Immun.* **62:** 4632–4636.

179. Wheeler, C. M., J. C. Garcia-Monco, M. G. Golightly, G. S. Habicht, and A. C. Steere. 1993. Nonprotein antigens of *Borrelia burgdorferi*. *J. Infect. Dis.* **167:**665–674.

180. Wilske, B., A. G. Barbour, S. Bergstrom, N. Burman, B. I. Restrepo, P. A. Rosa, T. Schwan, E. Soutschek, and R. Wallich. 1992. Antigenic variation and strain heterogeneity in *Borrelia* spp. *Res. Microbiol.* **143:**583–596.

181. Wilske, B., V. Preac-Mursic, S. Jauris, A. Hofman, I. Pradel, E. Soutschek, E. Schwab, E. Will, and G. Wanner. 1993. Immunological and molecular polymorphisms of OspC, an immunodominant major outer surface protein of *Borrelia burgdorferi*. *Infect. Immun.* **61:** 2182–2191.

182. Wooten, R. M., V. R. Modur, T. M. McIntyre, and J. J. Weis. 1996. *Borrelia burgdorferi* outer membrane protein A induces nuclear translocation of nuclear factor-κB and inflammatory activation in human endothelial cells. *J. Bacteriol.* **178:**4584–4590.

183. Zhang, J.-R., J. M. Hardham, A. G. Barbour, and S. J. Norris. 1997. Antigenic variation in Lyme disease borreliae by promiscuous recombination of VMP-like sequence cassettes. *Cell* **89:**1–20.

184. Zhang, J. R., and S. J. Norris. 1998. Kinetics and in vivo induction of genetic variation of *vlsE* in *Borrelia burgdorferi*. *Infect. Immun.* **66:** 3689–3697.

185. Zhong, W., T. Stehle, C. Museteanu, A. Siebers, L. Gern, M. Kramer, R. Wallich, and M. M. Simon. 1997. Therapeutic passive vaccination against chronic Lyme disease in mice. *Proc. Natl. Acad. Sci. USA* **94:** 12533–12538.

186. Zung, J., S. Lewengrub, M. Rudzinska, A. Spielman, S. Telford, and J. Piesman. 1989. Fine structural evidence for the penetration of the Lyme disease spirochete *Borrelia burgdorferi* through the gut and salivary tissues of *Ixodes dammini*. *Can. J. Zool.* **67:**1717–1748.

nov. (Borrelia genomic groups VS116 and M19). *Int. J. Syst. Bacteriol.* **47:**926–932.

PSEUDOMONAS AERUGINOSA
INFECTIONS

V. Deretic

15

Pseudomonas aeruginosa remains a significant threat to human health despite continuing medical advances. This ubiquitous gram-negative bacterium is notorious for its nutritional and ecological flexibility and recalcitrance to both antibiotic treatments and control by sanitary measures. These properties contribute to its prominence as a leading source of opportunistic nosocomial (hospital-acquired) and community-acquired infections. *P. aeruginosa* has been recognized as an infectious agent associated with a variety of breaches in the innate and adaptive defense mechanisms of the host, such as burns, neutropenia, and cystic fibrosis (CF).

P. aeruginosa is a serious problem in clinical practice. In contrast to some overt human pathogens capable of causing disease in healthy individuals, which have proved to be more amenable to control, *P. aeruginosa* has remained a difficult organism to treat and in some instances is impossible to eradicate. During the recent changes in the landscape of opportunistic pathogenesis, *P. aeruginosa* has retained its significance despite the fact that it is not a dominant pathogen in AIDS. The continuing notoriety of *P. aeruginosa* as a pathogen in affluent societies is based in part on its prominence in CF. It appears that the stubborn persistence of *P. aeruginosa* in nosocomial and community-acquired infections in individuals with predisposing conditions is here to stay unless some new radical measures are developed. Such status has already earned this bacterium the dubious honor of being recognized as the prototypical opportunistic pathogen. In this chapter, the spectrum of infections caused by *P. aeruginosa* will be surveyed first. This will be followed by examples of persistent infections associated with CF. Some of the unique adaptation mechanisms in CF, including the *P. aeruginosa* conversion to a mucoid phenotype, will also be covered. Major emphasis will be placed on the relationship between the genetic and physiological basis of CF and colonization with *P. aeruginosa* and on the inflammatory processes in the host with CF.

INFECTIONS CAUSED BY *P. AERUGINOSA*

P. aeruginosa causes a variety of infections, which are listed in Table 1. In addition to the now-familiar link with CF (41), *P. aeruginosa* is typically associated with nosocomial infections, but community-acquired infections also contribute a substantial number of cases (1, 4, 11, 12, 14, 82, 97, 101, 107, 121, 126). These in-

V. Deretic, Department of Microbiology and Immunology, University of Michigan, Ann Arbor, MI 48109.

Persistent Bacterial Infections, Edited by J. P. Nataro, M. J. Blaser, and S. Cunningham-Rundles, © 2000 ASM Press, Washington, D.C.

TABLE 1 *Pseudomonas aeruginosa* infections

Respiratory infections in CF
Nosocomial infections
Bacteremia
Pneumonia
Urinary tract infections
Burn infections
Ocular infections
Malignant or simple external otitis
Folliculitis and other skin infections
Chronic otitis media
Osteomyelitis
Septic arthritis
Endocarditis
Brain abscesses
Meningitis
Decubitus ulcer
Green nails

fections range from minor inconveniences, such as a self-limiting folliculitis ("jacuzzi rash") in individuals with no known predisposing conditions, to lethal acute or chronic infections in burned or neutropenic patients and individuals with CF. While rather benign, the hot-tub-acquired skin rash is an infection which illustrates both the difficulty of killing *P. aeruginosa* by sanitary measures and the need for hydration of the infection sites (e.g., the stratum corneum of the skin) to promote *P. aeruginosa* multiplication. *P. aeruginosa* grows in water (e.g., swimming pools and spas) with scarce nutrient sources, which also attests to its impressive nutritional flexibility. This organism can exceed 10^5/ml in improperly maintained jacuzzi or swimming pool water once free chlorine levels drop (below 0.5 mg/liter due to inadequate chlorination or secondary to alkalization due to improperly balanced chemicals), illustrating the high resistance of *P. aeruginosa* to germicides. Another example of difficulties in controlling *P. aeruginosa* is hospitals—environments that are under the most rigorous sanitary rules. Control efforts in hospitals focused on air and surfaces are not sufficient (44). The best results are achieved

only with direct and strict control of devices used for endotracheal intubation and other forms of respiratory therapy (nebulizers), hemodialysis machines, and urinary tract catheters.

ACUTE INFECTIONS

Nosocomial Infections
P. aeruginosa is one of the predominant pathogens in hospital-acquired infections (6, 11), which are defined as those infections that are not present or incubating prior to or at the time of hospital admission. *P. aeruginosa* is not a commensal bacterium and is not a part of normal flora. During hospitalization, colonization gradually increases as a prelude to overt infection. Hospital-acquired pneumonias, urinary tract infections, surgical-site infections, and bacteremias are among the nosocomial infections frequently caused by *P. aeruginosa*. The more recent trend of subtle but continuing reduction in *P. aeruginosa* nosocomial infections has been attributed to the increased significance of gram-positive pathogens in hospital-acquired infections.

Pneumonia
P. aeruginosa is the most common cause of hospital-acquired pneumonia in intensive-care units (11, 47, 92, 102, 113, 122). Of all *P. aeruginosa* infections, pneumonia is associated with the highest mortality rate. Patients on ventilators or using nebulizers are at increased risk. Injury to the tracheal and bronchial lining during intubation contributes to the susceptibility of patients in intensive care. The mechanical or saliva-associated enzymatic injury to the airway mucosa, which otherwise displays natural resistance to *P. aeruginosa*, allows its increased adherence and colonization (92).

Bacteremia
The persons at risk of developing *P. aeruginosa* bacteremia reflect a typical spectrum of *P. aeruginosa* infections: burned or neutropenic patients and individuals with indwelling devices in the urinary or respiratory tract (5). *P. aerugi-*

nosa bacteremias are among the infections most feared by physicians, as they are associated with high mortality. Bacteremias can be the result of hospital- and community-acquired infections.

Urinary Tract Infections

Urinary catheters are inserted in 10% of all hospitalized patients in the United States, resulting in a large number of patients at risk of developing nosocomial urinary tract infections. While *Escherichia coli* and enterococci are the most common causes, *P. aeruginosa* is a major contributor, accounting for over 10% of the cases (67). *P. aeruginosa* is introduced during urological procedures and grows well in urine. It causes urinary tract infections in individuals with hydrodynamically obstructed urine flow. *P. aeruginosa* urinary tract infections are considered pathognomonic for structural or physiological abnormalities of the urinary tract. Interestingly, *P. aeruginosa* isolates from the urinary tract can sometimes be mucoid, similar to the phenotype observed during chronic infections in CF (77). Mutations causing conversion to mucoidy in *P. aeruginosa* urinary tract isolates are similar to those selected for during chronic respiratory infections in CF (10).

Burn Infections and Other Skin Infections

The traditional association of *P. aeruginosa* with burn infections is very strong. The most typical answer of physicians or medical students asked to name an infection caused by *P. aeruginosa* is the characteristic response: "burns." Burn infections and associated sepsis are the cause of more than 50% of fatalities in seriously burned patients (109). In addition to destruction of skin as a local barrier, burns have immunosuppressive effects. In deep-tissue injury, the necrotic tissue is the site of uncontrolled replication of bacteria in the immediate vicinity of healthy tissue. Bloodstream invasion is facilitated at the margins between the nonperfused (burned) and perfused (healthy) tissues. The preseptic state of immunosuppression induced by the burn (impaired tumor necrosis factor alpha (TNF-α) production, defects in neutro-

phil chemotaxis, etc.) can be reversed promptly by surgical removal of the thermally injured mass. The initially localized proliferation of *P. aeruginosa* in the burn wound is followed by systemic invasion (once the number of organisms exceeds 10^5/g of tissue). Ecthyma gangrenosum (starting as a large erythematous macular rash and progressing quickly into large vesicles and necrotic ulcers, which coalesce, forming eschar) is a cutaneous manifestation of burn infections but can be seen in other serious disseminated infections, such as bacteremia.

There are other skin and soft-tissue infections. Maintaining skin dryness is a factor in preventing *P. aeruginosa* infections. Under normal circumstances, the water necessary for growth of *P. aeruginosa* is missing from the skin surface. The predisposing factor for folliculitis in healthy individuals appears to be overhydration of the stratum corneum.

Ocular Infections

P. aeruginosa has the ability to destroy ocular tissue and has emerged as a significant ophthalmological infectious agent (136). The spectrum of ocular infections caused by *P. aeruginosa* is broad and includes corneal ulceration, scleritis, endophthalmitis, and vitritis. The incidence of corneal infections has increased dramatically with the use of contact lenses. Corneal ulceration starts with abrasions but can also be secondary to excessive exposure and drying conditions, such as Bell's palsy. Unlike some other ocular pathogens, *P. aeruginosa* does not cause infection unless the corneal epithelium is damaged, as shown in experimental models with intact corneas flooded with *P. aeruginosa* organisms but remaining uninfected. However, even superficial epithelial abrasions, as with manipulation or extended wear of contact lenses, can initiate the infection. *P. aeruginosa* does not adhere to intact epithelial cells but attaches to the basal lamina in a fibronectin-inhibitable fashion. When contact lenses become covered with protein and mucus, this also promotes adherence of *P. aeruginosa* to the organic films. *P. aeruginosa* in turn makes bacterial biofilm, with the associated increased resistance to clearance mechanisms. The proteases elaborated by *P. aeruginosa* (elastase, alkaline protease, and other toxins) contribute to rapid corneal melting, but some of the process is attributed to infiltrating neutrophils and proteases released by the inflammatory cells. More recent studies have focused on detailed analyses of the role of host factors in the pathogenesis of ocular *P. aeruginosa* infections (17, 18, 29, 52, 134).

Endocarditis

P. aeruginosa endocarditis is manifested as infection of the heart valves or endocardial and endovascular linings (54). The predisposing factors are artificial valves, but the infection can also be secondary to cancer chemotherapy and neutropenia. *P. aeruginosa* endocarditis has also been associated with intravenous (i.v.) drug abuse, as *P. aeruginosa* is often present in nonsterile tap water used by drug users as a solvent for narcotics.

Bone and Joint Infections

P. aeruginosa osteomyelitis has been associated with i.v. drug abuse, diabetes, and other conditions (70, 80, 119). *P. aeruginosa* used to be an overwhelmingly predominant pathogen causing osteomyelits in i.v. drug users, but recent trends indicate that streptococci and staphylococci have become the predominant pathogens in this context. In i.v. drug abusers, *P. aeruginosa* characteristically causes infections of unusual joints, such as sternoclavicular and axial skeleton joints.

P. aeruginosa Infections in Patients with AIDS

One of the first reports of *P. aeruginosa* in AIDS was in 1987 (127), with a small percentage of patients having *P. aeruginosa* bacteremia, or lung infection along with the bacteremia. Subsequent studies reported similar low incidence of *P. aeruginosa* bacteremia in human immunodeficiency virus (HIV)-infected patients and a limited correlation between overt AIDS symptoms and susceptibility to *P. aeruginosa*. It is not clear whether HIV significantly increases the risk of *P. aeruginosa* infections, as among 400 HIV-positive individuals monitored over a year in one study carried out in Houston, only 3 patients were found with *P. aeruginosa* pneumonia (61). However, *P. aeruginosa* was identified in some studies as one of the most common causes of bacterial pneumonia (1) and hospital-acquired infections (33) in HIV-positive individuals. Curiously, serum sensitivity and serotype loss have been noted among isolates from chronically infected patients with AIDS, resembling phenotypic changes with the loss of lipopolysaccharide (LPS) O side chains typical of CF isolates. *P. aeruginosa* has also been reported as a major cause of relatively infrequent but serious lung cavitary disease in AIDS (4, 103).

Other Infections

In addition to pneumonia, *P. aeruginosa* causes other respiratory tract infections, such as sinusitis (which is rare in the general population but is a frequent feature of CF) and bronchitis. *P. aeruginosa* causes infections of the ear (simple or malignant external otitis and chronic otitis media) and is a rare but important cause of central nervous system infections manifested as meningitis, brain abscesses, and vertebral osteomyelitis with spinal epidural abscesses compressing the spinal cord. Vertebral osteomyelitis is sometimes a complication of ascending urinary tract infections. *P. aeruginosa* can also cause septic arthritis, which is usually monarticular, and can be a part of decubitus ulcer. This organism also causes a condition referred to as "green nails," the color coming from the pigment pyocyanin.

VIRULENCE FACTORS

Multifactorial Nature of Host-Pathogen Interactions in *P. aeruginosa* Infections

A multitude of virulence factors have been identified in *P. aeruginosa*. The broad repertoire of toxins and other virulence determinants attests to the fact that *P. aeruginosa* is adapted to many niches and hosts. Similar to the situation in other organisms with multiple virulence factors, *P. aeruginosa* adhesins, toxins, and persistence determinants are well researched. As with staphylococci and other examples where virulence is clearly multifactorial, it becomes difficult to identify a decisive virulence factor in disease caused by *P. aeruginosa*, with some exceptions. A case in point appears to be alginate production by CF strains (41). In other instances, a subset of factors may be more critical, i.e., exotoxin A and protease production during ophthalmic infections. Frequently, host factors and associated tissue necrosis are important if not primary contributors to pathology in *P. aeruginosa* infections (59, 68).

Classical Virulence Factors of *P. aeruginosa*

P. aeruginosa virulence factors have been studied for a long time. The traditional virulence determinants have recently been reviewed (128) and will only be listed here.

1. Adhesins and motility factors. Pilus and nonpilus adhesins and twitching motility factors, flagella, and chemotaxis have been identified as determinants allowing migration towards chemoattractants, attachment, and colonization and spread on surfaces.

2. Proteases. These products are responsible for necrotic and hemorrhagic effects. Over 90% of *P. aeruginosa* strains produce alkaline protease and elastase.

3. Exotoxin A. Exotoxin A is produced by almost all strains of *P. aeruginosa*, but a very small percentage of clinical strains lack the gene for it. It plays a role in corneal infection models, and exotoxin A mutant strains are less virulent in the burned-mouse infection model.

4. Cytotoxin. *P. aeruginosa* cytotoxin is carried on a temperate phage, and the incidence of cytotoxin-positive *P. aeruginosa* varies, depending on the detection method. Cytotoxin acts similarly to staphylococcal α toxin and introduces pores in host cell membranes.

5. Hemolysins. *P. aeruginosa* makes a heat-stable glycolipid hemolysin referred to as rhamnolipid, which can emulsify eukaryotic membranes. The heat-labile hemolysin phospholipase C is produced by all *P. aeruginosa* strains. *P. aeruginosa* produces another phospholipase C, referred to as a nonhemolitic phospholipase.

6. Endotoxin. *P. aeruginosa* LPS has low intrinsic endotoxin activity compared to that of other gram-negative pathogens, and the role of LPS has been recognized in the context of antigens and protective antibodies in some instances.

7. Polysaccharide alginate. The role of alginate as a prominent persistence determinant in CF is covered below. Of further importance is the demonstrated effect of alginate on inhibiting tobramycin action by limiting its diffusion. This is significant, as tobramycin is gaining popularity in the treatment of CF in special formulations, such as the tobramycin solution for inhalation (TOBI).

8. Exoenzyme S. This toxin appears to play a role in burn infection models, but its role in other infections may be underappreciated. The role of exoenzyme S (ExoS) is covered below in the context of the type III secretion system.

Newly Identified *P. aeruginosa* Factors Delivered to Host Cells by the Type III Secretion Apparatus

As with other gram-negative pathogens, recent investigations have focused on the type III secretion system and products delivered to the host cell via direct bacterium-host cell interactions (32). Type III secretion transfer is stimulated by contact between the bacterium and the host cell, and the bacterial effector proteins are delivered into the host cell cytosol without cleavage of a signal sequence which appears to be embedded somewhere within the N-terminal sequences of the proteins. One of the products delivered via the type III secretion system is ExoS. Recent analyses of the bacterial-eukaryotic-cell coculture system have demonstrated that one of the previously identified in vitro targets (16), Ras, is modified during in vivo interactions, thus substantiating the role of ExoS as a toxin (85). ExoS reduces proliferation and viability of host cells (78, 85). In addition to its ADP-ribosylating domain, the N-terminal segment of 234 amino acids has additional activities, manifested by disruption of actin filaments and cell rounding (34), which can be overridden by constitutively activating a small GTPase (e.g., treating cells with the Rho-activating toxin CNF-1) (91). ExoS also interacts with the host protein FAS (factor that activates exoenzyme S), a member of the 14-3-3 family of proteins (35), which bind to ligands via phosphoserine motifs. Although ExoS association with the zeta isoform of 14-3-3 does not involve a phosphorylated serine, the binding is very tight (76). As 14-3-3 proteins regulate apoptosis by sequestering the phosphorylated BAD, which in its free, nonphosphorylated form associates with Bcl-xL, leading to apoptosis (123), there may be an interesting connection between ExoS activities, apoptosis, and cell cycle processes.

Other type III secretion-delivered products include the following. (i) ExoT, which has 76% homology with ExoS, displays only 0.2% of the ADP-ribosylating activity of ExoS (130). ExoT has also been proposed to be the *Pseudomonas* anti-internalization factor, preventing uptake by epithelial cells (in contrast to *Salmonella* and *Shigella*, in which the type III secretion apparatus promotes internalization) (48). (ii) ExoU (PepA) has been described as an acute cytotoxin affecting cell viability and is associated with acute epithelial injury (30, 49). (iii) ExoY, a recently identified adenylate cyclase, is activated in eukaryotic cells (via a mechanism different from calmodulin, a factor which has been implicated in a *Bordetella* adenylate cyclase toxin that is homologous to ExoY) (131). In addition, the recently described protection in animals vaccinated with a critical component of the *P. aeruginosa* type III secretion system, PcrV, suggests potential novel strategies in preventing (active immunization) or treating (passive immunization) lung injury and inflammation (105).

Biofilm Formation

The biofilm mode of growth, which is the preferred form of existence for *P. aeruginosa* in the environment (20), should be considered a viru-lence factor. Whether the exopolysaccharides elaborated by *P. aeruginosa* in ecological sites are exclusively alginate or a combination of polymers is not known. The development of biofilms involves microcolony formation, and such morphological features have been observed in the lungs of patients with CF (69). Biofilms have been regarded as a protective mode of growth, which serves as a barrier against effective killing by phagocytic cells (55). The Biofilm mode of growth may also confer additional antibiotic resistance properties, either as a polyanionic shield (84) or through the slow metabolism and growth of bacteria in biofilms relative to those of the free swimming planktonic forms (3). Recent genetic studies of biofilm development (23) have uncovered a potential link between biofilm formation and quorum-sensing systems (88), which affect the expression of other virulence factors (elastase, exotoxin A, and alkaline protease) in *P. aeruginosa*. The relatively high densities of *P. aeruginosa* in some infection sites (e.g., sometimes seen in the lumen of the respiratory tract in CF) may play a role in the concerted production of potentially damaging exoproducts and antigens via this mechanism.

Animal Models of Infection

A compilation of animal models used to study *P. aeruginosa* is given in Table 2. This list is focused on the use of mice, as the availability of inbred strains, the broad repertoire of immunological reagents, and, most importantly, the continuing development of transgenic mice make this animal the most versatile model. However, some historically important models, such as the rat agar bead model of chronic respiratory infection (13), are included. The agar bead model has now been applied in the mouse, and recent studies have frequently used this approach to study chronic infection. As an alternative to this forced persistent infection, a model of repeated respiratory challenge in mice has recently been developed (133). Figure 1 shows the aerosol equipment used in this model.

One advantage of the repeated-respiratory-

TABLE 2 Murine[a] models in use for analysis of *P. aeruginosa* virulence[b]

Animal model	Application	Comment	Reference(s)
Burned mouse model	Burn infections	Thermal injury followed by subcutaneous injection of *P. aeruginosa*	115
Neutropenic mouse model of fatal *P. aeruginosa* sepsis	Septicemia in experimental neutropenia	Cyclophosphamide-induced neutropenia; intraperitoneal or surgical incision challenge with *P. aeruginosa*	21, 46, 129
Aerosol infection model in mice	Aerosol challenge	Initial development and parameters of *P. aeruginosa* aerosol infection	100, 112, 120
Lethal pulmonary challenge in granulocytopenic mice	Mice rendered neutropenic by cyclophosphamide	Aerosol challenge	111
Mouse agar bead model	Chronic respiratory infection	Agar beads protect *P. aeruginosa* from rapid clearance	114
Endobronchial infection in susceptible mice	Analysis of inflammatory cytokines	DBA/2 mice reported to be highly sensitive to *P. aeruginosa*	81
Neonatal-mouse model of acute pneumonia	Acute pneumonia in infant mice	Intranasal instillation; 7-day-old mice	118
Repeated aerosol exposure[c]	Chronic inflammation	12-week course of repeated exposures to *P. aeruginosa* aerosols; cytokines (TNF-α; MIP-2)	133
Murine model of chronic mucosal colonization	Colonization of the intestinal tract	Suppression of normal gastrointestinal flora with streptomycin	93
Mouse corneal infection model	Corneal damage	Inoculation of corneal incision	37
Eye infection model in cyclophosphamide-treated mice	Ocular infections	Animals rendered neutropenic by cyclophosphamide	50
Rat agar bead model of chronic respiratory infection	Chronic respiratory infection	Intratracheal instillation of bacteria embedded in agar beads	13
Guinea pig model of experimental pneumonia	Clearance upon aerosol exposure	Comparison of mucoid and nonmucoid *P. aeruginosa*	8

[a] Some frequently employed models in other animals are included (e.g., the rat chronic agar bead infection model [13]), but their coverage is not comprehensive. The emphasis on mice is due to the increasing availability of transgenic mice with various defects, which is expected to promote further investigations in this species.
[b] Modified with permission from Yu et al. (132).
[c] This model is similar to the one used for *B. cepacia* and *S. aureus* aerosol exposure in normal and CF transgenic mice (22).

challenge model in mice is that it permits studies of inflammation parameters. Since the mouse is quite efficient in removing *P. aeruginosa* from the respiratory tract, repeated exposure to bacterial aerosols is needed to mimic chronic infection. A similar effect can be achieved by instilling agar- or agarose-embedded bacteria into the tracheae, but this procedure is invasive and usually involves significant variation. The utility of the repeated-exposure model is evidenced by the experiments using interleukin 10 (IL-10) knockout mice, deficient in this important anti-inflammatory cytokine (133). Upon single exposure, no differences between control and IL-10 knockout animals can be detected in lung histopathology

(albeit IL-10 animals show some mortality upon initial exposure to *P. aeruginosa* that normally does not occur with control mice). However, following eight exposures, there are significant differences in the lung pathologies of C57BL/6J and IL-10T knockout mice (Fig. 2 and 3).

Alternative Models for Investigation of *P. aeruginosa* Virulence Determinants

PLANT AND NEMATODE MODELS
A model using the plant *Aradopsis thaliana* as a nonmammalian host has been reported (98, 99), with the strain *P. aeruginosa* 14, which is virulent in both plants and animals. It has been shown in this model that some virulence fac-

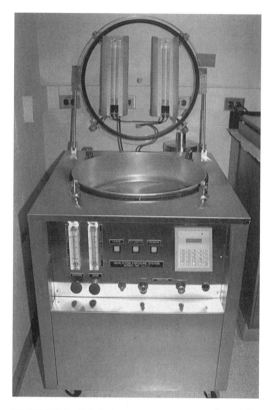

FIGURE 1 Inhalation exposure system adapted for use with *P. aeruginosa* aerosols. The system (Glas Col) is a whole-body exposure chamber for quantitative infection of animals by inhalation of airborne *P. aeruginosa*. The system has a nebulizer-Venturi unit in which bacterial suspension is introduced. The suspension is atomized and mixed with filtered room air, and a bacterial cloud is introduced into the exposure chamber kept under negative pressure. A programmable control is used to preheat, nebulize, expose, and control bacterial decay. The exhaust air is filtered through a HEPA filter and passed through an incinerator in the back of the unit. Germicidal UV lamps are used for decontamination of the chamber. The five-compartment cage can accommodate up to 100 mice for simultaneous exposure. The initial deposition in the lungs is exceptionally uniform, and the variation from mouse to mouse is similar to sampling errors usually seen with bacterial plating. The system has been used for single-inhalation exposure to demonstrate reduced pulmonary clearance of mucoid *P. aeruginosa* (10) and for the development of the repeated-respiratory-exposure inflammation model (133).

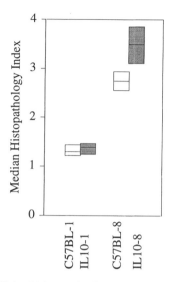

FIGURE 2 Eight-week-old (at the inception of the experiment) C57BL/6J (*n* = 12) (open boxes) and IL-10T (*n* = 8) (shaded boxes) mice were exposed to *P. aeruginosa* once (-1) or 8 (-8) times. Pairwise comparison (Student-Newman-Keuls test) indicated that the histopathology indices relative to unexposed controls were significant ($P < 0.005$). Histopathology scores were as described in Yu et al. (133). (Reproduced with permission from Yu et al. [133].)

tors, such as exotoxin A, may apply to both animal and plant infection models. This rather imaginative idea that simpler, nonmammalian surrogate models can be used to investigate *P. aeruginosa* virulence was next extended to the nematode *Caenorhabditis elegans* (72, 117). This approach also allowed a demonstration of the role of the *P. aeruginosa* redox-active pigment pyocyanin, which generates reactive oxygen intermediates, in toxicity to the worms, where it causes fast killing (within 24 h) (72). Other *P. aeruginosa* factors may be involved in the additional processes of slow killing of the nematodes (117). This innovative approach seems appealing and could aid in the search for new virulence factors, ensuring many years of interesting investigations. However, there are some a priori limitations of the plant and nematode models, as they do not take into account the effects of innate or acquired immunity. Related to this issue is the dominant role of host inflam-

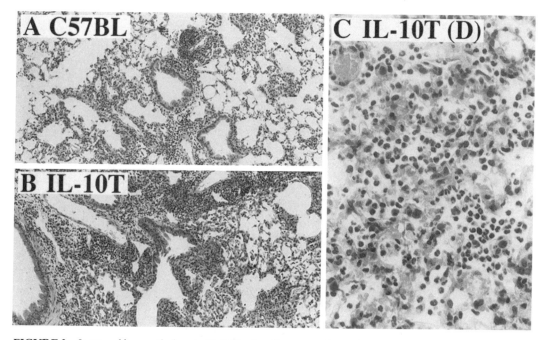

FIGURE 3 Increased lung pathology in IL-10T mice after repeated exposure to *P. aeruginosa*. Note perivascular, peribronchial, and intestinal inflammation and increased inflammatory changes in IL-10T (knockout) mice (B) relative to C57BL/6J mice (A). (C) Postmortem appearance of the lung from an IL-10T transgenic mouse (note numerous neutrophils) that succumbed after two exposures to *P. aeruginosa*. (Reproduced with modifications from Yu et al. [133].)

matory mediators in diseases caused by *P. aeruginosa*.

APPLICATION OF IVET TECHNOLOGY

In a recent study, a global approach for identification of in vivo-expressed genes adopted from enteric organisms (73) has been applied to isolate a group of 22 *P. aeruginosa* genes in a mouse septicemia model (124).

PERSISTENT RESPIRATORY INFECTIONS IN CF

P. aeruginosa and Respiratory Complications in CF

The major cause of high morbidity and mortality in CF is chronic respiratory infection with *P. aeruginosa* (41). Today, CF is the most common lethal genetic disorder in the United States, where approximately 30,000 children, adolescents, and adults are affected. The median age of survival, as listed on the Cystic

Fibrosis Foundation Web site (http://www.cff.org), is 31 years. The disease is characterized by a variety of symptoms, the most common being salty-tasting sweat and skin, persistent cough, wheezing, and appetite sometimes described as "ravenous" while at the same time the patient fails to thrive (due to intestinal defects, malnutrition, and anorexia). The usual complications in the respiratory tract are hemoptysis (blood in the sputum); pneumothorax (collapsed lung) due to mucus-plugged bronchioles, which then act as one-way "ball-valves," causing overinflated distal alveoli to burst; atelectasis, in CF almost invariably caused by complete mucus plugging, resulting in air resorbtion which leaves the lobe or segment airless; bronchiolectasis and bronchiectasis, with bronchioles and bronchi dilated and with weakened walls as the result of recurring infection and inflammation; fibrosis (scar tissue); low oxygen level; and, ultimately, respiratory failure. Respiratory failure can occur for various reasons, but in CF it is usually the end of a long process. Placing a terminal CF patient with respiratory failure on a mechanical ventilator does not always reverse the process, as it is not only the exchange of oxygen that matters (O_2 can be delivered by placing the patient on ventilator support, but there frequently is not enough healthy lung tissue to eliminate CO_2) (86). It is widely believed that the respiratory sequelae in CF and the progressive deterioration of respiratory function are the result of recurring infections culminating with chronic *P. aeruginosa* colonization that cannot be eradicated even with the most aggressive treatments.

P. aeruginosa colonizes the lung in CF after a succession of other pathogens. The initial bacterial pathogens in CF are *Staphylococcus aureus* and *Haemophilus influenzae*. These organisms are eventually supplanted by *P. aeruginosa*. Another important CF pathogen is *Burkholderia* (formerly *Pseudomonas*) *cepacia*, which can sometimes cause fatal acute infections usually not seen with *P. aeruginosa* (41). According to a recent comprehensive report by FitzSimmons (31), the incidence of *P. aeruginosa* in the age group over 26 years exceeded 80% while only 21% of patients under 12 months of age were colonized. The relationship between *P. aeruginosa* and CF has been the subject of numerous studies, but the reasons for this unusually firm association are still not fully understood. Some of the possible underlying causes are discussed below. However, it is essential to remember that *P. aeruginosa* is not the sole pathogen in CF and that its prevalence is not only the result of predisposing genetic and physiological factors but is also based on the unique recalcitrance of the organism to antibiotic treatments and its evasion of immune mechanisms, possibly related to the biofilm mode of growth and selection of mucoid variants in the lung in CF.

CFTR and Genetic and Physiological Basis of CF

CF is caused by mutations in the gene encoding a protein termed CF transmembrane conduc-

tance regulator (CFTR), which functions as an apical membrane chloride channel (125). Various CFTR mutations affect the processing, intracellular localization, and function of this chloride channel. Mutations in CFTR also have pleiotropic effects on the functioning of other ion transport processes (e.g., the amiloride-sensitive sodium channel, the outwardly rectifying chloride channel, the Na-H$^+$ exchanger, and bicarbonate conductance). The most common mutant *CFTR* allele, ΔF508, probably arose in an individual over 50,000 years ago. Because it potentially conferred selective advantage on the heterozygotes, this individual's progeny now number between 20 and 50 million (94). Although the ΔF508 mutation is the most common alteration (accounting for 70% of the cases), it is not the only mutation, and there are more than 500 CF-causing alleles of *CFTR* described thus far. The apparent selective advantage of a heterozygous state with one mutant *CFTR* allele may be based on resistance to cholera toxin (36) or *Salmonella enterica* serovar Typhi infections (95).

Undersialylation of Epithelial Glycoconjugates and Increased Adherence of *P. aeruginosa* to CF Respiratory Epithelium

It has been noted that glycoproteins and glycolipids on the apical membranes of CF cells display reduced sialylation, and expression of ΔF508 in heterologous cells results in decreased sialylation of glycoconjugates on the plasma membrane (28). CFTR and chloride transport could play a role in facilitating acidification of intracellular compartments, such as endosomes and the *trans*-Golgi network (TGN), by maintaining charge neutrality as protons are pumped into the lumens of these organelles. This hypothesis (2) appeared to be a plausible explanation for reduced sialylation of glycoconjugates, as loss of CFTR could result in increased pH and sialyltransferase in the TGN has an acidic pH optimum (6.0). However, several attempts have failed to detect reduced acidification of the TGN (106). Nevertheless, CFTR has been found associated with endosomes (71) and plays a role in endosome fusion (7), suggesting that it may function in intracellular membrane trafficking. In this model, which remains to be fully explored, CFTR as a putative regulator of vesicular trafficking could affect the time that membrane proteins spend in relevant compartments, such as the TGN, where they are exposed to sialyltransferase. Regardless of the exact mechanism, the increased levels of asialoganglioside 1 (aGM1) on CF epithelia promote adherence and colonization by *P. aeruginsoa* (53, 104). *P. aeruginsoa* pilin and whole bacilli (53, 104) bind better to aGM1 than to the sialylated ganglioside GM1 (66).

Reduced Uptake of *P. aeruginosa* by CF Respiratory Epithelial Cells

In the reduced-uptake model (96), *P. aeruginosa* is envisioned as being normally taken up by the respiratory epithelial cells and eliminated from the respiratory tract by cell desquamation. The work by Pier et al. (96) suggests that CFTR itself (its first extracellular loop) acts as a receptor for *P. aeruginosa* in its uptake by the epithelial cells. In this scenario, ΔF508 CFTR, which is not properly folded and remains trapped in the endoplasmic reticulum (ER), never traffics to the plasma membrane. This in turn eliminates the receptor for *P. aeruginosa* uptake by the epithelial cells. If one assumes that epithelial uptake of the bacterium could be part of the clearance process, the lack of CFTR could then translate into less efficient elimination of *P. aeruginosa*.

Impaired *P. aeruginosa* Killing by Airway Epithelium-Derived Antibiotic Peptides (Defensins) in Secretions with Abnormally High Salt Concentrations

The genetic defect in CF results in defective chloride channels and abnormal chloride and sodium transport across the epithelial cell membrane. This has led to intuitive predictions that the electrolyte content of the respiratory epithelium fluid is different (e.g., 170 mM chloride in CF versus the normal 85 mM [38]). Based on the premise that salt concentration is increased in airway fluids in CF, as observed in sweat secretions in CF, two reports (39, 108) have indicated that there may be a link between the altered electrolytes and infections in CF. Using a CF epithelium xenograft or epithelium monolayers grown in contact with air to mimic respiratory epithelium conditions, these groups have demonstrated that small antimicrobial peptides (e.g., human beta-defensins 1 and 2), which are capable of eliminating very small inocula of *P. aeruginosa*, fail to do so under conditions of increased salt concentration. However, the electrolyte composition of the airway surface fluid, according to other reports, seems not to differ between normal and CF respiratory epithelia and may even be hypotonic (62). Thus, the proposal that increased salt in the lung fluid in CF interferes with the action of antimicrobial peptides awaits the resolution of this controversy.

Reduced Inducible Nitric Oxide Synthase and NO Production in CF and *P. aeruginosa* Colonization

Nasal NO levels in CF are reduced relative to those in healthy controls, and orally exhaled NO output in CF is lower in comparison with that of patients with other inflammatory conditions (42). Calcium-independent nitric oxide synthase, also known as inducible nitric oxide synthase (iNOS), which has been traditionally associated with the bactericidal repertoire of the macrophages, is constitutively expressed in normal airway epithelial cells (43, 63). In contrast, both the human airways in CF and the *CFTR*-mutant transgenic murine airway epithelial cells are deficient in iNOS (57, 79). The gene for iNOS appears normal in CF, as its induction can be detected in submucosal inflammatory cells (most likely neutrophils) (79). The lack of iNOS production in CF may have two important repercussions. First, the reduced NO levels have been linked to the hyperabsorption of sodium in CF (57). NO stimulates soluble guanylate cyclase, and cyclic GMP (cGMP) production downregulates amiloride-sensitive sodium absorption. Thus, the lower NO production in CF respiratory epithelia results in diminished cGMP and further contributes to increased sodium absorption, already affected by altered interactions between CFTR and the epithelial sodium channel (116). The ensuing increased absorption of airway surface fluid contributes to altered mucus hydration and impaired mucocilliary clearance.

Second, nitric oxide has also been directly implicated as a bactericidal and bacteristatic agent (24). The lack of iNOS production and reduced NO output have been shown to play a role in susceptibility to *P. aeruginosa* (57). Excised murine lungs challenged with low inoculum (500 CFU) show a 25-fold reduction in survival of *P. aeruginosa* in normal mice relative to the ΔF508/ΔF508 homozygotes measured under conditions (high-salt Ringer's solution) that eliminate the contribution of the antibacterial peptides (defensins) discussed above. The lungs of normal mice treated with S-methylisothiourea, an inhibitor of iNOS, clear low-dose *P. aeruginosa* inocula 10-fold less efficiently than the untreated control. In vitro, sodium nitroprusside (a compound releasing NO) is bactericidal for *P. aeruginosa*, an activity that is abrogated by the addition of the NO scavenger N-methyl-D-glucamine dithiocarbamate. Data obtained in our laboratory with iNOS knockout transgenic mice support the role of NO in the innate defense against *P. aeruginosa*, as the iNOS knockout animals display an approximately 3-fold-reduced clearance in the aerosol infection model (133a).

Inflammation in CF

The major causes of high morbidity and mortality presently associated with CF are chronic inflammation and the resulting respiratory tissue destruction. A hallmark of the inflammatory processes in CF is an increased presence of polymorphonuclear leukocytes, although lymphocytes and macrophages can also be seen (60). Anti-inflammatory therapy is beneficial and slows down deterioration due to lung disease (65). Significantly elevated levels of TNF-α, IL-1, and IL-8 and reduced amounts of the major anti-inflammatory cytokine IL-10 in bronchoalveolar lavage fluid are typical of CF

(9). In the experimental model of repeated exposure to *P. aeruginosa* aerosols, mimicking chronic infection, the continuing presence of the pathogen results in increased pathology of the lung in the IL-10 knockout mice relative to identically exposed control animals (133). These findings support a critical role of this anti-inflammatory cytokine in preventing excessive damage to lung tissue.

In addition to the inflammation provoked by infections, it appears that some level of spontaneous inflammation in CF possibly exists even before colonization by infectious agents (60). Bronchoalveolar lavage fluids from children with CF aged between 3 months and 7 years and showing minimal or no clinical lung disease displayed increased levels of neutrophils, IL-8, and TNF-α (133). It is not known whether and how the mutations in *CFTR* are related to decreased production of anti-inflammatory cytokines, increased expression of proinflammatory cytokines, and altered response to exogenous stimuli (e.g., infection). Some of the hyperexcitability of CF tissues can be attributed to activation of NF-κB (a transcriptional factor necessary for expression of many proinflammatory cytokines) (27), as exogenous stimuli (e.g., TNF-α and IL-1) appear to strongly activate NF-κB in CF epithelial cells relative to those in normal controls. However, the reported elevated basal levels of NF-κB activation in CF cells have recently been attributed to growth in serum, which increases the basal levels of IL-8 and perhaps NF-κB. The exact mechanism underlying the hyperreactivity of CF cells is not known, but ER retention and ER overload response (87) to misfolded CFTR in ΔF508 cells may be one of the contributing factors. Alternatively, or in addition, a defective CFTR (or its absence) may have effects on apical scaffolding and the cortical cytoskeleton. CFTR has been shown (45) to interact with a PDZ domain containing ERM-binding protein, EBP50, localized in apical membranes and interacting with the actin-binding protein ezrin. The predicted alterations in the cytoskeleton could be a source of signals for the overexuberant response via the NF-κB pathway.

Enhanced expression of other molecules participating in migration of inflammatory cells, such as intracellular adhesion molecules (ICAM-1), secondary to production of proinflammatory cytokines in CF could also contribute to the recruitment and accumulation of neutrophils. It has also been reported that T cells from patients with CF may have a defect in IL-10 production (83), which is in keeping with the observation that epithelial cells from individuals with CF produce less IL-10 than those from healthy controls (9). Whether or not the imbalance between pro- and anti-inflammatory cytokines in CF is due to intrinsic properties directly linked to *CFTR* mutations, the binding of *P. aeruginosa* to CF epithelial cells, enhanced due to undersialylation of glycolipids in CF, has been shown to induce NF-κB activation and IL-8 production and lead to an overexuberant inflammatory response (27).

Establishment of Chronic Infections in CF and Conversion to Mucoidy in *P. aeruginosa*

In the majority of patients with CF (>80% [31]), *P. aeruginosa* becomes established as the predominant colonizer of the lung after a succession of other pathogens, as discussed above. The establishment of chronic *P. aeruginosa* infection is associated with a poor outlook for CF patients (90). There appear to be two stages in colonization with *P. aeruginosa*. The first phase is an insidious infection, with intermittent isolation of *P. aeruginosa* from the lungs of the patient with CF (64). This phase of the infection does not cause significant decline in pulmonary function and can last for various periods (0 to 5.5 years) (56). The transition to chronic infection is the next stage. This has been defined as a continuous isolation of *P. aeruginosa* for at least 6 months, along with increased antibody response to *P. aeruginosa* antigens (as opposed to the initial, intermittent phase with antibodies to no more than two *P. aeruginosa* precipitins in the serum) (56). The establishment of chronic infection coincides

with the conversion of *P. aeruginosa* to the mucoid phenotype (64, 89). Once a chronic infection is established, this condition becames almost permanent (41, 89). The persistence of the same strain of *P. aeruginosa* over many years in the same patient has been documented by different fingerprinting techniques.

There is no clearly defined time interval that can be assigned to the transition between intermittent infections (characterized by the nonmucoid form of *P. aeruginosa*) and chronic infections (dominated by isolates with the mucoid phenotype). The periods can vary, depending on the study, from less than a month to almost 5 years (41). According to one report, the mean duration of infection until isolation of mucoid forms was 3.37 (± 1.76) years (74). The mucoid phenotype of *P. aeruginosa* is rarely seen in infections other than CF, although mucoid strains can be isolated during chronic urinary tract infections (10, 77), but all mucoid isolates produce chemically similar polymers based on the polyuronic acid exopolysaccharide alginate. Alginate is a linear polymer of ($1{\rightarrow}4$)-linked β-D-mannuronic acid and its C-5 epimer α-L-guluronic acid in varying proportions and with additional modifications (i.e., acetylation). This chemically nontoxic compound is highly hydrophilic and generates a loosely structured capsule-like matrix which gels in the presence of calcium. The biochemistry, genetics, and physiology of alginate biosynthesis has been extensively reviewed (41). The switch from nonmucoid to mucoid forms is caused by point mutations which inactivate the *mucA* gene (10, 25, 26, 41, 75). MucA acts as a negative regulator of the alternative sigma factor AlgU, which directs transcription of the alginate biosynthetic genes. When *mucA* is inactivated, AlgU is no longer inhibited, and this results in the overproduction of alginate and the mucoid phenotype.

mucA mutants are selected for during chronic infections in CF, and alterations in *mucA* account for approximately 80% of mucoid strains. The remaining balance of 20% of the clinical strains undergo conversion via another pathway (9a). Regardless of the path of conversion to mucoidy (although there appear to be some differences in other virulence properties between the *mucA* and non-*mucA* strains), alginate has been widely accepted as a persistence factor (41). The majority of the support for such a role of alginate in allowing *P. aeruginosa* to persist in the CF lung comes from in vitro studies that have previously been extensively reviewed (41). The multitude of proposed functions can be divided into two groups: (i) the mucoid capsule-like material serves as a direct barrier against phagocytic cells and effective opsonization and (ii) alginate may play a role in biofilm-related phenomena, such as adhesion and antibiotic resistance. It is interesting, however, that evidence for an in vivo role for alginate was missing (with the exception of the fact that there is selective pressure in the lung for the emergence of *mucA* mutants) until very recently. Using several sets of isogenic strains in the mouse model of aerosol infection, Boucher et al. have recently demonstrated that alginate-producing forms are cleared less efficiently from the murine lung (10) (Table 3). Note that the differences in the clearance of mucoid versus nonmucoid strains are rather subtle, and only in experiments with carefully matched isogenic strains was it possible to demonstrate the advantage of mucoid forms. However, mucoid strains are eventually cleared (albeit more slowly than the nonmucoid isogenic strains) from the murine lung in contrast to the typical permanent colonization in CF.

TABLE 3 Decreased clearance of mucoid *P. aeruginosa* from the murine lung[a]

Strain[b]	Genotype[c]	NaCl (mM) in medium[d]	Phenotype[e]	% *P. aeruginosa* survival[f]		
				DBA/2NHsd ($n = 20$)	C57BL/6J ($n = 60$)	BALB/c ($n = 20$)
CF40	*mucA* Ins T_{295} $\Delta G440$		NM	ND	14.8 ± 0.7	ND
CF40	*mucA* Ins T_{295} $\Delta G440$	100	M	ND	45.2 ± 4.2	ND
CF45	*mucA* $\Delta G440$		NM	35.4 ± 11.7	7.5 ± 1.3	6.4 ± 0.7
CF45	*mucA* $\Delta G440$	60	M	72.4 ± 4.7	25.1 ± 4.4	5.5 ± 0.7
PAO381	*mucA*$^+$		NM	3.7 ± 0.8	20.5 ± 5.6	10.5 ± 1.3
PAO578I	PAO381 *mucA22*		M	17.2 ± 0.6	38.9 ± 8.9	41.6 ± 8.5
PAO381	*mucA*$^+$	60	NM	ND	24.8 ± 4.8	ND
PAO578II	PAO578I *sup-2*		NM	ND	21.0 ± 3.3	ND
PAO578II	PAO578I *sup-2*	60	NM	ND	20.6 ± 12.9	ND
PAO578II	PAO578I *sup-2*	300	M	ND	43.7 ± 4.5	ND
PAO6888	PAO578II *algD*::GM^r	300	NM	ND	12.8 ± 2.2	ND

[a] Reproduced from Boucher et al. (10).
[b] PAO578I is a constitutive mucoid derivative of PAO381. PAO578II is a derivative of PAO578I with a suppressor mutation (*sup-2*) which attenuates the mucoid phenotype and renders it dependent on the salt concentration in the medium.
[c] Known alterations in *mucA* are listed.
[d] NaCl concentration was optimized for maximal alginate production by individual CF isolates.
[e] M and NM, mucoid phenotype and nonmucoid phenotype, respectively, on the medium used to grow *P. aeruginosa* for clearance studies (see the text). Strain phenotypes on Luria-Bertani (LB) and *Pseudomonas* isolation agar (PIA) media were as follows: CF45, NM (LB) and M (PIA); CF40, NM (LB) and M (PIA); PAO381, NM on both media; PAO578I, M on both media; PAO578II, NM (LB) and M (PIA).
[f] Survival at 4 h is expressed as the percentage ($\pm$ standard deviation) of the initial CFU deposited in the lung. Initial bacterial depositions were as follows: BALB/c, 5.3×10^5 to 3.7×10^6; C57BL/6J, 2.2×10^5 to 3.5×10^6; and DBA/2NHsd, 7.0×10^5 to 9.5×10^6. The numbers of remaining bacteria were determined by plating of total-lung homogenate after 4 h. *n*, number of animals per mouse strain used in determining initial deposition and 4-h clearance. The *P* values (*t* test) were as follows: DBA/2NHsd, $P = 4.33 \times 10^{-2}$ for the two forms of CF45 and $P = 3.91 \times 10^{-2}$ for PAO381 versus PAO578I; C57BL/6J, $P = 2.10 \times 10^{-3}$ for the two forms of CF40, $P = 1.92 \times 10^{-2}$ for the two forms of CF45, $P = 1.64 \times 10^{-4}$ for PAO381 versus PAO578I, $P = 1.57 \times 10^{-2}$ for PAO578II and PAO578II at 0.3 M NaCl, and $P = 3.59 \times 10^{-3}$ for PAO578II at 0.3 M NaCl and PAO6888; BALB/c, $P = 2.20 \times 10^{-2}$ for PAO381 versus PAO578I. ND, not determined.

Models of Respiratory Infection in *CFTR* Transgenic Mice

The *CFTR* knockout mice, while displaying many characteristics of intestinal disease in CF, fail to develop respiratory infections or other signs of overt lung disease. This disappointing limitation of the *CFTR* transgenics, which had been expected to provide a model for infection and inflammation in CF, has been linked to the presence of alternative Cl^- and Na^+ channels in mice that could compensate for the lack of a functional *CFTR* gene (15). When the mutant *CFTR*^{m1UNC}/*CFTR*^{m1UNC} (carrying the S489X nonsense mutation [110]) has been back-crossed repeatedly into a C57BL/6J background, the resulting congenic mice (58) (strain designation, C57BL/6J *CFTR*^{m1UNC}/ *CFTR*^{m1UNC}) have developed some features of respiratory disease in CF: e.g., acinar and alveolar hyperinflation has been noted, possibly secondary to a buildup of mucus causing the ball valve obstruction effect discussed in "*P. aeruginosa* and Respiratory Complications in CF," above. These effects, seen in the congenic mice, have been attributed to a loss of epithelial response to UTP, an agonist of a P_{2U}-type purinergic receptor causing IP_3 production and associated release of Ca^{2+} intracellular stores. As manifested by the lack of nasal potential difference response in congenic mice upon stimulation by UTP, it is possible that these phenomena are related to a loss of the BAPTA-inhibitable Ca^{2+}-activated Cl^- channel. Alternatively, the C57BL/6J *CFTR*^{m1UNC}/ *CFTR*^{m1UNC} congenic mice may have an amiloride-insensitive Na^+ channel (other than the epithelial sodium channel), involved in constitutive sodium hyperabsorption. The congenic mice also developed detectable fibrosis and early increase in neutrophils which subsided with time, while the modest increase in the number of interstitial macrophages and fibroblasts remained statistically significant with age. However, no spontaneous colonization with the typical CF pathogens, including *P. aeruginosa*, has been observed in congenic animals.

Several studies (40, 51) have been reported using *CFTR* knockout mice carrying the S489X mutation (*CFTR*^{m1UNC} [110]) and forced *P. aeruginosa* infections via instillation of agar beads containing bacteria into the respiratory tract. In one of these reports, no differences in *P. aeruginosa* CFU recovered from the lungs were noted between *CFTR* and normal mice (51), but more inflammation was observed in the *CFTR* knockouts. In another report (40), similar lung pathology was observed in both groups of mice, but the mice with CF showed increased *P. aeruginosa* CFU recoverable from the lung. The differences between these two reports can be ascribed to the use of congenic animals in the latter study. Both groups of investigators have nevertheless observed increased mortality among mice with CF infected with *P. aeruginosa* embedded in agar beads (58 to 82% mortality in mice with CF versus 12 to 23% mortality in controls), possibly reflecting excessive inflammatory response in CF transgenics. The excessive inflammatory response has been validated by the reported twofold increase in MIP2 and KC, the putative murine functional equivalents of human IL-8 (the mouse does not have IL-8). TNF-α was also increased in the lungs of infected animals with CF relative to colonized controls. However, the overall increase in inflammatory cells in infected *CFTR* animals was relatively modest compared to that in infected normal controls (40), although as expected the percentage of neutrophils in bronchoalveolar lavage fluid went from the very low fraction of less than 5% to over 40% in infected animals.

In our own studies (133a) using the aerosol delivery model (133), we have observed peculiar variability among CF knockout mice in their ability to clear *P. aeruginosa*. For example, we noted that *CFTR*^{m1UNC}/*CFTR*^{m1UNC} mice either clear or do not clear *P. aeruginosa*, depending upon their nutritional status. Furthermore, the FABP-human CFTR *CFTR*^{m1UNC}/ *CFTR*^{m1UNC} bitransgenic mice, which have their gastrointestinal defect corrected (135), clear *P. aeruginosa* from the lung quite efficiently (133a). In pursuit of the potential relationship between nutrition and pulmonary clearance of *P. aeruginosa* in CF, we have recently shown that malnourished normal mice show reduced capacity to clear *P. aeruginosa*. This defect can be promptly restored by placing the malnourished mice on a complete and well-balanced diet. In keeping with our observations, the severity of intestinal disease is intensified in back-crossed congenic C57BL/6J $CFTR^{m1UNC}/CFTR^{m1UNC}$ animals versus $CFTR^{m1UNC}/CFTR^{m1UNC}$ mice, which correlates with signs of pulmonary disease in the congenics (58). In another study (40), congenic C57BL/6J $CFTR^{m1UNC}/CFTR^{m1UNC}$ mice that showed a 10-fold-increased burden of *P. aeruginosa* CFU were also 25 to 30% underweight relative to C57BL/6J controls. Although the authors of the study reported no correlation between animal weight and *P. aeruginosa* clearance, the same animals were used to establish higher *P. aeruginosa* numbers in the lungs of mice with CF, and all *CFTR* transgenic mice, without exception, were of lower body weight than any of the normal controls. Based on these considerations and our own observations with malnourished animals, we propose that the unusual susceptibility of the lung in CF to bacterial infections, including those with *P. aeruginosa*, may be secondary to intestinal problems and the generally poor nutritional status of individuals with CF. This proposal is further substantiated by the fact that aggressive nutritional intervention improves the clinical outlook for patients with CF (19).

CONCLUDING REMARKS

P. aeruginosa is an important opportunistic pathogen and a significant cause of nosocomial infections. *P. aeruginosa* causes life-threatening infections in patients with compromised innate immune defenses, such as burn victims, neutropenic individuals undergoing chemotherapy, and persons with CF. The *P. aeruginosa* infections in CF have earned this organism a celebrity status among pathogens, not only due to the obvious clinical significance but also because this area poses challenges that exceed our current scientific and medical knowledge of both the host and the pathogen. Many ques-

tions remain. Will future studies based on the complete genome of *P. aeruginosa* (http://www.pseudomonas.com) uncover something new about the organism and give us a decisive advantage in treating infections with this pathogen? Will better antibiotics and better delivery systems be sufficient? Can useful and innovative vaccines be developed? Is gene therapy in CF an answer? Can better animal (e.g., primate) models of CF be developed? These and additional questions have been the force behind contemporary CF research, which in addition to being pervaded by practical issues, has also fostered many fundamental scientific developments. The principle of positional cloning, developed in the course of identification of the *CFTR* gene, is one such example. It is my belief that the outlook is good and that CF research efforts will continue to yield important fundamental scientific and applied medical advances of interest to the research community and benefiting patients and their families.

ACKNOWLEDGMENTS

I thank past and present graduate students, postdoctoral fellows, and other professional colleagues for their scientific contributions.

The research on *P. aeruginosa* and CF in my laboratory is supported by NIH grant AI31139 and a grant from the Cystic Fibrosis Foundation.

REFERENCES

1. **Afessa, B., W. Green, J. Chiao, and W. Frederick.** 1998. Pulmonary complications of HIV infection: autopsy findings. *Chest* **113:**1225–1229.
2. **Al-Awqati, Q., J. Barasch, and D. Landry.** 1992. Chloride channels of intracellular organelles and their potential role in cystic fibrosis. *J. Exp. Biol.* **172:**245–266.
3. **Anwar, H., J. L. Strap, and J. W. Costerton.** 1992. Establishment of aging biofilms: possible mechanism of bacterial resistance to antimicrobial therapy. *Antimicrob. Agents Chemother.* **36:** 1347–1351.
4. **Asboe, D., V. Gant, H. M. Aucken, D. A. Moore, S. Umasankar, J. S. Bingham, M. E. Kaufmann, and T. L. Pitt.** 1998. Persistence of *Pseudomonas aeruginosa* strains in respiratory infection in AIDS patients. *AIDS* **12:**1771–1775.
5. **Baltch, A. L.** 1994. *Pseudomonas aeruginosa* bacteremia, p. 73–128. *In* A. L. Baltch and R. P.

Smith (ed.), *Pseudomonas aeruginosa. Infections and Treatment.* Marcel Dekker, New York, N.Y.

6. **Beck-Sague, C. M., S. N. Banerjee, and W. R. Jatvis.** 1994. Epidemiology and control of *Pseudomonas aeruginosa* in US hospitals, p. 51–71. *In* A. L. Baltch and R. P. Smith (ed.), *Pseudomonas aeruginosa. Infections and Treatment.* Marcel Dekker, New York, N.Y.

7. **Biwersi, J., N. Emans, and A. S. Verkman.** 1996. Cystic fibrosis transmembrane conductance regulator activation stimulates endosome fusion in vivo. *Proc. Natl. Acad. Sci. USA* **93:**12484–12489.

8. **Blackwood, L. L., and J. E. Pennington.** 1981. Influence of mucoid coating on clearance of *Pseudomonas aeruginosa* from lungs. *Infect. Immun.* **32:**443–448.

9. **Bonfield, T. L., J. R. Panuska, M. W. Konstan, K. A. Hillard, J. B. Hillard, H. Ghnaim, and M. Berger.** 1995. Inflammatory cytokines in cystic fibrosis lungs. *Am. J. Respir. Crit. Care Med.* **152:**2111–2118.

9a. **Boucher, J. C., M. J. Schurr, and V. Deretic.** Dual regulation of mucoidy in *P. aeruginosa* and sigma factor antagonism. *Mol. Microbiol.,* in press.

10. **Boucher, J. C., H. Yu, M. H. Mudd, and V. Deretic.** 1997. Mucoid *Pseudomonas aeruginosa* in cystic fibrosis: characterization of *muc* mutations in clinical isolates and analysis of clearance in a mouse model of respiratory infection. *Infect. Immun.* **65:**3838–3846.

11. **Bowton, D. L.** 1999. Nosocomial pneumonia in the ICU—year 2000 and beyond. *Chest* **115**(Suppl. 3):28S–33S.

12. **Cainzos Fernandez, M.** 1998. Skin and soft-tissue infections caused by *Pseudomonas aeruginosa. Rev. Clin. Esp.* **198**(Suppl. 2):21–24. (In Spanish.)

13. **Cash, H. A., D. E. Woods, B. McCullough, W. G. Johanson, and J. A. Bass.** 1979. A rat model of chronic respiratory infection with *Pseudomonas aeruginosa. Am. Rev. Resp. Dis.* **119:**453–459.

14. **Cisneros Herreros, J. M., E. Canas Garcia-Otero, J. Caballero Granado, and B. Becerril Carral.** 1998. Bacteremia, endocarditis and meningitis caused by *Pseudomonas aeruginosa. Rev. Clin. Esp.* **198**(Suppl. 2):25–29. (In Spanish.)

15. **Clarke, L. L., B. R. Grubb, J. R. Yankaskas, C. U. Cotton, A. McKenzie, and R. C. Boucher.** 1994. Relationship of a non-cystic fibrosis transmembrane conductance regulator-mediated chloride conductance to organ-level disease in Cftr($-/-$) mice. *Proc. Natl. Acad. Sci. USA* **91:**479–483.

16. **Coburn, J., and D. M. Gill.** 1991. ADP-ribosylation of p21ras and related proteins by *Pseudomonas aeruginosa* exoenzyme S. *Infect. Immun.* **59:**4259–4262.

17. **Cole, N., S. Bao, M. Willcox, and A. J. Husband.** 1999. Expression of interleukin-6 in the cornea in response to infection with different strains of *Pseudomonas aeruginosa. Infect. Immun.* **67:**2497–2502.

18. **Cole, N., S. Bao, M. Willcox, and A. J. Husband.** 1999. TNF-alpha production in the cornea in response to *Pseudomonas aeruginosa* challenge. *Immunol. Cell Biol.* **77:**164–166.

19. **Corey, M., F. J. McLaughlin, M. Williams, and H. Levison.** 1988. A comparison of survival, growth, and pulmonary function in patients with cystic fibrosis in Boston and Toronto. *J. Clin. Epidemiol.* **41:**583–591.

20. **Costerton, J. W., P. S. Stewart, and E. P. Greenberg.** 1999. Bacterial biofilms: a common cause of persistent infections. *Science* **284:**1318–1322.

21. **Cryz, S. J., Jr., E. Fürer, and R. Germanier.** 1983. Simple model for the study of *Pseudomonas aeruginosa* infections in leukopenic mice. *Infect. Immun.* **39:**1067–1071.

22. **Davidson, D. J., J. R. Dorin, G. McLachlan, V. Ranaldi, D. Lamb, C. Doherty, J. Govan, and D. J. Porteous.** 1995. Lung disease in the cystic fibrosis mouse exposed to bacterial pathogens. *Nat. Genet.* **9:**351–357.

23. **Davies, D. G., M. R. Parsek, J. P. Pearson, B. H. Iglewski, J. W. Costerton, and E. P. Greenberg.** 1998. The involvement of cell-to-cell signals in the development of a bacterial biofilm. *Science* **280:**295–298.

24. **De Groote, M. A., and F. C. Fang.** 1995. NO inhibitions: antimicrobial properties of nitric oxide. *Clin. Infect. Dis.* **21**(Suppl. 2):S162–S165.

25. **Deretic, V.** 1996. Molecular biology of mucoidy in *Pseudomonas aeruginosa*, p. 223–244. *In* J. A. Dodge, D. J. H. Brock, and J. H. Widdicombe (ed.), *Cystic Fibrosis—Current Topics,* vol. 3. John Wiley & Sons Ltd., Chichester, United Kingdom.

26. **Deretic, V., M. J. Schurr, J. C. Boucher, and D. W. Martin.** 1994. Conversion of *Pseudomonas aeruginosa* to mucoidy in cystic fibrosis: environmental stress and regulation of bacterial virulence by alternative sigma factors. *J. Bacteriol.* **176:**2773–2780.

27. **DiMango, E., A. J. Ratner, R. Bryan, S. Tabibi, and A. Prince.** 1998. Activation of NF-κB by adherent *Pseudomonas aeruginosa* in normal and cystic fibrosis respiratory epithelial cells. *J. Clin. Investig.* **101:**2598–2605.

28. **Dosanjh, A., W. Lencer, D. Brown, D. A. Ausiello, and J. L. Stow.** 1994. Heterologous expression of delta F508 CFTR results in decreased sialylation of membrane glycoconjugates. *Am. J. Physiol.* **266:**C360–C366.

29. **Er, H., Y. Turkoz, I. H. Ozerol, and E.**

Uzmez. 1998. Effect of nitric oxide synthase inhibition in experimental *Pseudomonas* keratitis in rabbits. *Eur. J. Ophthalmol.* **8:**137–141.

30. Finck-Barbancon, V., J. Goranson, L. Zhu, T. Sawa, J. P. Wiener-Kronish, S. M. Fleiszig, C. Wu, L. Mende-Mueller, and D. W. Frank. 1997. ExoU expression by *Pseudomonas aeruginosa* correlates with acute cytotoxicity and epithelial injury. *Mol. Microbiol.* **25:**547–557.

31. FitzSimmons, S. C. 1993. The changing epidemiology of cystic fibrosis. *J. Pediatr.* **122:**1–9.

32. Frank, D. W. 1997. The exoenzyme S regulon of *Pseudomonas aeruginosa.* *Mol. Microbiol.* **26:** 621–629.

33. Frank, U., F. D. Daschner, G. Schulgen, and J. Mills. 1997. Incidence and epidemiology of nosocomial infections in patients infected with human immunodeficiency virus. *Clin. Infect. Dis.* **25:**318–320.

34. Frithz-Lindsten, E., Y. Du, R. Rosqvist, and A. Forsberg. 1997. Intracellular targeting of exoenzyme S of *Pseudomonas aeruginosa* via type III-dependent translocation induces phagocytosis resistance, cytotoxicity and disruption of actin microfilaments. *Mol. Microbiol.* **25:**1125–1139.

35. Fu, H., J. Coburn, and R. J. Collier. 1993. The eukaryotic host factor that activates exoenzyme S of Pseudomonas aeruginosa is a member of the 14-3-3 protein family. *Proc. Natl. Acad. Sci. USA* **90:**2320–2324.

36. Gabriel, S. E., K. N. Brigman, B. H. Koller, R. C. Boucher, and M. J. Stutts. 1994. Cystic fibrosis heterozygote resistance to cholera toxin in the cystic fibrosis mouse model. *Science* **266:** 107–109.

37. Gerke, J. R., and M. V. Magliocco. 1981. Experimental *Pseudomonas aeruginosa* infection of the mouse cornea. *Infect. Immun.* **3:**209–216.

38. Gilljam, H., A. Ellin, and B. Strandvik. 1997. Increased bronchial chloride concentrations in cystic fibrosis. *Scand. J. Clin. Lab. Investig.* **49:** 2588–2595.

39. Goldman, M. J., G. M. Anderson, E. D. Stolzenberg, U. P. Kari, M. Zasloff, and J. M. Wilson. 1997. Human beta-defensin-1 is a salt-sensitive antibiotic in lung that is inactivated in cystic fibrosis. *Cell* **88:**553–560.

40. Gosselin, D., M. M. Stevenson, E. A. Cowley, U. Griesenbach, D. H. Eidelman, M. Boule, M. F. Tam, G. Kent, E. Skamene, L. C. Tsui, and D. Radzioch. 1998. Impaired ability of Cftr knockout mice to control lung infection with *Pseudomonas aeruginosa.* *Am. J. Respir. Crit. Care Med.* **157:**1253–1262.

41. Govan, J. R. W., and V. Deretic. 1996. Microbial pathogenesis in cystic fibrosis: mucoid *Pseu-* *domonas aeruginosa* and *Burkholderia cepacia.* *Microbiol. Rev.* **60:**539–574.

42. Grasemann, H., E. Michler, M. Wallot, and F. Ratjen. 1997. Decreased concentration of exhaled nitric oxide (NO) in patients with cystic fibrosis. *Pediatr. Pulmonol.* **24:**173–177.

43. Guo, F. H., H. R. De Raeve, T. W. Rice, D. J. Stuehr, F. B. Thunnissen, and S. C. Erzurum. 1995. Continuous nitric oxide synthesis by inducible nitric oxide synthase in normal human airway epithelium in vivo. *Proc. Natl. Acad. Sci. USA* **92:**7809–7813.

44. Haley, R. W., and R. H. Shachtman. 1980. The emergence of infection surveillance and control programs in US hospitals: an assessment, 1976. *Am. J. Epidemiol.* **111:**574–591.

45. Hall, R. A., L. S. Ostedgaard, R. T. Premont, J. T. Blitzer, N. Rahman, M. J. Welsh, and R. J. Lefkowitz. 1998. A C-terminal motif found in the beta2-adrenergic receptor, P2Y1 receptor and cystic fibrosis transmembrane conductance regulator determines binding to the Na+/H+ exchanger regulatory factor family of PDZ proteins. *Proc. Natl. Acad. Sci. USA* **95:** 8496–8501.

46. Hatano, K., J. B. Goldberg, and G. B. Pier. 1995. Biologic activities of antibodies to the neutral-polysaccharide component of the *Pseudomonas aeruginosa* lipopolysaccharide are blocked by O side chains and mucoid exopolysaccharide (alginate). *Infect. Immun.* **63:**21–26.

47. Hauer, T., M. Lacour, P. Gastmeier, G. Schulgen, M. Schumacher, H. Ruden, and F. Daschner. 1996. Nosocomial infections intensive care units. A nation-wide prevalence study. *Anaesthesist* **45:**1184–1191. (In German.)

48. Hauser, A. R., S. Fleiszig, P. J. Kang, K. Mostov, and J. N. Engel. 1998. Defects in type III secretion correlate with internalization of *Pseudomonas aeruginosa* by epithelial cells. *Infect. Immun.* **66:**1413–1420.

49. Hauser, A. R., P. J. Kang, and J. N. Engel. 1998. PepA, a secreted protein of Pseudomonas aeruginosa, is necessary for cytotoxicity and virulence. *Mol. Microbiol.* **27:**807–818.

50. Hazlett, L. D., D. D. Rosen, and R. S. Berk. 1977. *Pseudomonas* eye infections in cyclophosphamide-treated mice. *Investig. Ophthalmol. Vis. Sci.* **16:**649.

51. Heeckeren, A., R. Walenga, M. W. Konstan, T. Bonfield, P. B. Davis, and T. Ferkol. 1997. Excessive inflammatory response of cystic fibrosis mice to bronchopulmonary infection with *Pseudomonas aeruginosa.* *J. Clin. Investig.* **100:** 2810–2815.

52. Hobden, J. A., S. Masinick-McClellan, R. P. Barrett, K. S. Bark, and L. D. Hazlett. 1999.

Pseudomonas aeruginosa keratitis in knockout mice deficient in intercellular adhesion molecule 1. *Infect. Immun.* **67:**972–975.

53. **Imundo, L., J. Barasch, A. Prince, and Q. Al-Awqati.** 1995. Cystic fibrosis epithelial cells have a receptor for pathogenic bacteria on their apical surface. *Proc. Natl. Acad. Sci. USA* **92:** 3019–3023. (Erratum, **92:**11322.)

54. **Jackson, G. G.** 1994. Infective endocarditis caused by *Pseudomonas aeruginosa*, p. 129–158. *In* A. L. Baltch and R. P. Smith (ed.), *Pseudomonas aeruginosa. Infections and Treatment.* Marcel Dekker, New York, N.Y.

55. **Jensen, E. T., A. Kharazmi, K. Lam, J. W. Costerton, and N. Hoiby.** 1990. Human polymorphonuclear leukocyte response to *Pseudomonas aeruginosa* grown in biofilms. *Infect. Immun.* **58:** 2383–2385.

56. **Johansen, H. K., and N. Hoiby.** 1992. Seasonal onset of initial colonisation and chronic infection with *Pseudomonas aeruginosa* in patients with cystic fibrosis in Denmark. *Thorax* **47:**109–111.

57. **Kelley, T. J., and M. L. Drumm.** 1998. Inducible nitric oxide synthase expression is reduced in cystic fibrosis murine and human airway epithelial cells. *J. Clin. Investig.* **102:**1200–1207.

58. **Kent, G., R. Iles, C. E. Bear, L. J. Huan, U. Griesenbach, C. McKerlie, H. Frndova, C. Ackerley, D. Gosselin, D. Radzioch, H. O'Brodovich, L. C. Tsui, M. Buchwald, and A. K. Tanswell.** 1997. Lung disease in mice with cystic fibrosis. *J. Clin. Investig.* **100:**3060–3069.

59. **Kernacki, K. A., D. J. Goebel, M. S. Poosch, and L. D. Hazlett.** 1998. Early cytokine and chemokine gene expression during *Pseudomonas aeruginosa* corneal infection in mice. *Infect. Immun.* **66:**376–379.

60. **Khan, T. Z., J. S. Wagener, T. Bost, J. Martinez, F. J. Accurso, and D. W. Riches.** 1995. Early pulmonary inflammation in infants with cystic fibrosis. *Am. J. Respir. Crit. Care Med.* **151:** 1075–1082.

61. **Kielhofner, M., R. L. Atmar, R. J. Hamill, and D. M. Musher.** 1992. Life-threatening Pseudomonas aeruginosa infections in patients with human immunodeficiency virus infection. *Clin. Infect. Dis.* **14:**403–411.

62. **Knowles, M. R., J. M. Robinson, R. E. Wood, C. A. Pue, W. M. Mentz, G. C. Wager, J. T. Gatzy, and R. C. Boucher.** 1997. Ion composition of airway surface liquid of patients with cystic fibrosis as compared with normal and disease-control subjects. *J. Clin. Investig.* **100:** 2588–2595. (Erratum, **101:**285, 1998.)

63. **Kobzik, L., D. S. Bredt, C. J. Lowenstein, J. Drazen, B. Gaston, D. Sugarbaker, and J. S. Stamler.** 1993. Nitric oxide synthase in human

and rat lung: immunocytochemical and histochemical localization. *Am. J. Respir. Cell. Mol. Biol.* **9:**371–377.

64. **Koch, C., and N. Hoiby.** 1993. Pathogenesis of cystic fibrosis. *Lancet* **341:**1065–1069.

65. **Konstan, M. W., P. J. Byard, C. L. Hoppel, and P. B. Davis.** 1995. Effect of high-dose ibuprofen in patients with cystic fibrosis. *N. Engl. J. Med.* **332:**848–854.

66. **Krivan, H. C., D. D. Roberts, and V. Ginsburg.** 1988. Many pulmonary pathogenic bacteria bind specifically to the carbohydrate sequence GalNAc beta 1-4Gal found in some glycolipids. *Proc. Natl. Acad. Sci. USA* **85:**6157–6161.

67. **Kunin, C. M.** 1994. Infections of the urinary tract due to *Pseudomonas aeruginosa*, p. 237–256. *In* A. L. Baltch and R. P. Smith (ed.), *Pseudomonas aeruginosa. Infections and Treatment.* Marcel Dekker, New York, N.Y.

68. **Kwon, B., and L. D. Hazlett.** 1997. Association of CD4 + T cell-dependent keratitis with genetic susceptibility to Pseudomonas aeruginosa ocular infection. *J. Immunol.* **159:**6283–6290.

69. **Lam, J., R. Chan, K. Lam, and J. W. Costerton.** 1980. Production of mucoid microcolonies by *Pseudomonas aeruginosa* within infected lungs in cystic fibrosis. *Infect. Immun.* **28:**546–556.

70. **Lavery, L. A., S. C. Walker, L. B. Harkless, and K. Felder-Johnson.** 1995. Infected puncture wounds in diabetic and nondiabetic adults. *Diabetes Care* **18:**1588–1591. (Erratum, **19:**549, 1996.)

71. **Lukacs, G. L., X. B. Chang, N. Kartner, O. D. Rotstein, J. R. Riordan, and S. Grinstein.** 1992. The cystic fibrosis transmembrane regulator is present and functional in endosomes. Role as a determinant of endosomal pH. *J. Biol. Chem.* **267:** 14568–14572.

72. **Mahajan-Miklos, S., M. W. Tan, L. G. Rahme, and F. M. Ausubel.** 1999. Molecular mechanisms of bacterial virulence elucidated using a *Pseudomonas aeruginosa-Caenorhabditis elegans* pathogenesis model. *Cell* **96:**47–56.

73. **Mahan, M. J., J. M. Slauch, and J. J. Mekalanos.** 1993. Selection of bacterial virulence genes that are specifically induced in host tissues. *Science* **259:**686–688.

74. **Mahenthiralingam, E., M. E. Campbell, and D. P. Speert.** 1994. Nonmotility and phagocytic resistance of *Pseudomonas aeruginosa* isolates from chronically colonized patients with cystic fibrosis. *Infect. Immun.* **62:**596–605.

75. **Martin, D. W., M. J. Schurr, M. H. Mudd, J. R. W. Govan, B. W. Holloway, and V. Deretic.** 1993. Mechanism of conversion to mucoidy in *Pseudomonas aeruginosa* infecting cystic fi-

brosis patients. *Proc. Natl. Acad. Sci. USA* **90:** 8377–8381.

76. **Masters, S. C., K. J. Pederson, L. Zhang, J. T. Barbieri, and H. Fu.** 1999. Interaction of 14-3-3 with a nonphosphorylated protein ligand, exoenzyme S of *Pseudomonas aeruginosa. Biochemistry* **38:**5216–5221.

77. **McAvoy, M. J., V. Newton, A. Paull, J. Morgan, P. Gacesa, and N. J. Russell.** 1989. Isolation of mucoid strains of *Pseudomonas aeruginosa* from non-cystic-fibrosis patients and characterisation of the structure of their secreted alginate. *J. Med. Microbiol.* **28:**183–189.

78. **McGuffie, E. M., D. W. Frank, T. S. Vincent, and J. C. Olson.** 1998. Modification of Ras in eukaryotic cells by *Pseudomonas aeruginosa* exoenzyme S. *Infect. Immun.* **66:**2607–2613.

79. **Meng, Q. H., D. R. Springall, A. E. Bishop, K. Morgan, T. J. Evans, S. Habib, D. C. Gruenert, K. M. Gyi, M. E. Hodson, M. H. Yacoub, and J. M. Polak.** 1998. Lack of inducible nitric oxide synthase in bronchial epithelium: a possible mechanism of susceptibility to infection in cystic fibrosis. *J. Pathol.* **184:**323–331.

80. **Miskew, D. B., M. A. Lorenz, R. L. Pearson, and A. M. Pankovich.** 1983. Pseudomonas aeruginosa bone and joint infection in drug abusers. *J. Bone Joint Surg. Am.* **65:**829–832.

81. **Morissette, C., E. Skamene, and F. Gervais.** 1995. Endobronchial inflammation following *Pseudomonas aeruginosa* infection in resistant and susceptible strains of mice. *Infect. Immun.* **63:** 1718–1724.

82. **Morrison, V. A.** 1998. The infectious complications of chronic lymphocytic leukemia. *Semin. Oncol.* **25:**98–106.

83. **Moss, R. B., R. C. Bocian, Y. P. Hsu, Y. J. Dong, M. Kemna, T. Wei, and P. Gardner.** 1996. Reduced IL-10 secretion by CD4 + T lymphocytes expressing mutant cystic fibrosis transmembrane conductance regulator (CFTR). *Clin. Exp. Immunol.* **106:**374–388.

84. **Nichols, W. W., S. M. Dorrington, M. P. Slack, and H. L. Walmsley.** 1988. Inhibition of tobramycin diffusion by binding to alginate. *Antimicrob. Agents Chemother.* **32:**518–523.

85. **Olson, J. C., E. M. McGuffie, and D. W. Frank.** 1997. Effects of differential expression of the 49-kilodalton exoenzyme S by *Pseudomonas aeruginosa* on cultured eukaryotic cells. *Infect. Immun.* **65:**248–256.

86. **Orenstein, D. A.** 1989. *Cystic Fibrosis: A Guide for Patient and Family.* Raven Press, New York, N.Y.

87. **Pahl, H. L., and P. A. Baeuerle.** 1995. A novel signal transduction pathway from the endoplasmic reticulum to the nucleus is mediated by transcription factor NF-kappa B. *EMBO J.* **14:**2580–2588.

88. **Parsek, M. R., D. L. Val, B. L. Hanzelka, J. E. Cronan, Jr., and E. P. Greenberg.** 1999. Acyl homoserine-lactone quorum-sensing signal generation. *Proc. Natl. Acad. Sci. USA* **96:** 4360–4365.

89. **Pedersen, S. S.** 1992. Lung infection with alginate-producing, mucoid *Pseudomonas aeruginosa* in cystic fibrosis. *APMIS* **100**(Suppl. 28):1–79.

90. **Pedersen, S. S., N. Hoiby, F. Espersen, and C. Koch.** 1992. Role of alginate in infection with mucoid Pseudomonas aeruginosa in cystic fibrosis. *Thorax* **47:**6–13.

91. **Pederson, K. J., A. J. Vallis, K. Aktories, D. W. Frank, and J. T. Barbieri.** 1999. The amino-terminal domain of *Pseudomonas aeruginosa* ExoS disrupts actin filaments via small-molecular-weight GTP-binding proteins. *Mol. Microbiol.* **32:** 393–401.

92. **Pennington, J. E.** 1994. *Pseudomonas aeruginosa* pneumonia and other respiratory tract infections, p. 159–182. *In* A. L. Baltch and R. P. Smith (ed.), *Pseudomonas aeruginosa. Infections and Treatment.* Marcel Dekker, New York, N.Y.

93. **Pier, B. B., G. Meluleni, and E. Neuger.** 1992. A murine model of chronic mucosal colonization by *Pseudomonas aeruginosa. Infect. Immun.* **60:**4768–4776.

94. **Pier, G. B.** 1999. Evolution of the F508 CFTR mutation: response. *Trends Microbiol.* **7:**56–58.

95. **Pier, G. B., M. Grout, T. Zaidi, G. Meluleni, S. S. Mueschenborn, G. Banting, R. Ratcliff, M. J. Evans, and W. H. Colledge.** 1998. Salmonella typhi uses CFTR to enter intestinal epithelial cells. *Nature* **393:**79–82.

96. **Pier, G. B., M. Grout, T. S. Zaidi, J. C. Olsen, L. G. Johnson, J. R. Yankaskas, and J. B. Goldberg.** 1996. Role of mutant CFTR in hypersusceptibility of cystic fibrosis patients to lung infections. *Science* **271:**64–67.

97. **Pruitt, B. A., Jr., A. T. McManus, S. H. Kim, and C. W. Goodwin.** 1998. Burn wound infections: current status. *World J. Surg.* **22:**135–145.

98. **Rahme, L. G., E. J. Stevens, S. F. Wolfort, J. Shao, R. G. Tompkins, and F. M. Ausubel.** 1995. Common virulence factors for bacterial pathogenicity in plants and animals. *Science* **268:** 1899–1902.

99. **Rahme, L. G., M. W. Tan, L. Le, S. M. Wong, R. G. Tompkins, S. B. Calderwood, and F. M. Ausubel.** 1997. Use of model plant hosts to identify *Pseudomonas aeruginosa* virulence factors. *Proc. Natl. Acad. Sci. USA* **94:** 13245–13250.

100. **Rehm, S. R., G. N. Gross, and A. K. Pierce.** 1980. Early bacterial clearance from murine lungs. *J. Clin. Investig.* **66:**194–199.

101. **Rello, J., and M. Ricart.** 1998. Respiratory tract infections by *Pseudomonas aeruginosa* in patients under intubation. *Rev. Clin. Esp.* **198**(Suppl. 2):17–20. (In Spanish.)

102. **Richards, M. J., J. R. Edwards, D. H. Culver, and R. P. Gaynes.** 1999. Nosocomial infections in pediatric intensive care units in the United States. National Nosocomial Infections Surveillance System. *Pediatrics* **103:**e39.

103. **Rodriguez Arrondo, F., M. A. von Wichmann, J. Arrizabalaga, J. A. Iribarren, G. Garmendia, and P. Idigoras.** 1998. Pulmonary cavitation lesions in patients infected with the human immunodeficiency virus: an analysis of a series of 78 cases. *Med. Clin. (Barc).* **111:**725–730. (In Spanish.)

104. **Saiman, L., and A. Prince.** 1993. *Pseudomonas aeruginosa* pili bind to asialoGM1 which is increased on the surface of cystic fibrosis epithelial cells. *J. Clin. Investig.* **92:**1875–1880.

105. **Sawa, T., T. L. Yahr, M. Ohara, K. Kurahashi, M. A. Gropper, J. P. Wiener-Kronish, and D. W. Frank.** 1999. Active and passive immunization with the *Pseudomonas* V antigen protects against type III intoxication and lung injury. *Nat. Med.* **5:**392–398.

106. **Seksek, O., J. Biwersi, and A. S. Verkman.** 1996. Evidence against defective trans-Golgi acidification in cystic fibrosis. *J. Biol. Chem.* **271:**15542–15548.

107. **Siegman-Igra, Y., R. Ravona, H. Primerman, and M. Giladi.** 1998. Pseudomonas aeruginosa bacteremia: an analysis of 123 episodes, with particular emphasis on the effect of antibiotic therapy. *Int. J. Infect. Dis.* **2:**211–215.

108. **Smith, J. J., S. M. Travis, E. P. Greenberg, and M. J. Welsh.** 1996. Cystic fibrosis airway epithelia fail to kill bacteria because of abnormal airway surface fluid. *Cell* **85:**229–236. (Erratum, **87:**following 355.)

109. **Smith, R. P.** 1994. Skin and soft tissue infections due to *Pseudomonas aeruginosa*, p. 326–370. *In* A. L. Baltch and R. P. Smith (ed.), *Pseudomonas aeruginosa. Infections and Treatment.* Marcel Dekker, New York, N.Y.

110. **Snouwaert, J. N., K. K. Brigman, A. M. Latour, N. N. Malouf, R. C. Boucher, O. Smithies, and B. H. Koller.** 1992. An animal model for cystic fibrosis made by gene targeting. *Science* **257:**1083–1088.

111. **Sordelli, D. O., V. E. Garcia, C. M. Cerequetti, P. A. Fontan, and A. M. Hooke.** 1992. Intranasal immunization with temperature sensitive mutants protects granulocytopenic mice

from lethal pulmonary challenge with *Pseudomonas aeruginosa. Curr. Microbiol.* **24:**9–14.

112. **Southern, P. M., A. K. Pierce, and J. P. Sanford.** 1968. Exposure chamber for 66 mice suitable for use with Henderson aerosol apparatus. *Appl. Microbiol.* **16:**540–542.

113. **Spencer, R. C.** 1996. Predominant pathogens found in the European Prevalence of Infection in Intensive Care Study. *Eur. J. Clin. Microbiol. Infect. Dis.* **15:**281–285.

114. **Starke, J. R., M. S. Edwards, C. Langston, and C. J. Baker.** 1987. A mouse model of chronic pulmonary infection with *Pseudomonas aeruginosa* and *Pseudomonas cepacia. Pediatr. Res.* **22:**698–702.

115. **Stieritz, D. D., and I. A. Holander.** 1975. Experimental studies of the pathogenesis of infections due to *Pseudomonas aeruginosa*: description of a burned mouse model. *J. Infect. Dis.* **131:**688–691.

116. **Stutts, M. J., C. M. Canessa, J. C. Olsen, M. Hamrick, J. A. Cohn, B. C. Rossier, and R. C. Boucher.** 1995. CFTR as a cAMP-dependent regulator of sodium channels. *Science* **269:**847–850.

117. **Tan, M. W., S. Mahajan-Miklos, and F. M. Ausubel.** 1999. Killing of Caenorhabditis elegans by *Pseudomonas aeruginosa* used to model mammalian bacterial pathogenesis. *Proc. Natl. Acad. Sci. USA* **96:**715–20.

118. **Tang, H., M. Kays, and A. Prince.** 1995. Role of *Pseudomonas aeruginosa* pili in acute pulmonary infection. *Infect. Immun.* **63:**1278–1285.

119. **Tierney, M. R., and A. S. Baker.** 1995. Infections of the head and neck in diabetes mellitus. *Infect. Dis. Clin. N. Am.* **9:**195–216.

120. **Toews, G. B., G. N. Gross, and A. K. Pierce.** 1979. The relationship of inoculum size to lung bacterial clearance and phagocytic cell response in mice. *Am. Rev. Resp. Dis.* **120:**559–566.

121. **Vidal Marsal, F., and J. Mensa Pueyo.** 1998. *Pseudomonas aeruginosa* as a pathogen in patients with human immunodeficiency virus infection. *Rev. Clin. Esp.* **198**(Suppl. 2):37–43. (In Spanish.)

122. **Wang, F. D., Y. Y. Chen, and C. Y. Liu.** 1998. Prevalence of nosocomial respiratory tract infections in the surgical intensive care units of a medical center. *Chung Hua I Hsueh Tsa Chih* (Taipei). **61:**589–595.

123. **Wang, H. G., N. Pathan, I. M. Ethell, S. Krajewski, Y. Yamaguchi, F. Shibasaki, F. McKeon, T. Bobo, T. F. Franke, and J. C. Reed.** 1999. Ca2+ -induced apoptosis through calcineurin dephosphorylation of BAD. *Science* **284:**339–343.

124. **Wang, J., A. Mushegian, S. Lory, and S. Jin.** 1996. Large-scale isolation of candidate virulence genes of *Pseudomonas aeruginosa* by in vivo selection. *Proc. Natl. Acad. Sci. USA* **93**: 10434–10439.

125. **Welsh, M. J., L.-C. Tsui, T. F. Boat, and A. L. Beaudet.** 1995. Cystic fibrosis, p. 3799–3876. *In* C. R. Scriver, A. L. Beaudet, W. S. Sly, and D. Valle (ed.), *The Metabolic and Molecular Basis of Inherited Disease*, vol. III. McGraw-Hill, Inc., New York, N.Y.

126. **Wilson, R., and R. B. Dowling.** 1998. Lung infections. 3. *Pseudomonas aeruginosa* and other related species. *Thorax* **53**:213–219.

127. **Witt, D. J., D. E. Craven, and W. R. McCabe.** 1987. Bacterial infections in adult patients with the acquired immune deficiency syndrome (AIDS) and AIDS-related complex. *Am. J. Med.* **82**:900–906.

128. **Woods, D. E., and M. L. Vasil.** 1994. Pathogenesis of *Pseudomonas aeruginosa* infections, p. 21–50. *In* A. L. Baltch and R. P. Smith (ed.), *Pseudomonas aeruginosa. Infections and Treatment.* Marcel Dekker, New York, N.Y.

129. **Wretlind, B., and T. Kronevi.** 1977. Experimental infections with protease-deficient mutants of *Pseudomonas aeruginosa* in mice. *J. Med. Microbiol.* **11**:145–154.

130. **Yahr, T. L., J. T. Barbieri, and D. W. Frank.** 1996. Genetic relationship between the 53- and 49-kilodalton forms of exoenzyme S from *Pseudomonas aeruginosa. J. Bacteriol.* **178**:1412–1419.

131. **Yahr, T. L., A. J. Vallis, M. K. Hancock, J. T. Barbieri, and D. W. Frank.** 1998. Exo Y, an adenylate cyclase secreted by the *Pseudomonas aeruginosa* type III system. *Proc. Natl. Acad. Sci. USA* **95**:13899–13904.

132. **Yu, H., J. C. Boucher, and V. Deretic.** 1998. Molecular analysis of *Pseudomonas aeruginosa* virulence. *Methods Microbiol.* **27**:383–393.

133. **Yu, H., M. Hanes, C. E. Chrisp, J. C. Boucher, and V. Deretic.** 1998. Microbial pathogenesis in cystic fibrosis: pulmonary clearance of mucoid *Pseudomonas aeruginosa* and inflammation in a mouse model of respiratory challenge. *Infect. Immun.* **66**:280–288.

133a.**Yu, H., S. Z. Nasr, and V. Deretic.** 2000. Innate lung defenses and compromised *Pseudomonas aeruginosa* clearance in the malnourished mouse model of respiratory infections in cystic fibrosis. *Infect. Immun.* **68**:2142–2147.

134. **Zaidi, T. S., J. Lyczak, M. Preston, and G. B. Pier.** 1999. Cystic fibrosis transmembrane conductance regulator-mediated corneal epithelial cell ingestion of *Pseudomonas aeruginosa* is a key component in the pathogenesis of experimental murine keratitis. *Infect. Immun.* **67**: 1481–1492.

135. **Zhou, L., C. R. Dey, S. E. Wert, M. D. DuVall, R. A. Frizzell, and J. A. Whitsett.** 1994. Correction of lethal intestinal defect in a mouse model of cystic fibrosis by human CFTR. *Science* **266**:1705–1708.

136. **Zloty, P., and M. W. Belin.** 1994. Ocular infections caused by *Pseudomonas aeruginosa*, p. 371–400. *In* A. L. Baltch and R. P. Smith (ed.), *Pseudomonas aeruginosa. Infections and Treatment.* Marcel Dekker, New York, N.Y.

MYCOBACTERIUM INFECTIONS

Michele Trucksis

16

M. TUBERCULOSIS

Tuberculosis kills 3 million people each year, more than any other infectious agent (15). This number, however, accounts for only a fraction of the individuals who are infected with *Mycobacterium tuberculosis,* as one-third of the world population (1.7 billion people) is estimated to be infected (4). The World Health Organization estimates that the worldwide mortality due to tuberculosis has remained unchanged since Robert Koch first cultured the tubercle bacillus in 1882 (6). Despite the discovery and use of antimycobacterial agents, which reduced tuberculosis in developed countries, there has been little effect globally. The failure to control tuberculosis is due to the ability of *Mycobacterium* to exist in a persistent, latent, or dormant form. In spite of a century of study, we still know surprisingly little about the mechanisms through which *M. tuberculosis* establishes a persistent infection within the host tissues or, once established, what signals allow it to escape this dormant state and resurface to incite active infection. The ability to transform into a persistent or dormant form may be an intrinsic adaptive property of *M. tuberculosis* which it utilizes

in response to the hostile environment of host tissue. This dormant state appears dynamic in that the organisms, upon cues from the environment, are able to reenter a replicative form with the potential to cause active disease. The host's cellular immune response appears to determine the fate of the organisms escaping the dormant state. Experience with human immunodeficiency virus (HIV)-infected patients dually infected with *M. tuberculosis* has revealed that the CD4 cell appears to be the most important member of the immune surveillance team. It is the depletion of these cells which leads to the increased rate of reactivation of latent tuberculosis infection in patients dually infected with HIV and tuberculosis. In this chapter, mechanisms responsible for these phenomena will be discussed and the methods of studying dormancy will be described.

PATHOGENESIS

Tuberculosis is a chronic infection caused by *M. tuberculosis*. *M. tuberculosis* predominantly causes disease in the lungs, although it can affect any organ in the body. The respiratory tract is the most common portal of entry for the infectious droplet nuclei made airborne by coughing or sneezing. These small particles, containing one to three bacilli (11), reach the terminal air spaces, where primary infection

Michele Trucksis, Medical Service, Veterans Affairs Medical Center, and Center for Vaccine Development, Department of Medicine, University of Maryland, Baltimore, MD 21201.

Persistent Bacterial Infections, Edited by J. P. Nataro, M. J. Blaser, and S. Cunningham-Rundles, © 2000 ASM Press, Washington, D.C.

occurs. The areas most commonly infected are those with the greatest airflow, which is where the bacilli are most likely to be deposited. These areas include the lower division of the lower lobe, the middle lobe, the lingula, and the anterior segment of the upper lobe of the lung.

When the tubercle bacilli enter the lung, they are ingested by alveolar macrophages. Several receptors (reviewed in reference 17) have been implicated in entry, including complement receptors CR1 (41), CR3 (46), and CR4 (22, 41, 42), the mannose receptor (40), and the surfactant protein A receptor (SPA-R) (16). The choice of receptor for entry by *M. tuberculosis* may determine the fate of the organism. Binding of *M. tuberculosis* to CR3 by a nonopsonic mechanism results in a diminished or absent respiratory burst (3, 57) and thus may be a preferred portal of entry. Another theoretical advantage to the use of CR3 by *M. tuberculosis* is that ligation of CR3 may drive the immune response to a TH2 (pathogen-favorable) response by suppressing the production of interleukin 12 (IL-12) by macrophages (29), although there is no experimental data to support this. Once ingested, most of the bacilli are killed by the partially activated alveolar macrophages, but the remainder multiply within these phagocytes, eventually destroying them. The mycobacteria survive by disrupting normal macrophage defense mechanisms through sabotage of phagosome maturation pathways (21, 47).

The infected macrophages spread through the lymphatic channels to regional lymph nodes and then metastasize throughout the body. In the nonimmune host, progressive disease may develop at either the primary or metastatic site. Whether the outcome of the battle between host and invader results in the development of active disease or initial control and development of a latent infection depends on the initial bacillary load and on the interplay of tissue-damaging and macrophage-activating immune responses, which are host mechanisms to control bacillary multiplication (11). Most infected individuals become tuberculin reac-

tion positive, at the same time developing sufficient cell-mediated immunity (macrophage-activating immune response) to limit the further growth of the pathogen, a response that leads to a persistent carrier state that frequently lasts for the lifetime of the host. However, 5% of immunocompetent persons who are infected fail to control the organisms and develop early disease (during the first 5 years after infection), and an additional 5% develop reactivated disease at some point during their lifetimes.

The interplay of tissue-damaging and macrophage-activating immune responses results in either the development of a lung lesion (granuloma) that progresses to caseous necrosis if the tissue-damaging response dominates or regression of the lesion and resolution of the infection if the macrophage-activating immune response dominates. The bacilli in the solid caseous center of the granuloma are inhibited from replicating (the nonreplicating persistence [NRP] state in the Wayne model described below) but are not killed. If the granuloma progresses to necrosis, with the destruction of the host cells as a consequence of the immune response, the bacteria are released into an extracellular environment where they again multiply. Partially activated macrophages at the periphery of the granuloma are able to ingest and destroy some bacteria but are unable to completely sterilize the lesion. Nonactivated macrophages throughout the body can phagocytize the released bacilli, but the organisms can proliferate within these cells. The host again responds with an immune response, which causes further tissue destruction but which also kills at least some bacillus-laden macrophages. If the infection and the tissue-damaging response continue, tuberculosis progresses, causing liquefaction and cavity formation; the bacilli multiply extensively, spread to other parts of the lung, and are released into the environment, where they may infect another host.

The interactions of macrophages, lymphocytes, and the *M. tuberculosis* organism result in regulation of the immune response in tuberculosis (Fig. 1). The macrophage has a central role, producing a variety of toxic substances

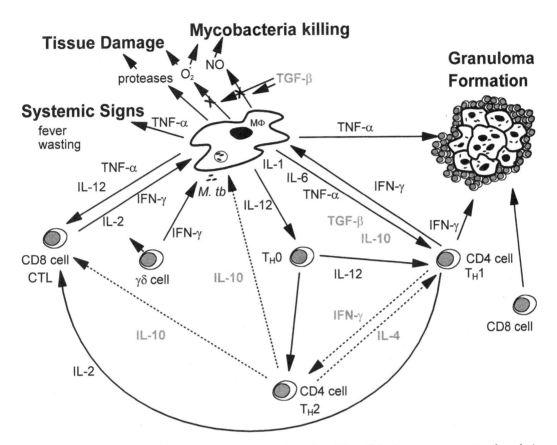

FIGURE 1 Model of the cellular immune response to tuberculosis. The cellular immune response to tuberculosis infection involves a complex network of bidirectional cellular and cytokine interactions. The dashed arrows and mediators shown in gray represent inhibitory pathways. TNF-α, tumor necrosis factor alpha; *M. tb*, *M. tuberculosis*; Mφ, macrophage; CTL, cytotoxic T lymphocyte.

which are involved in killing mycobacteria but which may also cause host tissue destruction. Secretion of tumor necrosis factor alpha is responsible for systemic effects, including fever and weight loss.

Granulomas form when the mycobacterium cannot be totally eliminated, as a host response to limit the spread of the infection. The state of the mycobacterium in the center of the granuloma is unclear; however, it may be unable to replicate but may remain viable in a dormant state. This immune response to tuberculosis has been most extensively studied using the murine model, but experimental data involving human tuberculosis infection have identified some significant differences from the

murine model. The first is that gamma interferon (IFN-γ) may not activate human macrophages as it does in the murine model (38); the factor responsible for macrophage activation in humans is not known. Downstream of IFN-γ action in the murine model is the induction of nitric oxide synthase, leading to production of nitric oxide, which plays a role in mycobacterial killing in mice (8, 19). Whether this mechanism of mycobacterial killing is functional in human monocytes is controversial. One study of human alveolar macrophages failed to demonstrate either production of nitric oxide synthase mRNA or nitrous oxide following stimulation of the macrophages by mycobacteria (2). However, in another study of human alveolar macrophages obtained from bronchopulmonary lavage of patients with clinically active *M. tuberculosis* infection, human nitric oxide synthase was identified (35).

The human immune response to mycobacteria is decidedly a TH1-like response and is characteristic of the cellular immune response to intracellular pathogens. Some investigators interpret the lack of a protective cell-mediated response in patients who develop active disease as a deviation of the immune response from a TH1 to a TH2 pattern or a shift in balance favoring TH2. But there is little evidence for a TH2 cytokine profile in human pulmonary tuberculosis. More likely it is secretion of inhibitory cytokines by macrophages which accounts for the dysfunction (5) or an imbalance between the inflammatory cytokine response (tissue damaging) and the TH1-type protective response (macrophage activating), resulting in active disease (25). A variety of cytokines which act as positive and negative regulators of lymphocyte and macrophage activity are illustrated in Fig. 1.

CLINICAL PERSISTENCE

Clinical persistence is the hallmark of tuberculosis. The majority of persons (approximately 90% of immunocompetent individuals) who become infected with *M. tuberculosis* develop latent or persistent disease. This condition is characterized by a positive skin test to purified protein derivative but no radiological, clinical, or microbiological evidence of active disease. The disease can remain dormant in the human host for many years only to reactivate (27) when immune senescence, immunosuppressive therapy, or an immunosuppressive condition allows the dormant organisms to escape immune surveillance and reestablish active disease. Since the advent of chemotherapy for tuberculosis, the problem of persistence has been manifested by clinical relapse following treatment. Most of the relapses that occur in compliant patients are due to organisms that are still susceptible to the antibiotics whose use in treatment failed. The most widely accepted hypothesis for this phenomenon is that the organisms assumed a state in which they became insusceptible to drug action and thus persisted.

Several investigators who have studied surgical resection in patients with pulmonary tuberculosis have commented on the number of cases where persistent organisms have been found to be viable. In a study by Wayne and Salkin (54) published in 1956, the majority of lung specimens from patients with tuberculosis contained acid-fast bacilli that could be seen microscopically but could not be grown in culture. These lesions were from resected lung tissue where air could not penetrate due to the dense content of the lesion and the lack of a patent bronchus leading to the lesion. But, more surprising, at least 20% of blocked lesions from patients whose sputa no longer contained organisms yielded colonies of *M. tuberculosis* on culture, leading to the hypothesis that these organisms, which were considered obligate aerobes, are capable of surviving under anaerobic conditions. These observations led to the development of the Wayne in vitro model of dormancy (50).

MECHANISMS OF PERSISTENCE

Many workers in the field have offered definitions of mycobacterial persistence. McCune et al. wrote "microbial persistence is the term used to signify the phenomenon whereby microbes that are susceptible to a drug in vitro can nevertheless survive long continued exposure to it in vivo" (30). However, exposure to an antimicrobial agent is not required for the organism to enter this state; a latent infection occurs naturally in the majority of persons who become infected. Clinically, latency is a phase during which the infection is identified by a positive skin test to an intradermal inoculation of purified protein derivative in the absence of a clinically active infection demonstrated by microbiological or radiological methods. In such a phase, the bacilli conceivably could be present in some altered form or they could be unaltered but so few in number that they escape detection (30). In an altered form the organisms may no longer be acid fast and may thus be invisible (26). Most researchers believe that the persistent organisms exhibit reduced or altered metabolism forced upon them through adaptation to an adverse environment. The adaptive process may then involve a switchover to a reduced metabolic state or to a spore-like state (13) that becomes insusceptible to drug action. What then are the hypotheses regarding the mechanisms of persistence in *Mycobacterium*?

PERSISTENCE IS THE ABILITY OF THE *M. TUBERCULOSIS* ORGANISM TO ASSUME A NONCULTURABLE STATE

The Cornell model developed by McCune et al. (30) illustrates the state of latent tuberculosis infection. In this model, mice were inoculated with *M. tuberculosis* and then treated with isoniazid and pyrazinamide for 12 weeks. During the subsequent 12 weeks, no drugs were administered but the mice remained free of active disease. Although acid-fast organisms were detectable (by microscopic examination) in small numbers in tissue homogenates, the mice were in a "sterile state" as defined by the inability to detect the organisms by cell-free culture, tissue culture, and blind animal passage. Following this sterile interval, one-third of the animals suffered reactivation of their disease and developed active infection. If, however, the period of treatment was extended to 26 weeks, no reactivation of disease was seen for a follow-up period of 6 months (31). The ability to form the sterile state is most likely due to both microbial and host factors. If the host is treated with cortisone during the sterile state, reactivation occurs more promptly. In a more recent study using the Cornell model (13), de Wit showed that despite negative cultures during the immediate drug-free period, quantitative PCR consistently detected about 10^5 to 10^6 organisms. The PCR results were confirmed by dot blot analysis (13). Whether the DNA represented dead bacilli, released DNA, or dormant forms could not be determined.

In a study of human surgical lung biopsy specimens from patients with tuberculosis, *M. tuberculosis* was found in closed lung cavities (48). Although histology of specimens revealed acid-fast bacilli, isolation of the organisms from the material required a prolonged incubation time (3 to 10 months) compared to the usual period of 8 weeks. Interestingly, the bacilli isolated were not resistant to the antibiotics the patients had been treated with prior to the surgical removal of tissue. The authors remarked that the long incubation time suggested that the bacilli were in a low metabolic state and thus needed a period of readjustment (48) before regrowth could occur. In this state the organisms appeared resistant to treatment with antibiotics to which they were sensitive in vitro (48).

PERSISTENCE IS THE ABILITY OF *M. TUBERCULOSIS* TO BE PRESENT IN AN ALTERED FORM

Khomenko defined persistence as the presence of an altered form of *M. tuberculosis* that was no longer acid fast (26). He showed in a guinea pig model that 3 to 6 months after the start of chemotherapy, ultrafine (filterable) forms of *M. tuberculosis* with electron-dense cell walls could be isolated from lung cavity walls (26). These forms were not acid fast and failed to grow from the pathological material. However, if these ultrafine forms were passed in animals, the organisms reverted to typical tubercle bacilli capable of multiplication (26).

Recently, other investigators have examined the ultrastructural morphology by transmission electron microscopy of *M. tuberculosis* cultured under microaerobic or anaerobic conditions and identified a strikingly thickened cell wall in these but not in aerobically grown organisms (10). The thickened cell wall was associated with high expression of the 16-kDa heat shock protein, α-crystallin homolog (10). They hypothesized that reduced oxygen tension may trigger the tubercle bacillus to enter a state of dormancy. This environment may be experienced in the internal milieu of the granuloma, a hostile, acidic environment with low O_2 and high CO_2 levels. The thickened cell wall may protect against the hostile environment associated with granulomas and may preclude the necessity for these bacteria to sporulate. Localization studies suggested that the α-crystallin protein has several targets throughout the cell and that it may be integral to the stabilization of cellular structure (i.e., a chaperone function) during the dormant state (10). The chaperone activity of this protein, like that of other members of the small-heat-shock-protein family with which it shares sequence homology, lies in its ability to suppress the thermally induced denaturation of other proteins (32). In addition, overexpression of the M. tuberculosis α-crystallin protein conferred a phenotype of resistance to autolysis at the end of log-phase growth (59). Unlike the findings of Khomenko, the organisms studied by Cunningham still retained the acid-fast staining property.

PERSISTENCE IS THE RESULT OF ALTERED OR REDUCED METABOLISM OF THE M. TUBERCULOSIS ORGANISM

Stationary-phase growth and strict anaerobic incubation may precipitate the shutdown of protein synthesis in the dormant M. tuberculosis (23). Hu et al. (23) have quantitated the change in protein synthesis in M. tuberculosis organisms as they enter stationary phase. They estimate that the rate of protein synthesis decreased to 2% of the logarithmic growth rate. The organisms in this state were still viable and capable of responding to environmental stimuli, such as repletion of oxygen or heat shock, by resuming normal protein synthesis. The biochemical and genetic bases of altered protein synthesis are unknown. Investigation of mycobacterial cells which pass from an actively multiplying state to a low-metabolic nonmultiplying state identified a switch in metabolism to the glyoxalate cycle, which permits adaptation to the usually lethal effects of anaerobiosis (53). The observation by Wayne et al. (55) that M. tuberculosis organisms that have become persistent are susceptible to killing by the antibacterial activity of metronidazole, a drug specific for anaerobes, but display partial or complete resistance to iso-

niazid and rifampin suggests that these organisms are dormant.

PERSISTENCE MAY INVOLVE A SPORE-LIKE FORM

The identification of an M. tuberculosis sigma factor (SigF) related to sporulation sigma factors from Streptomyces coelicolor and Bacillus subtilis raises the question of whether the tubercle bacilli enter a spore-like state that allows them to survive in the environment or in the host during persistent infection (12). Further evidence for a spore-like state may be the presence of the non-acid-fast forms described by Khomenko (26) and Hans Much (45).

PERSISTENCE MAY BE THE RESULT OF A HOST-PATHOGEN INTERACTION WHICH FAVORS IMMUNE SURVEILLANCE ESCAPE

Some investigators argue that the foci of "latent" tuberculosis are not dormant but instead activate repeatedly, creating a state of dynamic balance between the organism and host cells (18). They contend that the cell-mediated immunity maintains the inactivity of latent foci through active immunological surveillance. This is most convincingly illustrated by the patient dually infected with HIV and tuberculosis who, depleted of CD4 cells, develops active tuberculosis disease at a rate 170 times that of a latently infected HIV-negative individual (18). The tubercle bacillus is the same in both patients, but the HIV-positive patient's immune dysfunction allows the organism to escape immune surveillance and develop an active disease state. Other evidence pointing to an active bacterial turnover is the 65% efficacy of 6 months of isoniazid prophylaxis in latent tuberculosis infection (9); antimycobacterial agents are highly effective against tubercle bacilli only when the bacilli are growing. In contrast, the observation that relapses of M. tuberculosis disease occur in a finite group of individuals who have received adequate antimycobacterial chemotherapy supports the alternative hypothesis that the organisms remaining viable are not actively dividing.

MARKERS OF THE PERSISTENT STATE

How the tubercle bacillus survives during the dormant state of infection is unknown. However, markers of the persistent state are being described, and these point increasingly to the existence of a dormant state. These markers include the change in tolerance to anaerobiosis (51), production of the 16-kDa α-crystallin homolog (10), an increase in glycine dehydrogenase production (51), and expression of the antigen 85 complex (49).

Most actively replicating organisms are killed early in therapy, but prolonged treatment is required to eradicate persisting organisms exhibiting reduced or altered metabolism. In a study by Wallis et al. (49), induction of *M. tuberculosis* antigen 85 complex in the sputa of patients with active pulmonary tuberculosis who were undergoing treatment predicted the patients who were likely to steadily produce sputum with viable *M. tuberculosis* and thus be at high risk of treatment failure. The antigen 85 complex, a group of three 30- to 32-kDa mycolyl transferase proteins, is essential for the integrity of a partially damaged mycobacterial cell wall. These investigators hypothesized that induction of this complex might be part of an adaptive transition to a persistent state that is induced by isoniazid treatment (49).

METHODS OF STUDYING LATENCY

Animal models have been used to demonstrate both immunologically induced latency (7, 36, 37) and posttreatment latency (13) with reactivation disease. In vitro models of dormancy of *M. tuberculosis* use a self-generated oxygen depletion gradient in unagitated cultures (50).

At least three groups of investigators have developed a mouse model of latent tuberculosis which, unlike the Cornell model described above, mimics natural latent infection by avoiding the use of antimycobacterial drugs. In the model developed by Phyu et al. (37), mice were given 10^4 to 10^5 CFU of *M. tuberculosis* intraperitoneally and remained clinically healthy. Although colony counts increased initially in the lungs and spleens, between the 21st

and 52nd weeks the counts were stable. Corticosterone challenge was used to reactivate the latent infection.

Orme (36), in contrast, gave a low-dose aerosol of *M. tuberculosis* to mice at 3 months of age. These mice had no clinical signs of disease until 24 months of age, when they died of overwhelming infection. The control mice, who were uninfected, lived 3 to 6 months longer. The old mice appeared unable to generate acquired resistance to the reactivated infection.

Brown et al. (7) gave a dose of 100 *M. tuberculosis* organisms intravenously and established latency by 65 days postinfection. Activation of the hypothalamic-pituitary-adrenal axis by restraint of the mice caused reactivation of *M. tuberculosis* infection, manifested by an increase in CFU in the lungs and spleens. Adams et al. (1) gave a dose of 10^5 *M. tuberculosis* organisms intravenously and 6 months later achieved reactivation by the administration of a recombinant adenovirus encoding a fusion protein of the tumor necrosis factor receptor extracellular domain and the mouse immunoglobulin G heavy chain domain (AdTNFR). Following AdTNFR treatment, the chronically infected mice developed a 3-$\log_{10}$ increase of *M. tuberculosis* in the lungs and tuberculous bronchopneumonia. Each of these models should allow an examination of the host-parasite interaction and the question of whether the reactivation of disease is due to an environmental signal to the microbe or is dependent on host characteristics.

The Wayne model of *M. tuberculosis* persistence is an in vitro–culture model based on adaptation of bacilli in liquid medium to different levels of O_2 depletion (52). In this model, two stages of NRP were seen. The first stage, NRP1, occurred when the dissolved O_2 level approached 1% saturation, corresponding to a microaerophilic state. In this state, there was no apparent change in CFU or synthesis of DNA. While the tubercle bacilli were in this state, there was a shift in metabolism to the glyoxylic acid cycle with an increase in glycine dehydrogenase activity. With further depletion of O_2, the bacilli shifted into a second stage, NRP2, corresponding to an anaerobic state. This state was characterized by a marked decrease in glycine dehydrogenase activity and tolerance to anaerobiosis. These states may reflect the environments in which the tubercle bacilli exist in the necrotic granuloma tissue of the mammalian host. With resumption of aeration, the dormant bacteria undergo synchronized cell division. This requires RNA synthesis but not DNA synthesis, and so it is assumed that during adaptation to the nonreplicative form, the dormant bacteria have replicated their DNA but have not divided. The model is being used to identify both the molecular events responsible for the ability of the organism to become dormant and the triggers responsible for reactivation.

SUMMARY

Unlike many other bacteria which persist by colonization of an accessible body site, persistence in *M. tuberculosis* infection is truly a quiescent state. Many questions remain. The site where the organism persists is not clearly known: some believe it to be the lung, and others believe small foci occur throughout the infected host. What determines which patient develops primary active disease, latent disease which reactivates at a distant time point, or latent infection which does not reactivate? Is tuberculosis persistence due to host or microbial factors? What are the triggers that determine latency or reactivation? Is the dormant state a result of an adaptive response of the organism to avoid host immune detection and elimination? Is this form an altered non–acid-fast or spore-like form? Is the dormant form due to altered metabolism? Does isoniazid treatment actually result in induction to a latent state? Can we predict (using antigen 85 complex) those patients who are at high risk of treatment failure and thus make it possible to individualize therapy? Can we improve the outcome of treatment by using adjunctive therapy with immunomodulating cytokines? Should we be designing treatment strategies that target both actively replicating and non-replicating organisms?

M. LEPRAE

Mycobacterium leprae is the causative agent of leprosy, an apparently ancient mycobacterial disease. *M. leprae* infection is characterized by the existence of two classical clinical forms, although most patients have features of both (20). At one end of the clinical spectrum is lepromatous leprosy, which is characterized by the presence of skin nodules and plaques. Patients typically have involvement of the cooler areas of the body, such as the nares, ear lobes, and testes. High-level bacteremia is present in some severely affected patients. *M. leprae* displays a tropism for peripheral nerve cells, and lepromatous patients may have severe symmetrical peripheral neuropathy. Tuberculoid leprosy is generally less severe and is characterized by the presence of focal anesthetic skin lesions, marked histologically by the presence of granulomata.

Lepromatous and tuberculoid leprosy represents distinct pathological and pathogenetic entities. Tuberculoid patients apparently mount a TH1-type response, as seen in tuberculosis. IFN-γ and IL-2 release is characteristically demonstrated (14, 24). Lepromatous leprosy is apparently marked by a failure of the patient to develop the TH1-type response that is necessary for the control of both *M. leprae* and *M. tuberculosis* infections. Lesions of lepromatous leprosy demonstrate reduced levels of IFN-γ and IL-2 and increased levels of TH2-type cytokines, IL-4, IL-5, and IL-10 (58).

The pathogenesis of leprosy is not as well understood as that of tuberculosis, due in part to difficulty in cultivating the causative organism. *M. leprae* is invasive and is capable of entering macrophages, epithelial cells, and Schwann cells lining the axons of peripheral nerves (43). The ability to enter cells that are relatively poor killers of intracellular pathogens may serve to promote the persistence of *M. leprae*; however, entry into nonphagocytic cells is generally sufficient to elicit a major histocompatibility complex type I restricted response, and therefore, further modulation of the immune response is required to ensure persistence of the infection. Indeed, it has long been recognized that *M. leprae* is capable of inducing a suppression of T-cell proliferation, although the precise bacterial products responsible for this phenomenon are still controversial (33). Additional features of *M. leprae* have also been suggested to play roles in the persistence of the organism (reviewed in reference 44). The thioredoxin-thioreductase gene has been shown to confer increased intracellular survival in mononuclear phagocytes via the scavenging of reactive oxygen species (56). The phenolic glycolipid PGL-1 has also been suggested to scavenge reactive oxygen species (34), and the production of superoxide dismutase by *M. leprae* may serve to scavenge O_2^- (28). Other genes are likely to be involved as well (39). Thus, like *M. tuberculosis*, *M. leprae* has evolved a strategy of persistent infection that is mediated by multiple factors, based fundamentally on the ability of the organism to thwart productive immune-mediated responses.

ACKNOWLEDGMENT

I thank JoAnne Flynn for helpful discussion and critical review of the manuscript.

REFERENCES

1. **Adams, L. B., C. M. Mason, J. K. Kolls, D. Scollard, J. L. Krahenbuhl, and S. Nelson.** 1995. Exacerbation of acute and chronic murine tuberculosis by administration of a tumor necrosis factor receptor-expressing adenovirus. *J. Infect. Dis.* **171:**400–405.

2. **Aston, C., W. N. Rom, A. T. Talbot, and J. Reibman.** 1998. Early inhibition of mycobacterial growth by human alveolar macrophages is not due to nitric oxide. *Am. J. Respir. Crit. Care Med.* **157:**1943–1950.

3. **Berton, G., C. Laudanna, C. Sorio, and F. Rossi.** 1992. Generation of signals activating neutrophil functions by leukocyte integrins: LFA-1 and gp150/95, but not CR3, are able to stimulate the respiratory burst of human neutrophils. *J. Cell Biol.* **116:**1007–1017.

4. **Bloom, B. R., and C. J. L. Murray.** 1992. Tuberculosis: commentary on a reemergent killer. *Science* **257:**1055–1064.

5. **Boom, W. H.** 1996. The role of T-cell subsets in *Mycobacterium tuberculosis* infection. *Infect. Agents Dis.* **5:**73–81.

6. **Brennan, P. J.** 1997. Tuberculosis in the context of emerging and reemerging diseases. *FEMS Immunol. Med. Microbiol.* **18:**263–269.

7. **Brown, D. H., B. A. Miles, and B. S. Zwilling.** 1995. Growth of *Mycobacterium tuberculosis* in BCG-resistant and -susceptible mice: establishment of latency and reactivation. *Infect. Immun.* **63:**2243–2247.

8. **Chan, J., K. Tanaka, D. Carroll, J. Flynn, and B. R. Bloom.** 1995. Effects of nitric oxide synthase inhibitors on murine infection with *Mycobacterium tuberculosis*. *Infect. Immun.* **63:**736–740.

9. **Comstock, G. W., and S. F. Woolpert.** 1972. Preventive treatment of untreated, nonactive tuberculosis in an Eskimo population. *Arch. Environ. Health* **25:**333–337.

10. **Cunningham, A. F., and C. L. Spreadbury.** 1998. Mycobacterial stationary phase induced by low oxygen tension: cell wall thickening and localization of the 16-kilodalton α-crystallin homology. *J. Bacteriol.* **180:**801–808.

11. **Dannenberg, A. M., and G. A. W. Rook.** 1994. Pathogenesis of pulmonary tuberculosis: an interplay of tissue-damaging and macrophage-activating immune responses—dual mechanisms that control bacillary multiplication, p. 459–483. *In* B. R. Bloom (ed.), *Tuberculosis: Pathogenesis, Protection, and Control.* American Society for Microbiology, Washington, D.C.

12. **DeMaio, J., Y. Zhang, C. Ko, D. B. Young, and W. R. Bishai.** 1996. A stationary-phase stress-response sigma factor from *Mycobacterium tuberculosis*. *Proc. Natl. Acad. Sci. USA* **93:**2790–2794.

13. **De Wit, D., M. Wootton, J. Dhillon, and D. A. Mitchison.** 1995. The bacterial DNA content of mouse organs in the Cornell model of dormant tuberculosis. *Tuber. Lung Dis.* **76:**555–562.

14. **Dockrell, H. M., S. K. Young, K. Britton, P. J. Brennan, B. Rivoire, M. F. R. Waters, S. B. Lucas, F. Shahid, M. Dojki, T. J. Chiang, Q. Ehsan, K. P. W. J. McAdam, and R. Hussain.** 1996. Induction of Th1 cytokine responses by mycobacterial antigens in leprosy. *Infect. Immun.* **64:**4385–4389.

15. **Dolin, P. J., M. C. Raviglione, and A. Kochi.** 1994. Global tuberculosis incidence and mortality during 1990–2000. *Bull. W. H. O.* **72:**213–220.

16. **Downing, J. F., R. Pasula, J. R. Wright, H. L. Twigg III, and W. J. Martin II.** 1995. Surfactant protein A promotes attachment of *Mycobacterium tuberculosis* to alveolar macrophages during infection with human immunodeficiency virus. *Proc. Natl. Acad. Sci. USA* **92:**4848–4852.

17. **Ehlers, M. R. W., and M. Daffé.** 1998. Interac-

tions between *Mycobacterium tuberculosis* and host cells: are mycobacterial sugars the key? *Trends Microbiol.* **6:**328–335.

18. **Ellner, J. J.** 1997. Review: the immune response in human tuberculosis—implications for tuberculosis control. *J. Infect. Dis.* **176:**1351–1359.

19. **Flynn, J. L., C. A. Scanga, K. E. Tanaka, and J. Chan.** 1998. Effects of aminoguanidine on latent murine tuberculosis. *J. Immunol.* **160:**1796–1803.

20. **Gelber, R. H.** 1995. Leprosy (Hansen's disease), p. 2243–2250. *In* G. L. Mandell, J. E. Bennett, and R. Dolin (ed.), *Principles and Practice of Infectious Diseases.* Churchill Livingstone, New York, N.Y.

21. **Gordon, A. H., P. D'Arcy Hart, and M. R. Young.** 1980. Ammonia inhibits phagosome-lysosome fusion in macrophages. *Nature* **286:**79–80.

22. **Hirsch, C. S., J. J. Ellner, D. G. Russell, and E. A. Rich.** 1994. Complement receptor-mediated uptake and tumor necrosis factor-α-mediated growth inhibition of *Mycobacterium tuberculosis* by human alveolar macrophages. *J. Immunol.* **152:**743–753.

23. **Hu, Y. M., P. D. Butcher, K. Sole, D. A. Mitchison, and A. R. M. Coates.** 1998. Protein synthesis is shut down in dormant *Mycobacterium tuberculosis* and is reversed by oxygen or heat shock. *FEMS Microbiol. Lett.* **158:**139–145.

24. **Kaplan, G.** 1994. Cytokine regulation of disease progression in leprosy and tuberculosis. *Immunobiology* **191:**564–568.

25. **Kaplan, G., and V. H. Freedman.** 1996. The role of cytokines in the immune response to tuberculosis. *Res. Immunol.* **147:**565–572.

26. **Khomenko, A. G.** 1987. The variability of *Mycobacterium tuberculosis* in patients with cavitary pulmonary tuberculosis in the course of chemotherapy. *Tubercle* **68:**243–253.

27. **Korovessis, P., E. Papadaki, M. Repanti, and M. Stamatakis.** 1995. Latent solitary tuberculous psoas abscess 52 years after healed thoracolumbar tuberculous spondylitis. *Spine* **15:**1709–1712.

28. **Lygren, S. T., O. Closs, H. Bercouvier, and L. G. Wayne.** 1986. Catalases, peroxidases, and superoxide dismutase in *Mycobacterium leprae* and other mycobacteria studied by cross immunoelectrophoresis and polyacrylamide gel electrophoresis. *Infect. Immun.* **54:**666–671.

29. **Marth, T., and B. L. Kelsall.** 1997. Regulation of interleukin-12 by complement receptor 3 signaling. *J. Exp. Med.* **185:**1987–1995.

30. **McCune, R. M., F. M. Feldmann, H. P. Lambert, and W. McDermott.** 1966. Microbial persistence. I. The capacity of tubercle bacilli to survive sterilization in mouse tissues. *J. Exp. Med.* **123:**445–468.

31. **McCune, R. M., F. M. Feldmann, and W.**

McDermott. 1966. Microbial persistence. II. Characteristics of the sterile state of tubercle bacilli. *J. Exp. Med.* **123:**469–486.

32. **Mehlen, P., J. Briolay, L. Smith, C. Diaz-Latoud, N. Fabre, D. Pauli, and A. P. Arrigo.** 1993. Analysis of the resistance to heat and hydrogen peroxide stresses in COS cells transiently expressing wild type or deletion mutants of the *Drosophila* 27-kDa heat-shock protein. *Eur. J. Biochem.* **215:**277–284.

33. **Molloy, A., G. Gaudernack, W. R. Levis, Z. A. Cohn, and G. Kaplan.** 1990. Suppression of T-cell proliferation by *Mycobacterium leprae* and its products: the role of lipopolysaccharide. *Proc. Natl. Acad. Sci. USA* **87:**973–977.

34. **Neill, M. A., and S. J. Klebanoff.** 1988. The effect of phenolic glycolipid-1 from *Mycobacterium leprae* on the antimicrobial activity of human macrophages. *J. Exp. Med.* **167:**30–42.

35. **Nicholson, S., M. G. Bonecini-Almeida, J. R. Lapa e Silva, C. Nathan, Q. W. Xie, R. Mumford, J. R. Weidner, J. Calaycay, J. Geng, and N. Boechat.** 1996. Inducible nitric oxide synthase in pulmonary alveolar macrophages from patients with tuberculosis. *J. Exp. Med.* **183:**2293–2302.

36. **Orme, I. M.** 1988. A mouse model of the recrudescence of latent tuberculosis in the elderly. *Am. Rev. Respir. Dis.* **137:**716–718.

37. **Phyu, S., T. Mustafa, T. Hofstad, R. Nilsen, R. Fosse, and G. Bjune.** 1998. A mouse model for latent tuberculosis. *Scand. J. Infect. Dis.* **30:**59–68.

38. **Rook, G. A. W., J. Taverne, C. Leveton, and J. Steele.** 1987. The role of gamma-interferon, vitamin D_3 metabolites and tumor necrosis factor in the pathogenesis of tuberculosis. *Immunology* **62:**229–234.

39. **Sathish, M., and T. M. Shinnick.** 1994. Identification of genes involved in resistance of mycobacteria to killing by macrophages. *Ann. N. Y. Acad. Sci.* **730:**26–36.

40. **Schlesinger, L. S.** 1993. Macrophage phagocytosis of virulent but not attenuated strains of *Mycobacterium tuberculosis* is mediated by mannose receptors in addition to complement receptors. *J. Immunol.* **150:**2920–2930.

41. **Schlesinger, L. S., C. G. Bellinger-Kawahara, N. R. Payne, and M. A. Horwitz.** 1990. Phagocytosis of *Mycobacterium tuberculosis* is mediated by human monocyte complement receptors and complement component C3. *J. Immunol.* **144:**2771–2780.

42. **Schorey, J. S., M. C. Carroll, and E. J. Brown.** 1997. A macrophage invasion mechanism of pathogenic mycobacteria. *Science* **277:**1091–1093.

43. **Schorey, J. S., Q. Li, D. W. McCourt, M. Bong-Mastek, J. E. Clark-Curtiss, T. L. Ratliff, and E. J. Brown.** 1995. A *Mycobacterium leprae* gene encoding a fibronectin binding protein is used for efficient invasion of epithelial cells and Schwann cells. *Infect. Immun.* **63:**2652–2657.

44. **Shinnick, T. M., H. King, and F. D. Quinn.** 1995. Molecular biology, virulence and pathogenicity of mycobacteria. *Am. J. Med. Sci.* **309:**92–98.

45. **Stanford, J. L.** 1987. Much's granules revisited. *Tubercle* **68:**241–242.

46. **Stokes, R. W., I. D. Haidl, W. A. Jefferies, and D. P. Speert.** 1993. Mycobacteria-macrophage interactions: macrophage phenotype determines the nonopsonic binding of *Mycobacterium tuberculosis* to murine macrophages. *J. Immunol.* **151:**7067–7076.

47. **Sturgill-Koszycki, S., P. H. Schlesinger, P. Chakraborty, P. L. Haddix, H. L. Collins, A. K. Fok, R. D. Allen, S. L. Gluck, J. Heuser, and D. G. Russell.** 1994. Lack of acidification in *Mycobacterium* phagosomes produced by exclusion of the vesicular proton-ATPase. *Science* **263:**678–681.

48. **Vandiviere, H. M., W. E. Loring, I. Melvin, S. Willis, et al.** 1956. The treated pulmonary lesion and its tubercle bacillus. II. The death and resurrection. *Am. J. Med. Sci.* **232:**30–37.

49. **Wallis, R. S., M. Perkins, M. Phillips, M. Joloba, B. Demchuk, A. Namale, J. L. Johnson, D. Williams, K. Wolski, L. Teixeira, R. Dietze, R. D. Mugerwa, K. Eisenach, and J. J. Ellner.** 1998. Induction of the antigen 85 complex of *Mycobacterium tuberculosis* in sputum: a determinant of outcome in pulmonary tuberculosis treatment. *J. Infect. Dis.* **178:**1115–1121.

50. **Wayne, L. G.** 1976. Dynamics of submerged growth of *Mycobacterium tuberculosis* under aerobic and microaerophilic conditions. *Am. Rev. Respir. Dis.* **114:**807–811.

51. **Wayne, L. G.** 1994. Dormancy of *Mycobacterium tuberculosis* and latency of disease. *Eur. J. Clin. Microbiol. Infect. Dis.* **13:**908–914.

52. **Wayne, L. G., and L. G. Hayes.** 1996. An in vitro model for sequential study of shiftdown of *Mycobacterium tuberculosis* through two stages of nonreplicating persistence. *Infect. Immun.* **64:**2062–2069.

53. **Wayne, L. G., and K. Y. Lin.** 1982. Glyoxylate metabolism and adaptation of *Mycobacterium tuberculosis* to survival under anaerobic conditions. *Infect. Immun.* **37:**1042–1049.

54. **Wayne, L. G., and D. Salkin.** 1956. The bacteriology of resected tuberculous pulmonary lesions. I. The effect of interval between reversal of infectiousness and subsequent surgery. *Am. Rev. Tuber.* **74:**376–387.

55. **Wayne, L. G., and H. A. Sramek.** 1994. Metronidazole is bactericidal to dormant cells of *Mycobacterium tuberculosis*. *Antimicrob. Agents Chemother.* **38:**2054–2058.

56. **Weiles, B., T. H. M. Ottenhoff, T. M. Steenwijk, K. L. M. C. Franken, R. R. P. DeVries, and J. A. M. Langerman.** 1997. Increased intracellular survival of *Mycobacterium smegmatis* containing the *Mycobacterium leprae* thioredoxin-thioredoxin reductase gene. *Infect. Immun.* **65:**2537–2541.

57. **Wright, S. D., and S. C. Silverstein.** 1983. Receptors for C3b and C3bi promote phagocytosis but not the release of toxic oxygen from human phagocytes. *J. Exp. Med.* **158:**2016–2023.

58. **Yamamura, M., K. Uyemura, R. J. Deans, K. Weinberg, T. H. Rea, B. R. Bloom, and R. L. Modlin.** 1991. Defining protective responses to pathogens: cytokine profiles in leprosy patients. *Science* **254:**277–279.

59. **Yuan, Y., D. D. Crane, and C. E. Barry III.** 1996. Stationary phase-associated protein expression in *Mycobacterium tuberculosis*: function of the mycobacterial α-crystallin homolog. *J. Bacteriol.* **178:**4484–4492.

BARTONELLA SPECIES

Jane E. Koehler

17

OVERVIEW OF PATHOGENESIS

The majority of *Bartonella* species and infections have been described only in the past decade or even the past few years. This chapter will provide an introduction to the rapidly expanding but still very limited knowledge about the interactions of these *Bartonella* species and their reservoirs and vectors and the adaptations these bacteria have developed to maintain persistent infection in the host mammalian species. Bartonellae are extremely fastidious, small gram-negative alpha proteobacteria that are hemin dependent. These bacilli are extraordinarily well-adapted to the niches that they occupy: the bloodstreams of mammalian reservoirs and the intestinal tracts of obligately hematophagous arthropod vectors. *Bartonella* species are so well-adapted that they can coexist in the bloodstreams of mammals at astonishingly high counts of thousands to millions of CFU per milliliter of blood for an indefinite period of time, even perhaps for the life of the animal.

This host adaptation by bartonellae is so exquisitely developed that a pathogenic response probably occurs in only a small percentage of

infected mammals, and death of the host appears to be extremely unusual. The most dramatic diseases caused by bartonellae occur when a *Bartonella* species is introduced into an accidental host to which it is not adapted or into a host with a severely compromised immune system. The recognition of *Bartonella* infections in contemporary North America was the direct result of the latter, when the AIDS epidemic dramatically increased the number of individuals with severe immunocompromise. Patients in the late stages of human immunodeficiency virus (HIV) infection developed striking lesions of bacillary angiomatosis (BA), highly vascular skin lesions sometimes resembling Kaposi sarcoma, when infected with one of two species, *Bartonella henselae* or *Bartonella quintana* (34). The first such patient was identified early in the AIDS epidemic, in 1983 (64), and the dramatic appearance of these BA lesions led to the identification of additional cases and the search for the causative bacillus.

The disease BA was named in 1989 (46), and the causative genus of bacilli was identified in the early 1990s (54). These discoveries launched an intensive investigation that subsequently uncovered the long-sought etiologic agent of cat scratch disease (CSD) and, more recently, the extensive diversity of *Bartonella* species that interact with numerous mamma-

Jane E. Koehler, Division of Infectious Diseases, Department of Medicine, 521 Parnassus Ave., Room C-443, University of California at San Francisco, San Francisco, CA 94143-0654.

Persistent Bacterial Infections, Edited by J. P. Nataro, M. J. Blaser, and S. Cunningham-Rundles, © 2000 ASM Press, Washington, D.C.

lian reservoirs and vectors. Dozens of mammalian species serve as reservoir hosts from which lice, fleas, sandflies, and possibly ticks transmit an expanding number of *Bartonella* species. The study of *Bartonella*-host interactions has just begun, with very few studies addressing either in vitro or in vivo interactions with the host.

CLINICAL AND EPIDEMIOLOGICAL CHARACTERISTICS

Human Infection

Bartonella bacilliformis was the first and sole species in the genus *Bartonella* until 1992, when the genus *Rochalimaea*, comprising *Rochalimaea quintana*, *Rochalimaea henselae*, and *Rochalimaea vinsonii*, was combined with the genus *Bartonella* (8). There are now at least 13 named species and probably an equal number of unnamed species. Of these, only four have been definitively associated with human disease: *B. henselae*, *B. quintana*, *B. bacilliformis*, and *Bartonella elizabethae* (Table 1). The general categories of syndromes produced by infection of humans with these species include persistent bacteremia (all four species), granulomatous lymphadenitis (CSD; *B. henselae*), endocarditis (*B. quintana* > *B. henselae* > *B. elizabethae*), and vascular proliferative lesions (*B. quintana*, *B. henselae*, and *B. bacilliformis*) (31).

PERSISTENT OR RELAPSING BACTEREMIA

Chronic, asymptomatic bacteremia has been reported in infections with most *Bartonella* species, but in humans it most frequently occurs with two species, *B. quintana* and *B. bacilliformis*. Initial infection with *B. bacilliformis* may be asymptomatic, may result in rapid, fatal anemia due to hemolysis of red blood cells (RBC), or may cause immunosuppression and death due to intercurrent *Salmonella* or *Mycobacterium tuberculosis* infection (69). Asymptomatic bacteremia with *B. bacilliformis* is frequently noted: sampling of individuals in one area of endemicity in the Peruvian Andes (*B. bacilliformis* occurs only in the Peruvian Andes because of the distribution of the sandfly vector) revealed a prevalence of bacteremia of 5 to 10% (71).

B. quintana infection may be asymptomatic or may be characterized by high fever, severe shin pain, and relapsing symptoms over weeks to months. Soldiers in World War I who developed trench fever were noted to have relapsing fever and other symptoms at 5-day (quintan) intervals (Fig. 1), hence the species designation, *B. quintana* (66, 67). Although tens of thousands of soldiers were infected with *B. quintana*, the infection was not lethal; symptoms, and apparently bacteremia, resolved without antibiotic treatment (66). Persistent *B. quintana* bacteremia can also be asymptomatic, and the experimental infection of humans with *B. quintana* during and after World War I revealed that the organism was present in the blood of humans as many as 300 and 443 days after the onset of disease (66). In contemporary times, a study of 71 homeless people presenting at an emergency department in 1997 in France

TABLE 1 *Bartonella* species and human infection[a]

Classification		Human infection		
Bartonella species	Previous genus	Bacteremic syndrome	Chronic lymphadenopathy	Chronic vascular lesions
B. bacilliformis	*Bartonia*	Oroya fever		Verruga peruana
B. henselae	*Rochalimaea*	Relapsing fever Endocarditis	CSD (immunocompetent)	BA (immunocompromised)
B. quintana	*Rickettsia* *Rochalimaea*	Trench fever Endocarditis		BA (immunocompromised)
B. elizabethae	*Rochalimaea*	Endocarditis		

[a] Reprinted from reference 31, with permission.

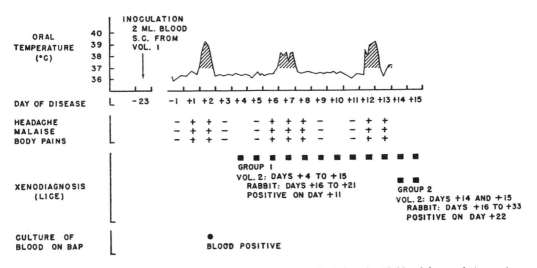

FIGURE 1 Pattern of fever in a volunteer (vol. 2) experimentally infected with blood from vol. 1, a patient infected with *B. quintana*. Prolonged bacteremia is present, diagnosed by positive xenodiagnosis and isolation of *B. quintana* from the patient's blood. BAP, blood agar plates; S. C., subcutaneous; +, present; −, absent. (Reprinted from reference 67 with permission of the publisher.)

identified *B. quintana* bacteremia in 14%, and of those bacteremic patients, 80% were afebrile (10). An unusually large number of bacteria (>1,000 CFU/ml) can be present chronically in the blood of humans in the absence of sepsis or major symptoms (34).

Persistent asymptomatic bacteremia with *B. henselae* has also been reported in several immunocompetent humans, despite treatment with antibiotics. In one patient (48), *B. henselae* could be isolated from blood cultures for 14 weeks, 8 weeks after treatment with doxycycline and ceftriaxone, two antibiotics likely to have good antimicrobial activity against *B. henselae*. Another patient developed bacteremia with *B. henselae* complicated by fever and painless loss of vision in the left eye (neuroretinitis) (72). The patient was treated with two first-line antibiotics for 4 weeks, and all symptoms resolved, but *B. henselae* bacteremia was demonstrated subsequently. Thus, in humans, as in other mammals (see below), infection with *Bartonella* species can be prolonged and relapsing, although neither the proportion of humans who develop persistent bacteremia after infection nor the usual duration of bacteremia is known at present.

ENDOCARDITIS

Endocarditis, or heart valve infection, develops as a complication in some patients with *Bartonella* bacteremia; the majority of these individuals have preexisting valvular heart abnormalities (52). It is presumed that the prolonged bacteremia in the presence of valvular lesions results in seeding of the valves with bacteria. This often leads to formation of valvular vegetations that break off and embolize. *Bartonella* endocarditis usually follows a subacute course, with a diagnosis made after months of symptoms (20). The species most commonly associated with endocarditis in humans is *B. quintana*, and most patients with *Bartonella* endocarditis require replacement of the infected cardiac valve (52, 63).

GRANULOMATOUS LYMPHADENITIS AND OTHER GRANULOMATOUS INFLAMMATORY DISEASES

Granulomatous inflammatory disease (CSD), most commonly of the lymph nodes, occurs in immunocompetent humans infected with *B. henselae*. This infection usually begins at the site of a cat scratch, with subsequent involvement of the lymph nodes draining the scratch. Histopathologically, these lesions are characterized by necrotizing granulomatous inflammation and infiltration with neutrophils, eosinophils, and histiocytes (51). Extracellular (only very rarely, if ever, intracellular) *B. henselae* bacilli can occasionally be seen (51), but few bacteria are present in the granulomatous lesions in contrast to the large numbers seen in the lesions of BA. These *B. henselae* infections resolve slowly over several months, and antibiotic therapy probably has no impact on the resolution of granulomatous lymphadenitis. Of note, although *Bartonella clarridgeiae* infects a substantial proportion of cats in some regions, e.g., Europe, the species has not been isolated, nor has its DNA been amplified, from tissue of CSD patients (5).

VASCULAR PROLIFERATIVE DISEASES

The vascular proliferative manifestations of *Bartonella* infection in humans differ dramatically from the granulomatous lesions of CSD. Three species of *Bartonella* have been associated with these lesions, *B. bacilliformis*, *B. quintana*, and *B. henselae*. After acute hemolytic (Oroya fever) or asymptomatic *B. bacilliformis* infection, some individuals develop an eruptive, chronic phase of *B. bacilliformis* infection known as verruga peruana. This phase of the infection is often without systemic symptoms and is characterized by warty, usually painless, vascular cutaneous lesions that can occur in crops or singly, localized to the face and extremities but occasionally scattered over the entire body (11). Infection in the form of verruga peruana can persist for several months to several years, but rarely causes death (50). Although many other mammals are infected chronically with many different *Bartonella* species, vascular proliferative lesions have been described only in humans.

Histopathological examination of these chronic lesions reveals a lobular vascular proliferation consisting of plump endothelial cells with a predominantly lymphocytic and plasmacytic infiltration (50). Some pathologists have reported observing Rocha-Lima inclusions, which appear to be intracytoplasmic in-

clusions containing bacteria in endothelial cells, but their exact nature remains unknown. *B. bacilliformis* bacilli can be visualized by electron microscopy and are localized to the extracellular space just adjacent to the proliferating endothelial cells (50). Histopathologic studies therefore indicate that virtually all of the bacteria are localized extracellularly.

Infection of immunocompromised patients with *B. henselae* and *B. quintana* can result in formation of chronic vascular proliferative lesions (i.e., BA) that are clinically and histopathologically similar to those of verruga peruana caused by *B. bacilliformis*. These lesions occur almost exclusively in the profoundly immunocompromised patient, usually with a CD4 cell count of $<50/mm^3$. Although *B. henselae* and *B. quintana* most frequently cause cutaneous BA lesions, they can also cause invasive, vascular proliferative lesions of other organs, including soft tissue, bone, lymph nodes, brain, liver, lung, and gastrointestinal tract (37). The invasive nature of these BA lesions and their high degree of vascularity are features common to malignant lesions, and thus BA is often misdiagnosed as cancer. There appears to be a species-specific tropism of *B. henselae* to the liver, lymph nodes, and central nervous system and of *B. quintana* to bone and subcutaneous tissue (36), the basis for which is completely unknown.

BA is a systemic disease, and $\geq 50\%$ of patients have concomitant bacteremia (36). As with verruga peruana, BA represents a chronic, persistent infection, even in severely immunocompromised patients with AIDS. In one study, the median time from onset of BA symptoms to time of diagnosis was approximately 8 to >12 months (34). During this time, patients experienced intermittent fevers and gradual increase in the size and/or number of BA lesions. Although relapse is common in immunocompetent patients after antibiotic treatment, relapse of BA (often at a different site or with bacteremia) is even more common in immunocompromised patients. It is frequently necessary to administer lifelong suppressive antibiotics to these patients to prevent subsequent relapse of *Bartonella* infection. In recent years, immune reconstitution with highly active anti-retroviral therapy has led to a marked decrease in the incidence of BA in HIV-infected patients.

The lesions of cutaneous BA appear quite similar to those of verruga peruana histopathologically, with lobular vascular proliferation of vessels. The cellular infiltrate is somewhat different in BA than in verruga peruana: more neutrophils and leukocytoclastic debris are visualized in BA lesions, with fewer plasma cells and lymphocytes. Additionally, an increased number of bacteria are present in BA lesions, and these bacteria often form microcolonies in the tissue. The bacilli in BA lesions are usually extracellular, as noted in lesions of verruga peruana (45).

Domestic Feline and Canine *Bartonella* Infection

In 1994, *B. henselae* bacteremia was identified in the seven pet cats (*Felis domesticus*) of four patients who developed BA due to *B. henselae* (32). In this study, feline *B. henselae* bacteremia was found to be very common in the San Francisco Bay area (41% of cats), and persistent bacteremia of >1 year was evident (32). Subsequently, at least four *Bartonella* species or subspecies have been isolated from domestic cats, the most common being two subspecies of *B. henselae* (referred to as *B. henselae* type I and type II) and the species *B. clarridgeiae*. The prevalence of infection with the two species differs according to the geographic region: a significantly greater proportion of cats in Europe are infected with *B. clarridgeiae* than in the United States. In the Netherlands, 36% of bacteremic cats were infected with *B. clarridgeiae*, 28% were infected with *B. henselae* type I, and 56% were infected with *B. henselae* type II (6). In France, 30% of the cats with *Bartonella* bacteremia had positive cultures for *B. clarridgeiae*, 34% were positive for *B. henselae* type I, and 36% were positive for *B. henselae* type II (25). However, in the United States, the prevalence of *B. clarridgeiae* bacteremia is probably about 10% or less (36, 41). The subspecies *B.*

henselae type I and type II were only very recently described, and most studies have not identified *B. henselae* isolates to the subspecies level; however, prevalence also apparently varies among geographic regions (6, 14, 25, 61; A. N. Gurfield, H. J. Boulouis, B. B. Chomel, R. Heller, R. W. Kasten, K. Yamamoto, and Y. Piemont, presented at the 8th Symposium of the International Society for Veterinary Epidemiology and Economics, Paris, France, 1997). Inoculation of cats with *B. quintana* did not result in bacteremia (53), providing evidence for a host species specificity for bartonellae.

Simultaneous feline infection with different *Bartonella* species and subspecies also occurs: coinfection with *B. henselae* and *B. clarridgeiae* has been reported (6; Gurfield et al., 8th Symp. Int. Soc. Vet. Epidemiol. Econ.), and coinfection with type I and type II *B. henselae* has been identified in several cats (Gurfield et al., 8th Symp. Int. Soc. Vet. Epidemiol. Econ.). Additionally, Yamamoto et al. (74) demonstrated that cats experimentally infected with *B. henselae* type II could subsequently be infected with heterologous strains (*B. henselae* type I or *B. clarridgeiae*) but not with a homologous strain of *B. henselae* type II. In addition to these two types of *B. henselae*, multiple subtypes of the species have been identified by enterobacterial repetitive intergenic consensus sequence and repetitive extragenic palindromic sequence PCR (57), and it appears that there is substantial diversity among *B. henselae* isolates, unlike *B. quintana*, for which only two groups have been demonstrated (58) by the most sensitive *Bartonella* typing method identified to date, pulsed-field gel electrophoresis.

Although most studies of naturally and experimentally infected cats identified no symptoms accompanying *B. henselae* inoculation and bacteremia, in one study, experimental intravenous infection was associated with fever, anorexia, generalized lymphadenopathy, and granulomatous lesions in different tissues of the experimentally infected cats (24). Vertical transmission was not observed in domestic cats experimentally infected with *B. henselae* (1), leading to the hypothesis that arthropod vectors might be involved in cat-to-cat transmission of *B. henselae* (see "Vectors" below). In several studies, bacteremia recurred or failed to resolve in cats treated with antibiotics to which *B. henselae* showed in vitro susceptibility (41, 53), as has been observed for humans. Finally, vascular proliferative lesions have not been identified in immunocompromised cats with feline immunodeficiency virus or feline leukemia virus or in any mammalian reservoir species except immunocompromised humans.

Canine infection with *Bartonella vinsonii* subsp. *berkhoffii* was first reported by Kordick et al. (42). The prevalence of this subspecies in domestic and wild dogs is not known, but persistent, relapsing infection with *B. vinsonii* subsp. *berkhoffii* was documented in one pet dog over a 15-month period (39). Intradermal inoculation of dogs with a cat-specific species of *Bartonella*, *B. henselae*, did not result in bacteremia, but seroconversion did occur (12). *B. vinsonii* subsp. *berkhoffii* has never been isolated from cats, again underscoring the specificity of *Bartonella* species to infect and persist almost exclusively in their cognate hosts.

Rodent and Other Wildlife Mammalian *Bartonella* Infections

Wild rodents apparently constitute a tremendous reservoir of *Bartonella* species. A prevalence study of *Bartonella* (formerly *Grahamella*) species in small woodland mammals in the United Kingdom found that 62% of these mammals (representing different species of voles and mice) were bacteremic with one of three different, new species: *Bartonella grahamii*, *Bartonella taylorii*, and *Bartonella doshiae* (7). A larger study in the southeastern United States found *Bartonella* spp. bacteremia in 42% of rodents tested (44). The diversity of these rodent isolates was striking, and the isolates could be divided into four phylogenetic groups of 14 genotypic variants based on citrate synthase gene sequences. Unlike the felines, where the majority develop *Bartonella* antibodies (13), 98.5% of rodents did not have detectable *Bartonella* antibodies (44). Also unlike the feline res-

ervoir, *Bartonella* spp. could be isolated from embryos and neonatal mice or rats, indicating potential vertical transmission of *Bartonella* in these rodents (43). Several wild rat species are also apparently infected with *Bartonella* species, and a new species, *Bartonella tribocorum*, was isolated recently from *Rattus norvegicus* in rural France (27).

In addition to the domestic cat, wild felids also serve as a reservoir for *Bartonella* species. In a recent study by Yamamoto et al. (75), 53% of California wild bobcats (*Felis rufus*) were seropositive for *B. henselae*, as were 35% of California mountain lions (*Felis concolor*). Antibodies were also found in 30% of the captive felids in California zoos, and seroprevalence was more than twofold greater for cats of the *Felis* genus compared with the genus *Panthera* (lions, tigers, leopards, and jaguars) (75). *F. domesticus* (the domestic cat) could be productively infected with the mountain lion strain of *Bartonella* and could subsequently be infected with *B. henselae* but not with the same (as yet unnamed) mountain lion strain (74). Thus, these *Bartonella* species infecting wild and domestic felids would appear to be closely related but distinct, but little is known about these newest wild-felid-specific species. One additional new *Bartonella* species, *Bartonella alsatica*, was described in 1999. This species was isolated from the blood of 30% of the wild rabbits tested in France (26), further broadening the range of reservoir animals infected with *Bartonella* species.

Vectors

For many years, arthropods have been known to be competent vectors for two species, *B. quintana* and *B. bacilliformis* (Fig. 2). The arthropod vector for *B. bacilliformis* is *Lutzomyia*, the sandfly, and human infection with *B. bacilliformis* is restricted to the geographic distribution of the sandfly, between the altitudes of 2,500 and 8,000 feet in the Peruvian Andes (70). For *B. quintana*, intensive investigation during and after World War I identified the human body louse, *Pediculus humanus*, as the arthropod vector responsible for transmission

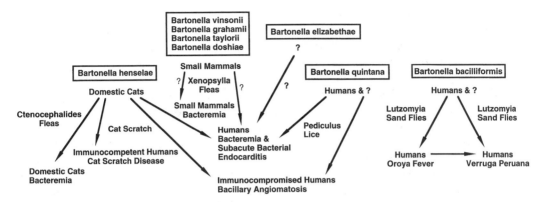

FIGURE 2 Reservoirs, vectors, and mammalian infections associated with *Bartonella* species. The *Bartonella* species are shown in boxes, with the respective mammalian reservoir just below each box. The mode of transmission (arthropod vector or cat scratch) is shown next to each arrow, and the resultant mammalian infection is shown at the end of each arrow. (Reprinted from reference 31 with permission of the publisher.)

(65). The body louse has been implicated as the vector of *B. quintana* in contemporary times as well: patients with BA due to *B. quintana*, but not *B. henselae*, were significantly more likely to have had infestation with body lice and to be homeless than their matched controls (36). Similarly, in Russia, *B. quintana* DNA could be detected in body lice collected from homeless persons (59).

The domestic cat has also been known for decades to be the principal vector for transmission of the agent of CSD to humans (49). However, when a large proportion of domestic cats was found to be bacteremic with *B. henselae*, the mechanism by which cats become infected was unknown but was suspected to be the cat flea, *Ctenocephalides felis*. Initial experiments found that *B. henselae* could be cultured from the fleas combed from bacteremic cats (32) and that *Bartonella* DNA could be amplified from 34% of fleas combed from infected cats and tested individually by PCR (15). In addition, the highest seroprevalence of *B. henselae* in cats was found to be positively correlated with climates most favorable to flea survival in various regions of the United States (30). In 1996, the cat flea was identified as an extremely efficient vector of *B. henselae* from cat to cat (15). As few as five fleas removed from bacteremic cats and placed on specific-

pathogen-free (SPF) kittens could infect the recipient (15). Another flea species, *Xenopsylla cheopis*, has been implicated as the vector of *Bartonella* (formerly *Grahamella*) species among the wild rodent population (68). Finally, ticks are another potential vector for transmission of *Bartonella* infections to humans and wildlife. In the United States, two patients developed bacteremia with *B. henselae* after sustaining tick bites (48). In the Netherlands, Schouls et al. found that *Bartonella* DNA could be detected in at least 60% of *Ixodes ricinus* ticks removed from roe deer (62).

At present, very little is known about the mechanism of transmission of *B. bacilliformis* from sandfly to human. The bacterium has been identified in the mouthparts and intestinal tracts of sandflies (69). In contrast, studies have shown that *B. quintana* (29) and *B. henselae* (28) multiply extracellularly in the lumen of the gut of their respective invertebrate hosts. Transmission of *B. quintana*, *B. henselae*, and wildlife-specific *Bartonella* species probably involves mechanical inoculation of the mammal with feces excreted from the infected arthropod. For instance, the body louse defecates at the bite site while taking a blood meal, and the human unwittingly self-inoculates the *B. quintana*-infected louse feces into the bite wound while scratching the bite (65). Similarly, feces of fleas fed on cats bacteremic with *B. henselae* are infectious when injected into uninfected cats (22), and feces of *Bartonella*-infected *X. cheopis* were infectious to voles (68).

In summary, in the past 12 years, the human syndromes associated with *Bartonella* species infection (especially in the immunocompromised patient) have been elucidated. In the past 5 years the feline and canine reservoirs for *Bartonella* species have been identified, and in the past 2 years there has been a tremendous increase in our knowledge about the number and heterogeneity of *Bartonella* species and subspecies that infect a large number of wild and domestic mammalian reservoir species, transmitted via a number of different arthropod vector species (Fig. 2). The clinical and epidemiological data gathered thus far provide compelling evidence that *Bartonella* species have a unique ability to persist in their respective mammalian host (and probably in invertebrate arthropod host) species.

MECHANISM OF PERSISTENCE AND POTENTIAL AREAS OF INVESTIGATION

Although the first two *Bartonella* species were described and isolated decades ago, very few studies of *Bartonella* pathogenesis have been published. From the clinical and epidemiological data described above, several common themes emerge for the bartonellae and their interactions with mammals and arthropods. First, bartonellae are hemin dependent and have adapted to persist in alternating niches that provide the bacilli with constant access to blood and hemin in the bloodstreams of mammals or the guts of hematophagous arthropods. Second, bartonellae are able to adapt to survive in these niches for prolonged periods of time, even for the life span of the animal or arthropod. Third, these bacteria are able to adapt to evade the mammalian host immune system and to multiply to very high numbers in the bloodstream while eliciting minimal symptoms or pathogenic response. Fourth, bartonellae have adapted to infect many different mammalian species, and each mammalian reservoir species

has one *Bartonella* species or a cluster of closely related species that can establish a productive and persistent infection. Of the mammalian species tested to date, it is evident that a large proportion, usually the majority, of wild mammals are infected with bartonellae and that very few animals have overt illness; some animals resolve the infection. Fifth, relapse of *Bartonella* infection occurs frequently, but reinfection, especially with very closely related species or subspecies, can occur, as can simultaneous coinfection with at least two species or subspecies of *Bartonella*. The bartonellae persist in the arthropod vectors as well and do not appear to cause lethal sequelae in these invertebrate hosts, unlike other bacilli (e.g., *Yersinia pestis*, which causes lethal infection in the flea *X. cheopis*). Virtually nothing is known about the mechanism of persistence of bartonellae in these host reservoir and vector species. This ability of bartonellae to persist and relapse is likely multifactorial, and there are a number of diverse processes that could be involved.

Lack of Elimination of *Bartonella* Infection by the Immune System

Humoral immune response does not appear to eliminate the infecting *Bartonella* species from the cognate host. In humans and cats, *B. quintana* and *B. henselae* bacteremia, respectively, persist despite the development of a humoral antibody response (13). In heterologous infections, however, e.g., humans or dogs infected with the feline *B. henselae*, bacteremia rarely occurs, an antibody response is elicited (16), and the bartonellae are usually eliminated without antibiotic therapy. Other reservoir hosts, e.g., rodents, do not appear to develop an antibody response to the infecting *Bartonella* species. The mechanism by which bartonellae circumvent the host immune response is not known.

Although some bacteria evade complement activation and induction of phagocyte-mediated killing by production of a capsule or S-layer, neither of these structures has been identified for *Bartonella* species. A study of the human humoral immune response to *B.*

henselae revealed that the organism was very sensitive to serum-mediated cytolysis (56). Sera from patients without *Bartonella* infection had a bactericidal effect on *B. henselae*, and heat-inactivated sera were not bactericidal, suggesting a complement-mediated serum sensitivity. This bactericidal activity was not affected by the addition of *B. henselae*-specific antibodies. Although the *B. henselae* strain tested was serum sensitive with human sera, it would be instructive to investigate the serum sensitivity and resistance of other *B. henselae* blood isolates, as well as *B. quintana* strains. The authors of this study also found that phagocytosis and generation of reactive oxygen products were significantly enhanced in the presence of *B. henselae*-specific antibodies, although the leukocytes from patients with AIDS did not phagocytize the bacilli as efficiently as polymorphonuclear leukocytes from immunocompetent donors or asymptomatic HIV-infected patients (56).

Extensive bleb-like structures of the outer membrane have been described for *B. quintana* (9). Blebbing of the outer membrane occurs with some bacteria, e.g., *Borrelia burgdorferi*, releasing vesicles of surface antigens, such as OspA and OspB. This has been proposed as a potential "decoy" strategy to bind host antibodies directed against these surface antigens in blebs, conferring some protection on the bacterium (60). Another potential mechanism of immune evasion utilized by some bacteria is the binding of host proteins, such as iron-binding proteins, to the bacterial surface; binding of proteins such as transferrin would be an attractive strategy for a bacterium that resides in the mammalian bloodstream.

Alteration of T-cell-mediated response has also been implicated in persistent bacterial infections. Induction of CD4-CD8 inversion and immunosuppression has been reported in patients infected with *B. bacilliformis*; these patients often succumb to intercurrent infection with intracellular pathogens, especially *Salmonella* spp. and *M. tuberculosis*. A similar phenomenon has not been reported for human infections with other *Bartonella* species. Guptill et al. (24) investigated whether an immunosup-

pressive effect could be identified in SPF kittens experimentally infected with *B. henselae*. They found that CD4/CD8 ratios for *B. henselae*-infected kittens were similar to those reported for SPF kittens without infection. They also found no change in blastogenic responses to concanavalin A and pokeweed mitogen prior to and after experimental infection of SPF kittens with *B. henselae*. Cells secreting antibodies specific for *B. henselae* were identified in the bone marrow, spleen, and peripheral lymph nodes of infected but not control kittens. They concluded that there was no evidence for suppression of T-cell-mediated immune response in association with *B. henselae* infection (24).

Another striking feature is the very high level of *Bartonella* bacteremia (10^3 to 10^6 CFU per milliliter of blood) found in mammals, e.g., humans and cats, in the absence of a sepsis syndrome. This may be due to the ability of bartonellae to suppress the host cytokine response to lipopolysaccharide (LPS) or to block the activity of one or more components of this response. Alternatively, production of an LPS molecule that fails to induce the host immune response could be a successful strategy for achieving persistence of bartonellae in the bloodstream. Another member of the alpha proteobacteria, *Rhodobacter*, synthesizes a nontoxic LPS that incorporates both short and unsaturated fatty acids; this LPS can even antagonize the adverse effects of *Escherichia coli* LPS (23). It will be important to characterize the LPS of bartonellae and to investigate the mammalian cytokine response to *Bartonella* LPS in vivo.

Phenotypic (Antigenic and Phase) Variation

Antigenic variation most commonly involves bacterial surface structures, including pili, flagella, LPS, capsules, S-layers and outer membrane proteins (OMP) (21). Antigenic variation is a common strategy associated with relapsing bacteremia and has been employed by a number of bacterial species. *B. henselae* and *B. quintana* do not have flagella, the pilin gene has not yet been identified for bartonellae (and *B. quintana* has few pili), and no *Bartonella* species has been reported to have a capsule or S-layer; thus, initial evaluation of antigenic variation has been directed toward OMP. The relapsing bacteremia documented with *B. bacilliformis* and *B. quintana* in humans, and *B. henselae* in cats, is similar to that of *Borrelia hermsii*. In this spirochete, variable OMP genes (*vmp*) recombine to generate recombinant OMP of different molecular masses that can be readily visualized by gel electrophoresis (2). For *Bartonella* species, only a few OMP have been identified, and no antigenically variant OMP have been reported. Additionally, gel electrophoresis failed to reveal any evidence of size shifts in the protein profile of sequential isolates from *B. henselae*-infected cats (40).

Variation of pilus expression also has been noted for some *Bartonella* species, but whether this represents true phase variation (reversible gain or loss of a defined structure [55]) is not clear because only in vitro rough-to-smooth variation has been reported. *B. henselae* strains, when first isolated from blood or tissue, have a rough phenotype that correlates with the presence of a large number of pili. With successive passaging on agar, the pili, and the rough phenotype, are gradually lost (3). Whether there is phase variation in vivo and whether it might contribute to persistence is not known.

Some of the initial clinical observations provided support for variation of the *Bartonella* phenotype in vivo compared with that in vitro. A marked discrepancy between the in vivo and in vitro antibiotic susceptibilities was noted, particularly for the cell–wall-active antibiotics (35). In vitro, there is usually susceptibility to penicillin, yet treatment of patients with BA lesions with penicillin does not result in improvement, and we have observed the formation of new lesions during penicillin treatment of one patient (33). Additionally, isolation of *B. henselae* from the blood of patients (a minimum of 8 days for appearance of colonies) is more difficult than isolation from the blood of cats (a minimum of 3 days) (36), and cocultivation of human blood or tissue with eukaryotic

cells facilitates the isolation of *Bartonella* species from humans (34). Finally, generation of penicillin-resistant L forms of *B. bacilliformis* in vitro was described briefly in one publication, although further documentation was not provided (69). Unusually shaped bacterial forms have also been observed in association with RBC in blood smears from humans infected with *B. bacilliformis* (69). These observations may indicate that there are changes in cell wall structure in vivo (that may or may not be reversible) that eliminate or alter the target site for cell-wall-active antibiotics. These altered forms may have a unique ability to persist, as has been proposed for L forms (19). Alternatively, the lack of response to antibiotics may reflect inaccessibility of the bartonellae, e.g., sequestration and protection from antibiotics (see below).

The above-mentioned examples represent only preliminary investigations, and additional *Bartonella* isolates from different animal reservoirs should be evaluated for temporal changes in cell wall and cell surface structures. Evaluation of antigenic variation will require the development of animal models and experimental inoculation with well-characterized *Bartonella* strains. Identification of the genes for *Bartonella* cell surface proteins, including flagella, OMP, and pili, and characterization of these proteins will also be essential for understanding the mechanisms by which *Bartonella* species cause persistent infection.

Sequestration in a Sanctuary Site

Persistence of *Bartonella* may be a consequence of sequestration in a site protected from the immune system. Although there is no evidence that bartonellae survive intracellularly in professional phagocytes, two sites of sequestration have been suggested on the basis of intimate associations visualized microscopically: the RBC and the endothelial cell (EC). For *B. bacilliformis*, a specific, epicellular association between the bacterium and RBC can be observed by scanning electron microscopy (4). Deformation of the RBC membrane can be visualized, and a factor has been purified from culture supernatant that deforms RBC (73). In acute, severe cases of bartonellosis, more than 90% of the cells become infected with ≥6 bacilli. These forms then gradually undergo morphological changes, decrease in number, and disappear (69). In more chronically infected mammals, such as rodents, the epicellular association of *Bartonella* species with RBC is more persistent, but for any given RBC it must presumably be limited by the lifespan of the RBC.

For *B. henselae*, *B. quintana*, and *Bartonella* species infecting rodents, the bacilli also apparently have an epicellular association with RBC, but whether the deformation seen with *B. bacilliformis* occurs with these other *Bartonella* species has not been established. Whether a significant percentage of bacilli are actually intracellularly localized is controversial. Although one study found intracellular *B. henselae* (38), another did not identify any intraerythrocytic *B. henselae* in experimentally infected cats (24). This probably reflects the difficulty in assessing intracellular versus epicellular bacilli using light or transmission electron microscopy. A gentamicin protection assay or confocal microscopy would probably be more sensitive methods to determine the proportion of viable bacilli residing intracellularly in RBC. The exact nature of this association between bacilli and RBC and the role of this interaction in persistent infection are not known but are currently under investigation.

Present data are also inconclusive as to whether *Bartonella* bacilli have a relevant intracellular phase in ECs in vivo. Very few, if any, *B. henselae* bacilli can be visualized in the lymph nodes of patients with CSD. In contrast, numerous organisms (often forming microcolonies in the tissue) can be seen in BA lesions of patients with AIDS, and the majority of these *B. henselae* or *B. quintana* bacilli appear to be extracellularly localized in vivo. Occasional intracellular organisms can be visualized in BA lesions, but these bacilli often appear to be in a degenerating state. The verruga peruana lesions associated with *B. bacilliformis* have fewer bacilli present than in BA lesions, and there are clumps of bacilli known as Rocha-Lima bodies

(45). These bodies appear to be clumps of bacilli that may lie within phagolysosomes or perhaps labyrinthine cisterns formed from invaginated cell membrane (45). The metabolic state of bacilli in the Rocha-Lima bodies and their role in the pathogenesis and persistence of *Bartonella* in infected humans are not clear.

In vitro studies, however, have identified unique intracellular interactions between *Bartonella* bacilli and several eukaryotic cell lines. Batterman et al. (3) used a gentamicin protection assay to demonstrate that a highly piliated *B. henselae* strain entered an epithelial cell line (HEp-2) two or three log units more frequently than *E. coli*. The type strain of *B. quintana* did not adhere to or invade this cell line (3). Broqui and Raoult (9) found that *B. quintana* could invade an EC line (ECV), and Dehio et al. (18) observed invasion of another EC line (HuVEC) by *B. henselae* in vitro. In the last two studies, the bacteria were centrifuged against the ECs, and uptake of bacteria, either singly or in clumps, was observed to begin within hours. Dehio et al. (18) noted a second mechanism of invasion: the EC appeared to direct bacterial aggregation on the cell surface with subsequent engulfment and internalization of the bacterial aggregate, termed the invasome. This process evolved over 24 h and was cytochalasin D dependent. The role of this process in vivo and in the pathogenesis of BA lesions is not clear at present, but even if only a small percentage of bacteria establish intracellular infection, this could serve as a site of sequestration and a mechanism for persistence of bartonellae.

QUESTIONS FOR FURTHER STUDY

The study of *Bartonella* pathogenesis is still in its infancy, and although there is a tractable system for genetic manipulation (via conjugation [17, 47]), it will be essential to identify and characterize virulence factors. To date, no plasmids, transposable elements, pathogenicity islands, or active transducing phage have been identified or associated with virulence genes. Nothing is known about the sensing or regulatory functions in bartonellae, but it is obvious that an organism occupying two such diverse niches, arthropod gut and mammalian bloodstream, must have an efficient sensing and global regulatory system. The availability of the *B. henselae* genome sequence in the near future (S. G. E. Andersson, C. M. U. Alsmark, B. Canbäck, and C. G. Kurland, presented at the First International Conference on *Bartonella* as Emerging Pathogens, Tübingen, Germany, 1999) will greatly enhance these studies, and the next phase of comparative genomics and microarrays will provide further insight into the mechanisms of pathogenesis and persistence of *Bartonella* bacilli.

ACKNOWLEDGMENT

This work was supported by NIH grant R01 AI 43703.

REFERENCES

1. **Abbott, R. C., B. B. Chomel, R. W. Kasten, K. A. Floyd-Hawkins, Y. Kikuchi, J. E. Koehler, and N. C. Pedersen.** 1997. Experimental and natural infection of cats with *Bartonella henselae*. *Comp. Immunol. Microbiol. Infect. Dis.* **20:** 41–51.

2. **Barbour, A. G.** 1993. Linear DNA of *Borrelia* species and antigenic variation. *Trends Microbiol.* **1:**236–239.

3. **Batterman, H. J., J. A. Peek, J. S. Loutit, S. Falkow, and L. S. Tompkins.** 1995. *Bartonella henselae* and *Bartonella quintana* adherence to and entry into cultured human epithelial cells. *Infect. Immun.* **63:**4553–4556.

4. **Benson, L. A., S. Kar, G. McLaughlin, and G. M. Ihler.** 1986. Entry of *Bartonella bacilliformis* into erythrocytes. *Infect. Immun.* **54:**347–353.

5. **Bergmans, A. M., J. W. Groothedde, J. F. Schellekens, J. D. van Embden, J. M. Ossewaarde, and L. M. Schouls.** 1995. Etiology of cat scratch disease: comparison of polymerase chain reaction detection of *Bartonella* (formerly *Rochalimaea*) and *Afipia felis* DNA with serology and skin tests. *J. Infect. Dis.* **171:**916–923.

6. **Bergmans, A. M. C., C. M. A. de Jong, G. van Amerongen, C. S. Schot, and L. M. Schouls.** 1997. Prevalence of *Bartonella* species in domestic cats in the Netherlands. *J. Clin. Microbiol.* **35:**2256–2261.

7. **Birtles, R. J., T. G. Harrison, and D. H. Molyneux.** 1994. *Grahamella* in small woodland mammals in the U.K.: isolation, prevalence and host specificity. *Ann. Trop. Med. Parasitol.* **88:** 317–327.

8. **Brenner, D. J., S. P. O'Connor, H. H. Winkler, and A. G. Steigerwalt.** 1993. Proposals to unify the genera *Bartonella* and *Rochalimaea*, with descriptions of *Bartonella quintana* comb. nov., *Bartonella vinsonii* comb. nov., *Bartonella henselae* comb. nov., and *Bartonella elizabethae* comb. nov., and to remove the family *Bartonellaceae* from the order *Rickettsiales*. *Int. J. Syst. Bacteriol.* **43:** 777–786.

9. **Broqui, P., and D. Raoult.** 1996. *Bartonella quintana* invades and multiplies within endothelial cells in vitro and in vivo and forms intracellular blebs. *Res. Microbiol.* **147:**719–731.

10. **Brouqui, P., B. Lascola, V. Roux, and D. Raoult.** 1999. Chronic *Bartonella quintana* bacteremia in homeless patients. *N. Engl. J. Med.* **340:** 184–189.

11. **Caceres-Rios, H., J. Rodriguez-Tafur, F. Bravo-Puccio, C. Maguina-Vargas, C. S. Diaz, D. C. Ramos, and R. Patarca.** 1995. Verruga peruana: an infectious endemic angiomatosis. *Crit. Rev. Oncog.* **6:**47–56.

12. **Chomel, B. B.** 1996. Cat-scratch disease and bacillary angiomatosis. *Rev. Sci. Tech.* **15:** 1061–1073.

13. **Chomel, B. B., R. C. Abbott, R. W. Kasten, K. A. Floyd-Hawkins, P. H. Kass, C. A. Glaser, N. C. Pedersen, and J. E. Koehler.** 1995. *Bartonella henselae* prevalence in domestic cats in California: risk factors and association between bacteremia and antibody titers. *J. Clin. Microbiol.* **33:**2445–2450.

14. **Chomel, B. B., E. T. Carlos, R. W. Kasten, K. Yamamoto, C.-C. Chang, R. S. Carlos, M. V. Abenes, and C. M. Pajares.** 1999. *Bartonella henselae* and *Bartonella clarridgeiae* infection in domestic cats from the Philippines. *Am. J. Trop. Med. Hyg.* **60:**593–597.

15. **Chomel, B. B., R. W. Kasten, K. Floyd-Hawkins, B. Chi, K. Yamamoto, J. Roberts-Wilson, A. N. Gurfield, R. C. Abbott, N. C. Pedersen, and J. E. Koehler.** 1996. Experimental transmission of *Bartonella henselae* by the cat flea. *J. Clin. Microbiol.* **34:**1952–1956.

16. **Dalton, M. J., L. E. Robinson, J. Cooper, R. L. Regnery, J. G. Olson, and J. E. Childs.** 1995. Use of *Bartonella* antigens for serologic diagnosis of cat-scratch disease at a national referral center. *Arch. Intern. Med.* **155:**1670–1676.

17. **Dehio, C., and M. Meyer.** 1997. Maintenance of broad-host-range incompatibility group P and group Q plasmids and transposition of Tn5 in *Bartonella henselae* following conjugal plasmid transfer from *Escherichia coli*. *J. Bacteriol.* **179:**538–540.

18. **Dehio, C., M. Meyer, J. Berger, H. Schwarz, and C. Lanz.** 1997. Interaction of *Bartonella henselae* with endothelial cells results in bacterial

aggregation on the cell surface and the subsequent engulfment and internalisation of the bacterial aggregate by a unique structure, the invasome. *J. Cell Sci.* **110:**2141–2154.

19. **Domingue, G. J., Sr., and H. B. Woody.** 1997. Bacterial persistence and expression of disease. *Clin. Microbiol. Rev.* **10:**320–344.

20. **Drancourt, M., J. L. Mainardi, P. Brouqui, F. Vandenesch, A. Carta, F. Lehnert, J. Etienne, F. Goldstein, J. Acar, and D. Raoult.** 1995. *Bartonella* (*Rochalimaea*) *quintana* endocarditis in three homeless men. *N. Engl. J. Med.* **332:**419–423.

21. **Finlay, B. B., and S. Falkow.** 1997. Common themes in microbial pathogenicity revisited. *Microb. Mol. Biol. Rev.* **61:**136–169.

22. **Foil, L., E. Andress, R. L. Freeland, A. F. Roy, R. Rutledge, P. C. Triche, and K. L. O'Reilly.** 1998. Experimental infection of domestic cats with *Bartonella henselae* by inoculation of *Ctenocephalides felis* (Siphonaptera: Pulicidae) feces. *J. Med. Entomol.* **35:**625–628.

23. **Golenbock, D. T., R. Y. Hampton, N. Qureshi, K. Takayama, and C. R. H. Raetz.** 1991. Lipid A-like molecules that antagonize the effects of endotoxins on human monocytes. *J. Biol. Chem.* **226:**19490–19498.

24. **Guptill, L., L. Slater, C.-C. Wu, T.-L. Lin, L. T. Glickman, D. F. Welch, and H. Hogen-Esch.** 1997. Experimental infection of young specific pathogen-free cats with *Bartonella henselae*. *J. Infect. Dis.* **176:**206–216.

25. **Heller, R., M. Artois, V. Xemar, D. De Briel, H. Gehin, B. Jaulhac, H. Monteil, and Y. Piemont.** 1997. Prevalence of *Bartonella henselae* and *Bartonella clarridgeiae* in stray cats. *J. Clin. Microbiol.* **35:**1327–1331.

26. **Heller, R., M. Kubina, P. Mariet, P. Riegel, G. Delacour, C. Dehio, F. Lamarque, R. Kasten, H.-J. Boulouis, H. Monteil, B. Chomel, and Y. Piemont.** 1999. *Bartonella alsatica* sp. nov., a new *Bartonella* species isolated from the blood of wild rabbits. *Int. J. Syst. Bacteriol.* **49:** 283–288.

27. **Heller, R., P. Riegel, Y. Hansmann, G. Delacour, D. Bermond, C. Dehio, F. Lamarque, H. Monteil, B. Chomel, and Y. Piemont.** 1998. *Bartonella tribocorum* sp. nov., a new *Bartonella* species isolated from the blood of wild rats. *Int. J. Syst. Bacteriol.* **48:**1333–1339.

28. **Higgins, J. A., S. Radulovic, D. C. Jaworski, and A. F. Azad.** 1996. Acquisition of the cat scratch disease agent *Bartonella henselae* by cat fleas (Siphonaptera: Pulicidae). *J. Med. Entomol.* **33:** 490–495.

29. **Ito, S., and J. W. Vinson.** 1965. Fine structure of *Rickettsia quintana* cultivated in vitro and in the louse. *J. Bacteriol.* **89:**481–495.

30. **Jameson, P., C. Greene, R. Regnery, M. Dryden, A. Marks, J. Brown, J. Cooper, B. Glaus, and R. Greene.** 1995. Prevalence of *Bartonella henselae* antibodies in pet cats throughout regions of North America. *J. Infect. Dis.* **172:** 1145–1149.

31. **Koehler, J. E.** 1998. *Bartonella:* an emerging human pathogen, p. 147–163. *In* W. M. Scheld, D. Armstrong, and J. M. Hughes (ed.), *Emerging Infections I.* ASM Press, Washington, D.C.

32. **Koehler, J. E., C. A. Glaser, and J. W. Tappero.** 1994. *Rochalimaea henselae* infection. A new zoonosis with the domestic cat as reservoir. *JAMA* **271:**531–535.

33. **Koehler, J. E., P. E. LeBoit, B. M. Egbert, and T. G. Berger.** 1988. Cutaneous vascular lesions and disseminated cat-scratch disease in patients with the acquired immunodeficiency syndrome (AIDS)-related complex. *Ann. Intern. Med.* **109:**449–455.

34. **Koehler, J. E., F. D. Quinn, T. G. Berger, P. E. LeBoit, and J. W. Tappero.** 1992. Isolation of *Rochalimaea* species from cutaneous and osseous lesions of bacillary angiomatosis. *N. Engl. J. Med.* **327:**1625–1631.

35. **Koehler, J. E., and D. A. Relman.** 1999. *Bartonella* species, p. 578–583. *In* V. L. Yu, T. C. Merigan, Jr., and S. L. Barriere (ed.), *Antimicrobial Therapy and Vaccines.* Williams and Wilkins, Baltimore, Md.

36. **Koehler, J. E., M. A. Sanchez, C. S. Garrido, M. J. Whitfeld, F. M. Chen, T. G. Berger, M. C. Rodriguez-Barradas, P. E. LeBoit, and J. W. Tappero.** 1997. Molecular epidemiology of *Bartonella* infections in patients with bacillary angiomatosis-peliosis. *N. Engl. J. Med.* **337:** 1876–1883.

37. **Koehler, J. E., and J. W. Tappero.** 1993. Bacillary angiomatosis and bacillary peliosis in patients infected with human immunodeficiency virus. *Clin. Infect. Dis.* **17:**612–624.

38. **Kordick, D. L., and E. B. Breitschwerdt.** 1995. Intraerythrocytic presence of *Bartonella henselae*. *J. Clin. Microbiol.* **33:**1655–1656.

39. **Kordick, D. L., and E. B. Breitschwerdt.** 1998. Persistent infection of pets with three *Bartonella* species. *Emerg. Infect. Dis.* **4:**325–328.

40. **Kordick, D. L., T. T. Brown, K. Shin, and E. B. Breitschwerdt.** 1999. Clinical and pathologic evaluation of chronic *Bartonella henselae* or *Bartonella clarridgeiae* infection in cats. *J. Clin. Microbiol.* **37:**1536–1547.

41. **Kordick, D. L., M. G. Papich, and E. B. Breitschwerdt.** 1997. Efficacy of enrofloxacin or doxycycline for treatment of *Bartonella henselae* or

Bartonella clarridgeiae infection in cats. *Antimicrob. Agents Chemother.* **41:**2448–2455.

42. **Kordick, D. L., B. Swaminathan, C. E. Greene, K. H. Wilson, A. M. Whitney, S. O'Connor, D. G. Hollis, G. M. Matar, A. G. Steigerwalt, G. B. Malcolm, P. S. Hayes, T. L. Hadfield, E. B. Breitschwerdt, and D. J. Brenner.** 1996. *Bartonella vinsonii* subsp. *berkhoffii* subsp. nov., isolated from dogs; *Bartonella vinsonii* subsp. *vinsonii*; and emended description of *Bartonella vinsonii*. *Int. J. Syst. Bacteriol.* **46:**704–709.

43. **Kosoy, M. Y., R. L. Regnery, O. I. Kosaya, D. C. Jones, E. L. Marston, and J. E. Childs.** 1998. Isolation of *Bartonella* spp. from embryos and neonates of naturally infected rodents. *J. Wildl. Dis.* **34:**305–309.

44. **Kosoy, M. Y., R. L. Regnery, T. Tzianabos, E. L. Marston, D. C. Jones, D. Green, G. O. Maupin, J. G. Olson, and J. E. Childs.** 1997. Distribution, diversity, and host specificity of *Bartonella* in rodents from the southeastern United States. *Am. J. Trop. Med. Hyg.* **57:**578–588.

45. **LeBoit, P. E.** 1997. Bacillary angiomatosis, p. 407–415. *In* D. H. Connor, F. W. Chandler, H. J. Manz, D. A. Schwartz, and E. E. Lack (ed.), *Pathology of Infectious Diseases*, vol. 1. Appleton and Lange, Stamford, Conn.

46. **LeBoit, P. E., T. G. Berger, B. M. Egbert, J. H. Beckstead, T. S. B. Yen, and M. H. Stoler.** 1989. Bacillary angiomatosis: the histopathology and differential diagnosis of a pseudoneoplastic infection in patients with human immunodeficiency virus disease. *Am. J. Surg. Pathol.* **13:**909–920.

47. **Lee, A. K., and S. Falkow.** 1998. Constitutive and inducible green fluorescent protein expression in *Bartonella henselae*. *Infect. Immun.* **66:**3964–3967.

48. **Lucey, D., M. J. Dolan, C. W. Moss, M. Garcia, D. G. Hollis, S. Wegner, G. Morgan, R. Almeida, D. Leong, K. S. Greisen, et al.** 1992. Relapsing illness due to *Rochalimaea henselae* in immunocompetent hosts: implication for therapy and new epidemiological associations. *Clin. Infect. Dis.* **14:**683–688.

49. **Margileth, A. M.** 1993. Cat scratch disease. *Adv. Pediatr. Infect. Dis.* **8:**1–21.

50. **Montgomery, E. A., and F. U. Garcia.** 1997. Bartonellosis—infection by *Bartonella bacilliformis*, p. 431–439. *In* D. H. Connor, F. W. Chandler, H. J. Manz, D. A. Schwartz, and E. E. Lack (ed.), *Pathology of Infectious Diseases*, vol. 1. Appleton and Lange, Stamford, Conn.

51. **Osborne, B. M., J. J. Butler, and B. Mackay.** 1987. Ultrastructural observations in cat scratch disease. *Am. J. Clin. Pathol.* **87:**739–744.

52. **Raoult, D., P. E. Fournier, M. Drancourt,** **T. J. Marrie, J. Etienne, J. Cosserat, P. Cacoub, Y. Poinsignon, P. Leclercq, and A. M. Sefton.** 1996. Diagnosis of 22 new cases of *Bartonella* endocarditis. *Ann. Intern. Med.* **125:**646–652.

53. **Regnery, R. L., J. A. Rooney, A. M. Johnson, S. L. Nesby, P. Manzewitsch, K. Beaver, and J. G. Olson.** 1996. Experimentally induced *Bartonella henselae* infections followed by challenge exposure and antimicrobial therapy in cats. *Am. J. Vet. Res.* **57:**1714–1719.

54. **Relman, D. A., J. S. Loutit, T. M. Schmidt, S. Falkow, and L. S. Tompkins.** 1990. The agent of bacillary angiomatosis: an approach to the identification of uncultured pathogens. *N. Engl. J. Med.* **323:**1573–1580.

55. **Robertson, B. D., and T. F. Meyer.** 1992. Genetic variation in pathogenic bacteria. *Trends Genet.* **8:**422–428.

56. **Rodriguez-Barradas, M. C., J. C. Bandres, R. J. Hamill, J. Trial, J. E. R. Clarridge, R. E. Baughn, and R. D. Rossen.** 1995. In vitro evaluation of the role of humoral immunity against *Bartonella henselae*. *Infect. Immun.* **63:**2367–2370.

57. **Rodriguez-Barradas, M. C., R. J. Hamill, E. D. Houston, P. R. Georghiou, J. E. Clarridge, R. L. Regnery, and J. E. Koehler.** 1995. Genomic fingerprinting of *Bartonella* species by repetitive element PCR for distinguishing species and isolates. *J. Clin. Microbiol.* **33:**1089–1093.

58. **Roux, V., and D. Raoult.** 1995. Inter- and intraspecies identification of *Bartonella* (*Rochalimaea*) species. *J. Clin. Microbiol.* **33:**1573–1579.

59. **Rydkina, E. B., V. Roux, E. M. Gagua, A. B. Predtechenski, I. V. Tarasevich, and D. Raoult.** 1999. *Bartonella quintana* in body lice collected from homeless persons in Russia. *Emerg. Infect. Dis.* **5:**176–178.

60. **Salyers, A. A., and D. D. Whitt.** 1994. *Bacterial Pathogenesis: a Molecular Approach*, p. 290–300. American Society for Microbiology, Washington, D.C.

61. **Sander, A., C. Buhler, K. Pelz, E. von Cramm, and W. Bredt.** 1997. Detection and identification of two *Bartonella henselae* variants in domestic cats in Germany. *J. Clin. Microbiol.* **35:**584–587.

62. **Schouls, L. M., I. Van De Pol, S. G. T. Rijpkema, and C. S. Schot.** 1999. Detection and identification of *Ehrlichia*, *Borrelia burgdorferi* sensu lato, and *Bartonella* species in Dutch *Ixodes ricinus* ticks. *J. Clin. Microbiol.* **37:**2215–2222.

63. **Spach, D. H., A. S. Kanter, N. A. Daniels, D. J. Nowowiejski, A. M. Larson, R. A. Schmidt, B. Swaminathan, and D. J. Brenner.** 1995. *Bartonella* (*Rochalimaea*) species as a

cause of apparent "culture-negative" endocarditis. *Clin. Infect. Dis.* **20:**1044–1047.

64. **Stoler, M. H., T. A. Bonfiglio, R. T. Steigbigel, and M. Pereira.** 1983. An atypical subcutaneous infection associated with acquired immune deficiency syndrome. *Am. J. Clin. Pathol.* **80:** 714–718.

65. **Strong, R. P.** 1918. *Trench Fever: Report of Commission, Medical Research Committee, American Red Cross.* Oxford University Press, Oxford, England.

66. **Swift, H. F.** 1920. Trench fever. *Arch. Intern. Med.* **26:**76–98.

67. **Varela, G., J. W. Vinson, and C. Molina-Pasquel.** 1969. Trench fever. II. Propagation of *Rickettsia quintana* on cell-free medium from the blood of two patients. *Am. J. Trop. Med. Hyg.* **18:** 708–712.

68. **von Krampitz, H. E.** 1962. Weitere Untersuchungen an Grahamella Brumpt 1911. *Z. Tropenmed. Parasitol.* **13:**34–53.

69. **Weinman, D.** 1968. Bartonellosis, p. 3–24. *In* D. Weinman and M. Ristoc (ed.), *Infectious Blood Diseases of Man and Animals.* Academic Press, Inc., New York, N.Y.

70. **Weinman, D., and J. P. Kreier.** 1977. *Bartonella* and *Grahamella*, p. 197–233. *In* J. P. Kreier (ed.), *Parasitic Protozoa*, vol. 4. Academic Press, Inc., New York, N.Y.

71. **Weinman, D., and H. Pinkerton.** 1937. Carrion's disease. IV. Natural sources of bartonella in the endemic zone. *Proc. Soc. Exp. Biol. Med.* **37:** 596–598.

72. **Wong, M. T., M. J. Dolan, C. P. Lattuada, Jr., R. L. Regnery, M. L. Garcia, E. C. Mokulis, R. A. LaBarre, D. P. Ascher, J. A. Delmar, J. W. Kelly, et al.** 1995. Neuroretinitis, aseptic meningitis, and lymphadenitis associated with *Bartonella (Rochalimaea) henselae* infection in immunocompetent patients and patients infected with human immunodeficiency virus type 1. *Clin. Infect. Dis.* **21:**352–360.

73. **Xu, Y. H., Z. Y. Lu, and G. M. Ihler.** 1995. Purification of deformin, an extracellular protein synthesized by *Bartonella bacilliformis* which causes deformation of erythrocyte membranes. *Biochim. Biophys. Acta* **1234:**173–183.

74. **Yamamoto, K., B. B. Chomel, R. W. Kasten, C. C. Chang, T. Tseggai, P. R. Decker, M. Mackowiak, K. A. Floyd-Hawkins, and N. C. Pedersen.** 1998. Homologous protection but lack of heterologous protection by various species and types of *Bartonella* in specific pathogen-free cats. *Vet. Immunol. Immunopathol.* **65:** 191–204.

75. **Yamamoto, K., B. B. Chomel, L. J. Lowenstine, Y. Kikuchi, L. G. Phillips, B. C. Barr, P. K. Swift, K. R. Jones, S. P. D. Riley, R. W. Kasten, J. E. Foley, and N. C. Pedersen.** 1998. *Bartonella henselae* antibody prevalence in free-ranging and captive wild felids from California. *J. Wildl. Dis.* **34:**56–63.

PATHOGENESIS OF PERSISTENT CLINICAL SYNDROMES

IV

PERSISTENCE OF INFECTIVE ENDOCARDITIS

Mark C. Herzberg

18

Infective endocarditis describes a family of persistent microbial infections of the heart valves. Typically targeting previously damaged or diseased valves, infecting microbes colonize within a thrombus-like mass of platelets and fibrin. The platelet-fibrin "vegetations" sequester and protect the microbial colonies from both the innate and adaptive immune systems and from therapeutic intervention with antibiotics. After successful antibiotic therapy, sterile vegetations typically persist and are detected by echocardiography (129). Prophylactic and therapeutic regimens for bacterial endocarditis may be complicated by the emergence of antibiotic-resistant bacteria. For example, children who have been treated for otitis media with common antibiotic protocols develop antibiotic-resistant streptococci in dental plaque that can persist for years (46). These viridans streptococci are of particular interest in infective endocarditis, since they are commensals that can behave as pathogens. This chapter will explore their ability to behave as endogenous pathogens and will hopefully be instructive as we try to understand persistence of the larger constellation of endocarditis-associated pathogens.

The clinical presentation of infective endocarditis usually includes nonspecific symptoms of malaise, fever, sweats, myalgia, weight loss, and sustained elevations of C-reactive protein, erythrocyte sedimentation rate, and other inflammatory markers (11, 107, 131). Sustained fever is associated with the persistence of cardiac valve infection, while sustained C-reactive protein levels reflect the complexity of the pathologic process. At presentation, cardiac murmur, tachycardia, vascular phenomena, and a change in mental state are usually noted. Anemia is present in about 50% of patients, and renal and liver dysfunction is present in about one-third. Myocardial abscesses occur in about 50% of cases associated with viridans streptococci, about 30% of cases associated with *Staphylococcus aureus*, and 20% of culture-negative cases (83).

PATHOGENESIS

Infective endocarditis generally occurs in individuals with previously diseased or damaged heart valves, most frequently after bacteremia containing viridans streptococci or *S. aureus* (37, 38). Oral and dental infections appear to be the most common portals of entry for infecting bacteria, with viridans streptococci the most frequent etiological agents and streptococci as-

Mark C. Herzberg, Department of Preventive Sciences, School of Dentistry, University of Minnesota, Minneapolis, MN 55455.

Persistent Bacterial Infections, Edited by J. P. Nataro, M. J. Blaser, and S. Cunningham-Rundles, © 2000 ASM Press, Washington, D.C.

sociated twice as frequently as staphylococci (131).

The most common viridans streptococci implicated in endocarditis are *Streptococcus sanguis* sensu stricto (31.9%), *Streptococcus oralis* (29.8%), and *Streptococcus gordonii* (12.7%) (30). Although often considered to be nonpathogenic commensals in their native niches, some species of viridans streptococci are associated with severe endocardial infection. In a recent study, *Streptococcus bovis* (*Streptococcus gallolyticus*) was associated with more complicated infective endocarditis than other streptococci or staphylococci (80). Patients infected with *S. bovis* were older, frequently had underlying gastrointestinal lesions, showed higher mortality with fewer embolic events, and more frequently required cardiac surgery than those infected with other microorganisms. Multiple affected valves, infectious myocardial infiltration of the left ventricle, and severe regurgitation occurred more often in *S. bovis* endocarditis than with other organisms. Species that induce expression of enzymes and transport proteins that facilitate metabolism of mammalian oligopeptides (21) and oligosaccharides with nonreducing terminal sialic acid (16, 71) are those most commonly associated with persistent intravascular infections. The viridans streptococci generally cause endocarditis with a milder clinical course than that caused by the staphylococci (72, 131).

Bacteremic patients commonly show thromboembolic complications (87, 127). Although infective endocarditis associated with intravenous drug abuse can occur without a history of valve disease, the risk of infective endocarditis greatly increases in individuals with a past history of rheumatic heart disease or other valvular injury. The risk is also associated with the frequency or severity of bacteremia (37) but does not appear to increase appreciably as a consequence of the treatment of dental infections, which often promotes polymicrobial bacteremias (121). Subclinical bacteremias also occur commonly during chronic oral and dental infections, such as periodontitis.

Recently, a new causal model of infective endocarditis was proposed based on a comprehensive review of the epidemiological data (35). The data suggest that bacteremias that may recur for years before the appearance of clinical signs of disease stimulate a proinflammatory state on the endothelial surfaces of the heart valves. Within 2 to 3 weeks of the onset of clinical disease, a late bacteremia promotes colonization of the valve and a characteristic fulminant infection.

Endocarditis marks the culmination of an unusual odyssey for the infecting microbes. In general, the causative microorganisms originate on the skin or mucous membranes, enter the blood through breached integument, circulate and survive in the blood by resisting reticuloendothelial clearance, adhere selectively to damaged heart valves, and colonize within thrombotic, degranulated platelets. Most often, the causative microorganisms are sessile commensals in the oral cavity that subsequently adapt to several changes in environment. The microbes must adjust to the breached epithelial tissues, followed by entry and turbulent transit in the circulation. In the blood, these sessile colonizers must survive as planktonic cells. Within several minutes, a few bacterial cells or colony fragments will bind to the damaged heart valve, reestablishing a sessile existence.

Microbes can bind to altered endothelial cells, immobilized platelets, or damaged connective tissue cells and proteins of the heart valve surface. Bacteria may also adhere to circulating platelets, which then aggregate on the injured valve during the formation of the thrombotic vegetation. The microbes must survive in the interior milieu of a thrombus in the presence of platelet microbicidal protein and in the absence of preferred carbon sources, such as sucrose. Many of the most common microorganisms associated with infective endocarditis are considered to be of low virulence, often causing no known disease in their native niches. Yet these microbes show a remarkable capacity to adapt to changing environments and colonize foreign sites, where they also show unexpected pathogenicity.

How can a benign commensal, which may

serve a protective function on dental and mucosal epithelial tissues, behave as a pathogen and cause disease in the endovascular environment? It is unlikely that endocarditis represents a state toward which its pathogens have specifically evolved. Endocarditis and other infections more likely represent an imbalance in the host-commensal equilibrium. The development of pathology is a function of the genetic complement of the infecting microbe and the likelihood that the host response will be accompanied by tissue damage (17). There is no evidence that endovascular infection provides an evolutionary advantage to endocarditis pathogens. Most likely, the virulence factors that will be discussed below evolved to serve some other purpose for the bacterium.

Modestly virulent microbes may infect or colonize abnormal heart valves only briefly to cause "bland" vegetations or may colonize and persist yet cause subclinical disease (Fig. 1). More virulent pathogens may colonize even normal valves briefly, but cause large thrombotic vegetations resulting in abnormal valvular function, or they may colonize, persist, and cause septic thrombotic vegetations, valve destruction and insufficiency, and febrile disease. The ability to colonize, therefore, is a virulence trait which must be accompanied by expression of pathogenic (i.e., damaging) characteristics to cause disease. The persistence of endocarditis is a function of the host's dichotomous ability to promote and also resolve and sterilize the vegetative lesion weighed against the virulence of the infecting microbes.

Promotion of the Vegetation

Disseminated intravascular coagulation and shock can be triggered during episodes of bacteremia (86) in association with microorganisms most frequently associated with infective endocarditis. For example, disseminated intravascular coagulation and shock are caused by *S. aureus* (87, 106) and *S. sanguis* (3, 13, 40) in individuals not generally considered to be at risk of infective endocarditis. Hence, it is not surprising that the active stage of infective endocarditis is characterized by dynamic changes in coagulation and platelet aggregation that are accompanied by an increase in acute-phase reactants (126) and a tendency towards complicating thrombotic events (52). Indeed, a small initiating stimulus can also activate the coagulation cascade in discrete segments of the vascular tree, such as the heart valves, to promote a large fibrin clot (113).

Patients with infective endocarditis show elevated anti-phospholipid antibodies associ-

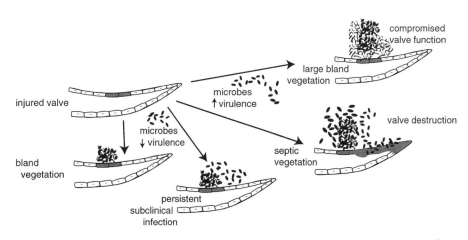

FIGURE 1 Tripartite model of infective endocarditis. The persistence of endocarditis reflects the balance between the host's ability to repair an injured valve and promote or support a bland nonbacterial thrombotic vegetation and the virulence of the infecting microbe.

ated with endothelial-cell activation, thrombin generation, and impairment of fibrinolysis (81). Embolic events are common and severe complications of infective endocarditis. Strains that activate coagulation through (i) thrombin- and Hageman factor-like enzymes (93), (ii) promotion of expression of tissue factor by endothelial cells (33) or monocytes (5, 6), or (iii) induction of platelet aggregation (29, 61, 63, 122) would be expected to trigger formation of larger vegetations, causing disease with a more complicated clinical course. In contrast, strains producing hydrolytic proteases can cause necrosis of the vegetations and, with progression, valvular destruction and insufficiency. For example, proteolytic strains of *Enterococcus faecalis* cause partial dissolution of experimental vegetations in rabbits, resulting in high levels of bacteremia; small, soft, friable vegetations; a high frequency of kidney infarcts; and shorter survival times (55).

The septic vegetation forms primarily by accumulation of masses of platelets within a fibrin scaffold, as observed in rabbits by using light, immunofluorescent, and electron microscopy (36). On the periphery, vegetations are surrounded by bound mononuclear phagocytes. These phagocytes retain phagocytic function, since they contain large numbers of streptococci 30 min after intravenous inoculation. Fewer circulating streptococci adhere directly to the vegetation, but *Proteus* and *Staphylococcus albus* adhere directly in high numbers and without phagocytosis. The adherent bacteria form colonies within capsules of fibrin, which apparently provide protection from phagocytosis. Layers of fibrin and platelets accumulate in apparent cycles of thrombosis. The bacterial colonies become further enclosed in thrombi, and the vegetations increase in mass. Cycles of thrombosis and reseeding by circulating bacteria continue, and 2 days after initiation, the colonies increase perceptibly in size.

Using ^{111}In-labeled platelets as tracers, platelet accumulation can be seen to contribute to the increasing mass of experimental vegetations, which increases directly with the duration of endocarditis (65). A strain of *S. sanguis*

which induced aggregation of rabbit platelets in vitro (Agg[+]) causes endocarditis characterized by significantly larger vegetations, febrile episodes, hematological changes, signs of myocardial ischemia, gross lesions in major organs, and greater mortality than an Agg[−] strain, saline, or the Agg[+] strain pretreated with monospecific rabbit antibodies or Fab fragments against its platelet aggregation-associated protein (PAAP). The PAAP is strongly suggested to promote the formation and development of vegetations. Furthermore, an Agg[+] strain was recovered in higher numbers than an Agg[−] strain from experimental vegetations in a rat model (92). In contrast to the Agg[+] strain, the Agg[−] strain binds effectively to insoluble fibrinogen and fibronectin or preformed platelet-fibrin clots, suggesting that adhesion mechanisms are sufficient to promote infection.

PLATELET ADHESION AND AGGREGATION

The ability to interact with platelets and promote their aggregation in vitro and in vivo appears to be linked directly to the mass of the vegetation and the severity of the clinical signs (reviewed in reference 67). Indeed, the ability of *S. aureus* to bind platelets in vitro is directly related to pathogenicity in the rabbit model (124). Certain strains of *S. aureus* (19) and *S. sanguis* (29, 61, 63, 122) induce human platelets in plasma to aggregate in vitro. The ability of strains to induce platelet aggregation generally depends on their ability to adhere to platelets (54, 61, 62) and to bind to platelet receptors (53, 118).

Platelet aggregation induced by many strains of *S. sanguis* requires expression of PAAP on fibrils of the cell wall (42, 62). The PAAP is synthesized as a rhamnose-rich glycoprotein of 115 kDa (43, 64) and contains a collagen-like platelet-interactive domain (41), which contains a functional suprasecondary structural motif in the sequence Pro-Gly-Glu-Gln-Gly-Pro-Lys (44, 47). The PAAP apparently interacts with a signal-transducing receptor complex on platelets. The receptor complex includes glycoprotein Ia-IIa, an α2β1 integrin (53, 118); CD26, which is expressed in low copy numbers; CD31; and CD36 (K. Gong, T. Ouyang, and M. C. Herzberg, unpublished data). The signal transduction pathway appears to be independent of G proteins, but the platelet response to *S. sanguis* is potentiated by (i) endogenous catecholamines through α2-adrenoreceptors (66) and (ii) an *S. sanguis* ecto-ATPase, which hydrolyzes released dense granule adenosine triphosphate, an inhibitor of platelet aggregation, to ADP, an agonist (60, 90).

Platelet aggregation induced by bacteria generally involves a fibrinogen–dependent mechanism. Binding of fibrinogen by platelet glycoprotein IIb-IIIa, an αIIbβ3 integrin, cross-links platelets during aggregation and thrombus formation. *S. aureus* appears to bind fibrinogen but to induce aggregation of platelets without cross-linking by glycoprotein IIb-IIIa (8).

Some viridans streptococci appear to interact with platelets by PAAP-independent mechanisms. These strains bind glycoprotein Ib (49, 51) or the glycoprotein Ib-IX-V complex colocalizing with the Fc receptor, FcγRIIA (51, 123, 125). Glycoprotein Ib is suggested to bind an uncharacterized ligand or adhesin on the streptococcal surface, while FcγRIIA binds the Fc domain of specific immunoglobulin G (IgG) antibodies bound to antigens on viridans streptococci. The platelet FcγRIIA has been implicated in signal transduction in platelets in response to other agonists, including collagen (130). Furthermore, activation of complement may also promote signaling in platelets. A platelet-aggregating strain of *S. sanguis* promotes more rapid assembly of the C5b-9 complex on the cell wall than a nonaggregating strain, suggesting a correlation with the lag time (50).

Resolution of the Thrombotic Vegetation

FIBRINOLYSIS

In the thrombus-like vegetation, fibrinogen polymerizes to fibrin, often trapping and sequestering microbes. The infected thrombus-like compartment of the vegetation may be dis-aggregated by exogenous fibrinolytic enzymes, rendering some vegetations bland or otherwise asymptomatic for years. For example, tissue plasminogen activator (tPA) promotes fibrinolysis by generating plasmin, which digests fibrin. When used to disaggregate preformed platelet-fibrin clots in vitro, tPA digested ^{125}I-labeled fibrin, released incorporated *Staphylococcus epidermidis*, and reduced the mass of the clots (14). In the rabbit model, recombinant human tPA cleared 5-fold more ^{111}In-labeled platelets from the heart than were cleared in untreated rabbits within 50 min and 1.4-fold more after 3 days (101). Combined treatment with recombinant human tPA and penicillin was more effective in reducing the mass of vegetations and clinical signs of *S. sanguis* experimental endocarditis than penicillin or recombinant tPA alone, which in turn were more effective than saline controls. As is known for coronary thrombosis, administration of tPA to experimental rabbits was less effective in clearing platelets from older vegetations. Experimental vegetations in rabbits accumulate fibrin continuously after infection in the absence of therapeutic doses of tPA (M. Yokota, personal communication). The effectiveness of exogenous tPA in experimental endocarditis suggests that the endogenous enzymes could contribute to healing of incipient or early valvular vegetations.

HEALING

In human endocarditis, an increase in vegetation size during antibiotic therapy predicts a prolonged healing phase associated with a significantly increased risk of thromboembolic events, independent of blood culture results (111, 112). In experimental rabbits, antibiotic treatment is associated with an increased inflammatory cell response at the surface of the vegetation and within the vasculature of the supporting tissue of the valve (48). Later, healing is associated with endothelialization of the vegetative lesions, which corresponds to the histological appearance in experimental rabbits and, upon sterilization, is accompanied by organization of the interior (36). When sequestered from host defenses and diffusing antibiotics, "persistent" bacteria appear within surrounding thrombi.

Sterilization of the Infected Vegetation

ANTIBIOTIC THERAPY
Infecting microbes may become embedded to colonize within the dense platelet-fibrin matrix of the vegetations. Microbes are more inaccessible to systemic antibiotics when embedded than when attached at the periphery (102). In the presence of otherwise-effective antibiotics, survival of staphylococci, for example, is better within the fibrin core than when they are colonizing the periphery of the vegetation.

PLATELET MICROBICIDAL PROTEINS
Platelet microbicidal proteins are small cationic peptides that are released by aggregated platelets. While the ability of S. aureus, for example, to adhere or to induce platelet aggregation in vitro is independent of sensitivity to the platelet microbicidal proteins, sensitive blood-borne pathogens may be killed in vitro (134). In contrast, staphylococci and viridans group streptococci isolated from blood cultures obtained from patients with confirmed cases of infective endocarditis are generally resistant to platelet microbicidal proteins in vitro (10, 133). Resistance is associated with more aggressive development of valvular lesions and blood-borne spread of sepsis in experimental endocarditis in rabbits (28). Microbial toxins, such as staphylococcal alpha toxin, which would be expected to lyse cells and tissues, actually appear to increase the availability of platelet microbicidal proteins in experimental vegetations (9). As a result, elevated local levels of platelet microbicidal proteins reduce the pathogenicity of S. aureus in the rabbit model of experimental endocarditis.

POLYMORPHONUCLEAR CELLS AND MONOCYTES
Phagocytosis appears to be inefficient in clearing certain bacterial species from within experimental vegetations (6) or from preformed platelet-fibrin matrices in vitro (7). While they may be mobilized to the vegetation, monocytes unable to accomplish phagocytosis might upregulate tissue factor. Susceptibilities to polymorphonuclear leukocytes and monocytes may also differ among infecting species. Available granulocytes strongly potentiated the action of cloxacillin against S. epidermidis, while monocytes contributed modestly in rabbits treated to develop selective granulocytopenia or monocytopenia as a background for experimental endocarditis (99). While monocytes appeared to contribute little protection against S. sanguis or Escherichia coli, granulocytes were modestly effective (97, 98). In experimental endocarditis, polymorphonuclear cells and monocytes vary, therefore, in efficacy and the stage of disease in which protection can be provided against different microbial species.

NATURALLY OCCURRING ANTIBODIES
Rheumatic fever is a major cause of heart valve disease and scarring that creates a risk of infective endocarditis. The host response to rheumatic carditis includes expression of anti-myosin antibodies that cross-react with group A streptococci. Monoclonal anti-myosin antibodies from patients with rheumatic carditis were found to react with specific peptides from the light meromyosin region of the human cardiac myosin molecule (1). While related anti-meromyosin specificities may occur naturally, these human antibodies cross-react strongly with N-acetyl-β-D-glucosamine, the dominant epitope of the group A streptococcal carbohydrate.

Many species associated with infective endocarditis show immunologic mimicry between cell surface antigens and the sialyl-Lewis(x) [sLe(x)] oligosaccharide (70). sLe(x) cross-reactive bacteria include S. sanguis and virtually all other viridans streptococci, Streptococcus pyogenes, Actinobacillus actinomycetemcomitans, Eikenella corrodens, and Porphyromonas gingivalis. These oral bacteria would be expected to react with naturally occurring IgM and IgG anti-sLe(x) antibodies in the blood (22). In the absence of naturally occurring specific antibody, sLe(x)-cross-reactive strains may react directly with the selectin family of host adhesive proteins, which could promote binding to endothelial cells and platelets in the proximity of the vegetative lesion.

PASSIVE IMMUNITY

Staphylococcal polysaccharides have been used to elicit protective antibodies against infective endocarditis (85). Capsular antibodies were elicited by immunization of rabbits with a polysaccharide-protein conjugate vaccine. The rabbit antibodies protected experimental rats against serotype 5 *S. aureus* infection in a model of endocarditis.

Colonization-Recolonization and Adaptation

In human endocarditis, the formation of bland and septic vegetations occurs at sites of previous heart valve injury or disease. In this environment, infecting microbes encounter the damaged heart valve, which presents as exposed extracellular matrix, adherent and "activated" endothelium, aggregated platelets, and fibrin. Platelets and fibrin accumulate in response to the tissue injury. Platelets, fibrin, endothelium, and extracellular matrix may each serve as specific binding sites for infecting microbes.

EXPRESSION OF ADHESINS

Adhesion to platelets and preformed platelet-fibrin clots would appear intuitively to be associated with the ability of microbes to infect platelet vegetations and cause infective endocarditis. For the viridans streptococci, persistence in the oral cavity is crucial to their potential as endocarditis pathogens. Strains of viridans streptococci that bind to both platelets and saliva-coated hydroxylapatite, a model of the tooth surface, use the same adhesin and binding site epitopes (54). Strains that do not adhere to platelets rely on other adhesin specificities to bind to saliva-coated hydroxylapatite, suggesting constitutive expression of adhesins for platelet and tooth binding sites on the tooth.

Dextran synthesis by viridans streptococci has been suggested to be a virulence factor in infective endocarditis, promoting adhesion and persistence. When 21 streptococcal isolates from patients with infective endocarditis were compared, dextran formation did not promote adhesion (23). Nonetheless, adhesion was necessary, but not sufficient, to explain why strains caused disease. Furthermore, expression of extracellular or cell-associated glucosyltransferase, fructosyltransferase, and soluble or insoluble dextrans was independent of the platelet interactivity phenotype of *S. sanguis* (63). Since sucrose, the required substrate for dextran biosynthesis, is not present in the endovascular environment, other adhesion mechanisms are essential.

While initial adhesion was unaffected, the ability of *S. aureus* to bind to collagen in vitro increases the potential to infect and colonize damaged heart valves in a rat model of infective endocarditis (69). Alternative adhesins may be expressed as regulated tandem genes, such as the surface-located fibrinogen-binding proteins ClfA and ClfB of *S. aureus* (105) or SspA and SspB (26) and CshA and CshB (94) of *S. gordonii*. The CshA polypeptide is conserved among the sanguis group of viridans streptococci and serves as the structural and functional trunk of large adhesive fibrils (96). The endocarditis-associated nutritionally variant viridans streptococci express the high-molecular-weight fibrillar protein Emb. The N terminus of Emb contains an extracellular matrix binding domain (91). To accommodate the challenges of fickle environments, each species of infecting bacteria employs several adhesion strategies, each with a different molecular basis.

ENVIRONMENTAL REGULATION OF GENES IN NONNATIVE ENVIRONMENTS

Gram-positive and gram-negative species use different signaling molecules to communicate intercellularly and display multiple phenotypes (117). The intercellular signals and other environmental information are integrated by signal transduction networks. Through signal transduction, gene expression and cellular differentiation are modified to advance the survival of the bacteria in the community.

Genes expressed in vitro would not be expected to reflect the spectrum of genes expressed in vivo or that contribute to the microbe's ability to cause disease. For example, at least 13 *S. gordonii* genes are expressed uniquely in the platelet vegetation in experimental endocarditis in rabbits and not in vitro (68, 78). Identified tentatively by homology, genes expressed in vivo may be involved in oligosaccharide metabolism, amino acid transport, DNA synthesis and transcriptional regulation, adhesin maintenance, and other protective functions. In *S. aureus*, the *sar* locus controls the synthesis of both extracellular and cell wall virulence determinants (18). Expression of the individual *sar* promoters appears to depend on the specificity of pressors in different anatomic microenvironments formed in the vegetation in experimental infective endocarditis.

Genes encoding proteins needed for survival in challenging environments must be expressed for pathogenicity to be expressed. For example, the gene *putP* encodes the high-affinity transporter for proline uptake in *S. aureus*. An oligonucleotide signature-tagged insertional inactivation of *putP* reduced intravegetation density and in vivo survival in an infective-endocarditis model (12). In contrast, inactivation of loci encoding an oligopeptide transporter, a purine repressor, and lantibiotic biosynthesis, each of which was a candidate gene locus essential for survival in vivo (115), had no substantial impact on survival within vegetations.

Genes encoding the uptake of essential amino acids may be essential for virulence. Indeed, an *S. gordonii hppA* (oligopeptide permease) mutant shows altered transcriptional effects on *cshA* adhesin gene expression and reduced adhesion (95). HppA is suggested to be required for a signaling response of cells to an extracellular factor. Through HppA, *cshA* transcription is modulated to promote cell surface CshA expression and adhesion. A related ATP-binding cassette transport protein, FimA,

which is widely expressed on the cell surface among the oral streptococci, has also been tested in animals as a vaccine to prevent endocarditis (128). Immunized rats show significantly reduced infectivity in experimental endocarditis compared to unimmunized controls. While antibodies against FimA modestly inhibit in vitro adhesion to platelet-fibrin clots, antagonism to growth by interfering with the transporter functions of FimA may also occur.

Environmental exposure to certain extracellular matrix proteins may alter the expression of specific microbial proteins. Growth in the presence of laminin changes the ability of *S. gordonii* to express a collagen-like 145-kDa surface adhesin, which reacts with sera from patients with confirmed cases of endocarditis (119). Similarly, when *S. sanguis* is grown in the presence of collagen, the PAAP shows enhanced ability to induce aggregation of platelets (45).

INFECTED VEGETATIONS AS BIOFILMS

After infection, microbial colonies on heart valves adapt to communal life and behave differently than when observed in pure culture in vitro (20). The colonies are often polymicrobial, reflecting in part the predisposing bacteremia. The challenging environment and the need to coexist with microbial partners and competitors result in communal organization, with like species synthesizing an exopolymeric superstructure. The hydrated superstructure permits diffusion of water-soluble ions but separates colonies from one another and protects them from elements of the host defense system and therapeutic agents, such as antibiotics. The "persistence" phenotype of members of the microbial community may differ widely from that expected from observing bacteria in pure culture. While environmental conditions may alter gene expression, the apparent genotypes of community members may also change. In biofilms, there is a high rate of conjugal transfer of DNA (56).

SESSILE VERSUS PLANKTONIC PHENOTYPIC SWITCHES

Bacteria use peptide-like signaling molecules to communicate. In cell density-dependent regulation, the signal peptide is processed post-translationally and secreted by a dedicated ATP-binding-cassette exporter (79). This secreted peptide pheromone functions as a signaling ligand for a specific sensing receptor of a two-component signal-transduction system. The genes encoding the two-component system and the signaling peptide are generally located within an operon facilitating autoregulation of peptide-pheromone expression.

Using this system, gram-negative bacteria, such as *Pseudomonas aeruginosa*, communicate by diffusion of *N*-acyl homoserine lactone signals, controlling expression of extracellular virulence factors, the type II secretion apparatus, a stationary-phase sigma factor, and biofilm differentiation (2, 25, 110). Initial interactions of planktonic cells with the sessile biofilm surface may be promoted through motility mediated by flagella or twitching (108). With increasing biofilm density and cell starvation, cell-associated exopolymers degrade enzymatically, promoting detachment and a switch from sessile to planktonic cells (25).

Similar mechanisms may exist in dental plaque biofilms and within valvular vegetations on heart valves. *Streptococcus mutans* organisms grown in experimental biofilms differentially express genes associated with exopolysaccharide metabolism, including *gtfBC*, *ftf*, and *scrA* (15). Inactivation of the *gbpA* gene, which encodes a glucan-binding protein, changes the dental plaque biofilm from large to small sessile colonies and reduces virulence in an animal model of dental caries (59). Cell-to-cell communication among naturally transformable streptococcal and other gram-positive species may be mediated by competence-stimulating peptide (CSP) and related oligopeptides (87, 88, 89, 132). In *S. sanguis*, competence is regulated by the *com* operon, which contains three genes, *comC*, *comD*, and *comE*. The *comC* gene encodes a CSP which at a critical extracellular concentration may induce competence in the bacterial population. The receptor for CSP, a transmembrane histidine kinase, is encoded by *comD*; *comE* encodes the response regulator protein. Together, the products of *comD* and

comE form a two-component signal transduction system. DNA released into saliva is slowly degraded but can transform competent streptococci (100). Interspecies recombinational exchanges can occur, resulting in mosaic alleles of *comC* (58).

The hexaheptapeptide permease (Hpp) system in *S. gordonii* may also regulate competence and growth rate, as well as the expression of a major cell surface adhesin, CshA (95, 96). The *hppA* gene encodes an oligopeptide permease and appears to control the growth rate in complex medium, competence, and the efficiency of transformation (74). The surface lipoprotein HppA also appears to serve as a sensing receptor for an extracellular factor that modulates *cshA* transcription (95). The Hpp system links competence and cell density-dependent growth with the ability of *S. gordonii* to adhere through cell surface expression of CshA, perhaps serving as a sessile-planktonic switch.

Stress also regulates gene expression in oral streptococci and may alter platelet interactions. Heat shock regulation by CtsR is highly conserved in gram-positive bacteria, whereby the product of the *ctsR* gene represses the *clpC* operon, including *clpE*, which encodes a novel member of the Hsp100 Clp ATPase family (28). HSP65 is also upregulated by heat shock. In *S. sanguis*, HSP65 is highly homologous to GroEL of *E. coli* and HSP65 of *M. tuberculosis* and appears to inhibit platelet aggregation in vitro (P. Liu, K. Gong, and M. C. Herzberg, unpublished data). Hence, one may speculate that febrile episodes in endocarditis can upregulate streptococcal HSP65 and self-limit platelet aggregation into the thrombotic valvular vegetation.

TISSUE PROCESSING TO PROVIDE NUTRIENTS

Sucrose is the preferred carbon source for viridans streptococci. Given the availability of sucrose as a substrate, streptococci will generally synthesize a glucan- or fructan-rich exopolymer that enhances colonization of heart valves in a rat model of infective endocarditis (103). Since there is no sucrose in the blood, persistent species will likely induce expression of enzymes and other proteins that facilitate metabolism of mammalian proteins and glycoproteins in the blood and within vegetations. In carefully controlled chemostat conditions, pH was shown to be an important determinant for expression of viridans streptococcal glycosidases and proteases, including thrombin-like activity and Hageman factor (93). While thrombin-like activity, which is optimal at pH 7.5, may sequester growing streptococci by promoting platelet clots, the glycosidases are expressed optimally at pH 6.5 (93) and hydrolyze oligosaccharides in the vegetation environment to monosaccharides that can be metabolized (16, 71).

Responding to limited free amino acids, *S. gordonii* expresses and releases an extracellular serine-type protease with gelatinase and type IV collagenase activities (76). The purified protease cleaved bovine gelatin, human placental type IV collagen, and the Aα chain of fibrinogen but not albumin, fibronectin, laminin, or myosin. At higher initial concentrations of amino acids, the protease remained cell associated and the addition of an amino acid mixture to an actively secreting culture stopped further enzyme release. The gelatinase and type IV collagenase activities would enable *S. gordonii* to hydrolyze selected basement membrane and extracellular matrix proteins to provide essential amino acids, including proline. Growth in the presence of collagen changed the expression of *S. sanguis* PAAP (45), while expression of the high-affinity transporter for proline also appeared to be necessary for the survival of *S. aureus* in experimental vegetations (12).

Adaptation by the Host

INDUCTION OF TISSUE FACTOR

Tissue factor promotes activation of coagulation and the deposition of fibrin, contributing to hemostasis, thrombogenesis, and inflammation (116). Initiation of coagulation requires induced expression by intravascular cells (34) of mediators, including lipopolysaccharide (LPS), interleukin-1β (IL-1β), tumor necrosis factor alpha (TNF-α), and C5a (73). Conditions that

upregulate tissue factor or downregulate tissue factor pathway inhibitors may promote formation or persistence of thrombi, including valvular vegetations (4). Indeed, only low levels (~1% of normal) of tissue factor expression may be necessary to sustain hemostatic function, based on complementation studies of null mutants of murine tissue factor (109). Mammalian stressors, such as prolonged hypoxia, can upregulate tissue factor mRNA and protein to induce platelet accumulation and fibrin formation in the lungs of mice (84) and nonbacterial thrombotic vegetations in rats (104). Tissue factor-specific mRNA can be detected in foamy macrophages and endothelial cells, while the nascent protein localizes in the rough endoplasmic reticulum and in the thrombus. In humans, there is an elevated prevalence of cardiac valvular lesions in patients with solid tumors. Vegetations were associated with other thromboembolic events and were accompanied by a significantly increased level of plasma D dimer (39), a sign of fibrin polymerization.

Tissue factor expression in vegetations has been modeled in vitro (5, 7, 32, 33) and in vivo (6). By day 2 after experimental induction of enterococcal bacteremia in rabbits or after infection of excised aortic valves ex vivo, procoagulant activity was promoted on the valve surface (31). The activity appeared to be independent of granulocytes and monocytes. *S. aureus* promotes expression of tissue factor-like procoagulant activity by cultured human valvular endothelial cells (32), but upregulation by streptococci and enterococci appears indirect, requiring proinflammatory IL-1 or lipopolysaccharide LPS (33). Originating from dental plaque, the resultant bacteremia will be polymicrobial and include gram-positive streptococci and LPS-containing gram-negative bacteria. Hence, LPS and elicited IL-1 would probably be present in the blood. Binding of monocytes to fibrin matrices also promotes expression of tissue factor. Levels increase significantly when monocytes also interact with *S. sanguis*. Upregulation of monocyte tissue factor by *S. sanguis* appears to involve signaling mediated by adhesive integrins rather than through aborted phagocytic pathways. When etoposide treatment was used to deplete monocyte numbers in a rabbit model, tissue factor activity and severity of infection were reduced while the mass of the vegetations was unaffected (6). These data suggest that infected vegetations develop by tissue factor-dependent and -independent mechanisms of coagulation. Tissue factor-independent activation of coagulation is associated with low levels of infecting *S. sanguis*, which may promote the accumulation of platelets into the thrombus-like vegetation. The platelet-rich vegetations contain only a small fraction of monocytes by mass.

PLATELET ACCUMULATION AND FORMATION OF VEGETATION

The ability of microbes to induce platelet aggregation in vitro may be associated with the pathogenicity of those strains in infective endocarditis. Clinical isolates that induce rapid, irreversible platelet aggregation are strongly associated with subacute bacterial endocarditis and disseminated intravascular coagulation in vivo (77). Bacteria associated with clinical cases of infective endocarditis, however, may not adhere well to platelet-fibrin clots in vitro, although the viridans streptococci adhere better than other endocarditis-associated species (23). Accumulation of platelets to form vegetation in association with infecting bacteria may be aspirin sensitive, as modeled in experimental rabbits (82). After inoculation with *S. aureus*, an optimal dose of aspirin was associated with reduction in vegetation mass, growth, and final bacterial density, as well as frequency and extent of septic renal embolic lesions. After exposure to salicylic acid, *S. aureus* showed reduced induction of platelet aggregation and adhesion to sterile vegetations, platelets in suspension, fibrin matrices, or fibrin-platelet matrices. Hence, aspirin affects both platelets and *S. aureus*, reducing the severity and metastatic events in experimental *S. aureus* endocarditis.

INDUCTION OF CYTOKINE EXPRESSION

Lipoteichoic acid expressed by streptococci and staphylococci may play an important role in triggering the recruitment and activation of leukocytes to the platelet vegetation (24). The macrophage-activating and chemotactic cytokine macrophage inflammatory protein 1 alpha (MIP-1 alpha) was expressed by neutrophils, macrophages, and fibroblasts in specimens of human valvular vegetations. Lipoteichoic acid isolated from either *S. aureus* or *S. pyogenes* resulted in time- and dose-dependent expression of MIP-1 alpha mRNA and protein by human peripheral blood monocytes.

Aggregation substance and enterococcal binding substance stimulate human lymphocytes to express high levels of gamma interferon, TNF-α, and TNF-β, which is consistent with functional stimulation of T-lymphocyte proliferation and macrophage activation (114). Mutants defective in expression of either substance caused mild experimental endocarditis in rabbits when compared to the wild type, which caused large vegetations, splenomegaly, and lung congestion.

The viridans streptococci stimulate cytokine production by mononuclear cells in vitro. For example, *S. mutans* induced high levels of IL-12, gamma interferon, and TNF-α, all of which are associated with inflammation, enhanced monocyte function, and generation of a Th1 response (75). Supernatants of clinical blood culture isolates of viridans streptococci stimulated human blood monocytes to produce significantly more TNF-β and IL-8 than oral commensal isolates from the same subjects (120).

CONCLUDING REMARKS

While the endocarditis-associated oral streptococci prime and stimulate specific T cells, the humoral response is generally modest when compared to that in response to exogenous pathogens. The mucosal commensals survive in part because the secretory immune system is insufficient to prevent adhesion in preferred niches and to promote clearance by swallowing. During bacteremia and consequent valvular infection, the systemic immune response may be restrained. For example, *S. sanguis* induces transmucosal tolerance, which affects the

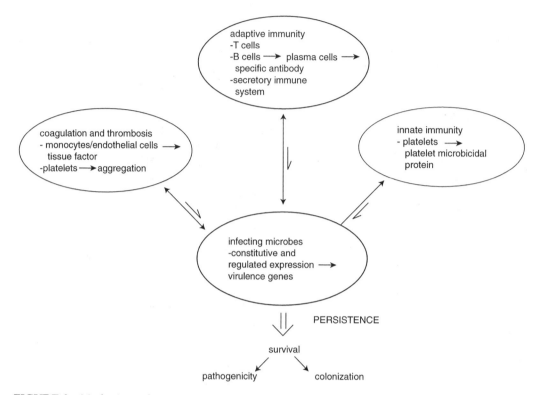

FIGURE 2 Mechanisms of microbial persistence in infective endocarditis.

systemic T-cell compartment and may minimize the T-helper cell response and specific antibody production (M. Costalonga and M.C. Herzberg, unpublished data). The host distinguishes the commensals from exogenous pathogens. When commensals breach the mucosa and infect the heart valves in infective endocarditis, the host immune repertoire against these endogenous pathogens is programmed for systemic tolerance. Infective endocarditis appears to persist because of the tolerant stance of the adaptive immune system, microbial resistance to innate immunity, and triggering of coagulation and thrombosis by the infecting microorganisms as a tissue response to injury (Fig. 2). The thrombus–like vegetation serves as a biofilm barrier against host defense, forming unique microenvironments that are regulatory for expression of specialized virulence genes in infecting microbes.

ACKNOWLEDGMENTS

I thank Maurice W. Meyer, professor emeritus and long-time collaborator, for helpful comments and suggestions and Urve Daigle for word processing support.

Work in my lab described here has been supported by NIH grants DE05501, DE08590, DE00270, and DE09737.

REFERENCES

1. **Adderson, E. E., A. R. Shikhman, K. E. Ward, and M. W. Cunningham.** 1998. Molecular analysis of polyreactive monoclonal antibodies from rheumatic carditis: human anti-N-acetylglucosamine/anti-myosin antibody V region genes. *J. Immunol.* **161:**2020–2031.
2. **Allison, D. G., B. Ruiz, C. SanJose, A. Jaspe, and P. Gilbert.** 1998. Extracellular products as mediators of the formation and detachment of *Pseudomonas fluorescens* biofilms. *FEMS Microbiol. Lett.* **167:**179–184.
3. **Arning, M., A. Gehrt, C. Aul, V. Runde, U. Hadding, and W. Schneider.** 1990. Septicemia due to *Streptococcus mitis* in neutropenic patients with acute leukemia. *Blut* **61:**364–368.

4. **Asada, Y., K. Marutsuka, K. Hatakeyama, Y. Sato, S. Hara, A. Kisanuki, and S. Sumiyoshi.** 1998. The role of tissue factor in the pathogenesis of thrombosis and atherosclerosis. *J. Atheroscler. Thromb.* **4:**135–139.

5. **Bancsi, M. J., J. Thompson, and R. M. Bertina.** 1994. Stimulation of monocyte tissue factor expression in an in vitro model of bacterial endocarditis. *Infect. Immun.* **62:**5669–5672.

6. **Bancsi, M. J., M. H. Veltrop, R. M. Bertina, and J. Thompson.** 1996. Influence of monocytes and antibiotic treatment on tissue factor activity of endocardial vegetations in rabbits infected with *Streptococcus sanguis*. *Infect. Immun.* **64:**448–451.

7. **Bancsi, M. J., M. H. Veltrop, R. M. Bertina, and J. Thompson.** 1996. Role of phagocytosis in activation of the coagulation system in *Streptococcus sanguis* endocarditis. *Infect. Immun.* **64:**5166–5170.

8. **Bayer, A. S., P. M. Sullam, M. Ramos, C. Li, A. L. Cheung, and M. R. Yeaman.** 1995. *Staphylococcus aureus* induces platelet aggregation via a fibrinogen-dependent mechanism which is independent of principal platelet glycoprotein IIb/IIIa fibrinogen-binding domains. *Infect. Immun.* **63:**3634–3641.

9. **Bayer, A. S., M. D. Ramos, B. E. Menzies, M. R. Yeaman, A. J. Shen, and A. L. Cheung.** 1997. Hyperproduction of alpha-toxin by *Staphylococcus aureus* results in paradoxically reduced virulence in experimental endocarditis: a host defense role for platelet microbicidal proteins. *Infect. Immun.* **65:**4652–4660.

10. **Bayer, A. S., D. Cheng, M. R. Yeaman, G. R. Corey, M. S. McClelland, L. J. Harrel, and V. G. Fowler, Jr.** 1998. In vitro resistance to thrombin-induced platelet microbicidal protein among clinical bacteremic isolates of *Staphylococcus aureus* correlates with an endovascular infectious source. *Antimicrob. Agents Chemother.* **42:**3169–3172.

11. **Bayer, A. S., A. F. Bolger, K. A. Taubert, W. Wilson, J. Steckelberg, A. W. Karchmer, M. Levison, H. F. Chambers, A. S. Dajani, M. H. Gurwitz, J. W. Newburger, et al.** 1998. Diagnosis and management of infective endocarditis. *Circulation* **98:**2936–2948.

12. **Bayer, A. S., S. N. Coulter, C. K. Stover, and W. R. Schwan.** 1999. Impact of the high-affinity proline permease gene (*putP*) on the virulence of *Staphylococcus aureus* in experimental endocarditis. *Infect. Immun.* **67:**740–744.

13. **Bochud, P. Y., T. Calandra, and P. Francioli.** 1994. Bacteremia due to viridans streptococci in neutropenic patients: a review. *Am. J. Med.* **97:**256–264.

14. **Buiting, A. G., J. Thompson, J. J. Emeis, H. Mattie, E. J. Brommer, and R. van Furth.** 1987. Effects of tissue-type plasminogen activator on *Staphylococcus epidermidis*-infected plasma clots as a model of infected endocardial vegetations. *J. Antimicrob. Chemother.* **19:**771–780.

15. **Burne, R. A., Y. Y. Chen, and J. E. Penders.** 1997. Analysis of gene expression in *Streptococcus mutans* in biofilms in vitro. *Adv. Dent. Res.* **11:**100–109.

16. **Byers, H. L., K. A. Homer, and D. Beighton.** 1996. Utilization of sialic acid by viridans streptococci. *J. Dent. Res.* **75:**1564–1571.

17. **Casadevall, A., and L.-A. Pirofski.** 1999. Host-pathogen interactions: redefining the basic concepts of virulence and pathogenicity. *Infect. Immun.* **67:**3703–3713.

18. **Cheung, A. L., C. C. Nast, and A. S. Bayer.** 1998. Selective activation of *sar* promoters with the use of green fluorescent protein transcriptional fusions as the detection system in the rabbit endocarditis model. *Infect. Immun.* **66:**5988–5993.

19. **Clawson, C. C., J. G. White, and M. C. Herzberg.** 1980. Platelet interaction with bacteria. VI. Contrasting the role of fibrinogen and fibronectin. *Am. J. Hematol.* **9:**43–53.

20. **Costerton, J. W., P. S. Stewart, and E. P. Greenberg.** 1999. Bacterial biofilms: a common cause of persistent infections. *Science* **284:**1318–1322.

21. **Coulter, S. N., W. R. Schwan, E. Y. Ng, M. H. Langhorne, H. D. Ritchie, S. Westbrock-Wadman, W. O. Hufnagle, K. R. Folger, A. S. Bayer, and C. K. Stover.** 1998. *Staphylococcus aureus* genetic loci impacting growth and survival in multiple infection environments. *Mol. Microbiol.* **30:**393–404.

22. **Cowles, J. W., S. L. Spitalnik, and N. Blumberg.** 1989. The fine specificity of Lewis blood group antibodies. Evidence for maturation of the immune response. *Vox Sang.* **56:**107–111.

23. **Crawford, I., and C. Russell.** 1986. Comparative adhesion of seven species of streptococci isolated from the blood of patients with sub-acute bacterial endocarditis to fibrin-platelet clots *in vitro*. *J. Appl. Bacteriol.* **60:**127–133.

24. **Danforth, J. M., R. M. Strieter, S. L. Kunkel, D. A. Arenberg, G. M. VanOtteren, and T. J. Standiford.** 1995. Macrophage inflammatory protein-1 alpha expression in vivo and in vitro: the role of lipoteichoic acid. *Clin. Immunol. Immunopathol.* **74:**77–83.

25. **Davies, D. G., M. R. Parsek, J. P. Pearson, B. H. Iglewski, J. W. Costerton, and E. P. Greenberg.** 1998. The involvement of cell-to-cell signals in the development of a bacterial biofilm. *Science* **280:**295–298.

26. **Demuth, D. R., Y. Duan, W. Brooks, A. R.**

Holmes, R. McNab, and H. F. Jenkinson. 1996. Tandem genes encode cell-surface polypeptides SspA and SspB which mediate adhesion of the oral bacterium *Streptococcus gordonii* to human and bacterial receptors. *Mol. Microbiol.* **20:** 403–413.

27. Derre, I., G. Rapoport, and T. Msadek. 1999. CtsR, a novel regulator of stress and heat shock response, controls *clp* and molecular chaperone gene expression in gram-positive bacteria. *Mol. Microbiol.* **31:**117–131.

28. Dhawan, V. K., A. S. Bayer, and M. R. Yeaman. 1998. In vitro resistance to thrombin-induced platelet microbicidal protein is associated with enhanced progression and hematogenous dissemination in experimental *Staphylococcus aureus* infective endocarditis. *Infect. Immun.* **66:** 3476–3479.

29. Douglas, C. W., P. R. Brown, and F. E. Preston. 1990. Platelet aggregation by oral streptococci. *FEMS Microbiol. Lett.* **60:**63–67.

30. Douglas, C. W., J. Heath, K. K. Hampton, and F. E. Preston. 1993. Identity of viridans streptococci isolated from cases of infective endocarditis. *J. Med. Microbiol.* **39:**179–182.

31. Drake, T. A., G. M. Rodgers, and M. A. Sande. 1984. Tissue factor is a major stimulus for vegetation formation in enterococcal endocarditis in rabbits. *J. Clin. Investig.* **73:**1750–1753.

32. Drake, T. A., and M. Pang. 1988. *Staphylococcus aureus* induces tissue factor expression in cultured human cardiac valve endothelium. *J. Infect. Dis.* **157:**749–756.

33. Drake, T. A., and M. Pang. 1989. Effects of interleukin-1, lipopolysaccharide, and streptococci on procoagulant activity of cultured human cardiac valve endothelial and stromal cells. *Infect. Immun.* **57:**507–512.

34. Drake, T. A., J. H. Morrissey, and T. S. Edgington. 1989. Selective cellular expression of tissue factor in human tissues. Implications for disorders of hemostasis and thrombosis. *Am. J. Pathol.* **134:**1087–1097.

35. Drangsholt, M. T. 1998. A new causal model of dental diseases associated with endocarditis. *Ann. Periodontol.* **3:**184–196.

36. Durack, D. T. 1975. Experimental bacterial endocarditis. IV. Structure and evolution of very early lesions. *J. Pathol.* **115:**81–89.

37. Durack, D. T. 1995. Prevention of infective endocarditis. *N. Engl. J. Med.* **332:**38–44.

38. Dyson, C., R. A. Barnes, and G. A. Harrison. 1999. Infective endocarditis: an epidemiological review of 128 episodes. *J. Infect.* **38:**87–93.

39. Edoute, Y., N. Haim, D. Rinkevich, B. Brenner, and S. A. Reisner. 1997. Cardiac valvular vegetations in cancer patients: a prospective echocardiographic study of 200 patients. *Am. J. Med.* **102:**252–258.

40. Elting, L. S., G. P. Bodey, and B. H. Keefe. 1992. Septicemia and shock syndrome due to viridans streptococci: a case-control study of predisposing factors. *Clin. Infect. Dis.* **14:**1201–1207.

41. Erickson, P. R., and M. C. Herzberg. 1987. A collagen-like immunodeterminant on the surface of *Streptococcus sanguis* induces platelet aggregation. *J. Immunol.* **138:**3360–3366.

42. Erickson, P. R., and M. C. Herzberg. 1990. Purification and partial characterization of a 65-kDa platelet aggregation-associated protein antigen from the surface of *Streptococcus sanguis*. *J. Biol. Chem.* **265:**14080–14087.

43. Erickson, P. R., and M. C. Herzberg. 1993. Evidence for the covalent linkage of carbohydrate polymers to a glycoprotein from *Streptococcus sanguis*. *J. Biol. Chem.* **268:**23780–23783.

44. Erickson, P. R., and M. C. Herzberg. 1993. The *Streptococcus sanguis* platelet aggregation-associated protein. Identification and characterization of the minimal platelet-interactive domain. *J. Biol. Chem.* **268:**1646–1649.

45. Erickson, P. R., and M. C. Herzberg. 1995. Altered expression of the platelet aggregation-associated protein from *Streptococcus sanguis* after growth in the presence of collagen. *Infect. Immun.* **63:**1084–1088.

46. Erickson, P. R., and M. C. Herzberg. 1999. Emergence of antibiotic resistant *Streptococcus sanguis* in dental plaque of children after frequent antibiotic therapy. *Pediatr. Dent.* **21:**181–185.

47. Erickson, P. R., M. C. Herzberg, and G. Tierney. 1992. Cross-reactive immunodeterminants on *Streptococcus sanguis* and collagen. Predicting a structural motif of platelet-interactive domains. *J. Biol. Chem.* **267:**10018–10023.

48. Ferguson, D. J., A. A. McColm, D. M. Ryan, and P. Acred. 1988. A morphological study of the effect of treatment with the antibiotic ceftazidime on experimental staphylococcal endocarditis and aortitis. *Br. J. Exp. Pathol.* **69:**551–561.

49. Ford, I., C. W. Douglas, F. E. Preson, A. Lawless, and K. K. Hampton. 1993. Mechanisms of platelet aggregation by *Streptococcus sanguis*, a causative organism in infective endocarditis. *Br. J. Haematol.* **84:**95–100.

50. Ford, I., C. W. Douglas, J. Heath, C. Rees, and F. E. Preston. 1996. Evidence for the involvement of complement proteins in platelet aggregation by *Streptococcus sanguis* NCTC 7863. *Br. J. Haematol.* **94:**729–739.

51. Ford, I., C. W. Douglas, D. Cox, D. G. Rees, J. Heath, and F. E. Preston. 1997. The role of immunoglobulin G and fibrinogen in platelet

aggregation by *Streptococcus sanguis*. *Br. J. Haematol.* **97**:737–746.

52. **Fukuda, Y., Y. Kuroiwa, H. Tabuchi, T. Ohshige, J. Sanada, Y. Minami, S. Takaoka, H. Kataoka, S. Furukawa, K. Miyahara, K. Nakamura, and S. Hashimoto.** 1982. A thrombotic tendency in patients with infective endocarditis. *Jpn. Circ. J.* **46**:460–467.

53. **Gong, K., D. Y. Wen, T. Ouyang, A. T. Rao, and M. C. Herzberg.** 1995. Platelet receptors for the *Streptococcus sanguis* adhesin and aggregation-associated antigens are distinguished by anti-idiotypical monoclonal antibodies. *Infect. Immun.* **63**:3628–3633.

54. **Gong, K., T. Ouyang, and M. C. Herzberg.** 1998. A streptococcal adhesion system for salivary pellicle and platelets. *Infect. Immun.* **66**: 5388–5392.

55. **Gutschik, E., S. Moller, and N. Christensen.** 1979. Experimental endocarditis in rabbits. 3. Significance of the proteolytic capacity of the infecting strains of *Streptococcus faecalis*. *Acta Pathol. Microbiol. Scand. Sect. B* **87**:353–362.

56. **Hausner, M., and S. Wuertz.** 1999. High rates of conjugation in bacterial biofilms as determined by quantitative in situ analysis. *Appl. Environ. Microbiol.* **65**:3710–3713.

57. **Havarstein, L. S., P. Gaustad, I. F. Nes, and D. A. Morrison.** 1996. Identification of the streptococcal competence-pheromone receptor. *Mol. Microbiol.* **21**:863–869.

58. **Havarstein, L. S., R. Hakenbeck, and P. Gaustad.** 1997. Natural competence in the genus *Streptococcus*: evidence that streptococci can change pherotype by interspecies recombinational exchanges. *J. Bacteriol.* **179**:6589–6594.

59. **Hazlett, K. R. O., J. E. Mazurkiewicz, and J. A. Banas.** 1999. Inactivation of the *gbpA* gene of *Streptococcus mutans* alters structural and functional aspects of plaque biofilm which are compensated by recombination of the *gtfB* and *gtfC* genes. *Infect. Immun.* **67**:3909–3914.

60. **Herzberg, M. C., and K. L. Brintzenhofe.** 1983. ADP-like platelet aggregation activity generated by viridans streptococci incubated with exogenous ATP. *Infect. Immun.* **40**:120–125.

61. **Herzberg, M. C., K. L. Brintzenhofe, and C. C. Clawson.** 1983. Aggregation of human platelets and adhesion of *Streptococcus sanguis*. *Infect. Immun.* **39**:1457–1469.

62. **Herzberg, M. C., K. L. Brintzenhofe, and C. C. Clawson.** 1983. Cell-free released components of *Streptococcus sanguis* inhibit human platelet aggregation. *Infect. Immun.* **42**:394–401.

63. **Herzberg, M. C., K. Gong, G. D. MacFarlane, P. R. Erickson, A. H. Soberay, P. H. Krebsbach, G. Manjula, K. Schilling, and W. H. Bowen.** 1990. Phenotypic characterization of *Streptococcus sanguis* virulence factors associated with bacterial endocarditis. *Infect. Immun.* **58**: 515–522.

64. **Herzberg, M. C., P. R. Erickson, P. K. Kane, D. J. Clawson, C. C. Clawson, and F. A. Hoff.** 1990. Platelet-interactive products of *Streptococcus sanguis* protoplasts. *Infect. Immun.* **58**: 4117–4125.

65. **Herzberg, M. C., G. D. MacFarlane, K. Gong, N. N. Armstrong, A. R. Witt, P. R. Erickson, and M. W. Meyer.** 1992. The platelet interactivity phenotype of *Streptococcus sanguis* influences the course of experimental endocarditis. *Infect. Immun.* **60**:4809–4818.

66. **Herzberg, M. C., L. K. Krishnan, and G. D. MacFarlane.** 1993. Involvement of alpha 2-adrenoreceptors and G proteins in the modulation of platelet secretion in response to *Streptococcus sanguis*. *Crit. Rev. Oral Biol. Med.* **4**:435–442.

67. **Herzberg, M. C.** 1996. Platelet-streptococcal interactions in endocarditis. *Crit. Rev. Oral Biol. Med.* **7**:222–236.

68. **Herzberg, M. C., M. W. Meyer, A. Kiliç, and L. Tao.** 1997. Host-pathogen interactions in bacterial endocarditis: streptococcal virulence in the host. *Adv. Dent. Res.* **11**:69–74.

69. **Hienz, S. A., T. Schennings, A. Heimdahl, and J. I. Flock.** 1996. Collagen binding of *Staphylococcus aureus* is a virulence factor in experimental endocarditis. *J. Infect. Dis.* **174**:83–88.

70. **Hirota, K., H. Kanitani, K. Nemoto, T. Ono, and Y. Miyake.** 1995. Cross-reactivity between human sialyl Lewis(x) oligosaccharide and common causative oral bacteria of infective endocarditis. *FEMS Immunol. Med. Microbiol.* **12**:159–164.

71. **Homer, K. A., S. Kelley, J. Hawkes, D. Beighton, and M. C. Grootveld.** 1996. Metabolism of glycoprotein-derived sialic acid and N-acetylglucosamine by *Streptococcus oralis*. *Microbiology* **142**:1221–1230.

72. **Huebner, J., and D. A. Goldmann.** 1999. Coagulase-negative staphylococci: role as pathogens. *Annu. Rev. Med.* **50**:223–236.

73. **Ikeda, K., K. Nagasawa, T. Horiuchi, T. Tsuru, H. Nishizaka, and Y. Niho.** 1997. C5a induces tissue factor activity on endothelial cells. *Thromb. Haemost.* **77**:394–398.

74. **Jenkinson, H. F., R. A. Baker, and G. W. Tannock.** 1996. A binding-lipoprotein-dependent oligopeptide transport system in *Streptococcus gordonii* essential for uptake of hexa- and heptapeptides. *J. Bacteriol.* **178**:68–77.

75. **Jiang, Y., L. Magli, and M. Russo.** 1999. Bacterium-dependent induction of cytokines in mononuclear cells and their pathologic consequences in vivo. *Infect. Immun.* **67**:2125–2130.

76. **Juarez, Z. E., and M. W. Stinson.** 1999. An extracellular protease of *Streptococcus gordonii* hydrolyzes type IV collagen and collagen analogues. *Infect. Immun.* **67**:271–278.

77. **Kessler, C. M., E. Nussbaum, and C. U. Tuazon.** 1987. In vitro correlation of platelet aggregation with occurrence of disseminated intravascular coagulation and subacute bacterial endocarditis. *J. Lab. Clin. Med.* **109**:647–652.

78. **Kiliç, A. O., M. C. Herzberg, M. W. Meyer, X. Zhao, and L. Tao.** 1999. Streptococcal reporter gene-fusion vector for identification of in vivo expressed genes. *Plasmid* **42**:67–72.

79. **Kleerebezem, M., L. E. Quadri, O. P. Kuipers, and W. M. de Vos.** 1997. Quorum sensing by peptide pheromones and two-component signal-transduction systems in Gram-positive bacteria. *Mol. Microbiol.* **24**:895–904.

80. **Kupferwasser, I., H. Darius, A. M. Muller, S. Mohr-Kahaly, T. Westermeier, H. Oelert, R. Erbel, and J. Meyer.** 1998. Clinical and morphological characteristics in *Streptococcus bovis* endocarditis: a comparison with other causative microorganisms in 177 cases. *Heart* **80**:276–280.

81. **Kupferwasser, L. I., G. Hafner, S. Mohr-Kahaly, R. Erbel, J. Meyer, and H. Darius.** 1999. The presence of infection-related antiphospholipid antibodies in infective endocarditis determines a major risk factor for embolic events. *J. Am. Coll. Cardiol.* **33**:1365–1371.

82. **Kupferwasser, L. I., M. R. Yeaman, S. M. Shapiro, C. C. Nast, P. M. Sullam, S. G. Filler, and A. S. Bayer.** 1999. Acetylsalicylic acid reduces vegetation bacterial density, hematogenous bacterial dissemination, and frequency of embolic events in experimental *Staphylococcus aureus* endocarditis through antiplatelet and antibacterial effects. *Circulation* **99**:2791–2797.

83. **Kurland, S., E. Enghoff, J. Landelius, S. O. Nystrom, A. Hambraeus, and G. Friman.** 1999. A 10-year retrospective study of infective endocarditis at a university hospital with special regard to the timing of surgical evaluation in *S. viridans* endocarditis. *Scand. J. Infect. Dis.* **31**:87–91.

84. **Lawson, C. A., S. D. Yan, S. F. Yan, H. Liao, Y. S. Zhou, J. Sobel, W. Kisiel, D. M. Stern, and D. J. Pinsky.** 1997. Monocytes and tissue factor promote thrombosis in a murine model of oxygen deprivation. *J. Clin. Investig.* **99**:1729–1738.

85. **Lee, J. C., J. S. Park, S. E. Shepherd, V. Carey, and A. Fattom.** 1997. Protective efficacy of antibodies to the *Staphylococcus aureus* type 5 capsular polysaccharide in a modified model of endocarditis in rats. *Infect. Immun.* **65**:4146–4151.

86. **Levi, M., and H. ten Cate.** 1999. Disseminated intravascular coagulation. *N. Engl. J. Med.* **341**:586–592.

87. **Libman, H., and R. D. Arbeit.** 1984. Complications associated with *Staphylococcus aureus* bacteremia. *Arch. Intern. Med.* **144**:541–545.

88. **Lunsford, R. D., and J. London.** 1996. Natural genetic transformation in *Streptococcus gordonii*: *comX* imparts competence on strain wicky. *J. Bacteriol.* **178**:5831–5835.

89. **Lunsford, R. D., and A. G. Roble.** 1997. *comYA*, a gene similar to *comGA* of *Bacillus subtilis*, is essential for competence factor-dependent DNA transformation in *Streptococcus gordonii*. *J. Bacteriol.* **179**:3122–3126.

90. **MacFarlane, G. D., D. E. Sampson, D. J. Clawson, C. C. Clawson, K. L. Kelly, and M. C. Herzberg.** 1994. Evidence for an ecto-ATPase on the cell wall of *Streptococcus sanguis*. *Oral Microbiol. Immunol.* **9**:180–185.

91. **Manganelli, R., and I. van de Rijn.** 1999. Characterization of *emb*, a gene encoding the major adhesin of *Streptococcus defectivus*. *Infect. Immun.* **67**:50–56.

92. **Manning, J. E., E. B. Hume, N. Hunter, and K. W. Knox.** 1994. An appraisal of the virulence factors associated with streptococcal endocarditis. *J. Med. Microbiol.* **40**:110–114.

93. **Mayo, J. A., H. Zhu, D. W. Harty, and K. W. Knox.** 1995. Modulation of glycosidase and protease activities by chemostat growth conditions in an endocarditis strain of *Streptococcus sanguis*. *Oral Microbiol. Immunol.* **10**:342–348.

94. **McNab, R., H. F. Jenkinson, D. M. Loach, and G. W. Tannock.** 1994. Cell-surface-associated polypeptides CshA and CshB of high molecular mass are colonization determinants in the oral bacterium *Streptococcus gordonii*. *Mol. Microbiol.* **14**:743–754.

95. **McNab, R., and H. F. Jenkinson.** 1998. Altered adherence properties of a *Streptococcus gordonii* *hppA* (oligopeptide permease) mutant result from transcriptional effects on *cshA* adhesin gene expression. *Microbiology* **144**:127–136.

96. **McNab, R., H. Forbes, P. S. Handley, D. M. Loach, G. W. Tannock, and H. F. Jenkinson.** 1999. Cell wall-anchored CshA polypeptide (259 kilodaltons) in *Streptococcus gordonii* forms surface fibrils that confer hydrophobic and adhesive properties. *J. Bacteriol.* **181**:3087–3095.

97. **Meddens, M. J., J. Thompson, H. Mattie, and R. van Furth.** 1984. Role of granulocytes in the prevention and therapy of experimental *Streptococcus sanguis* endocarditis in rabbits. *Antimicrob. Agents Chemother.* **25**:263–267.

98. **Meddens, M. J., J. Thompson, W. C. Bauer, and R. van Furth.** 1984. Role of granulocytes

and monocytes in experimental *Escherichia coli* endocarditis. *Infect. Immun.* **43**:491–496.

99. **Meddens, M. J., J. Thompson, H. Mattie, and R. van Furth.** 1985. Role of granulocytes and monocytes in the prevention and therapy of experimental *Staphylococcus epidermidis* endocarditis in rabbits. *J. Infect.* **11**:41–50.

100. **Mercer, D. K., K. P. Scott, W. A. Bruce-Johnson, L. A. Glover, and H. J. Flint.** 1999. Fate of free DNA and transformation of the oral bacterium *Streptococcus gordonii* DL1 by plasmid DNA in human saliva. *Appl. Environ. Microbiol.* **65**:6–10.

101. **Meyer, M. W., A. R. Witt, L. K. Krishnan, M. Yokota, M. J. Roszkowski, J. D. Rudney, and M. C. Herzberg.** 1995. Therapeutic advantage of recombinant human plasminogen activator in endocarditis: evidence from experiments in rabbits. *Thromb. Haemost.* **73**:680–682.

102. **Michiels, M. J., and M. G. Bergeron.** 1996. Differential increased survival of staphylococci and limited ultrastructural changes in the core of infected fibrin clots after daptomycin administration. *Antimicrob. Agents Chemother.* **40**:203–211.

103. **Munro, C. L., and F. L. Macrina.** 1993. Sucrose-derived exopolysaccharides of *Streptococcus mutans* V403 contribute to infectivity in endocarditis. *Mol. Microbiol.* **8**:133–142.

104. **Nakanishi K., F. Tajima, Y. Nakata, H. Osada, K. Ogata, T. Kawai, C. Torikata, T. Suga, K. Takishima, T. Aurues, and T. Ikeda.** 1998. Tissue factor is associated with the nonbacterial thrombotic endocarditis induced by a hypobaric hypoxic environment in rats. *Virchows Arch.* **433**:375–379.

105. **Ni Eidhin, D., S. Perkins, P. Francois, P. Vaudaux, M. Hook, and T. J. Foster.** 1998. Clumping factor B (ClfB), a new surface-located fibrinogen-binding adhesin of *Staphylococcus aureus*. *Mol. Microbiol.* **30**:245–257.

106. **O'Connor, D. T., M. H. Weisman, and J. Fierer.** 1978. Activation of the alternate complement pathway in *Staphylococcus aureus* infective endocarditis and its relationship to thrombocytopenia, coagulation abnormalities, and acute glomerulonephritis. *Clin. Exp. Immunol.* **34**:179–187.

107. **Olaison, L., H. Hogevik, and K. Alestig.** 1997. Fever, C-reactive protein, and other acute-phase reactants during treatment of infective endocarditis. *Arch. Intern. Med.* **157**:885–892.

108. **O'Toole, G. A., and R. Kolter.** 1998. Flagellar and twitching motility are necessary for *Pseudomonas aeruginosa* biofilm development. *Mol. Microbiol.* **30**:295–304.

109. **Parry, G. C., J. H. Erlich, P. Carmeliet, T.**

Luther, and N. Mackman. 1998. Low levels of tissue factor are compatible with development and hemostasis in mice. *J. Clin. Investig.* **101**:560–569.

110. **Pearson, J. P., C. Van Delden, and B. H. Iglewski.** 1999. Active efflux and diffusion are involved in transport of *Pseudomonas aeruginosa* cell-to-cell signals. *J. Bacteriol.* **181**:1203–1210.

111. **Rohmann, S., R. Erbel, H. Darius, G. Gorge, T. Makowski, R. Zotz, S. Mohr-Kahaly, U. Nixdorff, M. Drexler, and J. Meyer.** 1991. Prediction of rapid versus prolonged healing of infective endocarditis by monitoring vegetation size. *J. Am. Soc. Echocardiogr.* **4**:465–474.

112. **Rohmann, S., R. Erbel, H. Darius, T. Makowski, P. Jensen, T. Fischer, and J. Meyer.** 1992. Spontaneous echo contrast imaging in infective endocarditis: a predictor of complications? *Int. J. Card. Imaging* **8**:197–207.

113. **Rosenberg, R. D., and W. C. Aird.** 1999. Vascular-bed-specific hemostasis and hypercoagulable states. *N. Engl. J. Med.* **340**:1555–1564.

114. **Schlievert, P. M., P. J. Gahr, A. P. Assimacopoulos, M. M. Dinges, J. A. Stoehr, J. W. Harmala, H. Hirt, and G. M. Dunny.** 1998. Aggregation and binding substances enhance pathogenicity in rabbit models of *Enterococcus faecalis* endocarditis. *Infect. Immun.* **66**:218–223.

115. **Schwan, W. R., S. N. Coulter, E. Y. Ng, M. H. Langhorne, H. D. Ritchie, L. L. Brody, S. Westbrock-Wadman, A. S. Bayer, K. R. Folger, and C. K. Stover.** 1998. Identification and characterization of the PutP proline permease that contributes to in vivo survival of *Staphylococcus aureus* in animal models. *Infect. Immun.* **66**:567–572.

116. **Semeraro, N., and M. Colucci.** 1997. Tissue factor in health and disease. *Thromb. Haemost.* **78**:759–764.

117. **Shapiro, J. A.** 1998. Thinking about bacterial populations as multicellular organisms. *Annu. Rev. Microbiol.* **52**:81–104.

118. **Soberay, A. H., M. C. Herzberg, J. D. Rudney, H. K. Nieuwenhuis, J. J. Sixma, and U. Seligsohn.** 1987. Responses of platelets to strains of *Streptococcus sanguis*: findings in healthy subjects, Bernard-Soulier, Glanzmann's, and collagen-unresponsive patients. *Thromb. Haemost.* **57**:222–225.

119. **Sommer, P., C. Gleyzal, S. Guerret, J. Etienne, and J. A. Grimaud.** 1992. Induction of a putative laminin-binding protein of *Streptococcus gordonii* in human infective endocarditis. *Infect. Immun.* **60**:360–365.

120. **Soto, A., P. H. McWhinney, C. C. Kibbler, and J. Cohen.** 1998. Cytokine release and mito-

genic activity in the viridans streptococcal shock syndrome. *Cytokine* **10**:370–376.

121. **Strom, B. L., E. Abrutyn, J. A. Berlin, J. L. Kinman, R. S. Feldman, P. D. Stolley, M. E. Levison, O. M. Korzeniowski, and D. Kaye.** 1998. Dental and cardiac risk factors for infective endocarditis. A population-based, case-control study. *Ann. Intern. Med.* **129**:761–769.

122. **Sullam, P. M., F. H. Valone, and J. Mills.** 1987. Mechanisms of platelet aggregation by viridans group streptococci. *Infect. Immun.* **55**:1743–1750.

123. **Sullam, P. M., G. A. Jarvis, and F. H. Valone.** 1988. Role of immunoglobulin G in platelet aggregation by viridans group streptococci. *Infect. Immun.* **56**:2907–2911.

124. **Sullam, P. M., A. S. Bayer, W. M. Foss, and A. L. Cheung.** 1996. Diminished platelet binding in vitro by *Staphylococcus aureus* is associated with reduced virulence in a rabbit model of infective endocarditis. *Infect. Immun.* **64**:4915–4921.

125. **Sullam, P. M., W. C. Hyun, J. Szollosi, J. F. Dong, W. M. Foss, and J. A. Lopez.** 1998. Physical proximity and functional interplay of the glycoprotein Ib-IX-V complex and the Fc receptor FcgammaRIIA on the platelet plasma membrane. *J. Biol. Chem.* **273**:5331–5336.

126. **Taha, T. H., S. Durrant, J. Crick, S. Bowcock, A. Bradshaw, and C. M. Oakley.** 1991. Hemostatic studies in patients with infective endocarditis: a report on nine consecutive cases with evidence of coagulopathy. *Heart Vessels* **6**:102–106.

127. **Valtonen, V., A. Kuikka, and J. Syrjanen.** 1993. Thrombo-embolic complications in bacteraemic infections. *Eur. Heart J.* **14**(Suppl. K):20–23.

128. **Viscount, H. B., C. L. Munro, D. Burnette-Curley, D. L. Peterson, and F. L. Macrina.** 1997. Immunization with FimA protects against *Streptococcus parasanguis* endocarditis in rats. *Infect. Immun.* **65**:994–1002.

129. **Vuille, C., M. Nidorf, A. E. Weyman, and M. H. Picard.** 1994. Natural history of vegetations during successful medical treatment of endocarditis. *Am. Heart J.* **128**:1200–1209.

130. **Watson, S. P., and J. Gibbins.** 1998. Collagen receptor signaling in platelets: extending the role of the ITAM. *Immunol. Today* **19**:260–264.

131. **Wells, A. U., C. C. Fowler, R. B. Ellis-Pegler, R. Luke, S. Hannan, and D. N. Sharpe.** 1990. Endocarditis in the 80s in a general hospital in Auckland, New Zealand. *Q. J. Med.* **76**:753–762.

132. **Whatmore, A. M., V. A. Barcus, and C. G. Dowson.** 1999. Genetic diversity of the streptococcal competence (*com*) gene locus. *J. Bacteriol.* **181**:3144–3154.

133. **Wu, T., M. R. Yeaman, and A. S. Bayer.** 1994. In vitro resistance to platelet microbicidal protein correlates with endocarditis source among bacteremic staphylococcal and streptococcal isolates. *Antimicrob. Agents Chemother.* **38**:729–732.

134. **Yeaman, M. R., D. C. Norman, and A. S. Bayer.** 1992. *Staphylococcus aureus* susceptibility to thrombin-induced platelet microbicidal protein is independent of platelet adherence and aggregation in vitro. *Infect. Immun.* **60**:2368–2374.

OSTEOMYELITIS

M. E. Shirtliff and J. T. Mader

19

Osteomyelitis is defined as inflammation of the bone marrow and adjacent tissue; it is nearly always caused by bacterial infection. Persistence in osteomyelitis infection can take two forms: a chronic infection, in which living bacteria can be isolated from biopsy samples, and a latent, quiescent infection, in which biopsy does not readily detect living bacteria. Chronic osteomyelitis denotes infection of the bone in which multiple therapeutic attempts to eradicate the infection have failed. The classification of osteomyelitis as acute or chronic is often made clinically based on the duration of the infection. Recently, the duration of infection that defines chronicity has decreased significantly. Therefore, symptoms continuing for only 10 days can indicate a chronic infection (60). Chronic osteomyelitis is found mostly in adults and usually involves the axial, or long, bones, vertebral bodies and adjacent disks, and the small bones of the feet (115). The presence of infected necrotic bone surrounded by an envelope of infected soft tissue is the hallmark of chronic osteomyelitis (21). The terms acute and chronic, while useful concepts in denoting the onset of infection, are ambiguous in describing other aspects of the infection. Typically, chronic osteomyelitis is a more refractory infection and is often more difficult to eradicate. Aggressive debridement, dead-space management, and prolonged antibiotic therapy are necessary to resolve the infection.

Persistence may also take the form of a latent, quiescent infection that may reactivate years after apparently successful treatment of the disease. If the patient suffers trauma in the involved area and/or the host response to the infection is suppressed, the organism(s) may again proliferate and lead to an exacerbation of the infection. Therefore, in osteomyelitis treatment the infection is said to be "arrested" rather than "cured."

Normal bone is highly resistant to infection, which occurs only as a result of a very large organism inoculation, trauma leading to bone damage, or the presence of foreign bodies. Different types of osteomyelitis can be classified according to the source of the infection (i.e., hematogenous or contiguous focus) and the vascular capability of the host (i.e., with or without generalized vascular insufficiency).

Once the bone is colonized and an active acute infection occurs, the infection may resolve, may become a quiescent, persistent in-

M. E. Shirtliff, Department of Microbiology and Immunology, The University of Texas Medical Branch, Galveston, TX 77555-1115. J. T. Mader, The Marine Biomedical Institute and Division of Marine Medicine, Department of Internal Medicine, The University of Texas Medical Branch, Galveston, TX 77555-1115.

Persistent Bacterial Infections, Edited by J. P. Nataro, M. J. Blaser, and S. Cunningham-Rundles, © 2000 ASM Press, Washington, D.C.

fection, or may become a chronic infection with associated progressive bone deterioration. The balance among the outcomes of these infections is determined by properties of and interactions between the pathogenic microorganism and the host. Virulence determinants of the organisms, underlying disease, the use of implanted medical devices, the immune status of the host, and the type and location of the bone are some of the important factors.

TYPES OF OSTEOMYELITIS

Primary and Secondary Hematogenous Osteomyelitis

Hematogenous osteomyelitis can be divided into primary and secondary types. Primary hematogenous osteomyelitis is caused by direct seeding of bone by a bacterial species in the blood. Although found in adults, it is more predominant in infants and children, with 85% of cases occurring in patients less than 17 years of age (115). Hematogenous osteomyelitis accounts for 20% of the total cases of osteomyelitis. Recent studies have documented a decline in hematogenous osteomyelitis, especially in children, possibly due partly to the large reduction in osteomyelitis from *Haemophilus influenzae* brought about by the modern vaccination program (11, 28). In children, the bone infection usually affects the long bones, while in adults, the lesion is usually located in the thoracic or lumbar vertebrae (115). Secondary hematogenous infection is the more common presentation in adults. This represents more of a persistent-latent state, i.e., the reactivation of a quiescent focus of hematogenous osteomyelitis initially developed and arrested in infancy or childhood. Due to the abundant vascular supply, the most common sites of hematogenous osteomyelitis are the metaphyses of tubular bones. Hematogenous osteomyelitis is more common in males of any age (94). The major types of hematogenous osteomyelitis seen clinically include long-bone and vertebral osteomyelitis.

LONG-BONE HEMATOGENOUS OSTEOMYELITIS

The metaphyses of the long bones (tibia and femur) are most frequently involved in osteomyelitis (M. E. Shirtliff, M. W. Cripps, and J. T. Mader, *Abstr. 99th Gen. Meet. Am. Soc. Microbiol.*, abstr. C-410, 1999); the anatomy of the metaphyseal region seems to explain this clinical localization (108). The nutrient artery ends in the metaphyses as narrow capillaries that make sharp loops near the growth plate and enter a system of large venous sinusoids, where the blood flow becomes slow and turbulent. These capillary loops are essentially the "end artery" branches of the nutrient artery. This structure leads to a slowing of blood flow in the area and presumably allows bacteria to settle and initiate an inflammatory response. The histology of the region may also contribute. The metaphyseal capillaries lack phagocytic lining cells, and the sinusoidal veins contain functionally inactive phagocytic cells (46). This allows further growth of microorganisms. Any end capillary obstruction could lead to an area of avascular necrosis. Minor trauma probably predisposes the infant or child to infection by producing a small hematoma, vascular obstruction, and a subsequent bone necrosis that is susceptible to inoculation from a transient bacteremia. Acute infection initially produces a local cellulitis that results in a breakdown of leukocytes, increased bone pressure, decreased pH, and decreased oxygen tension. The cumulative effects of these physiological factors further compromise the medullary circulation and enhance the spread of infection. Infection may proceed laterally through the Haversian and Volkmann canal system, perforate the bony cortex, and lift the periosteum from the surface of the bone. When this occurs in the presence of medullary extension, the periosteal and endosteal circulations are compromised; capillaries are lost, and large segments of cortical and cancellous bone die. In infants, medullary infection may spread to the epiphysis and joint surfaces through capillaries that cross the growth plate (51). In the child over 1 year of age, the growth plate is avascular and the infection is confined to the metaphysis and diaphysis. The joint is spared unless the metaphysis is intracapsular. Thus, cortical perforation at the proximal radius, humerus, or femur enables the infection to migrate to the elbow, shoulder, or hip joint, regardless of the age of the patient.

A single pathogenic species is almost always recovered from the bone. Polymicrobial hematogenous osteomyelitis is rare (114–116). In infants, *Staphylococcus aureus*, *Streptococcus agalactiae*, and *Escherichia coli* are the most frequently recovered bone isolates, while in the child, *S. aureus*, *Streptococcus pyogenes*, and *H. influenzae* are the most common organisms isolated. After the age of 4, the incidence of *H. influenzae* osteomyelitis decreases. However, the overall incidence of *H. influenzae* as a cause of osteomyelitis is decreasing because of the new *H. influenzae* vaccine now given to children (11, 24). In adults, *S. aureus* is the most common organism isolated (Shirtliff et al., *Abstr. 99th Gen. Meet. Am. Soc. Microbiol.*).

Infants and children have clinically different presentations of osteomyelitis. Neonatal osteomyelitis is characterized by systemic and local findings (50). Local findings include decreased motion of a limb and edema. A joint effusion adjacent to the area of bone infection is present in 60 to 70% of cases. Classically, infants with hematogenous osteomyelitis present with abrupt fever, irritability, lethargy, and local signs of inflammation 3 weeks or less in duration (51). However, at least 50% of older children present with vague complaints, including pain in the involved limb 1 to 3 months in duration and minimal temperature elevation. Infants and children with hematogenous osteomyelitis usually have normal soft tissue enveloping the infected bone and are capable of a very efficient metabolic response to infection. They also have the potential to absorb large sequestra and generate a significant periosteal response to the infection. This feature leads to substantial formation of bone, called an involucrum, at the margin of the infection. The involucrum affords skeletal continuity and maintains function during the healing phase. If antimicrobial therapy directed at the responsible pathogen is begun prior to extensive bone necrosis, there is an excellent probability of an arrest of the infection.

Hematogenous osteomyelitis is also found in the adult population. Adults usually present with vague complaints of nonspecific pain in the area of infection and a few constitutional symptoms 1 to 3 months in duration (115). However, acute clinical presentations of fever, chills, swelling, and erythema over the involved bone are occasionally seen. The clinical signs resulting from soft tissue extension often dominate the clinical findings at presentation and can lead to inappropriate diagnostic and therapeutic measures unless the clinical suspicion of an osseous etiology is entertained. In long bones, the infection usually begins in the diaphysis but may spread to involve the entire medullary canal. Extension into the epiphysis and joint space may occur because the growth plate has disappeared and the medullary areas are contiguous. As the periosteum is firmly adherent to the bone, cortical penetration usually leads to a soft-tissue abscess. Subperiosteal abscesses and massive cortical devitalization rarely occur. In time, sinus tracts connecting the sequestered nidus of infection to the skin via soft-tissue extension may form.

In chronic hematogenous osteomyelitis, the existing cortex is usually viable. The involucrum contains the sequestered, necrotic marrow and endosteal bone. Sequestra are often found within the thickened cortex and are surrounded by reactive bone and chronic granulations. These sequestered, lamellar fragments are rarely responsible for an acute exacerbation of infection but can support a progressive compromise of ischemic soft tissues that results in chronic ulceration and drainage.

VERTEBRAL OSTEOMYELITIS

Vertebral osteomyelitis in the adult population is usually hematogenous in origin but may be secondary to trauma. A history of urinary tract infection or intravenous drug abuse often is present. An early involvement of the anterior-inferior edge of the vertebral body suggests spread from the bony entrance of the anterior spinal artery (22, 121). Retrograde infection via Batson's venous plexus is also postulated (7). The segmental arteries supplying the vertebrae usually bifurcate to supply two adjacent bony segments. Therefore, the disease usually involves two adjacent vertebrae and the intervertebral disc.

The lumbar region is affected in at least 50% of cases of hematogenous vertebral osteomyelitis, followed by the thoracic spine (35%) and the cervical spine (20%) (96). However, in intravenous drug abusers, the cervical vertebrae are involved much more often (27%) and the thoracic vertebrae much less frequently (4.5%).

In vertebral osteomyelitis, polymorphonuclear leukocytes are present due to the acute inflammatory response. The enzymes released from disintegrating polymorphonuclear leukocytes, bacterial products, and vascular ischemia can cause an extension of the infection into the cartilaginous end plate, disk, and/or adjacent areas. Posterior extension of the infection may lead to epidural and subdural abscesses or even to meningitis. Extension anteriorly or laterally may lead to paravertebral, retropharyngeal, mediastinal, subphrenic, or retroperitoneal abscesses. Also, spread to adjacent vertebral bodies may occur rapidly through the rich venous networks in the spine.

As elsewhere, vertebral osteomyelitis is usually monomicrobial when it is hematogenous in origin (94). In the normal host, *S. aureus* remains the most commonly isolated organism. However, aerobic gram-negative rods are often found when the urinary tract is the source of infection, as well as among intravenous drug users. *Pseudomonas aeruginosa* and *Serratia marcescens* have high incidences among intravenous drug users (47, 94). Vertebral osteomyelitis secondary to a contiguous focus is usually a polymicrobial infection in which anaerobes are often isolated. Other sources of infection include the genitourinary tract, skin and soft tissue, respiratory tract, infected intravenous-injection site, endocarditis, dental infection, and unknown sources (95). Positive cultures are very important for diagnosis, since other conditions, such as trauma and vertebral collapse, may simulate infection.

Clinically, the patient usually presents with vague symptoms and signs consisting of dull, constant back pain and spasm of the paravertebral muscles (95). Localized pain and tenderness of the involved bone segments are present in at least 90% of cases. The pain is usually insidious and slowly progresses over 3 weeks to 3 months. Chronic vertebral osteomyelitis arises most often in those patients that have predisposing factors, such as the use of nonsterile injection techniques by intravenous drug abusers, previous spinal surgery, or implanted hardware.

Contiguous-Focus Osteomyelitis without Generalized Vascular Insufficiency

In the past, chronic osteomyelitis resulting from acute penetrating trauma has been referred to as contiguous-focus osteomyelitis (115). Although the term contiguous focus implies that the infection is caused by an adjacent soft-tissue infection, chronic contiguous-focus osteomyelitis can also begin as an acute infection, with the organisms being directly inoculated into the bone at the time of trauma. The organisms can also be spread by nosocomial contamination during pre- or intraoperative procedures. Osteomyelitis secondary to contiguous foci of infection accounts for at least half of all cases (115). Two recent studies have documented a decline in hematogenous osteomyelitis accompanied by a rise in contiguous disease (28). In age distribution, contiguous-focus osteomyelitis is biphasic. The infection occurs in younger persons secondary to trauma and related surgery and in older adults secondary to surgical procedures and decubitus ulcers.

In contrast to hematogenous osteomyelitis, in contiguous-focus osteomyelitis multiple pathogenic species are usually isolated from the infected bone. *S. aureus* and coagulase-negative staphylococci account for 75% of the bacterial isolates (68). However, gram-negative bacilli and anaerobic organisms are frequently isolated. The infection usually manifests within 1 month after inoculation of the organisms by trauma, surgery, or a soft-tissue infection. Patients usually present with low-grade fever, pain, and drainage.

A common complication associated with this type of osteomyelitis is that debridement may result in bony defects ranging in severity from an infected nonunion to segmental bone loss. This often compromises bone stability, which must be restored with fixation devices before functional recovery can occur. The frequency of bone stability loss, bone necrosis, and soft-tissue damage make this form of osteomyelitis difficult to treat. Even after years of apparent eradication of an osteomyelitis infection, success is not assured. A quiescent focus of bacteria can be reactivated years later and cause a recurrence of infection.

In chronic osteomyelitis, there are usually large areas of devitalized cortical and cancellous bone within the wound. The dead areas must be completely debrided, including devitalized scar tissue, marrow, and cortex. The soft tissue covering the area of bone trauma must heal. If healing does not occur, the existing infection will persist or a new infection could form. Compromise of local soft tissue is a major reason for continued drainage.

Contiguous-Focus Osteomyelitis with Generalized Vascular Insufficiency

The presence of general vascular insufficiency makes appropriate therapy and management of chronic contiguous-focus osteomyelitis difficult. Most patients in this category have diabetes mellitus (15). The small bones of the feet, the talus, the calcaneus and distal fibula, and the tibia are commonly involved in this category of infection. Usually, the infection is initiated by minor trauma of the feet, such as infected nail beds, cellulitis, or a trophic skin ulceration. The patients in this group usually range from 35 to 70 years of age. Multiple organisms are found in patients with diabetic foot osteomyelitis, including *S. aureus*, coagulase-negative *Staphylococcus* spp., *Streptococcus* spp., *Enterococcus* spp., gram-negative bacilli, and anaerobes (15). Aerobic gram-negative bacilli are usually a part of mixed infection (15).

Osteomyelitis in vascularly compromised patients can be difficult to diagnose. The patient may present with an ingrown toenail, a perforating foot ulcer, cellulitis, or a deep space infection. Concurrent peripheral neuropathy mutes the patient's perception of pain. Fever and systemic toxicity are often absent. Examination shows decreased dorsal pedis and posterior tibia pulses, poor capillary refill, and decreased sensation. Although arrest of the infection is desirable, a more attainable treatment goal is to suppress the infection and maintain the functional integrity of the involved limb. Debridement and ablation are often necessary to treat the infection. The underlying host disorders (diabetes, poor nutrition, or peripheral vascular disease) optimally should be treated prior to surgery. The refractory nature of this kind of infection often leads to recurrent bone infections, even after appropriate therapy. Resection of the infected bone is almost always necessary.

Malignant external otitis, also called necrotizing external otitis, is an unusual but potentially fatal infection that may occur in elderly diabetics. The treatment consists of local debridement of the external auditory canal granulation tissue and an aggressive course of intravenous antibiotics, administered for at least 4 to 6 weeks (30). Since most of these infections are caused by *Pseudomonas* spp., the initial broad-spectrum antibiotic regimen should cover this bacterial genus (30). If necessary, the antibiotic regimen can be adjusted after culture results from samples obtained during debridement and subsequent antibiotic sensitivity results. With aggressive therapy, the cure rate has been found to be between 74 and 91% (53). Surgical intervention is currently used only as a last resort. Monitoring the response to therapy is best done with serial computed tomography or gallium-indium scans (99).

Once the bone is colonized and an active acute infection occurs, the infection may resolve, may become a quiescent persistent infection, or may become a chronic infection with

TABLE 1 Systemic and local factors that affect immune surveillance, metabolism, and local vascularity

Factor[a]
Systemic
Diabetes mellitus
Renal or hepatic failure
Malnutrition
Chronic hypoxia
Immunosuppression or immune deficiency
Malignancy
Immune disease
Extremes of age
CGD
Local
Major-vessel compromise
Small- and medium-vessel disease
Extensive scarring
Arteritis
Radiation fibrosis
Chronic lymphedema
Venous stasis
Neuropathy
Tobacco abuse ($\geq$2 packs per day)

associated bone deterioration. The balance among these outcomes is determined by properties of and interactions between the pathogenic microorganism and the host.

PROPERTIES OF THE HOST IN OSTEOMYELITIS

Clinically and histologically, acute osteomyelitis blends into chronic disease. Pathological features of chronic osteomyelitis are the presence of necrotic bone, the formation of new bone, and the exudation of polymorphonuclear leukocytes joined by large numbers of lymphocytes, histiocytes, and occasionally plasma cells. While a number of virulence factors of pathogenic microorganisms enable persistent infections, many host factors assume a significant role. Generally, any systemic or local factor of the host that affects immune surveillance, metabolism, and local vascularity will reduce the ability of the host to resolve the infection and may result in the development of chronic osteomyelitis (Table 1).

The Involucrum and Local Vascular Insufficiency

In normal tissues, necrosis is an important feature of infection. Dead bone is absorbed by the action of granulation tissue developing at its surface. Absorption takes place earliest and most rapidly at the junction of living and necrotic bone. If the area of dead bone is small, it is entirely destroyed by granulation tissue, leaving a cavity behind. The necrotic cancellous bone in localized osteomyelitis, even though extensive, is usually absorbed. Some of the dead cortex (cortical bone) is gradually detached from living bone to form a sequestrum. The organic elements in the dead bone are largely broken down by the action of proteolytic enzymes elaborated by host defense and mesenchymal cells (polymorphonuclear leukocytes, macrophages, or the osteoclasts). Cancellous bone is absorbed rapidly and may be completely sequestrated or destroyed in 2 to 3 weeks, but necrotic cortex may require 2 weeks to 6 months for separation. After complete separation, termed sequestration, the dead bone is slowly eroded by granulation tissue and absorbed.

When the area of dead bone is too large, or the host response is systemically or locally compromised (Table 1), the process of bone resorption may be inadequate and may result in the development of an involucrum. An involucrum may be defined as live, encasing bone that surrounds infected dead bone within a compromised soft tissue envelope (84). The involucrum is irregular and is often perforated by openings through which pus may track into the surrounding soft tissues and eventually drain to the skin surfaces, forming a drain sinus tract (68). This host-derived response is the hallmark of chronic osteomyelitis and is an attempt by the host to isolate the infection process. The development of the involucrum occurs once the infection is established and fibrous tissue and chronic inflammatory cells surround granulations and dead bone (84). New bone forms from the surviving fragments of periosteum, endosteum, and the cortex in the region of the infection and is produced by a vascular reaction to the infection. New bone may be formed along the intact periosteal and endosteal surfaces. New bone may also form from the periosteum. The involucrum may gradually increase in density and thickness to form part or all of a new shaft. New bone increases in amount and density for weeks or months, depending on the size of the bone and the extent and duration of infection. New endosteal bone may proliferate and obstruct the medullary canal. After the infection is contained, there is a decrease in vascularization, and the metabolic demands of an effective inflammatory response cannot be satisfied. The revascularization and resorption of the dead bone and scar tissue are similarly affected. The process of resorption eventually subsides, and the Haversian canals are sealed by scar tissue. The decrease in vascularization produces a low oxygen tension in infected tissue that interferes with the normal oxygen-dependent intracellular killing mechanisms of the polymorphonuclear leukocytes and the angiogenesis and wound-healing activity of fibroblasts (67).

The coexistence of infected, nonviable tissues and an ineffective host response leads to the chronicity of this disease. The nidus of the persistent contamination must be removed before the infection will begin to regress (56, 68). Therefore, a thorough debridement is mandatory for resolution of chronic osteomyelitis in situations where the removal of the sequestrum by the host defense is inadequate. Once the sequestrum has been surgically removed, the remaining cavity may fill with new bone, especially in children. However, in adults the cavity may persist, or the space may fill with fibrous tissue that connects with the skin surface through a sinus tract.

Generalized Vascular Insufficiency

Most patients presenting with chronic osteomyelitis with generalized vascular insufficiency suffer from diabetes (15). The diminished arterial blood supply has traditionally been considered to be the major predisposing factor in infection initiation and progression to a chronic state (15). Recent observation suggests that neuropathy may be an equally important factor (16). Identifiable neuropathy as a complication of diabetes mellitus is present in approximately 80% of patients with foot disease (16). Neuropathy may cause foot infection through three mechanisms. First, patients with decreased sensation suffer mechanical or thermal injuries without awareness, leading to skin ulcerations. Second, motor neuropathy affecting the intrinsic muscles of the foot predisposes to gait disturbances and foot deformities, such as hammer and claw toes and Charcot foot. These anatomic alterations may lead to a maldistribution of weight which elevates focal pressure over the bony prominences. The increase in focal pressure where the foot contacts the ground or footwear may lead to subsequent skin ulceration. Third, autonomic neuropathy contributes by interfering with sweating and causing dry, cracked skin, which breaches the integrity of the skin envelope, allowing entry of microorganisms into the soft tissue. All three mechanisms may cause skin ulceration with subsequent skin infection, which may lead to contiguous-focus osteomyelitis. A higher rate of nasal and skin colonization with *S. aureus*, defects in host immunity, and impaired wound healing all play roles in diabetic foot infection (100). Superficial fungal skin infections, which are common in diabetic patients, may also allow bacteria entry through macerated or broken skin. Inadequate tissue perfusion in the area of trauma allows the infection to persist to a chronic state.

Age and Osteomyelitis

There are basic differences among the pathological characteristics of osteomyelitis in infants, children, and adults. In infants, small capillaries cross the epiphyseal growth plate and permit the extension of infection into the epiphysis and joint space (13). The cortical bone of the neonate and infant is thin and loose, consisting predominantly of woven bone, which permits escape of the pressure caused by infection but promotes the rapid spread of the infection directly into the subperiosteal region. A large sequestrum is not produced because extensive infarction of the cortex does not occur, but large subperiosteal abscesses may form. In children older than 1 year of age, infection presumably starts in the metaphyseal sinusoidal veins and is contained by the growth plate. The joint is spared unless the metaphysis is intracapsular. The infection spreads laterally, where it breaks through the cortex and lifts the loose periosteum to form a subperiosteal abscess. In adults, the growth plate has resorbed and the infection may again extend to the joint spaces. Also, in adults the periosteum is firmly attached to the underlying bone, so subperiosteal-abscess formation and intense periosteal proliferation are less frequently seen. The infection may erode through the periosteum, forming a draining sinus tract(s). Adult hematogenous osteomyelitis localizes in the cancellous bones, particularly the lumbar and thoracic areas of the spines, more frequently than in the long bones (96).

The elderly are more susceptible to a number of infections than younger adults, and therefore, the aged may be considered immunocompromised. The decline in natural and induced immunity seen in the elderly results in generalized reduction in the immune response to foreign antigens. The greater susceptibility to infections is due to the effects of age upon the immune system and immune suppression caused by age-related illnesses. Specifically, the deficient immune response to foreign antigens results from the loss of thymic and T-lymphocyte function (mainly related to the production of and response to interleukin-2) and associated decrease in antibody production by B cells (9).

Implanted Medical Devices

The increased use of implanted medical devices, such as intramedullary rods, screws, plates, and artificial joints, has provided a physiological niche for pathogenic organisms to cause osteomyelitis. Some bacterial species may initially colonize these implants during surgical implantation or subsequently by hematogenous seeding. An inherent problem associated with implants is their propensity to be coated in host proteins, such as fibrinogen and fibro-

nectin, shortly after implantation (35). In the short term, fibrinogen or fibrin seems to be the dominant coating host protein, while fibronectin becomes dominant in the long term, since fibrinogen and fibrin are degraded. Implants can then act as a colonization surface to which bacteria readily adhere through the binding activity of fibrinogen and fibrin binding receptors of *S. aureus*. Also, implants are often responsible for reduced blood flow and local immune compromise by impairing natural killer, lymphocytic, and phagocytic-cell activities. These implanted devices have also been linked to decreases in the amount of superoxide, a mediator of bacterial killing within professional phagocytic blood cells (90). Another mechanism by which implanted medical devices produce local immune compromise is frustrated phagocytosis (90). In this case, professional phagocytes may undergo apoptosis when encountering a substrate of a size that is beyond their phagocytic capabilities. The resulting release of reactive products of oxygen and lysosomal enzymes may cause accidental host tissue damage and local vascular insufficiency, thereby increasing the predisposition for development of chronic osteomyelitis. Also, a portion of the normal phagocytic processes are devoted to the removal of the implanted foreign material (particularly metals, methylmethacrylate, and polyglycolic acid), thereby utilizing energy and resources of the immune system that would normally be used to fight infection (92, 93, 118). Therefore, prosthetic implants not only provide a substrate for bacterial adherence but also limit the ability of the host to adequately deal with the infection. Once colonized, bacteria (such as staphylococcal species) are able to synthesize a "slime" layer, termed the glycocalyx or biofilm (see chapter 22). This layer prevents the inward diffusion of a number of antimicrobials and host phagocytic cells, allowing the bacteria to escape the effects of antimicrobial therapy and host clearance (12). Once an implant is colonized and chronic osteomyelitis ensues, the only treatment option is implant removal.

The risk of implant infection and persistent

osteomyelitis may be increased by a number of factors. First, certain joint replacements are more susceptible to infection because they remain close to the surface and have poor soft tissue coverage (e.g., total elbow arthroplasties) (101). Second, certain patient populations are at increased risk because of underlying conditions or systemic disease, including those patients suffering from diabetis mellitus and rheumatoid arthritis (27). Also, patients who are elderly, obese, or malnourished or who have undergone prior surgery at the implantation site are also at risk. Third, polymethylmethacrylate bone cement may be inhibitory to the activity of white blood cells and complement function. Also, the heat released during polymethylmethacrylate polymerization may kill the juxtaposed cortical bone, thereby creating a nonvascularized area. This provides the bacteria with a lush growth environment sealed off from the circulating host defenses.

A Special Case: Inherited Forms of Phagocyte Defects

Defects of phagocyte function are due to alterations in which the normal oxidative burst of the phagocytes or their phagocytic adherence ability (required for exit from the vasculature to infected tissues and opsonization of complement-coated bacteria) are reduced. These inherited defects can result in inhibition of bacterial clearance and progression to chronic osteomyelitis. Three phagocyte defect syndromes that have been associated with the development of chronic osteomyelitis are chronic granulomatous disease (CGD), myeloperoxidase deficiency, and hyperimmunoglobulin-E recurrent infection (Job's) syndrome.

Patients with CGD have a defective cytochrome (b_{245}) in the electron transport chain used in the production of reactive oxygen molecules (36, 104). These reactive molecules are normally responsible for the oxidative burst in phagocytes that kill ingested microorganisms (104). Since catalase-positive pathogenic species (such as *Staphylococcus* spp., *E. coli*, *Pseudomonas* spp., *Aspergillus* spp., and *Candida* spp.) are able to degrade the low levels of hydrogen peroxide present in the phagocytes of these patients, they are usually associated with the deep infections encountered in CGD sufferers (120). Myeloperoxidase-deficient patients often go undetected, since they rarely have recurrent infections unless they have a concomitant disease, such as diabetes mellitus (120). However, they may be predisposed to recurrent *Candida* sp. infection (119). Patients with hyperimmunoglobulin-E recurrent infection have defective gamma interferon production by CD4$^+$ T helper cells, resulting in abnormal chemotaxis and elevated immunoglobulin E (IgE) levels (26). These patients are susceptible to skin infections with *S. aureus* (120). The absence of specific granules is rare, but these patients also have recurrent infections thought to be secondary to a chemotactic defect and a minor abnormality of neutrophilic killing of microbes. Other disorders that affect phagocyte function include diabetes mellitus, liver failure, glycogen storage disease, antibody deficiency (IgG and IgM), complement deficiency (complement proteins C3 and C3b), leukocyte adhesion deficiency types 1 and 2, glucose-6-phosphate dehydrogenase deficiency, and Chediak-Higashi syndrome.

BACTERIAL VIRULENCE FACTORS IN THE DEVELOPMENT OF PERSISTENT INFECTION

Cellular and molecular techniques provide new methods for determining the relative importance of potential bacterial virulence factors. In a recent prospective review of 164 patients suffering from long-bone osteomyelitis between 1994 and 1996, *Staphylococcus* spp. represented 53% of all isolated bacteria (Shirtliff et al., *Abstr. 99th Gen. Meet. Am. Soc. Microbiol.*). *S. aureus* represented nearly 80% of all *Staphylococcus* spp. isolated. *Staphylococcus* spp. are capable of causing osteomyelitis in immunologically normal children and adults as well as in immature and immunocompromised individuals. Other pathogenic microorganisms associated with osteomyelitis include *Enterococcus* spp., *Streptococcus* spp., *P. aeruginosa*, *Enterobacter* spp., *Mycobacterium* spp., and anaerobic and fungal species (specifically, *Candida* spp.). Overall, each of these pathogenic species individually represents a very small minority of infections. An immature or compromised host immune status is usually a requirement for initial infection and development into a persistent and chronic osteomyelitis infection by species other than *Staphylococcus* and *Streptococcus*.

Virulence Factors of *S. aureus* and Their Roles in Persistence

Staphylococcal products that have a role in osteomyelitis may be classified as virulence factors responsible for adherence, direct host damage, or immune avoidance. There are also a number of enzymes and extracellular proteins that may or may not have a role in virulence. The differential regulation of these virulence factors due to staphylococcal population levels and environmental factors is extremely important in the establishment and persistence of infection. Osteomyelitis itself may be considered a persistent infection, but we will pay particular attention to chronic forms of this infectious disease.

REGULATION

The pathogenesis of staphylococcal chronic osteomyelitis is multifactorial, and it is difficult to determine the precise role of any given factor in infection persistence. *S. aureus* produces a large number of extracellular and cell-associated products that may contribute to virulence and the development of persistent infections. Most of these virulence factors seem to be specifically adapted to survival and infection within the host.

During early exponential growth, when cell density is low, proteins that promote adherence and colonization (such as fibronectin binding protein, protein A, staphylokinase, and coagulase) are expressed. When cell growth reaches high densities, the production of the adherence and colonization factors is suppressed, while secreted toxins and enzymes are expressed. These include enterotoxins B, C, and D; epidermolytic (exfoliative) toxin A; alpha, beta, and delta hemolysins; serine protease; nuclease; type 5 capsular polysaccharide; clumping factor; leu-

kocidin; phosphatidyl-specific phospholipase C; fatty-acid-modifying enzyme; lipase; hyaluronate lyase (hyaluronidase); and toxic shock syndrome toxin 1 (TSST-1). Many of these post-exponential-phase proteins are involved in damaging the host and obtaining nutrients from the host for pathogen growth and dissemination after the staphylococci have adequately colonized and increased in number to promote an active infection.

The expression of most of these staphylococcal products is under the partial or complete control of the staphylococcal accessory regulator (*sar*) and the accessory gene regulator (*agr*) loci. Activation of the *agr* and *sar* regulatory loci causes increased transcription of a regulatory RNA molecule called RNAIII (which is a product of *agr*) (52). RNAIII immediately blocks transcription of surface protein genes and, via a hypothesized timing signal, upregulates transcription of extracellular pathogenicity factors (such as exotoxins). The primary regulatory function of RNAIII is at the level of transcription by an undetermined mechanism but may involve one or more regulatory proteins (76a). This regulatory RNA molecule also controls production of at least two virulence factors, alpha hemolysin (*hla*) and protein A (*spa*). The mechanism is as follows. At the beginning of exponential-phase growth, alpha hemolysin expression is normally inhibited through intramolecular base pairing that blocks the ribosomal binding site (74). Later in exponential-phase growth, RNAIII is expressed and folds into a stable but inactive regulatory molecule. After a significant lag, the secondary structure of RNAIII is modified by an unknown agent, and the 5′ region of RNAIII can then hybridize with a complementary 5′ untranslated region of alpha hemolysin mRNA, making the transcripts accessible for translation initiation (74). Conversely, the 3′ region of RNAIII contains sequences complementary to the *spa* leader sequence, and hybridization is believed to inhibit translation of protein A.

It has been hypothesized that the transcription of RNAIII is regulated through a population-sensing autocrine system (i.e., quorum sensing), the details of which are still being debated (6, 20, 37, 87). According to one hypothesis, an extracellular staphylococcal protein termed RNAIII-activating protein (RAP) is constitutively expressed by *S. aureus* and concentrates in the culture medium or the microenvironment of infection (87). As the population of staphylococci grows, the concentration of this autocrine protein increases to high enough levels to activate RNAIII, with subsequent increases in the expression of secreted toxins, enzymes, and capsule production and inhibition of the production of the adherence and colonization factors (6). The importance of this protein in the virulence of *S. aureus* was demonstrated when mice were significantly protected from the pathogenic effects of staphylococcal infection when vaccinated with purified RAP (20, 37). The other and more intricately elucidated quorum-sensing hypothesis involves the products of the *agr* locus. This locus consists of two divergent transcription units driven by promoters P2 and P3. The P2 operon contains four genes, *agrB*, *agrD*, *agrC*, and *agrA*, and the P3 operon codes for RNAIII (see above) (79a). An octapeptide with a unique thioester ring structure (referred to as the *agr* autoinducing peptide [AIP]) is generated from its precursor, AgrD, and secreted out of the cell through the action of the AgrB membrane protein (52). As the concentration of AIP increases in the extracellular microenvironment, the interaction between AIP and the histidine kinase receptor protein, AgrC, also increases. This interaction enables AgrC to phosphorylate and thereby activate an intracellular *agr*-encoded protein (AgrA) (76a). AgrA~P then increases transcription at the P2 promoter. With SarA (the major transcript of the *sar* operon), AgrA~P also increases the transcription at the P3 promoter, resulting in elevated intracellular levels of RNAIII (20, 37). Therefore, as AIP concentrates in the extracellular environment, the level of RNAIII increases, enabling the growth-phase-dependent reduction in adherence factor production and

increase in extracellular pathogenicity factor production.

Another regulatory locus, termed *S. aureus* exoprotein expression (*sae*), has been discovered recently (61). While the activity of this locus has not yet been adequately elucidated, it was found that *sae* and *agr* interact in a complex way in the control of the expression of the genes of several exoproteins. Several environmental signals have also been implicated in the *sar-agr*-dependent and -independent regulatory pathways. Some of these signals are pH (88), osmolarity (23, 81), glucose (107), and DNA topology (81).

sar and RNAIII homologs have been identified in a number of coagulase-negative *Staphylococcus* spp., including *Staphylococcus lugdunensis* (17), *Staphylococcus epidermidis* (62, 112), *Staphylococcus simulans*, and *Staphylococcus warneri* (112). Therefore, this regulation system may be used by the other members of the genus *Staphylococcus*.

ADHERENCE FACTORS

As stated earlier, *S. aureus* must adhere to its target tissue to initiate infection. *Staphylococcus* spp. have a variety of receptors for host proteins that mediate adherence to the bone matrix, the extracellular matrix, or implanted medical devices (44, 91, 122). Eight adhesin-related genes have been identified; they are the genes encoding fibrinogen binding proteins (*fib*, *clfA*, and *fbpA*) (10, 18, 70), fibronectin binding proteins (*fnbA* and *fnbB*) (54), a collagen receptor (*cna*) (83), an elastin binding protein (*ebpS*) (80), and a broad-specificity adhesin (*map*) that mediates low-level binding of several proteins (including osteopontin, collagen, bone sialoprotein, vitronectin, fibronectin, and fibrinogen) (72). Also, this microorganism has been shown to possess a number of other host protein-binding receptors the genes for which have not yet been identified. These include a laminin (52 kDa) (64), a lactoferrin (450 kDa) (77), and a transferrin (42 kDa) (75) binding protein. The staphylococcal receptor that binds laminin, a host glycoprotein occurring on the basement membrane, may be used during extravasation

(65). These receptors were found in *S. aureus* but were absent from the noninvasive pathogen *S. epidermidis* (65). The lactoferrin and transferrin receptors bind to these host iron acquisition proteins and may be used as adhesins and/or as iron acquisition mechanisms.

There is increasing evidence that staphylococcal surface components act as important virulence determinants by enabling initial colonization. Mutations in these receptors strongly reduced the ability of staphylococci to produce infection (25, 109, 113). In addition, there was significant binding of *S. aureus* to bone sialoprotein, fibronectin, and collagen type 1 in a mouse model, indicating that adherence remains a key phase in the early stages of infection (79).

The expression of adhesins permits the attachment of the pathogen to cartilage. Inoculation of mice with staphylococci containing a mutated collagen adhesin gene showed that septic arthritis occurred 43% less often than with the corresponding wild type (103). Collagen adhesin-positive strains were also associated with the production of high levels of IgG and interleukin-6 (103).

Fibronectin binding protein rapidly coats any foreign body implanted in a patient and adheres in vivo to biomaterials coated with host proteins. An in vivo study of endocarditis with a rat model showed that mutants deficient for fibronectin binding protein were 250-fold less adherent to traumatized heart valves (58). *S. aureus* adherence to miniplates from iliac bones of guinea pigs was three times higher than that of the adhesin-defective mutant strain (34). It is likely that fibronectin binding proteins play an important role in bone and joint infections, especially those associated with implanted medical devices (82).

FACTORS CAUSING DAMAGE TO THE HOST

S. aureus also secretes a number of enterotoxins (A, B, C1 to -3, D, E, G, and J) and TSST-1. The enterotoxins and TSST-1 have been shown to exert a profound effect on the immune system when administered parenterally (97). They act as superantigens by binding to the conserved lateral regions of the host major histocompatibility complex class II molecule and T-cell receptor. While only approximately 1 in 10,000 T cells is activated during normal presentation of a nonself antigen, 2 to 20% of all T cells may be activated by a superantigen (97). These activated T cells are then able to increase the release of a number of cytokines, such as interleukin-2 (97), gamma interferon, and tumor necrosis factor (63). This upregulated production of cytokines causes a significant systemic toxicity, suppression of the adaptive immune responses, and inhibition of plasma cell differentiation. Also, the stimulated T cells proliferate and then rapidly disappear, apparently due to apoptosis (89). Therefore, immune dysfunction may be due to generalized immunosuppression and T-cell deletion. Since enterotoxins are usually produced during the postexponential phase of an established infection, they may also aid in producing the local immune deficiency and host damage seen in osteomyelitis. In fact, animals infected with strains of *S. aureus* isogenic for TSST-1 developed frequent and severe arthritis (42). Since the enterotoxins and TSST-1 subvert the cellular and humoral immune systems, they may determine whether a local infection is eliminated or develops into chronic osteomyelitis.

Staphylococcal hemolysin expression is increased during postexponential-phase growth. Among other stimulatory signals, the *sar-agr* regulon plays a role in this postexponential expression. Alpha hemolysin is secreted as a monomer that attaches to host membranes and polymerizes into a hexameric ring channel (105). While this hemolysin binds to human erythrocytes only in a nonspecific manner, it can still mediate significant host cell lysis when produced in high concentrations in the infection environment (45). Also, alpha hemolysin promotes significant blood coagulation by neutrophil adhesion (55), platelet aggregation (via a fibrinogen-dependent mechanism) (8), and its nonlytic attack on human platelets (5). In addition, this hemolysin can form channels in nucleated cells (e.g., endothelial cells) through which calcium ions freely pass (39, 106). The calcium influx is responsible for the vasoregulatory process and inflammatory response disturbances seen in severe infection (40). Lastly, alpha hemolysin has been shown to interfere with lymphocyte DNA replication (55). These multiple effects of alpha hemolysin on the host contribute to the vascular disturbances and immunodeficiency seen in staphylococcal infections, thereby contributing to persistence.

Another type of hemolysin, sphingomyelinase (beta hemolysin), has only weak cytocidal effects on human granulocytes, fibroblasts, lymphocytes, and erythrocytes (117). Instead, this hemolysin specifically attacks and kills those cells with membranes rich in sphingomyelin, such as monocytes. The death of monocytes reduces the effectiveness of the immune response and stimulates the release of cytokines (interleukin 1β, interleukin 6, and soluble CD14). These cytokine-related events may be important in the progression and persistence of osteomyelitis.

Delta hemolysin, the translation product of RNAIII of the *agr* regulon, specifically binds to monocytes and neutrophils (98). Delta hemolysin promotes the production and release of tumor necrosis factor alpha in the monocyte (98) and the expression of neutrophil complement receptor 3. While this toxin was unable to directly prime neutrophils for an enhanced response, it enhanced neutrophil priming by lipopolysaccharide or tumor necrosis factor. Therefore, the simultaneous presence of monocytes, neutrophils, and delta hemolysin-producing staphylococci may overactivate the host inflammatory response, resulting in host tissue damage in the microenvironment of bone infection. However, the exact role of this toxin in infection remains to be adequately elucidated.

Leukocidin (LukSF-PV) and gamma hemolysin (HlgAB and HlgCB) specifically lyse leukocytes. Each of these toxins is composed of an interchangeable two-component system. The active toxin is formed by taking one protein from the S component family (LukS-PV, HlgA, and HlgC) and one from the F component family (LukF-PV and HlgB) (33, 57). The S component is most likely responsible for the specific cytopathic effect of each of the toxins, and the F component is responsible for the common leukocyte binding activity. While LukF and HlgA show very strong similarity, they have been shown to be encoded by different gene loci (86). Since these cytotoxins specifically interact with and lyse leukocytes, they contribute to inhibition of infection clearance by the host immune system, thereby enabling staphylococcal species to persist.

IMMUNE AVOIDANCE FACTORS

The difficulty in treating osteomyelitis and the ability of the bacteria to evade clearance by the host immune response are mediated by a number of staphylococcal defense mechanisms. Such characteristics are expressed at both the cellular and matrical levels. *S. aureus* expresses a 42-kDa protein, protein A, which is bound covalently to the outer peptidoglycan layer of its cell wall. Protein A binds to the Fc portion of IgG and presents the Fab fragment of the antibody to the external environment. Therefore, the Fc portion is unable to either bind complement or signal polymorphonuclear leukocytes, which interferes with staphylococcal opsonization and phagocytosis. This interference has been demonstrated in vitro and in animal models with subcutaneous abscesses and peritonitis. Also, protein A coats the staphylococcal cell in a coat of host Fab fragments; the ability of the immune system to recognize the pathogen as nonself is thereby hindered. Protein A production is repressed by the *sar* locus via both RNAIII-dependent and -independent mechanisms during post-exponential-phase growth (19).

Capsular polysaccharide may interfere with opsonization and phagocytosis. Among the 11 reported serotypes, capsule types 5 and 8 (microcapsule producers) compose the vast majority (75 to 94%) of clinical isolates (4, 29, 78). The capsules of these two serotypes were found to be much smaller than the capsules of other serotypes of *S. aureus* (such as capsule type 1) or pathogenic species such as *Streptococcus pneu-*

moniae. Unencapsulated and microencapsulated strains demonstrated a high rate of serum clearance compared to that of fully encapsulated strains (4). However, the thinner capsule may be necessary in early bone infection stages in order to allow the interaction of staphylococcal adhesion factors with host proteins (such as fibrin and fibronectin). In one study, it was shown that a small capsule was necessary for fibroblast attachment by protein A of *S. aureus*, and a fully encapsulated strain reduced binding efficiency (69). In another study, the thin capsule was shown to be necessary for binding to bone collagen type 1, since high capsular expression actually inhibited binding (14). Once these microorganisms adhere to solid surfaces (such as bone), both in vitro and in vivo, staphylococci produce larger quantities of cell-associated capsule than those grown in liquid cultures (59). Specifically, type 5 and type 8 capsule production was shown to be strongly upregulated during postexponential growth (i.e., after adhesion and colonization) by *agr* regulation and perhaps other regulatory systems (110). This upregulated capsule production makes the organisms resistant to antimicrobial treatment and host immune clearance. Therefore, once the infection is established by staphylococcal adherence proteins, the pathogen enters postexponential growth phase and begins producing a thicker capsule that covers and hides the highly immunogenic adherence proteins. This thicker type 5 or 8 capsule has been found to be serum resistant through inhibition of phagocytosis and opsonization (4).

Staphylococcus spp. can also produce a thick glycocalyx that has sometimes been called slime (41). The glycocalyx develops on bone (such as the involucrum) or medically implanted devices to produce a biofilm (1). The pathogen usually grows in coherent microcolonies in the adherent biofilm, which is often so extensive that the underlying infected bone or implant surface is obscured. The glycocalyx is mainly composed of teichoic acids (80%) and staphylococcal and host proteins (49). Host-derived proteins, such as fibrin, are derived from the conversion of fibrinogen by the staphylococcal coagulase-prothrombin complex (see below) (2). The biofilm produced by *S. epidermidis* also contains the capsular polysaccharide-adhesin, which mediates cell adherence to biomaterials, and a polysaccharide intercellular adhesin that may mediate bacterial accumulation cellular aggregates (43, 73). Polysaccharide-adhesin is a high-molecular-mass (>250-kDa) molecule composed of acid-stable polymers of beta-1,6-linked glucosamine, while polysaccharide intercellular adhesin is a polymer of beta-1,6-linked *N*-acetyl glucosamine residues with a molecular mass of <30 kDa (73). The presence of glycocalyx was noted in 76% of *S. aureus*, 57% of *S. epidermidis*, 75% of *E. coli*, and 50% of *P. aeruginosa* clinical isolates (3).

Clinical strains of *Staphylococcus* spp. are able to persist through a number glycocalyx properties. First, this layer has been shown to protect the embedded pathogens from the action of antimicrobial agents and the host immune system by forming a mechanical barrier (31). Second, local immune deficiency often occurs through frustrated phagocytosis, since the normal phagocytic processes are devoted to the removal of the glycocalyx and the implant, if present. Therefore, the energy and resources of the immune system that would normally be used to fight infection are subverted. Third, the glycocalyx may activate monocyte production of prostaglandin E2 to indirectly inhibit T-cell proliferation (102). Finally, the glycocalyx has been shown to directly inhibit polymorphonuclear leukocytes (32).

S. aureus has also been shown to survive intracellularly after internalization by cultured osteoblasts (48). Type 5 capsule production of in vivo-grown *S. aureus* (i.e., internalized in cultured osteoblasts) was recently shown to be upregulated compared to that of *S. aureus* grown in vitro (66). Therefore, the capsule may not only resist phagocytosis and opsonization but may also contribute to intracellular survival. In addition to osteoblasts, staphylococci have demonstrated internalization into other cultured mammalian cells, such as bovine mammary gland epithelial cells and human umbilical vein endothelial cells (58a, 74a). Specifically, initial adherence to glandular epithelial cells has been shown to be mediated by fibronectin receptors on this pathogen (58a), possibly using fibronectin as a bridge between the host cell and bacterial receptors for this host factor. After adherence, bacteria may be internalized by host mechanisms involving membrane pseudopod formation (seen in established bovine mammary epithelial cell lines) or through receptor-mediated endocytosis via clathrin-coated pits (seen in mouse osteoblasts and epithelial cells) (27a, 58a). In either case, the dependence on the action of host cytoskeletal rearrangements through microfilaments is evident. After internalization, staphylococci may induce apoptosis or survive intracellularly (8a, 58a, 74a). Induced apoptosis may exacerbate the host cell damage seen in osteomyelitis. Also, staphylococci may escape clearance by the immune system and antimicrobial therapy by persisting within these host cells. Further research into the importance of this internalization process in the development of persistent infection is warranted.

OTHER STAPHYLOCOCCAL ENZYMES

Staphylokinase binds to plasminogen, and this complex activates plasmin-like proteolytic activity which causes dissolution of fibrin clots. While the activity of this enzyme has not been directly related to virulence, the importance of escaping fibrin clots to invade surrounding tissue is apparent. Another enzyme, fatty-acid-modifying enzyme, enables the modification of host-derived antibacterial lipids in abscesses (38). Therefore, in the intramedullary abscesses associated with osteomyelitis (Brodie's abscess), this enzyme may be responsible for prolonged bacterial survival and the development of chronic osteomyelitis. Coagulase, while not an enzyme, is an extracellular protein that forms a complex called staphylothrombin by binding host prothrombin (71). This complex is able to convert host fibrinogen to fibrin in order to promote localized clotting. The protein is mainly expressed during the exponential growth phase. Coagulase also has fibrinogen

binding capacity in the absence of thrombin (85). No differences in virulence were observed between wild-type strains and coagulase mutants in several infection models (76, 111). However, one can speculate as to the benefits derived from locally impeding blood flow and promoting a fibrin-rich area for augmented colonization by *Staphylococcus* spp. This genus also possesses a number of other enzymes (lipase, nucleases, and serine protease and metalloprotease) that are used to acquire host nutrients, such as lipids, nucleotides, and amino acids. Staphylococcal iron acquisition is mediated through siderophores, such as the 42-kDa transferrin binding protein and the 450-kDa lactoferrin binding protein (composed of multimers of 62- and 67-kDa subunits).

VIRULENCE FACTORS AND THE HOST IMMUNE SYSTEM

During acute osteomyelitis, the innate immune system responds to the peptidoglycan wall (via *N*-formyl methionine proteins and teichoic acids) of *S. aureus* to produce proinflammatory cytokines (such as interleukin 1, interleukin 6, and tumor necrosis factor alpha) and C-reactive protein. These factors enable the host to mount a protective inflammatory response that contains this pathogen and often resolves the infection. However, *S. aureus* is well equipped to persist by a number of virulence factors and strategies, including but not limited to invading and surviving in mammalian cells, hiding within a biofilm, or producing a thick, antiphagocytic capsule. Also, the cell-mediated (TH$_1$) and humoral (TH$_2$) adaptive immune responses are often inadequate. In a recent study using a murine model of acute hematogenous osteomyelitis, the increase in the central cytokines of cell-mediated immunity (interleukin 2 and gamma interferon) seemed to be only transient, while the inflammatory cytokines remained at elevated levels in osteomyelitic bone (123). This cytokine profile resulted in an initial expansion and activation of T-cell subsets followed by apoptosis. Therefore, *S. aureus* seemed to interfere with the antibacterial immune response by downregulating both T-cell immunity and adaptive immune cytokine production. Also, while a staphylococcal infection usually directs the immune system toward a TH_1 response, the efficacy of this type of immune response is questionable in the low oxygen partial pressures of infected bone where immune cell function is inhibited. Lastly, the necessity of the TH_2 response to clear *S. aureus* infection has recently been questioned in a study using interleukin 4-deficient mice (48a). It seems that a TH_2 response is required for *S. aureus* infection clearance only in certain mice, depending on their genetic background.

CONCLUSION

The development of osteomyelitis requires at least a limited subversion of the body's defenses. Chronic osteomyelitis denotes infection of the bone in which multiple therapeutic attempts to eradicate the infection have failed. The classification of osteomyelitis as acute or chronic is often made clinically based on the duration of the infection. Symptoms persisting for as little as 10 days can indicate a chronic infection. Chronic osteomyelitis is found mostly in adults and usually involves the axial, or long, bones, vertebral bodies and adjacent disks, and the small bones of the feet. The presence of infected necrotic bone surrounded by an envelope of infected soft tissue is the hallmark of chronic osteomyelitis. Persistence may also take the form of a latent, quiescent infection that may reactivate years after apparently successful treatment of the disease. Therefore, in osteomyelitis treatment the infection is said to be arrested rather than cured.

Different types of chronic osteomyelitis can be classified according to the source of the infection (i.e., hematogenous or contiguous focus) and the vascular capability of the host (i.e., with or without generalized vascular insufficiency). Once the bone is colonized and an active acute infection occurs, the infection may resolve, may become a quiescent, persistent infection, or may become a chronic infection with associated progressive bone deterioration. The balance among the outcomes of these infections is determined by properties of

and interactions between the pathogenic microorganism and the host.

Some properties of the host that are associated with the development of chronic osteomyelitis include a low bone resorption rate, development of an involucrum, local vascular insufficiency, generalized vascular insufficiency, greater age, presence of an implanted medical device, and any host defect that results in immune dysfunction (e.g., CGD).

A number of bacterial species may cause osteomyelitis. These include *Staphylococcus* spp., *Enterococcus* spp., *Streptococcus* spp., *P. aeruginosa*, *Enterobacter* spp., and anaerobic and fungal species (specifically, *Candida* spp.). *Staphylococcus* spp. cause the majority of osteomyelitis cases, while all other pathogenic species individually represent a very small minority of infections overall. The immature or compromised immune status of the host is the primary cause of initial infection and development into a persistent and chronic osteomyelitis infection by these other species.

Thus, *S. aureus* appears well adapted to cause persistent infections of bone. Staphylococcal products that have a role in chronic osteomyelitis may be classified as virulence factors responsible for adherence, direct host damage, or immunoavoidance. There are also a number of enzymes and extracellular proteins that may or may not have a role in virulence. The differential regulation of these virulence factors due to staphylococcal population levels and environmental factors is extremely important in the development of chronic infection.

ACKNOWLEDGMENTS

We thank Richard Novick, Naomi Balaban, David Simmons, Michael Cripps, and Donna Milner Mader for manuscript review, reference research, and preparation.

REFERENCES

1. **Akiyama, H., R. Torigoe, and J. Arata.** 1993. Interaction of Staphylococcus aureus cells and silk threads in vitro and in mouse skin. *J. Dermatol. Sci.* **6:**247–257.
2. **Akiyama, H., M. Ueda, H. Kanzaki, J. Tada, and J. Arata.** 1997. Biofilm formation of Staphy-

lococcus aureus strains isolated from impetigo and furuncle: role of fibrinogen and fibrin. *J. Dermatol. Sci.* **16:**2–10.

3. **Alam, S. I., K. A. Khan, and A. Ahmad.** 1990. Glycocalyx positive bacteria isolated from chronic osteomyelitis and septic arthritis. *Ceylon Med. J.* **35:**21–23.

4. **Albus, A., R. D. Arbeit, and J. C. Lee.** 1991. Virulence of *Staphylococcus aureus* mutants altered in type 5 capsule production. *Infect. Immun.* **59:**1008–1014.

5. **Arvand, M., S. Bhakdi, B. Dahlback, and K. T. Preissner.** 1990. Staphylococcus aureus alphatoxin attack on human platelets promotes assembly of the prothrombinase complex. *J. Biol. Chem.* **265:**14377–14381.

6. **Balaban, N., T. Goldkorn, R. T. Nhan, L. B. Dang, S. Scott, R. M. Ridgley, A. Rasooly, S. C. Wright, J. W. Larrick, R. Rasooly, and J. R. Carlson.** 1998. Autoinducer of virulence as a target for vaccine and therapy against Staphylococcus aureus. *Science* **280:**438–440.

7. **Batson, O. V.** 1940. The function of the vertebral veins and their role in the spread of metastases. *Ann. Surg.* **112:**138–140.

8. **Bayer, A. S., P. M. Sullam, M. Ramos, C. Li, A. L. Cheung, and M. R. Yeaman.** 1995. Staphylococcus aureus induces platelet aggregation via a fibrinogen-dependent mechanism which is independent of principal platelet glycoprotein IIb/IIIa fibrinogen-binding domains. *Infect. Immun.* **63:**3634–3641.

8a. **Bayles, K. W., C. A. Wesson, L. E. Liou, L. K. Fox, G. A. Bohach, and W. R. Trumble.** 1998. Intracellular *Staphylococcus aureus* escapes the endosome and induces apoptosis in epithelial cells. *Infect. Immun.* **66:**336–342.

9. **Ben-Yehuda, A. and M. E. Weksler.** 1992. Host resistance and the immune system. *Clin. Geriatr. Med.* **8:**701–711.

10. **Boden, M. K., and J. I. Flock.** 1994. Cloning and characterization of a gene for a 19 kDa fibrinogen-binding protein from Staphylococcus aureus. *Mol. Microbiol.* **12:**599–606.

11. **Bowerman, S. G., N. E. Green, and G. A. Mencio.** 1997. Decline of bone and joint infections attributable to Haemophilus influenzae type b. *Clin. Orthop. Relat. Res.* **341:**128–133.

12. **Brause, B. D.** 1986. Infections associated with prosthetic joints. *Clin. Rheum. Dis.* **12:**523–536.

13. **Buckholz, J. M.** 1987. The surgical management of osteomyelitis: with special reference to a surgical classification. *J. Foot Surg.* **26:**S17–S24.

14. **Buxton, T. B., J. P. Rissing, J. A. Horner, K. M. Plowman, D. F. Scott, T. J. Sprinkle, and G. K. Best.** 1990. Binding of a Staphyloco-

cus aureus bone pathogen to type I collagen. *Microb. Pathog.* **8:**441–448.

15. **Calhoun, J. H., J. Cantrell, J. Cobos, J. Lacy, R. R. Valdez, J. Hokanson, and J. T. Mader.** 1988. Treatment of diabetic foot infections: Wagner classification, therapy, and outcome. *Foot Ankle* **9:**101–106.

16. **Caputo, G. M., P. R. Cavanagh, J. S. Ulbrecht, G. W. Gibbons, and A. W. Karchmer.** 1994. Assessment and management of foot disease in patients with diabetes. *N. Engl. J. Med.* **331:**854–860.

17. **Chan, P. F., and S. J. Foster.** 1998. Role of SarA in virulence determinant production and environmental signal transduction in Staphylococcus aureus. *J. Bacteriol.* **180:**6232–6241.

18. **Cheung, A. I., S. J. Projan, R. E. Edelstein, and V. A. Fischetti.** 1995. Cloning, expression, and nucleotide sequence of a *Staphylococcus aureus* gene (*fbpA*) encoding a fibrinogen-binding protein. *Infect. Immun.* **63:**1914–1920.

19. **Cheung, A. L., M. G. Bayer, and J. H. Heinrichs.** 1997. *sar* genetic determinants necessary for transcription of RNAII and RNAIII in the *agr* locus of *Staphylococcus aureus*. *J. Bacteriol.* **179:**3963–3971.

20. **Cheung, A. L., Y. T. Chien, and A. S. Bayer.** 1999. Hyperproduction of alpha-hemolysin in a *sigB* mutant is associated with elevated SarA expression in *Staphylococcus aureus*. *Infect. Immun.* **67:**1331–1337.

21. **Cierny, G., and J. T. Mader.** 1987. Approach to adult osteomyelitis. *Orthop. Rev.* **16:**259–270.

22. **Crock, H. V., and M. Goldwasser.** 1984. Anatomic studies of the circulation in the region of the vertebral end-plate in adult Greyhound dogs. *Spine* **9:**702–706.

23. **Dassy, B., T. Hogan, T. J. Foster, and J. M. Fournier.** 1993. Involvement of the accessory gene regulator (agr) in expression of type 5 capsular polysaccharide by Staphylococcus aureus. *J. Gen. Microbiol.* **139:**1301–1306.

24. **De Jonghe, M., and G. Glaesener.** 1995. Type B Haemophilus influenzae infections. Experience at the Pediatric Hospital of Luxembourg. *Bull. Soc. Sci. Med. Grand-Duche Luxemb.* **132:**17–20. (In French.)

25. **Deora, R., and T. K. Misra.** 1996. Characterization of the primary sigma factor of Staphylococcus aureus. *J. Biol. Chem.* **271:**21828–21834.

26. **Donabedian, H., and J. I. Gallin.** 1983. The hyperimmunoglobulin E recurrent-infection (Job's) syndrome. A review of the NIH experience and the literature. *Medicine* **62:**195–208.

27. **Dougherty, S. H., and R. L. Simmons.** 1989. Endogenous factors contributing to prosthetic de-

vice infections. *Infect. Dis. Clin. N. Am.* **3:** 199–209.

27a. Ellington, J. K., S. S. Reilly, W. K. Ramp, M. S. Smeltzer, J. F. Kellam, and M. C. Hudson. 1999. Mechanisms of *Staphylococcus aureaus* invasion of cultured osteoblasts. *Microb. Pathog.* **26:** 317–323.

28. Espersen, F., N. Frimodt-Moller, R. V. Thamdrup, P. Skinhoj, and M. W. Bentzon. 1991. Changing pattern of bone and joint infections due to Staphylococcus aureus: study of cases of bacteremia in Denmark, 1959–1988. *Rev. Infect. Dis.* **13:**347–358.

29. Essawi, T., T. Na'was, A. Hawwari, S. Wadi, A. Doudin, and A. I. Fattom. 1998. Molecular, antibiogram and serological typing of Staphylococcus aureus isolates recovered from Al-Makased Hospital in East Jerusalem. *Trop. Med. Int. Health* **3:**576–583.

30. Evans, P., and L. Hofmann. 1994. Malignant external otitis: a case report and review. *Am. Fam. Physician* **49:**427–431.

31. Evans, R. P., C. L. Nelson, W. R. Bowen, M. G. Kleve, and S. G. Hickmon. 1998. Visualization of bacterial glycocalyx with a scanning electron microscope. *Clin. Orthop. Relat. Res.* **347:**243–249.

32. Ferguson, D. A. J., E. M. Veringa, W. R. Mayberry, B. P. Overbeek, D. W. Lambe, Jr., and J. Verhoef. 1992. Bacteroides and Staphylococcus glycocalyx: chemical analysis, and the effects on chemiluminescence and chemotaxis of human polymorphonuclear leucocytes. *Microbios* **69:**53–65.

33. Ferreras, M., F. Hoper, S. M. Dalla, D. A. Colin, G. Prevost, and G. Menestrina. 1998. The interaction of Staphylococcus aureus bi-component gamma-hemolysins and leucocidins with cells and lipid membranes. *Biochim. Biophys. Acta* **1414:**108–126.

34. Fischer, B., P. Vaudaux, M. Magnin, Y. el Mestikawy, R. A. Proctor, D. P. Lew, and H. Vasey. 1996. Novel animal model for studying the molecular mechanisms of bacterial adhesion to bone-implanted metallic devices: role of fibronectin in Staphylococcus aureus adhesion. *J. Orthop. Res.* **14:**914–920.

35. Francois, P., P. Vaudaux, and P. D. Lew. 1998. Role of plasma and extracellular matrix proteins in the physiopathology of foreign body infections. *Ann. Vasc. Surg.* **12:**34–40.

36. Gill, P. J., E. Goddard, D. W. Beatty, and E. B. Hoffman. 1992. Chronic granulomatous disease presenting with osteomyelitis: favorable response to treatment with interferon-gamma. *J. Pediatr. Orthop.* **12:**398–400.

37. Gillaspy, A. F., C. Y. Lee, S. Sau, A. L.

Cheung, and M. S. Smeltzer. 1998. Factors affecting the collagen binding capacity of *Staphylococcus aureus*. *Infect. Immun.* **66:**3170–3178.

38. Giraudo, A. T., H. Rampone, A. Calzolari, and R. Nagel. 1996. Phenotypic characterization and virulence of a sae- agr- mutant of Staphylococcus aureus. *Can. J. Microbiol.* **42:**120–123.

39. Gouaux, E., M. Hobaugh, and L. Song. 1997. Alpha-hemolysin, gamma-hemolysin, and leukocidin from Staphylococcus aureus: distant in sequence but similar in structure. *Protein Sci.* **6:** 2631–2635.

40. Grimminger, F., F. Rose, U. Sibelius, M. Meinhardt, B. Potzsch, R. Spriestersbach, S. Bhakdi, N. Suttorp, and W. Seeger. 1997. Human endothelial cell activation and mediator release in response to the bacterial exotoxins Escherichia coli hemolysin and staphylococcal alpha-toxin. *J. Immunol.* **159:**1909–1916.

41. Gristina, A. G., M. Oga, L. X. Webb, and C. D. Hobgood. 1985. Adherent bacterial colonization in the pathogenesis of osteomyelitis. *Science* **228:**990–993.

42. Groll, A., and P. M. Shah. 1989. Teichoic acid antibody assay in infections of the bones and joints caused by Staphylococcus aureus. *Unfallchirurg* **92:** 414–418. (In German.)

43. Heilmann, C., O. Schweitzer, C. Gerke, N. Vanittanakom, D. Mack, and F. Gotz. 1996. Molecular basis of intercellular adhesion in the biofilm-forming Staphylococcus epidermidis. *Mol. Microbiol.* **20:**1083–1091.

44. Herrmann, M., P. E. Vaudaux, D. Pittet, R. Auckenthaler, P. D. Lew, F. Schumacher-Perdreau, G. Peters, and F. A. Waldvogel. 1988. Fibronectin, fibrinogen, and laminin act as mediators of adherence of clinical staphylococcal isolates to foreign material. *J. Infect. Dis.* **158:** 693–701.

45. Hildebrand, A., M. Pohl, and S. Bhakdi. 1991. Staphylococcus aureus alpha-toxin. Dual mechanism of binding to target cells. *J. Biol. Chem.* **266:**17195–17200.

46. Hobo, T. 1922. Zur Pathogenese der akuten haematogenen Osteomyelitis, mit Berücksichtigung der Vitalfarbungslehre. *Acta Sch. Med. Univ. Imp. Kioto* **4:**1–29.

47. Holzman, R. S., and F. Bishko. 1971. Osteomyelitis in heroin addicts. *Ann. Intern. Med.* **75:** 693–696.

48. Hudson, M. C., W. K. Ramp, N. C. Nicholson, A. S. Williams, and M. T. Nousiainen. 1995. Internalization of Staphylococcus aureus by cultured osteoblasts. *Microb. Pathog.* **19:**409–419.

48a. Hultgren, O., M. Kopf, and A. Tarkowski. 1999. Outcome of *Staphylococcus aureus*-triggered sepsis and arthritis in IL-4 deficient mice depends on the genetic background of the host. *Eur. J. Immunol.* **29:**2400–2405.

49. **Hussain, M., M. H. Wilcox, and P. J. White.** 1993. The slime of coagulase-negative staphylococci: biochemistry and relation to adherence. *FEMS Microbiol. Rev.* **10:**191–207.

50. **Ish-Horowicz, M. R., P. McIntyre, and S. Nade.** 1992. Bone and joint infections caused by multiply resistant Staphylococcus aureus in a neonatal intensive care unit. *Pediatr. Infect. Dis. J.* **11:**82–87.

51. **Jackson, M. A., and J. D. Nelson.** 1982. Etiology and medical management of acute suppurative bone and joint infections in pediatric patients. *J. Pediatr. Orthop.* **2:**313–323.

52. **Ji, G., R. Beavis, and R. P. Novick.** 1997. Bacterial interference caused by autoinducing peptide variants. *Science* **276:**2027–2030.

53. **Johnson, M. P., and R. Ramphal.** 1990. Malignant external otitis: report on therapy with ceftazidime and review of therapy and prognosis. *Rev. Infect. Dis.* **12:**173–180.

54. **Jonsson, K., C. Signas, H. P. Muller, and M. Lindberg.** 1991. Two different genes encode fibronectin binding proteins in Staphylococcus aureus. The complete nucleotide sequence and characterization of the second gene. *Eur. J. Biochem.* **202:**1041–1048.

55. **Khachapuridze, G. G., S. G. Nergadze, N. N. Lapiashvili, I. N. Panieva, L. S. Barenfel'd, N. M. Pleskach, and M. S. Imedadze.** 1991. The effect of staphylococcal alpha-toxin on DNA replication in human cells. *Tsitologiia* **33:**82–89. (In Russian.)

56. **Kharbanda, Y., and R. S. Dhir.** 1991. Natural course of hematogenous pyogenic osteomyelitis (a retrospective study of 110 cases). *J. Postgrad. Med.* **37:**69–75.

57. **Konig, B., G. Prevost, and W. Konig.** 1997. Composition of staphylococcal bi-component toxins determines pathophysiological reactions. *J. Med. Microbiol.* **46:**479–485.

58. **Kuypers, J. M., and R. A. Proctor.** 1989. Reduced adherence to traumatized rat heart valves by a low-fibronectin-binding mutant of *Staphylococcus aureus*. *Infect. Immun.* **57:**2306–2312.

58a.**Lammers, A., P. J. Nuijten, and H. E. Smith.** 1999. The fibronectin binding proteins of *Staphylococcus aureus* are required for adhesion to and invasion of bovine mammary gland cells. *FEMS Microbiol. Lett.* **180:**103–109.

59. **Lee, J. C., S. Takeda, P. J. Livolsi, and L. C. Paoletti.** 1993. Effects of in vitro and in vivo growth conditions on expression of type 8 capsular polysaccharide by *Staphylococcus aureus*. *Infect. Immun.* **61:**1853–1858.

60. **Lew, D. P., and F. A. Waldvogel.** 1997. Osteomyelitis. *N. Engl. J. Med.* **336:**999–1007.

61. **Li, S., S. Arvidson, and R. Mollby.** 1997. Variation in the agr-dependent expression of alpha-toxin and protein A among clinical isolates of Staphylococcus aureus from patients with septicaemia. *FEMS Microbiol. Lett.* **152:**155–161.

62. **Lina, G., S. Jarraud, G. Ji, T. Greenland, A. Pedraza, J. Etienne, R. P. Novick, and F. Vandenesch.** 1998. Transmembrane topology and histidine protein kinase activity of AgrC, the agr signal receptor in Staphylococcus aureus. *Mol. Microbiol.* **28:**655–662.

63. **Littlewood-Evans, A. J., M. R. Hattenberger, C. Luscher, A. Pataki, O. Zak, and T. O'Reilly.** 1997. Local expression of tumor necrosis factor alpha in an experimental model of acute osteomyelitis in rats. *Infect. Immun.* **65:**3438–3443.

64. **Lopes, J. D., G. F. Da-Mota, C. R. Carneiro, L. Gomes, F. Costa-e-Silva-Filho, and R. R. Brentani.** 1988. Evolutionary conservation of laminin-binding proteins. *Braz. J. Med. Biol. Res.* **21:**1269–1273.

65. **Lopes, J. D., M. dos Reis, and R. R. Brentani.** 1985. Presence of laminin receptors in Staphylococcus aureus. *Science* **229:**275–277.

66. **Lowe, A. M., D. T. Beattie, and R. L. Deresiewicz.** 1998. Identification of novel staphylococcal virulence genes by in vivo expression technology. *Mol. Microbiol.* **27:**967–976.

67. **Mader, J. T., G. L. Brown, J. C. Guckian, C. H. Wells, and J. A. Reinarz.** 1980. A mechanism for the amelioration by hyperbaric oxygen of experimental staphylococcal osteomyelitis in rabbits. *J. Infect. Dis.* **142:**915–922.

68. **Mader, J. T., M. Ortiz, and J. H. Calhoun.** 1996. Update on the diagnosis and management of osteomyelitis. *Clin. Podiatr. Med. Surg.* **13:**701–724.

69. **Martin, D., L. G. Mathieu, J. Lecomte, and J. deRepentigny.** 1986. Adherence of gram-positive and gram-negative bacterial strains to human lung fibroblasts in vitro. *Exp. Biol.* **45:**323–334.

70. **McDevitt, D., P. Francois, P. Vaudaux, and T. J. Foster.** 1994. Molecular characterization of the clumping factor (fibrinogen receptor) of Staphylococcus aureus. *Mol. Microbiol.* **11:**237–248.

71. **McDevitt, D., P. Vaudaux, and T. J. Foster.** 1992. Genetic evidence that bound coagulase of Staphylococcus aureus is not clumping factor. *Infect. Immun.* **60:**1514–1523.

72. **McGavin, M. H., D. Krajewska-Pietrasik, C. Ryden, and M. Hook.** 1993. Identification of a *Staphylococcus aureus* extracellular matrix-binding

protein with broad specificity. *Infect. Immun.* **61:** 2479–2485.

73. **McKenney, D., J. Hubner, E. Muller, Y. Wang, D. A. Goldmann, and G. B. Pier.** 1998. The *ica* locus of *Staphylococcus epidermidis* encodes production of the capsular polysaccharide/adhesin. *Infect. Immun.* **66:**4711–4720.

74. **Mempel, M., E. Muller, R. Hoffmann, H. Feucht, R. Laufs, and L. Gruter.** 1995. Variable degree of slime production is linked to different levels of beta-lactam susceptibility in Staphylococcus epidermidis phase variants. *Med. Microbiol. Immunol.* **184:**109–113.

74a.**Menzies, B. E., and I. Kourteva.** 1998. Internalization of *Staphylococcus aureus* by endothelial cells induces apoptosis. *Infect. Immun.* **66:** 5994–5998.

75. **Modun, B., D. Kendall, and P. Williams.** 1994. Staphylococci express a receptor for human transferrin: identification of a 42-kilodalton cell wall transferrin-binding protein. *Infect. Immun.* **62:** 3850–3858.

76. **Moreillon, P., J. M. Entenza, P. Francioli, D. McDevitt, T. J. Foster, P. Francois, and P. Vaudaux.** 1995. Role of *Staphylococcus aureus* coagulase and clumping factor in pathogenesis of experimental endocarditis. *Infect. Immun.* **63:** 4738–4743.

76a.**Morfeldt, E., K. Tegmark, and S. Arvidson.** 1996. Transcriptional control of the *agr*-dependent virulence gene regulator. *Mol. Microbiol.* **21:** 1227–1237.

77. **Naidu, A. S., M. Andersson, and A. Forsgren.** 1992. Identification of a human lactoferrin-binding protein in Staphylococcus aureus. *J. Med. Microbiol.* **36:**177–183.

78. **Na'was, T., A. Hawwari, E. Hendrix, J. Hebden, R. Edelman, M. Martin, W. Campbell, R. Naso, R. Schwalbe, and A. I. Fattom.** 1998. Phenotypic and genotypic characterization of nosocomial *Staphylococcus aureus* isolates from trauma patients. *J. Clin. Microbiol.* **36:**414–420.

79. **Nilsson, I. M., T. Bremell, C. Ryden, A. L. Cheung, and A. Tarkowski.** 1996. Role of the staphylococcal accessory gene regulator (*sar*) in septic arthritis. *Infect. Immun.* **64:**4438–4443.

79a.**Novick, R. P., S. Projan, J. Kornblum, H. Ross, B. Kreiswirth, and S. Moghazeh.** 1995. The *agr* P-2 operon: an autocatalytic sensory transduction system in *Staphylococcus aureus*. *Mol. Gen. Genet.* **248:**446–458.

80. **Park, P. W., J. Rosenbloom, W. R. Abrams, and R. P. Mecham.** 1996. Molecular cloning and expression of the gene for elastin-binding protein (ebpS) in Staphylococcus aureus. *J. Biol. Chem.* **271:**15803–15809.

81. **Patel, A. H., J. Kornblum, B. Kreiswirth, R.** Novick, and T. J. Foster. 1992. Regulation of the protein A-encoding gene in Staphylococcus aureus. *Gene* **114:**25–34.

82. **Patel, A. H., P. Nowlan, E. D. Weavers, and T. Foster.** 1987. Virulence of protein A-deficient and alpha-toxin-deficient mutants of Staphylococcus aureus isolated by allele replacement. *Infect. Immun.* **55:**3103–3110.

83. **Patti, J. M., H. Jonsson, B. Guss, L. M. Switalski, K. Wiberg, M. Lindberg, and M. Hook.** 1992. Molecular characterization and expression of a gene encoding a Staphylococcus aureus collagen adhesin. *J. Biol. Chem.* **267:** 4766–4772.

84. **Pesanti, E. L., and J. A. Lorenzo.** 1998. Osteoclasts and effects of interleukin 4 in development of chronic osteomyelitis. *Clin. Orthop. Rel. Res.* **355:**290–299.

85. **Piriz, D. S., F. H. Kayser, and B. Berger-Bachi.** 1996. Impact of sar and agr on methicillin resistance in Staphylococcus aureus. *FEMS Microbiol. Lett.* **141:**255–260.

86. **Prevost, G., B. Cribier, P. Couppie, P. Petiau, G. Supersac, V. Finck-Barbancon, H. Monteil, and Y. Piemont.** 1995. Panton-Valentine leucocidin and gamma-hemolysin from *Staphylococcus aureus* ATCC 49775 are encoded by distinct genetic loci and have different biological activities. *Infect. Immun.* **63:**4121–4129.

87. **Rao, L., R. K. Karls, and M. J. Betley.** 1995. In vitro transcription of pathogenesis-related genes by purified RNA polymerase from *Staphylococcus aureus*. *J. Bacteriol.* **177:**2609–2614.

88. **Regassa, L. B., R. P. Novick, and M. J. Betley.** 1992. Glucose and nonmaintained pH decrease expression of the accessory gene regulator (*agr*) in *Staphylococcus aureus*. *Infect. Immun.* **60:** 3381–3388.

89. **Renno, T., M. Hahne, and H. R. MacDonald.** 1995. Proliferation is a prerequisite for bacterial superantigen-induced T cell apoptosis in vivo. *J. Exp. Med.* **181:**2283–2287.

90. **Roisman, F. R., D. T. Walz, and A. E. Finkelstein.** 1983. Superoxide radical production by human leukocytes exposed to immune complexes: inhibitory action of gold compounds. *Inflammation* **7:**355–362.

91. **Ryden, C., H. S. Tung, V. Nikolaev, A. Engstrom, and A. Oldberg.** 1997. Staphylococcus aureus causing osteomyelitis binds to a nonapeptide sequence in bone sialoprotein. *Biochem. J.* **327:**825–829.

92. **Santavirta, S., Y. T. Konttinen, V. Bergroth, and M. Gronblad.** 1991. Lack of immune response to methyl methacrylate in lymphocyte cultures. *Acta Orthop. Scand.* **62:**29–32.

93. **Santavirta, S., Y. T. Konttinen, T. Saito, M.**

Gronblad, E. Partio, P. Kemppinen, and P. Rokkanen. 1990. Immune response to polyglycolic acid implants. *J. Bone Joint Surg. Br.* **72:** 597–600.

94. Sapico, F. L. 1996. Microbiology and antimicrobial therapy of spinal infections. *Orthop. Clin. N. Am.* **27:**9–13.

95. Sapico, F. L., and J. Z. Montgomerie. 1979. Pyogenic vertebral osteomyelitis: report of nine cases and review of the literature. *Rev. Infect. Dis.* **1:**754–776.

96. Sapico, F. L., and J. Z. Montgomerie. 1986. Vertebral osteomyelitis, p. 1479–1481. *In* A. I. Braude, C. E. Davis, and J. Fierer (ed.), *Infectious Diseases and Medical Microbiology.* W. B. Saunders Co., Philadelphia, Pa.

97. Schlievert, P. M. 1993. Role of superantigens in human disease. *J. Infect. Dis.* **167:**997–1002.

98. Schmitz, F. J., K. E. Veldkamp, K. P. Van Kessel, J. Verhoef, and J. A. Van Strijp. 1997. Delta-toxin from Staphylococcus aureus as a costimulator of human neutrophil oxidative burst. *J. Infect. Dis.* **176:**1531–1537.

99. Sharp, J. F., J. A. Wilson, L. Ross, and R. M. Barr-Hamilton. 1990. Ear wax removal: a survey of current practice. *BMJ* **301:**1251–1253.

100. Smith, J. A., and J. J. O'Connor. 1996. Nasal carriage of Staphylococcus aureus in diabetes mellitus. *Lancet* **ii:**776–777.

101. Sourmelis, S. G., F. D. Burke, and J. P. Varian. 1986. A review of total elbow arthroplasty and an early assessment of the Liverpool elbow prosthesis. *J. Hand Surg. (Br.)* **11:**407–413.

102. Stout, R. D., K. P. Ferguson, Y. N. Li, and D. W. Lambe, Jr. 1992. Staphylococcal exopolysaccharides inhibit lymphocyte proliferative responses by activation of monocyte prostaglandin production. *Infect. Immun.* **60:**922–927.

103. Switalski, L. M., J. M. Patti, W. Butcher, A. G. Gristina, P. Speziale, and M. Hook. 1993. A collagen receptor on Staphylococcus aureus strains isolated from patients with septic arthritis mediates adhesion to cartilage. *Mol. Microbiol.* **7:**99–107.

104. Tauber, A. I., N. Borregaard, E. Simons, and J. Wright. 1983. Chronic granulomatous disease: a syndrome of phagocyte oxidase deficiencies. *Medicine* **62:**286–309.

105. Tokunaga, H., and T. Nakae. 1992. Calcium ion-mediated regulation of the alpha-2 toxin pore of Staphylococcus aureus. *Biochim. Biophys. Acta* **1105:**125–130.

106. Tomita, T., and Y. Kamio. 1997. Molecular biology of the pore-forming cytolysins from Staphylococcus aureus, alpha- and gamma-hemolysins and leukocidin. *Biosci. Biotechnol. Biochem.* **61:**565–572.

107. Tremaine, M. T., D. K. Brockman, and M. J. Betley. 1993. Staphylococcal enterotoxin A gene (*sea*) expression is not affected by the accessory gene regulator (*agr*). *Infect. Immun.* **61:** 356–359.

108. Trueta, J., and J. D. Morgan. 1960. The vascular contribution to osteogenesis. Studies by the injection method. *J. Bone Joint Surg.* **42B:** 97–109.

109. Vakil, B. V., N. Ramakrishnan, and D. S. Pradhan. 1984. Identification of a heat-labile cellular nuclease in Staphylococcus aureus with properties similar to the extracellular nuclease. *Arch. Microbiol.* **139:**240–244.

110. Vandenesch, F., S. J. Projan, B. Kreiswirth, J. Etienne, and R. P. Novick. 1993. Agr-related sequences in Staphylococcus lugdunensis. *FEMS Microbiol. Lett.* **111:**115–122.

111. van der Vijver, J. M., M. M. van Es-Boon, and M. F. Michel. 1975. A study of virulence factors with induced mutants of Staphylococcus aureus. *J. Med. Microbiol.* **8:**279–287.

112. Van Wamel, W. J., G. van Rossum, J. Verhoef, C. M. Vandenbroucke-Grauls, and A. C. Fluit. 1998. Cloning and characterization of an accessory gene regulator (*agr*)-like locus from Staphylococcus epidermidis. *FEMS Microbiol. Lett.* **163:**1–9.

113. Veenstra, G. J., F. F. Cremers, H. van Dijk, and A. Fleer. 1996. Ultrastructural organization and regulation of a biomaterial adhesin of Staphylococcus epidermidis. *J. Bacteriol.* **178:**537–541.

114. Waldvogel, F. A., G. Medoff, and M. N. Swartz. 1970. Osteomyelitis: a review of clinical features, therapeutic considerations and unusual aspects. *N. Engl. J. Med.* **282:**260–266. (Second of three parts.)

115. Waldvogel, F. A., G. Medoff, and M. N. Swartz. 1970. Osteomyelitis: a review of clinical features, therapeutic considerations and unusual aspects. *N. Engl. J. Med.* **282:**198–206. (First of three parts.)

116. Waldvogel, F. A., G. Medoff, and M. N. Swartz. 1970. Osteomyelitis: a review of clinical features, therapeutic considerations and unusual aspects. 3. Osteomyelitis associated with vascular insufficiency. *N. Engl. J. Med.* **282:**316–322.

117. Walev, I., U. Weller, S. Strauch, T. Foster, and S. Bhakdi. 1996. Selective killing of human monocytes and cytokine release provoked by sphingomyelinase (beta-toxin) of *Staphylococcus aureus*. *Infect. Immun.* **64:**2974–2979.

118. Wang, J. Y., B. H. Wicklund, R. B. Gustilo, and D. T. Tsukayama. 1997. Prosthetic metals impair murine immune response and cytokine release in vivo and in vitro. *J. Orthop. Res.* **15:** 688–699.

119. **Weber, M. L., A. Abela, L. de Repentigny, L. Garel, and N. Lapointe.** 1987. Myeloperoxidase deficiency with extensive candidal osteomyelitis of the base of the skull. *Pediatrics* **80:**876–879.

120. **White, C. J., and J. I. Gallin.** 1986. Phagocyte defects. *Clin. Immunol. Immunopathol.* **40:**50–61.

121. **Wiley, A. M., and J. Trueta.** 195. The vascular anatomy of the spine and its relationship to pyogenic vertebral osteomyelitis. *J. Bone Joint Surg.* **41B:**796–804.

122. **Yacoub, A., P. Lindahl, K. Rubin, M. Wendel, D. Heinegard, and C. Ryden.** 1994. Purification of a bone sialoprotein-binding protein from Staphylococcus aureus. *Eur. J. Biochem.* **222:**919–925.

123. **Yoon, K. S., R. H. Fitzgerald, S. Sud, Z. Song, and P. H. Wooley.** 1999. Experimental acute hematogenous osteomyelitis in mice. II. Influence of *Staphylococcus aureus* infection on T-cell immunity. *J. Orthop. Res.* **17:**382–391.

ABSCESSES

Laurie E. Comstock and Arthur O. Tzianabos

20

Abscesses represent a serious clinical condition and can result in significant morbidity and sometimes lead to death. Although particular types of abscesses, such as those of the brain and myocardium, are rare, other types, such as those of the peritoneal cavity, are prevalent and represent a common postoperative complication. Patients with abscesses often require surgery, with treatment in the United States alone costing an estimated $500 million annually.

Abscess formation is a primitive and usually insufficient host response aimed at containing an infectious locus. Abscesses in different anatomic locations arise as a consequence of diverse predisposing conditions. The microbes present in an abscess vary depending on the contaminating site. This chapter will examine (i) the predisposing conditions that lead to abscess formation, (ii) the bacteria that predominate in various abscesses and their contribution to abscess formation, and (iii) the host response to the invading organisms and why that response is usually ineffective in eradicating the infection. Abscesses are persistent infections but are quite distinct from other such infections discussed elsewhere in this volume.

The formation of intra-abdominal abscesses will be used throughout the chapter as our model. Due to the prevalence of intra-abdominal abscesses, much research has been conducted to examine the molecular interactions between the invading microorganisms and the host that lead to abscess formation. These interactions, which will be described in detail, demonstrate that bacteria have more than a passive role in abscess formation.

BACTERIAL ETIOLOGY OF ABSCESSES

The majority of abscesses are secondary to a primary infection. The architectures of various abscesses are similar, although the organisms they contain may differ. Most abscesses have a polymicrobial composition that is dictated by the location and flora of the contaminating site. These microbes are often part of the normal flora or are regular pathogens of a particular site that gain access to normally sterile sites, where they initiate abscess formation. A discussion of the predisposing conditions and sources of the microorganisms found in particular types of abscesses follows.

Intra-Abdominal Abscesses

Abscesses of the peritoneal cavity form as the result of colonic perforation with subsequent

Laurie E. Comstock and Arthur O. Tzianabos, Channing Laboratory, Brigham and Women's Hospital, Harvard Medical School, Boston, MA 02115.

Persistent Bacterial Infections, Edited by J. P. Nataro, M. J. Blaser, and S. Cunningham-Rundles, © 2000 ASM Press, Washington, D.C.

spillage of colonic contents into the normally sterile cavity. Disruption of the bowel can occur following blunt or penetrating trauma; intrinsic disease, such as diverticulitis or cancer; or peritonitis following bowel or abdominal surgery. Unlike other types of abscesses, in which the organisms often originate from an infectious site and spread hematogenously, these abscesses contain microorganisms that are part of the normal host microflora. Although the colonic microflora contains hundreds of bacterial species, only a few species are consistently isolated from intra-abdominal abscesses; thus, it is possible to examine the virulence factors that these select organisms produce that allow for their predominance in abscesses. These issues are addressed in a later section of this chapter.

Renal Abscesses

Abscesses of the kidney fall into two categories, carbuncles and corticomedullary abscesses, which differ in both their microbial compositions and the sites of the contaminating organisms. Carbuncles usually develop following the spread of *Staphylococcus aureus* from a skin infection to the kidney via the blood. Unlike other types of abscesses that are predominantly polymicrobial, the majority of carbuncles contain only *S. aureus*. Renal corticomedullary abscesses often occur in individuals who have a predisposing urinary tract condition with subsequent urinary tract infection. Therefore, the organisms contained in these abscesses are *Escherichia coli* and other gram-negative organisms that are common etiologic agents of urinary tract infections.

Brain Abscesses

The multifactorial criteria necessary for their formation probably account for the infrequency of brain abscesses. These abscesses usually form in areas of ischemia or infarction, where there is reduced oxygen tension. Such areas may be more vulnerable to the development of brain abscesses because bacteria can more easily establish an infectious locus. Some of the more common contaminants include

bacteria from acute or chronic otitis media or sinus infections, infectious endocarditis, upper respiratory tract infection, and skin infections (30). The bacterial pathogens isolated from brain abscesses vary depending on the site of origin of the bacteria. Many brain abscesses are polymicrobial, containing both aerobes and anaerobes; however, others, such as those arising from skin infections, often contain *S. aureus* alone (30).

Lung Abscesses

Lung abscesses, like intra-abdominal abscesses, do not require the hematogenous spread of organisms. Lung abscesses usually contain microbes that originate from the gingival crevice; most are polymicrobial, with anaerobes predominating. The major predisposing conditions are aspiration and periodontal infections.

Skin Abscesses

The organisms present in skin abscesses depend on the flora in the area of the abscess; however, in approximately 25% of cases, *S. aureus* is the sole isolate (17). The isolation of *S. aureus* alone in diverse types of abscesses demonstrates the ability of this pathogen to cause abscesses without the contribution of other organisms. This ability is not shared by many pathogens, with an exception being *Bacteroides fragilis*. As described below, the capsular polysaccharides of *B. fragilis* confer this ability; however, the virulence factors that correlate with the ability of *S. aureus* to induce abscess formation are not fully understood.

GENERALIZED HOST RESPONSE LEADING TO ABSCESS FORMATION

The initial events of the host response leading to abscess formation may differ depending on the contaminating site and the location of the abscess. We will use as our model the formation of intra-abdominal abscesses, as these are the most prevalent and best studied. Intra-abdominal infection is caused by the leakage of gastrointestinal contents laden with bacteria. Following bacterial spillage, the majority of organisms are removed by the diaphragmatic lymphatics.

The resident peritoneal macrophage population is aided by a rapid influx of polymorphonuclear cells that phagocytize most of the remaining bacteria and debris.

In the peritoneal cavity, vasoreactive substances that cause an increase in vascular permeability are released, resulting in the influx of plasma and fibrin deposition. Fibrin matrices delimit necrotic material and residual bacteria. Studies have shown the importance of the entrapment of bacteria in fibrin to the development of abscesses. For example, 10^7 E. coli cells injected into the rat peritoneal cavity fail to cause abscess formation, yet as few as 10^2 E. coli cells initiate abscess formation when they are implanted in fibrin clots (1). In a rat model, the intraperitoneal administration of the fibrinolytic agent tissue plasminogen activator (tPA) has also been shown to significantly reduce the formation of abscesses due to sterile feces contaminated with either B. fragilis or B. fragilis and E. coli (41).

Intra-abdominal infection not only induces fibrin deposition but also reduces abdominal fibrinolytic activity. One study of fecal peritonitis showed that there is an increase in plasminogen activator inhibitor during fecal peritonitis (40), which inhibits the action of tPA, one of the main agents leading to fibrinolysis in the peritoneal fluid. This increase in plasminogen activator inhibitor may explain the reduced fibrinolysis in the abdominal cavity during intra-abdominal infection.

A mature abscess consists of a core, containing necrotic debris and bacteria surrounded by a ring of neutrophils and macrophages, and a peripheral ring of fibroblasts and smooth muscle cells within a collagen capsule. The bacteria within the abscess are susceptible to killing by the surrounding neutrophils and macrophages but are often able to combat it. The bacteria continue to release products through the abscess wall, resulting in a continued attempt by the host to resolve the abscess. The greatest threat posed to the host as a consequence of abscess formation comes when the abscess ruptures, releasing a population of bacteria well adapted for survival. Untreated abscesses can serve as a focus of bacterial contamination, leading to the formation of abscesses at distant sites, septicemia, and shock.

BACTERIAL VIRULENCE FACTORS NECESSARY FOR ABSCESS FORMATION

Not all bacteria released from a contaminating site are equally able to survive in the environment of a forming abscess. The colonic microflora comprises approximately 450 different species (13); however, only a few bacterial species are consistently isolated from intra-abdominal abscesses. The bacteria present in intra-abdominal abscesses are not those that are most abundant in the normal colonic flora. For example, non-fragilis Bacteroides species account for nearly half of all microorganisms in the colonic microflora, while B. fragilis makes up only 0.5% and yet is isolated from abscesses more frequently than all non-fragilis species combined. Likewise, the relative frequency of E. coli in abdominal infections exceeds its prevalence in the colonic microflora by about 300-fold. The characteristics of certain species are related to their recovery from intra-abdominal abscesses. The bacteria must be adaptable to survive in the environment of the peritoneal cavity, avoid clearance, and finally survive the adverse conditions of the abscess. Most of the bacterial products contributing to these characteristics are not the classic virulence factors but are what distinguish these species from the normal flora that do not survive.

Aerotolerance

The normal sterile peritoneal cavity has a higher partial O_2 pressure than the colon (2, 29). The obligate anaerobic species that thrive in the colon may undergo oxidative stress when released into the peritoneal cavity; thus, only the numerically minor population of facultative and aerotolerant anaerobic species will survive. Anaerobes that produce enzymes to combat reactive oxygen species are better adapted for survival. The anaerobe most frequently isolated from intra-abdominal abscesses, B. fragilis, is aerotolerant due to its production of various enzymes, including superoxide dismutase (10) and catalase (24). Exposure of B. fragilis to oxygen or hydrogen peroxide has been shown to induce the synthesis of 28 proteins (23), some of which may also aid in aerotolerance.

Adherence

Survival in the new environment is essential to abscess formation but is not sufficient, as factors that prevent clearance must also be synthesized. B. fragilis binds to the abdominal walls of rats more readily than do unencapsulated Bacteroides organisms (19). It has been hypothesized that the prevalence of B. fragilis in intra-abdominal infections is correlated with an enhanced ability to bind to the first cell boundary likely to be encountered in the peritoneal cavity following release from the colon: the peritoneal mesothelium. Studies conducted with primary mouse mesothelial cells (MMCs) grown in vitro showed that B. fragilis adhered more avidly to MMCs than an unencapsulated Bacteroides species, Bacteroides distasonis, which suggested that the capsular polysaccharide complex (CPC) of B. fragilis functions as an attachment factor (8). The role of the CPC in mediating attachment to MMCs was confirmed by experiments in which pretreatment of B. fragilis with CPC-specific antibody significantly reduced bacterial attachment. Adherence studies with purified CPC showed that this antigen rapidly saturated binding sites on MMCs and bound in a specific manner.

Other organisms that predominate in various types of abscesses similarly adhere to host tissues or fibrin-fibronectin. The protein adhesins of S. aureus that bind to the extracellular matrix have recently been reviewed (7). It is likely that adherence to host tissues to prevent mechanical clearance is a necessary feature of abscessogenic bacteria.

Local Factors Contributing to Microbial Persistence

The environment of a mature abscess is unfavorable to the growth or survival of many species. The surviving bacteria act synergistically to promote their growth and minimize the ability of the host to resolve the infection. This synergy may explain why most abscesses are polymicrobial, usually containing both aerobes and anaerobes. The facultative organisms, such as E. coli, consume the existing oxygen, making conditions favorable for the growth of obligate anaerobic species. The dividing bacteria produce metabolites, toxins, and enzymes, which with the proteolytic enzymes of the macrophage create an environment with high osmotic pressure and low pH. These alterations to the local environment favor microbial persistence by impairing neutrophil migration and killing. The short-chain fatty acids of B. fragilis have been shown to impair leukocyte function. Two groups have demonstrated the ability of B. fragilis short-chain fatty acids to behave as leukotoxins (3, 26), which inhibit the chemotaxis of polymorphonuclear cells (PMNs) and the phagocytosis of other organisms, including E. coli (27) and S. aureus (22).

Within staphylococcal abscesses, two types of bactericidal host-derived lipids have been identified, a group of long-chain unsaturated fatty acids and a monoglyceride (6). Staphylococcal lipase has been demonstrated to increase the bactericidal effect by augmenting the release of the long-chain fatty acids from glycerides (33). Using a murine renal-abscess model and in vivo-expression technology, Lowe et al. have demonstrated that staphylococcal lipase is preferentially expressed in renal abscesses rather than during in vitro growth (16). S. aureus produces another enzyme, fatty-acid-modifying enzyme (FAME), which enhances survival of the bacteria in abscesses. FAME has been shown to inactivate the host-derived lipids by esterifying them to alcohols (14).

Microbial persistence in abscesses is further aided by the ineffectiveness of most antibiotics in resolving these infections. This ineffectiveness is attributed to two major factors: resistance and inactivation. The Bacteroides species have been described as reservoirs of antibiotic resistance genes (28). Because of their natural location in the human intestine, they encounter many pathogenic species harboring various antibiotic resistance genes. *Bacteroides* species have been shown to both receive and transfer antibiotic resistance genes across genera (18, 32). *Bacteroides* species have been encountered that are resistant to tetracycline, clindamycin, 5-nitroimidazoles, and β-lactams, including carbapenems. Although the increasing resistance of abscessogenic bacteria contributes to the difficulty of treatment, the environment of the abscess also hinders the effect of the antimicrobials. The abscess itself may hinder the absorption of the antibiotics to its interior. Although a sufficient concentration of antibiotic is usually able to penetrate the abscess, bacterial enzymes and low pH are able to render some antibiotics inactive (4). In addition, the slow growth of the bacteria in abscesses diminishes their susceptibility to most antibiotics.

Despite the factors described above that allow bacteria to persist in an abscess, there is substantial evidence that the role bacteria play in abscess formation is more than passive. The capsular polysaccharides of *B. fragilis* have been shown to induce the formation of abscesses in the absence of bacteria. The interaction of the *B. fragilis* capsular polysaccharides with the cells of the host immune system leading to the formation of abscesses is the topic of the next section.

REGULATION OF INTRA-ABDOMINAL-ABSCESS FORMATION BY *B. FRAGILIS* CAPSULAR POLYSACCHARIDES

The reason that abscess formation occurs in only some clinical situations may be provided by the identity of the bacteria most often isolated from abscesses. Certain structural properties of these bacteria result in their initiating an abscess in the host. The best-studied system for understanding the molecular interactions between host and microorganism that lead to abscess formation is the induction of intra-abdominal abscesses by the CPC of *B. fragilis*.

Induction of Abscess Formation

B. fragilis is the predominant anaerobic isolate in clinical cases of intra-abdominal abscesses.

Early investigation of the pathogenic potential of *B. fragilis* has led to the finding that this organism has the singular ability to induce abscess formation in a rat model of intra-abdominal infection. Unencapsulated *Bacteroides* species, other anaerobes, or facultative organisms commonly isolated in clinical cases do not have this ability. Studies in which the purified capsular polysaccharide from *B. fragilis* induced abscesses in the absence of viable organisms demonstrated the importance of this virulence factor in abscess formation (19). Immunochemical examination of the CPC of *B. fragilis* NCTC 9343 revealed that this complex is actually composed of an aggregate of two distinct high-molecular-weight polysaccharides, termed PS A and PS B. Immunoelectron microscopy showed that PS A and PS B are coexpressed on the surface of *B. fragilis* (39). Structural elucidation of these polymers demonstrated that PS A and PS B are composed of sugars containing charged substituent groups not commonly associated with capsular polysaccharides. PS A is a tetrasaccharide repeating unit with a balanced positively charged amino group and negatively charged carboxyl group. PS B is a hexasaccharide repeating unit with a 2-aminoethylphosphonate substituent containing a free amino group and a negatively charged phosphonate group. An additional negative charge conferred by a galacturonic acid residue gives this repeating unit one positive and two negative charges. Of the many capsular polysaccharides whose structures have been determined, few possess this charge motif.

With the immunochemical techniques employed to decipher the structure of the 9343 CPC, it was shown that all of the strains examined (strains of both fecal and clinical origin) possessed a capsular complex consisting of at least two different polysaccharides (21). A majority of these strains were antigenically diverse, and half of them exhibited some cross-reactivity with the 9343 CPC. These results suggested that the dual-polysaccharide motif associated with the prototype strain is a common feature among *B. fragilis* strains and illustrated the complexity of the capsules associated with these strains.

With the structural information concerning strain 9343 CPC in hand, structure-function studies of the distinct biological properties associated with the capsule of *B. fragilis* could be pursued. The CPC of strain 9343 induces abscess formation when implanted in the peritoneal cavities of rats along with sterile cecal contents and barium sulfate. Inclusion of the adjuvant is required for abscess induction. Testing of the abscess-inducing ability of the component polysaccharides, PS A and PS B, was performed (37). Rats were challenged intraperitoneally with each polymer, and the dose required to induce abscesses in 50% of the animals (AD_{50}) was determined for each. In this assay, PS A was an order of magnitude more active ($AD_{50} = 0.67$ µg) than PS B ($AD_{50} = 25$ µg) or the CPC ($AD_{50} = 22$ µg). This finding was intriguing given the fact that PS A was the only polysaccharide tested that had a balance of positive and negative charges.

To determine whether specific structural aspects of the *B. fragilis* polysaccharides were responsible for abscess induction, PS A and PS B were chemically modified to neutralize or eliminate positively or negatively charged groups on each repeating unit (37). Modification of either of the charged groups reduced the biologic potency of PS A by 2 orders of magnitude, which strongly suggests that this polymer requires both amino (positive) and carboxyl (negative) groups to promote abscess induction in this animal model.

Other bacterial polysaccharides with both positively and negatively charged groups were also evaluated in the rat model. Among the few natural polysaccharides that have oppositely charged groups, C substance (the group polysaccharide from *Streptococcus pneumoniae*) and the capsular polysaccharide of *S. pneumoniae* type 1 strains were selected for testing. These studies showed that polymers with different repeating-unit structures that possessed both positively and negatively charged groups also induced abscesses. However, bacterial polysaccharides with repeating-unit structures

that lack charged groups or have one negatively charged group (carboxyl group) per repeating unit did not. Finally, a polysaccharide that possessed only one negatively charged group per repeat (the Vi antigen of *Salmonella enterica* serovar Typhi) was chemically modified to possess both positively and negatively charged groups, thus "activating" this previously inactive polysaccharide so that it induced abscesses in the animal model (37).

Proposed Model of Intra-Abdominal-Abscess Formation by *B. fragilis* CPC

The infiltration and sequestration of PMNs within the peritoneal cavity form the basis of intra-abdominal abscesses. Cell adhesion molecules (CAMs) expressed by eukaryotic cells are critical in the trafficking of white blood cells from the vasculature to sites of inflammation. The expression of CAMs on the surfaces of cells increases in response to proinflammatory cytokines and chemokines and mediates extravasation and localization of PMNs to host cell surfaces. The role of the *B. fragilis* CPC in regulating the production of cytokines in the peritoneal cavity and the expression of CAMs, such as intercellular adhesion molecule-1 (ICAM-1), on mesothelial cells was studied in vitro (8, 9). The CPC of *B. fragilis* stimulates both tumor necrosis factor alpha and interleukin 1α (IL-1α) from murine peritoneal macrophages; these cytokines interact with mesothelial cells and induce them to produce ICAM-1. The production of ICAM-1 by mesothelial cells served as a functional ligand for infiltrating PMNs and increased the binding of this cell type to MMCs grown in vitro.

The CPC also stimulates IL-8 production by human peripheral blood monocytes and PMNs, which suggests that the CPC can recruit PMNs to sites of infection. Many roles have been proposed for the CPC in coordinating events that lead to abscess formation in the peritoneal cavity, but the principal effects appear to be the following. (i) It allows the localization of *B. fragilis*, resulting in enhanced adherence to the mesothelial surface and the ability to resist clearance from the peritoneum.

(ii) It stimulates proinflammatory cytokines and chemokines, which increase the expression of CAMs on host cells and recruitment of PMNs to the abdominal cavity. CAMs, such as ICAM-1, facilitate the adherence of infiltrating PMNs to mesothelial tissue. The recruitment of PMNs to the peritoneal cavity and the subsequent adherence of these cells to inflamed mesothelial tissue are likely the first stage of intra-abdominal-abscess formation in the infected host. Figure 1 shows the proposed mechanism by which the CPC coordinates these events.

Prevention of Abscess Formation

Treatment of animals with the purified components of the CPC of *B. fragilis* confers protection against abscess formation by whole bacte-

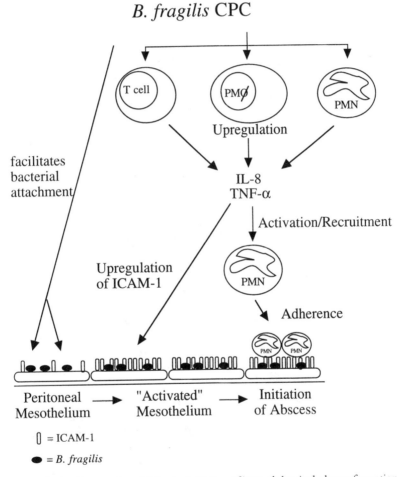

FIGURE 1 Proposed model for the initiation of intra-abdominal-abscess formation by *B. fragilis* CPC. The CPC binds to the peritoneal mesothelium, allowing bacterial attachment. The CPC also stimulates various immune cells to secrete IL-8 and tumor necrosis factor alpha. These factors have been shown to upregulate the expression of ICAM-1 on the mesothelial cells and recruit and activate PMNs. The upregulation of ICAM-1 allows for enhanced binding of PMNs to the mesothelium. This localization of bacteria and immune cells is necessary for the development of an abscess. PMφ, peritoneal macrophage.

ria. The more active component of the CPC, PS A, has recently been shown to act as an immunomodulator. Subcutaneous administration of PS A in the absence of any adjuvant mixtures protects against abscess formation following challenge with *B. fragilis* and also with an array of intestinal organisms capable of causing intra-abdominal abscesses (36). The presence of positively and negatively charged groups on the repeating-unit structure of PS A is necessary for the ability to prevent abscess formation in animals challenged with *B. fragilis*. Naturally occurring polysaccharides or polysaccharides chemically modified to possess these charged groups are also capable of protecting animals against challenge with *B. fragilis*. Further, these polysaccharides are capable of protecting against heterologous abscess-inducing bacteria. The ability to protect animals against abscess formation by antigenically distinct, heterologous bacterial species that induce this pathobiological host response indicated that PS A does not behave as a "classic" immunogen. Rather, it appears this polymer modulates the immune system to suppress a generalized host response leading to abscess formation, a finding that was further supported by the fact that PS A could be administered shortly before or even after challenge with *B. fragilis* and still protect against abscess formation.

The role of T cells in mediating protection against abscess formation by *B. fragilis* has been demonstrated in rodent models of intra-abdominal infection (20, 31, 36, 38). T cells taken from animals previously treated with PS A protect naïve T-cell recipient animals against abscess formation induced by either viable *B. fragilis* or *Fusobacterium varium* and *Enterococcus faecium*. Studies are currently under way to assess the subset of T cells that confers protection and the nature of this protective activity.

Studies of the role of *B. fragilis* and its purified capsule have delineated one mechanism by which abscess formation occurs in the infected host. It is clear that this host response is mediated by a distinct structural motif associated with polysaccharide antigens and is controlled by the cellular immune system. In the case of

B. fragilis, it is apparent that the capsule interacts with cells of the host immune system to initiate the cellular events that lead to abscess formation. The involvement of the capsular polysaccharides of other bacteria, such as *S. aureus*, which are often isolated from abscesses, clearly needs to be examined.

ABSCESS FORMATION—WHO BENEFITS?

Although abscesses represent a serious clinical condition, the medical community has long viewed their formation as somewhat beneficial to the host. Abscess formation is a primitive immune response to invading microorganisms that sequesters them and prevents their dissemination, possibly providing a teleological advantage by lessening early mortality. The data, however, are contradictory and do not support the notion that abscess formation functions primarily to prevent disseminated bacteremia and sepsis. Any benefit that the host may reap by forming abscesses would only be realized if the process allowed for a greater containment of an infection that the host was unable to resolve by other mechanisms or allowed for enhanced survival of the host when death was otherwise imminent. Studies that provide data addressing both sides of this issue are presented below.

Benefit to Host

Studies using bacteria enmeshed in fibrin clots to invoke the formation of abscesses provided some of the first evidence that abscess formation may decrease early mortality. When 2×10^8 *E. coli* cells contained in fibrin clots were implanted in the peritoneal cavity of a rat, the 24-h mortality rate was reduced from 100 to 0% compared with the implantation of bacteria in saline solution, and the survivors all developed abscesses (1). A later study of rats in which fibrin clots containing both *E. coli* and *B. fragilis* were used demonstrated that tPA, an agent that increases fibrinolysis, prevented abscess formation and significantly increased the early mortality rate (13). Although these studies demonstrate the importance of fibrin in abscess formation, they may be too artifactual to accurately address whether abscess formation reduces early mortality. The events that lead to rapid death of the host may be under way well before the bacteria become entrapped in fibrin. A system that more closely mimics the disease state is the peritoneal implantation of sterile feces contaminated with *E. coli* and *B. fragilis*. In this system, rats treated with tPA had a significantly higher mortality rate than controls (41), demonstrating again that abscess formation may decrease early mortality.

Another model that accurately depicts the disease process is the intraperitoneal implantation of cecal contents into rats. The inoculum mimics the release of colonic contents that precedes clinical cases of intra-abdominal infection and produces a biphasic disease process in animals. The first phase is associated with bacterial sepsis and a high mortality rate. The second phase of the disease is associated with the development of abscesses in surviving animals. With this model, subcutaneous administration of *B. fragilis* PS A significantly reduced abscesses and lowered the mortality rate (35). Therefore, prevention of abscess formation with the immunomodulator PS A did not lead to increased mortality but in fact resulted in the ability of the host to more effectively clear the bacterial insult from the peritoneal cavity.

Studies using the anticoagulant agent heparin also challenge the idea that abscess formation reduces early mortality. In rats, survival following induction of peritonitis by creating a closed ileal loop was drastically increased and abscess formation was considerably decreased in the heparin-treated group (5). The authors attributed the benefit to decreased fibrinogen deposits in the peritoneal cavity, which rendered the bacteria more susceptible to killing by the host immune system. Another study examining the effect of low-dose heparin in experimental peritonitis demonstrated that in dogs, heparin reduced both mortality and abscess formation (12). These studies suggest that inhibition of abscess formation does not increase early death. A recent study examining the effect of heparin on intra-abdominal infection of rats showed that heparin reduced early

death, average survival time, and abscess formation (34). Demonstration by histological study that the control group had a higher incidence of acute respiratory distress syndrome led the authors to conclude that the effect of heparin was to reduce pulmonary function deterioration. Because tPA, PS A, and heparin likely have effects other than to decrease abscess formation, assigning of teleological implications to these studies must be done with caution.

The ability of abscess formation to lessen early mortality may depend on the circumstances of each individual case. The severity of the contamination, the proportion of the bacterial insult that the abscess is walling off, the anatomic location of the abscess, and whether the containment process occurs early enough to prevent rapid death are all important contributors to any teleological advantage that abscesses may provide. It is generally agreed that in this era of antibiotic therapy, the prevention of abscess formation is much more beneficial to the host.

Detriment to Host

The consequences of abscess formation in most cases are detrimental to the host. Although abscesses may temporarily contain a bacterial population, their formation usually destroys the ability of the host to resolve an infection that otherwise might have been cleared. If abscess formation provides any benefit to the host, it is certainly not long term. On the contrary, abscesses can serve as foci releasing a host-adapted population of bacteria. While studies are inconclusive about whether the formation of abscesses reduces early mortality, clearly abscess formation increases overall mortality. Studies of rats demonstrating that abscess formation decreased early death also revealed that all animals that survived beyond 24 h formed abscesses, and the mortality rate at day 10 was 90% (1). In humans, untreated intra-abdominal abscesses were shown to lead to death of the host in the overwhelming majority of cases (15).

Due to the risk posed to the host by the presence of an abscess, resolution is a top clinical priority. With the exception of certain types of abscesses, such as those of the lung, which often drain spontaneously, the treatment is usually surgical removal or drainage. The advent of antimicrobial therapy has made it more beneficial to the host to have the organisms free in body fluids rather than sequestered where the drugs are ineffective. Studies of both rats and humans have shown that administration of agents that prevent abscess formation, coupled with antimicrobial therapy, lowers mortality (11, 25). This combination therapy is likely to be the most effective regimen for clinical cases, such as intra-abdominal infection, where abscess formation can be predicted.

Microbial Advantage

Studies with the capsular polysaccharides of *B. fragilis* clearly indicate that, at least in some instances, abscess formation is initiated by a particular bacterial structural motif, which suggests that the bacteria are inducing the host immune system to create abscesses as a pathogenic niche. The immediate advantage to the bacteria is obvious: they are sequestered from the host defenses that would otherwise be effective in their elimination. In the abscess, bacteria are able to create an environment that favors their persistence by rendering the local immune mechanisms and antibiotic therapy ineffective. Not only are the bacteria able to persist in the abscess, but their products often cause rupture of the abscess and the dissemination of the organisms to distant anatomic sites.

It is unlikely, however, that abscess formation provides a significant overall benefit to the microorganisms. In most cases, the presence of the microorganisms at the site where the abscess has formed is accidental. In addition, abscess formation leads not to transmission of the bacteria to another host but rather to the death of the host and themselves. The formation of abscesses, although likely providing a greater advantage to the bacteria than to the host, provides no long-term benefit to either. We propose that abscessogenic bacteria produce the structural components that induce the formation of abscesses because these structures serve

an important function in the organisms' normal niche rather than serving solely as a mechanism to enhance their persistence as pathogens.

REFERENCES

1. **Ahrenholz, D. H., and R. L. Simmons.** 1980. Fibrin in peritonitis. I. Beneficial and adverse effects of fibrin in experimental *E. coli* peritonitis. *Surgery* **88:**41–47.
2. **Bornside, G. H., G. W. Cherry, and M. B. Myers.** 1973. Intracolonic oxygen tension and in vivo bactericidal effect of hyperbaric oxygen on rat colonic flora. *Aerospace Med.* **44:**1282–1286.
3. **Botta, G. A., C. Eftimiadi, A. Costa, M. Tonetti, T. J. M. van Steenbergen, and J. de Graaff.** 1985. Influence of volatile fatty acids on human granulocyte chemotaxis. *FEMS Microbiol. Lett.* **27:**69–72.
4. **Bryant, R. E.** 1982. Effect of the suppurative environment on antibiotic activity, p. 313. *In* R. K. Root and M. A. Sande (ed.), *Contemporary Issues in Infectious Diseases*, vol. 1. Churchill Livingstone, New York, N.Y.
5. **Chalkiadakis, G., A. Kostakis, P. E. Karayannacos, H. Giamarellou, I. Dontas, I. Sakellariou, and G. D. Skalkeas.** 1983. The effect of heparin upon fibrinopurulent peritonitis in rats. *Surg. Gynecol. Obstet.* **157:**257–260.
6. **Engler, H. D., and F. A. Kapral.** 1992. The production of a bactericidal monoglyceride in staphylococcal abscesses. *J. Med. Microbiol.* **37:**238–244.
7. **Foster, T. J., and M. Hook.** 1998. Surface protein adhesins of *Staphylococcus aureus*. *Trends Microbiol.* **6:**484–488.
8. **Gibson, F. C., III, A. B. Onderdonk, D. L. Kasper, and A. O. Tzianabos.** 1998. Cellular mechanism of intraabdominal abscess formation by *Bacteroides fragilis*. *J. Immunol.* **160:**5000–5006.
9. **Gibson, F. C., III, A. O. Tzianabos, and A. B. Onderdonk.** 1996. The capsular polysaccharide complex of *Bacteroides fragilis* induces cytokine production from human and murine phagocytic cells. *Infect. Immun.* **64:**1065–1069.
10. **Gregory, E. M.** 1985. Characterization of the O_2-induced manganese-containing superoxide dismutase from *Bacteroides fragilis*. *Arch. Biochem. Biophys.* **238:**83–89.
11. **Grigoryev, E. G., A. S. Kogan, S. A. Kolmakov, E. V. Nechaev, S. A. Usov, and T. V. Fadeeva.** 1998. Immobilized proteinases in the treatment of diffuse purulent peritonitis. *Int. Surg.* **83:**245–249.
12. **Gupta, S., and P. K. Jain.** 1985. Low-dose heparin in experimental peritonitis. *Eur. Surg. Res.* **17:**167–172.
13. **Holdeman, L. V., I. J. Good, and W. E.**

Moore. 1976. Human fecal flora: variation in bacterial composition within individuals and a possible effect of emotional stress. *Appl. Environ. Microbiol.* **31:**359–375.

14. **Kapral, F. A., S. Smith, and D. Lal.** 1992. The esterification of fatty acids by *Staphylococcus aureus* fatty acid modifying enzyme (FAME) and its inhibition by glycerides. *J. Med. Microbiol.* **37:** 235–237.

15. **Levison, M. A.** 1992. Percutaneous versus open operative drainage of intra-abdominal abscesses. *Infect. Dis. Clin. N. Am.* **6:**525–544.

16. **Lowe, A. M., D. T. Beattie, and R. L. Deresiewicz.** 1998. Identification of novel staphylococcal virulence genes by in vivo expression technology. *Mol. Microbiol.* **27:**967–976.

17. **Meislin, H. W., S. A. Lerner, M. H. Graves, M. D. McGehee, F. E. Kocka, J. A. Morello, and P. Rosen.** 1977. Cutaneous abscesses: anaerobic and aerobic bacteriology and outpatient management. *Ann. Intern. Med.* **87:**145–149.

18. **Nikolich, M. P., G. Hong, N. B. Shoemaker, and A. A. Salyers.** 1994. Evidence for natural horizontal transfer of *tetQ* between bacteria that normally colonize humans and bacteria that normally colonize livestock. *Appl. Environ. Microbiol.* **60:**3255–3260.

19. **Onderdonk, A. B., D. L. Kasper, R. L. Cisneros, and J. G. Bartlett.** 1977. The capsular polysaccharide of *Bacteroides fragilis* as a virulence factor: comparison of the pathogenic potential of encapsulated and unencapsulated strains. *J. Infect. Dis.* **136:**82–89.

20. **Onderdonk, A. B., R. B. Markham, D. F. Zaleznik, R. L. Cisneros, and D. L. Kasper.** 1982. Evidence for T cell-dependent immunity to *Bacteroides fragilis* in an intraabdominal abscess model. *J. Clin. Investig.* **69:**9–16.

21. **Pantosti, A., A. O. Tzianabos, B. G. Reinap, A. B. Onderdonk, and D. L. Kasper.** 1993. *Bacteroides fragilis* strains express multiple capsular polysaccharides. *J. Clin. Microbiol.* **31:**1850–1855.

22. **Pirlo, P., A. Arzese, A. Cavallero, and G. A. Botta.** 1988. Inhibitory effect of short chain fatty acids produced by anaerobic bacteria on the phagocytosis of *Staphylococcus aureus* by human granulocytes, p. 223–234. *In* J. M. Hardie and S. P. Borriello (ed.), *Anaerobes Today.* John Wiley & Sons, Inc., New York, N.Y.

23. **Rocha, E. R., T. Selby, J. P. Coleman, and C. J. Smith.** 1996. The oxidative stress response in an anaerobe, *Bacteroides fragilis. J. Bacteriol.* **178:** 6895–6903.

24. **Rocha, E. R., and C. J. Smith.** 1995. Biochemical and genetic analysis of a catalase from the anaerobic bacterium *Bacteroides fragilis. J. Bacteriol.* **177:**3111–3119.

25. **Rotstein, O. D., and J. Kao.** 1988. Prevention

of intra-abdominal abscesses by fibrinolysis using recombinant tissue plasminogen activator. *J. Infect. Dis.* **158:**766–772.

26. **Rotstein, O. D., T. L. Pruett, and V. D. Fiegel.** 1985. Succinic acid, a metabolic byproduct of *Bacteroides* species, inhibits polymorphonuclear leukocyte functions. *Infect. Immun.* **48:**402–408.

27. **Rotstein, O. D., T. Vittorini, J. Kao, M. I. McBurney, P. E. Nasmith, and S. Grinstein.** 1989. A soluble *Bacteroides* by-product impairs phagocytic killing of *Escherichia coli* by neutrophils. *Infect. Immun.* **57:**745–753.

28. **Salyers, A. A., and N. B. Shoemaker.** 1996. Resistance gene transfer in anaerobes: new insights, new problems. *Clin. Infect. Dis.* **23**(Suppl. 1)**:**S36–S43.

29. **Sawyer, R. G., M. D. Spengler, R. B. Adams, and T. L. Pruett.** 1991. The peritoneal environment during infection. The effect of monomicrobial and polymicrobial bacteria on pO2 and pH. *Ann. Surg.* **213:**253–260.

30. **Seydoux, C., and P. Francioli.** 1992. Bacterial brain abscesses: factors influencing mortality and sequelae. *Clin. Infect. Dis.* **15:**394–401.

31. **Shapiro, M. E., D. L. Kasper, D. F. Zaleznik, S. Spriggs, A. B. Onderdonk, and R. W. Finberg.** 1986. Cellular control of abscess formation: role of T cells in the regulation of abscesses formed in response to *Bacteroides fragilis. J. Immunol.* **137:**341–346.

32. **Shoemaker, N. B., G. R. Wang, and A. A. Salyers.** 1992. Evidence for natural transfer of a tetracycline resistance gene between bacteria from the human colon and bacteria from the bovine rumen. *Appl. Environ. Microbiol.* **58:**1313–1320.

33. **Shryock, T. R., and F. A. Kapral.** 1992. The production of bactericidal fatty acids from glycerides in staphylococcal abscesses. *J. Med. Microbiol.* **36:**288–292.

34. **Sun, Y., C. H. Williams, R. M. Hardaway, and J. Shen.** 1997. The effect of heparinization on intra-abdominal infection and acute pulmonary failure. *Int. Surg.* **82:**367–370.

35. **Tzianabos, A. O., F. C. Gibson III, R. L. Cisneros, and D. L. Kasper.** 1998. Protection against experimental intraabdominal sepsis by two polysaccharide immunomodulators. *J. Infect. Dis.* **178:**200–206.

36. **Tzianabos, A. O., D. L. Kasper, R. L. Cisneros, R. S. Smith, and A. B. Onderdonk.** 1995. Polysaccharide-mediated protection against abscess formation in experimental intraabdominal sepsis. *J. Clin. Investig.* **96:**2727–2731.

37. **Tzianabos, A. O., A. B. Onderdonk, B. Rosner, R. L. Cisneros, and D. L. Kasper.** 1993. Structural features of polysaccharides that induce intra-abdominal abscesses. *Science* **262:** 416–419.

38. Tzianabos, A. O., A. B. Onderdonk, D. F. Zaleznik, R. S. Smith, and D. L. Kasper. 1994. Structural characteristics of polysaccharides that induce protection against intra-abdominal abscess formation. *Infect. Immun.* **62:**4881–4886.

39. Tzianabos, A. O., A. Pantosti, H. Baumann, J. R. Brisson, H. J. Jennings, and D. L. Kasper. 1992. The capsular polysaccharide of *Bacteroides fragilis* comprises two ionically linked polysaccharides. *J. Biol. Chem.* **267:**18230–18235.

40. van Goor, H., J. S. de Graaf, J. Grond, W. J. Sluiter, J. van der Meer, V. J. Bom, and R. P. Bleichrodt. 1994. Fibrinolytic activity in the abdominal cavity of rats with faecal peritonitis. *Br. J. Surg.* **81:**1046–1049.

41. van Goor, H., J. S. de Graaf, K. Kooi, W. J. Sluiter, V. J. Bom, J. van der Meer, and R. P. Bleichrodt. 1994. Effect of recombinant tissue plasminogen activator on intra-abdominal abscess formation in rats with generalized peritonitis. *J. Am. Coll. Surg.* **179:**407–411.

DENTAL PLAQUE

Cynthia Gove Bloomquist and William F. Liljemark

21

DENTAL PLAQUE

After tooth eruption, organic deposits form on the teeth. These deposits include the salivary pellicle, dental plaque, and calculus. Dental plaque is defined as bacterial communities or biofilms that are attached to the teeth or other solid oral structures (i.e., dental restorations or prostheses). The salivary pellicle is an organic film derived from the saliva and deposited on the tooth surface. It is, however, rapidly colonized by bacteria which make up the dental plaque. Calculus is calcified dental plaque covered by a layer of noncalcified plaque.

Based on the dental plaque's relationship to the gingival margin, it has been separated for microbiological studies into two different communities: supragingival and subgingival plaque. Supragingival plaque is sometimes further differentiated into coronal plaque (on the enamel surface of the tooth), or plaque in contact only with the tooth surface, and marginal plaque, in association with both the tooth surface and the gingival margin. Developing plaque generally refers to plaque less than 24 to 48 h old, which is the usual status of the coronal supragingival plaque community, as

Cynthia Gove Bloomquist and William F. Liljemark, Department of Oral Sciences, University of Minnesota School of Dentistry, Minneapolis, MN 55455.

mechanical removal via tooth brushing and eating is ongoing. Most developing plaque is less than 16 h old in the developed world. Subgingival plaque, which exists below the gingival margin, i.e., the gingival crevice or sulcus, is greatly influenced by the composition and quantity of the supragingival plaque from which it is derived. As the depth of the gingival sulcus increases, the resultant low E_h of the environment and lack of access to the host's diet also greatly affect the species composition.

SALIVARY PELLICLE

The salivary pellicle is composed of both human saliva and bacterial products. It is an acellular insoluble membranous layer ca. 0.1 to 1.0 micron thick which is tenaciously adherent to the enamel surfaces, or any exposed nonshedding surface present, and is derived primarily from the adsorption of mucinous glycoproteins from the saliva. The salivary pellicular structure, composition, and function have been widely studied (29, 55). The in vivo pellicle forms within seconds to minutes whenever an enamel surface is exposed to saliva. Secondary salivary constituents include (but are not limited to) proline-rich proteins, statherin, cystatins, histidine-rich proteins, lysozyme, amylase, secretory immunoglobulins A and G, and bacterially derived glucosyltransferases (GTFs) (4,

Persistent Bacterial Infections, Edited by J. P. Nataro, M. J. Blaser, and S. Cunningham-Rundles, © 2000 ASM Press, Washington, D.C.

54). In vitro and in vivo experiments comparing saliva-coated enamel (hydroxyapatite) to saliva-coated substratum other than enamel (glass, Teflon, dental composite materials, etc.) showed significant differences among pellicles, both in in vitro surface energetics and chemical composition and in vivo, as subsequent significantly different bacterial loads and species compositions (2, 46, 65).

SATURATION, ACCUMULATION, AND DENSITY-DEPENDENT GROWTH

Oral microbiologists were pioneers in recognizing that human pathogenic bacteria have surface or tissue tropisms to specific receptors (23). Specific adherence is now understood to be an essential mechanism in the colonization of any pathogenic or benign microorganism. Yet dental plaque, the most extensively studied biofilm in humans, is largely ignored by the medical community unless a "breakout" of its unique indigenous bacterial flora occurs.

In 1970, a short note published by Hillman et al. described the salivary influence on bacterial adherence to enamel powder (24). The in vitro salivary pellicle that formed on enamel powder significantly influenced the adherence of certain oral species. *Streptococcus salivarius* was strongly inhibited, and the adherence of *Streptococcus sanguis* was greatly enhanced. Subsequent experiments supported the observation that receptor specificity was central to adherence to the salivary pellicle in vivo (60, 61). *S. sanguis* receptor selectivity was evident immediately and persisted even to 7-day-old plaque. In contrast, two organisms of pathogenic interest—*Streptococcus mutans* and *Porphyromonas gingivalis*—exhibited relatively low affinity for experimental pellicle and were not generally present in high numbers in developing plaque.

These initial experiments provided a partial explanation for the observations that *S. salivarius* was not present in plaque in significant numbers and *S. sanguis* was present in high numbers. Prior to these experiments, nutritional, metabolic, and cooperative or antagonistic interactions among bacteria and among

host factors were suggested to be the controlling mechanisms (22). Most significant is the fact that the tropisms identified through these experiments were reflected in vivo in the relative proportions of bacteria in plaque that was 24 to 48 h old.

Saliva itself plays a major role in the recolonization of bacteria on oral surfaces by providing the molecules to form the pellicle, as the vehicle for the colonizing microbes, and by coating or adhering to the salivary bacteria already deposited in plaque. In itself it cannot be considered as a microhabitat or an ecological niche, as swallowing is frequent. Saliva plays two roles: it limits colonization of most surfaces in the oral cavity by a variety of mechanisms beyond the scope of this chapter, and it provides these surfaces with colonizing microorganisms shed primarily from the tongue, dental plaque, and other mucosal surfaces. Unstimulated saliva contains ca. 5×10^7 to 1.0×10^8 bacteria/ml.

Adherence plays a pivotal role, but in order to colonize an ecosystem, a species has to do more than adhere to a certain location. The definition of colonization includes both adherence and cell division (as true growth, not simply accumulation, usually via various adherence mechanisms). Initial colonization of enamel surfaces by bacteria occurs in three stages: (i) saturation of enamel pellicular binding sites followed by (ii) additional accumulation by a variety of adherence mechanisms and some growth until (iii) a critical density is reached, when density-dependent growth takes place (see below). These processes provide insight into the persistent infection caused by the indigenous microflora of dental plaque, which cause dental caries and the periodontal diseases.

Many specific bacterial adhesins and salivary pellicle receptors account for these adherence phenomena, and they have been extensively studied. There is extensive knowledge of the structures and functions of both the adhesins and the receptors. New information on the regulation and expression of these adhesins is rapidly being elucidated (8, 20).

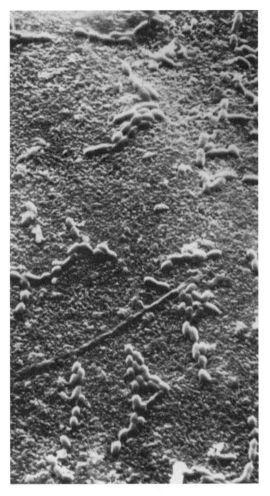

FIGURE 1 Adherent *S. gordonii* strain S7 on in vitro saliva pellicle–coated enamel; density of bacteria is low, similar to that seen initially in vivo (5, 30).

In vitro adherence assays with saliva-covered enamel or hydroxyapatite found the pellicle surfaces saturated, in studies of the predominant developing plaque species, most notably *S. sanguis* and *Streptococcus gordonii*, when 0.1 to 30% of the surface was covered (Fig. 1). The scanning electron micrograph is a representation of the distance between adhering pioneer bacteria on the salivary pellicle in vitro. Adherence becomes more complex as relationships form between bacteria themselves and the surfaces in the mouth. Coaggregation refers to adherence between different species or genera,

which specifically adhere to each other in liquids. Intergeneric species aggregations are perhaps better termed coadherence and studied as adherence to preformed plaque (6, 52). Although this phenomenon is usually studied in vitro, plaque photomicrographs clearly show these relationships between species (34).

When directly measured on inserted premeasured enamel pieces in vivo, bacterial adherence to saliva pellicle-coated enamel saturated pellicular sites at approximately 2.0×10^5 cells/mm^2 by 4 h and 3.6×10^7 to 8.7×10^7 bacteria/mm^2 after 24 h in the mouth (5). Approximately 1 million to 2 million bacteria 1 μm in diameter would completely cover 1 mm^2 of a flat surface (10^8 bacteria per cm^2).

Gibbons and Loesche suggested that bacteria divide four to six times in the first 24-h period of plaque formation in the mouth, and they saw this as a slow 4- to 6-hour generation time (21, 36). This was the basis of the prevailing view that biofilm bacteria grow (divide) slowly. However, new evidence obtained by directly measuring DNA synthesis in situ using intraoral enamel pieces with developing plaque has changed this view (5). Biofilm studies quantify the "growth rate" (i.e., accumulation) based solely on changing viable-cell counts. As most viable cells will form a colony on an appropriate agar medium, this does not give an indication of the stage of growth of the cells in a population. The combination of radiolabeled [*methyl*-^{3}H] thymidine with viable plate counts provided a useful method to measure the potential of biofilm bacteria for growth.

Similar to the in vitro measurements (Fig. 1), in vivo plaque formation began with rapid adherence of bacteria until ca. 12 to 32% of the enamel's salivary pellicle was saturated (ca. 250,000 to 630,000 cells per mm^2). At this density, which saturated the pellicle, the adherent bacteria had low levels of DNA synthesis. As bacterial numbers reached densities between 800,000 and 2 million cells/mm^2, there was an increased amount of DNA synthesis per cell. As densities approached 2 to 6 million cells/mm^2 of enamel surface, there was a significantly increased incorporation of radiolabeled nucleosides per cell, which appeared to be cell density dependent.

Thus, dental-biofilm bacteria do not divide or grow with a 4- to 6-h generation time but with a vigorous growth stage for three to four generations, which occurs at a certain cell density. It was thus hypothesized that when the plaque bacteria reach a high enough density (a "quorum"), they sense this density by determining the titer of a signal produced among the bacteria, which triggers the onset of rapid DNA synthesis in the population.

PHYSICAL STRUCTURE OF DENTAL PLAQUE

What does accumulated dental plaque look like? No single image can represent its physical structure. It ranges from several cells to many millimeters deep and comprises a range of organisms from streptococci to gram-negative anaerobes and treponeme species. However, it is unique in the human body, as it resides on a nonshedding surface, unlike the flora that inhabits the epithelium. Transmission and scanning electron microscopy has carefully documented the dehydrated structure of this biofilm over the last 30 years.

By 1976, Listgarten had carefully studied naturally formed dental plaques isolated from many locations and in conditions of health and disease (34). Figure 2 shows a section of dense plaque associated with gingivitis. Surprisingly, although confocal microscopy has documented a natural monospecies biofilm (13), there are no confocal micrographs of natural dental plaque available. Figure 3 shows an in vitro biofilm composed of uncharacterized dental plaque bacteria (44). Whether the transmission micrographs or the confocal micrographs represent a more accurate portrayal of plaque architecture remains to be seen.

It is clear, however, that despite the closeness of bacteria in plaque, diffusion is not limiting (62). It is also clear that after a certain time, when plaque has accumulated substantially, the biofilm itself becomes a community in its own right, resembling a multicellular tissue in some ways.

RELATIONSHIP BETWEEN MICROBIAL BIOFILM AND HOST

The human indigenous oral flora represents a complex microbe-host relationship ranging from commensal to pathogenic in nature. The presence of the normal supragingival oral flora generally results in oral health. Dental caries and periodontal diseases are conditional diseases, requiring both the presence of critical numbers of certain indigenous species and the response of the host. In the case of caries the condition is related to sugar consumption. Periodontal diseases require certain host and environmental conditions, including inadequate dental hygiene and specific local environmental factors. The ecology of the oral cavity is complex due to its anatomy, physiology, and varied microbial populations. Taxonomists have identified over 300 species which are now considered indigenous to the human oral cavity (40, 41). This complexity has presented a formidable barrier to the identification of possible pathogens from within this population, and many organisms remain uncultivable to this day.

Oral diseases fall between the commensal nonspecific variety ("any gross plaque causes disease") and diseases with specific etiologies, where the presence of a pathogen is equivalent to disease (16). However, dental plaque can be viewed either as intrinsically healthy or as disease producing. In microbial terms, the normal flora collectively describes the various microbial types frequently found by culture or microscopy on the surfaces in the oral cavities

FIGURE 2 Structure of a natural microbial dental plaque biofilm. Electron micrograph of a serial section of a sample from a subject with gingivitis. The most apically located microbial mass consists of a mixture of coccoid and filamentous bacteria, details of which are shown in the insert. Magnification, ×4,050 (34). (Reprinted with permission of the *Journal of Periodontology*.)

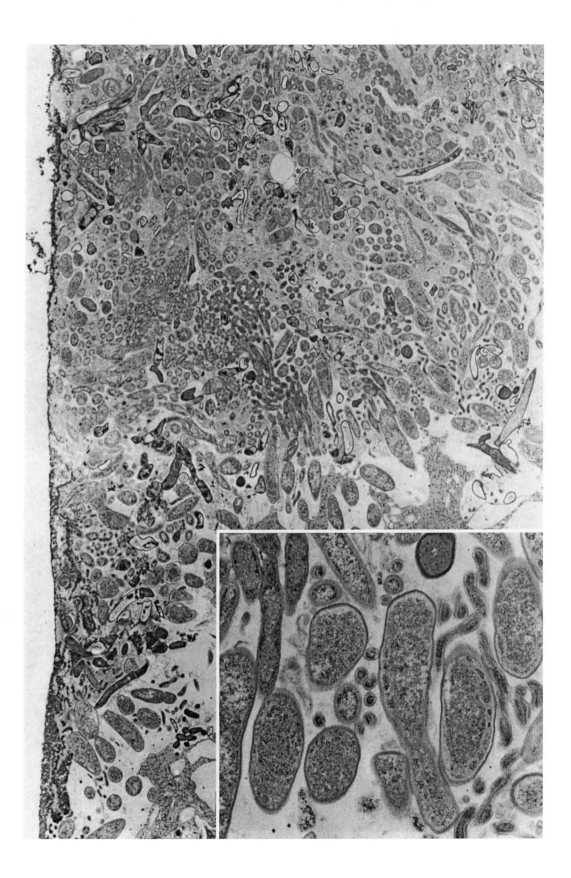

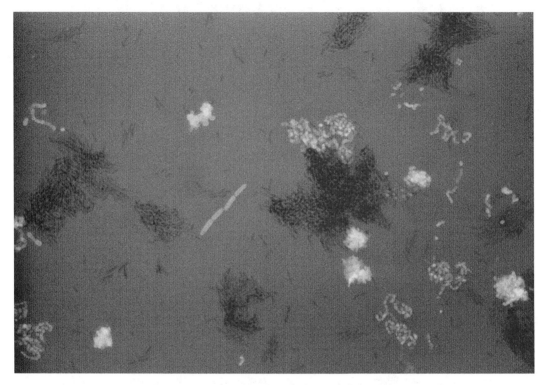

FIGURE 3 Microcolonial forms seen in an in vitro mixed-species biofilm grown in flow cells (44). The inoculum was whole saliva, and perfusion was done with sterile glucose-supplemented (1 mM) saliva. Staining was done with negative fluorescein, with imaging by fluorescein exclusion using scanning confocal laser microscopy. Four distinct morphologies were documented after 48 h of incubation in sterile saliva. (Reprinted with permission of the *Journal of Microbiological Methods*.)

of healthy individuals and is a synonym for the indigenous microflora (32). Indigenous species are frequently encountered in one or more typical human anatomic regions, are found at least as often in the absence of disease as in its presence, and have as their primary habitat the human species and, as described here, the oral cavity (33). Indigenous species, in relation to their host, are in a state between symbiosis (the living together of two dissimilar organisms, both benefiting) and pathogenicity (where one organism is harmed). The typical indigenous microbe is obligately parasitic (nonsaprophytic) and not overtly, actively, or obligately pathogenic in a particular host. The indigenous microbes that compose the normal flora will, when disturbed, promptly reestablish themselves in a similar ecosystem. Amphibionts have

the potential to produce disease but do not always express their virulence (45).

The pathogenicity of a microbe denotes its ability to cause disease. The indigenous flora usually protects against disease. Infection refers to the presence and multiplication of a pathogenic microorganism in body tissues to the extent that harm is done to the host. In the oral cavity, indigenous species become pathogenic when they leave microhabitats where they are harmless (e.g., tongue papillae) to reproduce in microhabitats where their by-products or presence causes disease (e.g., the subgingival crevice). Indigenous species also become pathogenic when they reproduce under certain conditions in certain locations and become a larger proportion of the population. Predominant indigenous species must constantly reestablish themselves in their microhabitats. This colonization requires a minimal infective dose of microbes per milliliter of saliva in the oral cavity or presence in supragingival plaque (31, 61). Colonization predominantly by nonpathogenic species results in dental health (37).

Dental plaque functions as a true biofilm community. Once established at a site, the species composition of this community appears somewhat stable over time, despite its exposure to outside (environmental) changes, such as oral hygiene, diet, and exogenous organisms. The stability is not due to metabolic simplicity but represents a highly dynamic balance held in place by many synergistic and antagonistic interactions among the component species and between flora and host. It is stable, as is any other ecosystem, as long as the system parameters do not change greatly.

PLASTICITY OF PHENOTYPES MAKES RAPID CHANGES WITHIN BIOFILMS POSSIBLE

An important characteristic of bacteria that distinguishes their behavior in complex ecosystems from that of multicellular organisms is their quick and efficient phenotypic response to environmental changes (11). Biofilm bacteria are distinguished from clonal cells in multicellular organisms by the ability to change phenotypically. The concept of bacteria as "single celled" comes from the time of Koch's postulates, and before that the demonstrations of Pasteur and others that pathogenic cultures could be grown reproducibly from isolated single bacterial cells. Today we know that multicellularity is the ubiquitous form for most natural bacteria, although examples of bacterial multicellular behavior in the *Myxobacteria*, and mobile swarm colonies, were previously considered exceptional specializations (51). The structure and organization of biofilm communities make us consider whether our focus on a few extremely well-studied species, such as *Escherichia coli*, might not have created an archetype not terribly common in the natural world. The organization of *E. coli* colonies on agar plates is a biofilm model (with excess nutrient) that can be visualized in the microscope, by macrophotography, and by using special dyes and genetic inserts to reveal patterns of differential gene expression (50). Similarly, cariogenic streptococci profoundly alter patterns in their gene expression and physiology and become more virulent under conditions of carbohydrate excess, shifting to lactate production (10). The expression of extracellular virulence-associated polymers, GTF, and fructosyltransferase is affected by pH, growth rate, and carbohydrate source (8).

The use of single-species in vitro biofilms has demonstrated the marked differences between planktonic and adherent populations (8, 12, 43). It is necessary to continue physiological and genetic studies to discover the molecular basis for organisms to grow and persist on surfaces. Dental plaque is a structurally organized community, and the response in planktonic or monospecies cultures is not necessarily applicable to their behavior within a biofilm. One clear example of gene expression which may affect dental biofilms is seen in the use of constructed strains of *S. mutans* which express the urease genes of *S. salivarius*. Clancy and Burne showed that the ability of these strains to modulate glycolytic acidification is directly related to the amount of urease they produce (11). The production of ammonia makes the environment more favorable for less aciduric species, e.g., sanguis group streptococci and actinomycetes, and provides an assimilable source of nitrogen for plaque bacteria. This and the arginine deiminase systems of the sanguis group streptococcal species help keep plaque pH buffered and prevent the aciduric caries-producing strains from increasing in proportion. Studying constructed strains such as this in biofilm models will in all probability confirm what animal studies with these strains have found—that the pH fall due to glycolysis is ameliorated by urease activity.

CARIES AS A CONDITIONAL DISEASE

In the 1940s and 1950s the prevailing view was that the indigenous oral microbiota was primarily commensally related to the human oral cavity, similar to the complex flora in the gut. During the 1950s and 1960s, indigenous microorganisms were finally implicated as the primary etiologic agents of dental caries and periodontal diseases (19, 26, 42). Microbial ecologists revealed through germfree (gnotobiotic) and conventional animal models that certain indigenous oral bacteria were more virulent than others and were able to cause gross disease in teeth (e.g., *S. mutans*) and in the periodontal supporting structures (e.g., *Actinomyces* species) (18, 27). These experiments signified an important breakthrough, suggesting that a single species, or a small group of species, caused oral diseases.

ROLE OF GLUCANS IN DENTAL BIOFILMS AND CARIES

A series of pivotal observations were published in the late 1960s and early 1970s. Only mutans group streptococcal strains which produced glucans (dextrans) from sucrose were found to be capable of causing caries in animal models. Additionally, only strains of mutans group streptococci which bound glucan caused animal caries (35). These observations were extended to suggest that glucans were the universal glue that also held plaque together (i.e., the plaque matrix), as mutans group streptococcal plaques in animals fed large amounts of sucrose were dispersed by glucanases (dextranases). These observations in animals did not hold true in human clinical trials. The task during the 1970s, then, was to search in longitudinal and cross-sectional studies to find amphibionts among individual microbial species (or groups of species) from the oral microorganisms associated with human dental caries or periodontal diseases.

In vitro studies have shown that glucan binds well to experimental pellicle (30). These studies also found that species of mutans group streptococci bind better to glucan-treated experimental pellicle than to control pellicles. More recent reports have located GTF in natural salivary pellicles and found that when sucrose is present, glucans are formed (48). Further, GTFs added to experimental pellicles, in the presence of sucrose, enhanced *S. gordonii* and mutans group streptococcal binding to the experimental pellicle (25, 49). However, many mutans group streptococci also possess adhesins which will bind, albeit with much less affinity than those of the sanguis group streptococci, to experimental pellicle. These adhesins are generally found on *S. mutans* strains and less often (at least so far) on *Streptococcus sobrinus* strains. It is generally accepted, however, that sucrose and glucans via their GTFs (bound to the mutans group streptococcal surface) and glucan-binding proteins (unique to mutans group streptococci) play an important role in the establishment of mutans group streptococci and, thus, in subsequent caries production.

The role of glucans in human plaque formation is only now beginning to be understood through in vivo studies. Data from our laboratory extend and confirm the observation that accumulation of streptococci is much more efficient in the presence of sucrose rinsing (14, 25, 49). It appears that in the presence of sucrose the rate increase of initial adherence is due to a measurably increased number of pellicle binding sites. Not only was mutans group streptococcal adherence promoted, but also that of most streptococcal species and *Veillonella* species. GTFs may not need to be tightly bound to cell surfaces; even if transiently bound they produce an increased rate of initial adherence to the tooth (9, 38; W. F. Liljemark and C. G. Bloomquist, submitted for publication).

Caries are associated with bacteria which are highly acid tolerant and acidogenic, such as the mutans group streptococci (which include the species *S. mutans* and *S. sobrinus*) and lactobacilli (7, 33). Overgrowth of these usually minor components of plaque is associated with the increased or high and frequent consumption of sugar (14, 39). Changes in species numbers and metabolic activities of these microbes are influenced by the environment, which affects the expression of virulence genes. The consensus among many scientists regarding the microbes related to these oral diseases is as follows: the primary etiologic agents of coronal caries and root caries are the mutans group streptococci, particularly *S. mutans* and *S. sobrinus* (7, 17, 35, 62–64); secondarily implicated are the *Lactobacillus* species and perhaps some non-mutans group streptococci in coronal caries, particularly the acid-tolerant strains *S. sanguis*, *S. gordonii*, and *Streptococcus oralis* (47, 63, 64).

PERIODONTAL DISEASES

Development of periodontal disease requires a gingival crevice deeper than 3 mm, after which there is an increase in the proportion of obligately anaerobic species, many of which are gram negative and proteolytic rather than saccharolytic. Primarily implicated in chronic periodontitis are several species, perhaps more appropriately described as risk indicators than etiologic agents, which include *P. gingivalis*, *Bacteroides forsythus*, the spirochetal *Treponema* and *Selenomonas* species, and secondarily *Wolinella recta* and *Fusobacterium* species (53). *Actinobacillus actinomycetemcomitans* is a pathogen not found ubiquitously in human mouths and is considered the primary etiologic agent of juvenile periodontitis. *Prevotella*, *Fusobacterium*, and *Actinomyces* species are associated with gingivitis (53). Periodontal diseases are also conditional diseases, but their appearance is multifactorial and, as with any mixed-species infection (with the exception of juvenile periodontitis), their study is limited by the methods available.

Until recently, pinpointing the total numbers and proportions of a possible periodontal pathogen in dental plaque was arduous and limited by the supplemented blood agar medium used. With standard plating, a species is not even noted unless it makes up >1% of the flora on blood agar medium (1 colony out of 100). Unlike septicemia or epidermal or mucosal diseases where the mere presence of certain pathogenic species can indicate disease, prevalence does not always correlate with dental disease. Plaque-sampling methods may not select the exact microhabitats where a pathogen predominates (Fig. 2) (3, 31). Periodontal pathogens have been chosen for virulence studies (comparing them to nonoral pathogens) and are implicated based on animal models rather than on strong correlations with a species' prevalence and proportion in humans.

WHY DO THESE ENDOGENOUS PATHOGENS SURVIVE?

The endogenous diseases dental caries and periodontitis are chronic, slowly progressing, and relatively painless to the majority of people affected. It is therefore essential that any methods to promote oral health not do more harm than good. Fortunately, we are usually not heavily colonized by these potentially pathogenic microbes. For example, mutans group streptococci are usually only found in high proportions immediately in apposition to initial decalcification sites on enamel (64). Mutans group streptococcal colonization of teeth is often localized to a few surfaces, predominantly the pits and fissures and adjacent areas, thus establishing primarily retentive habitats (35, 56).

Similarly, *P. gingivalis* and the other contributing potential periodontal pathogens are not found ubiquitously in the gingival crevice area but tend to prefer deeper sulci and are often not found in healthy sites even in people with chronic periodontitis (53). Caries and periodontal diseases are results of the constant recolonization of these more retentive sites. It has been demonstrated that scrupulous oral hygiene prevents both caries and chronic periodontitis (1). With good oral hygiene, these microbes must colonize to replace the predominant species even at those sites susceptible to disease. This is particularly true for countries whose populations have regular oral hygiene habits and return visits for professional tooth cleanings. As most of us are not edentulous, it is clear that the relationship between host and biofilm is usually benign.

From a microbial ecologist's point of view, mutans group streptococci, *P. gingivalis*, and the other pathogens are extremely disadvantaged. Mutans group streptococci can only colonize teeth themselves and are constantly being swept away and swallowed. *P. gingivalis* and other periopathogens are fastidious near-obligate anaerobes, which physiologically limits their dispersion from their primary reservoir in the deep crypts of the tongue dorsum. Both potential periopathogens and caries-producing microorganisms have adhesins specific for the oral sites they colonize, similar to the more predominant nonpathogenic species.

Why is it, then, with all the ecological mechanisms for recolonization, that these bacteria generally colonize with difficulty? Perhaps most important is the infective dose available. Except in caries-susceptible people and periodontally diseased mouths, very low numbers of these organisms are recovered from saliva (15). Secondly, except for glucan binding, the adhesive interactions of both mutans group streptococci and *P. gingivalis* with the pellicle are weak compared to those of the sanguis group streptococci and many other early colonizers. This may be due to the presence of fewer adhesins per cell, to adhesin molecules that are not easily stabilized into irreversible binding situations, or simply to competition for salivary pellicle receptors with the more predominant bacteria in saliva, i.e., sanguis group streptococci, *Veillonella*, and *Haemophilus*. Salivary agglutination and in vitro coaggregation phenomena are not likely to influence colonization and recolonization, as in our opinion, these organisms must recolonize close to their potential site of action or they will usually not establish a permanent habitat. Thus, in order for effective recolonization of tooth surfaces or the gingival crevice to occur, these microbes must use adhesins to attach to the pellicle and not be desorbed for some time (57). Mutans group streptococcal colonization is more effective in people with high-sucrose diets (28).

In the case of mutans group streptococci, de Stoppelaar et al. first noted that if sanguis group streptococci were very predominant, mutans group streptococci were found in very low numbers (14). The converse was also true. Recently, van der Hoeven and Schaeken found that sanguis group streptococci were replaced by mutans streptococci in animals pretreated with chlorhexidine varnish, at least those on low-sucrose diets (58). In fact, in order for mutans group streptococci to cause caries they must effectively colonize and produce glucans

to permit acid to diffuse freely to the enamel surface. Van Houte et al. used *S. mutans* cell masses of various cell densities (62). They showed experimentally that increased separation of cells by glucan increases their in vitro plaque porosity. This increased porosity caused a pronounced pH drop, especially in the deeper layers. This is also based on the diffusion of sugar (sucrose) through a more porous plaque, which then leads to an even higher rate of acid production and thus a larger pH drop. The application of their data makes it necessary to assume that natural plaque has such a high cell density that the cells prevent this diffusion in order to prevent maximum acid production, compared to the less dense extracellular glucan-rich matrix in *S. mutans* cell masses. *P. gingivalis*, on the other hand, must adhere initially close to the gingival sulcus and remain undisturbed. In order for it to survive, its niche must become rapidly anaerobic and its fastidious nutritional needs must be met by a not-too-healthy gingival sulcus, perhaps one suffering from gingivitis (a different etiology), where essential serum components become more available.

In conclusion, the multispecies dental plaque biofilm has taught and will continue to teach us about many fundamental mechanisms. It provides us with (i) an example of the ecological relationship between host and microbe in a multispecies biofilm, (ii) a model to study both the persistence and perturbation of biofilm physiology in response to host and/or environmental forces, and (iii) an opportunity to assess the efficacy of biofilm treatments in an easily accessed natural model.

REFERENCES

1. **Axelsson, P., J. Lindhe, and B. Nystrom.** 1991. On the prevention of caries and periodontal disease. Results of a 15-year longitudinal study in adults. *J. Clin. Periodontol.* **18:**182–189.
2. **Baier, R. E., and P.-O. Glantz.** 1978. Characterization of oral in vivo films formed on different types of solid surfaces. *Acta Odontol. Scand.* **36:** 289–301.
3. **Bandt, C. L., W. F. Liljemark, B. L. Pihlstrom, J. E. Hinrichs, E. M. Schaffer, and L. F. Wolff.** 1982. The use of selective media for

examining relationships between dental plaque microorganisms and periodontal disease in a large sample clinical investigation. *J. Periodontol. Res.* **17:**518–520.

4. **Bennick, A.** 1982. Salivary proline-rich proteins. *Mol. Cell. Biochem.* **45:**83–99.

5. **Bloomquist, C. G., B. E. Reilly, and W. F. Liljemark.** 1996. Adherence, accumulation, and cell division of a natural adherent bacterial population. *J. Bacteriol.* **178:**1172–1177.

6. **Bos, R., H. C. Van der Mei, H. J. Busscher, and J. M. Meinders.** 1994. A quantitative method to study co-adhesion of microorganisms in a parallel plate flow chamber: basic principles of the analysis. *J. Microbiol. Methods* **20:**289–305.

7. **Bowden, G. H. W.** 1990. Microbiology of root surface caries in humans. *J. Dent. Res.* **69:** 1205–1210.

8. **Burne, R. A., Z. T. Wen, Y. Y. Chen, and J. E. Penders.** 1999. Regulation of expression of the fructan hydrolase gene of *Streptococcus mutans* GS-5 by induction and carbon catabolite repression. *J. Bacteriol.* **181:**2863–2871.

9. **Carlsson, J., and J. Egelberg.** 1965. Effect of diet on early plaque formation in man. *Odontol. Rev.* **16:**112–125.

10. **Carlsson, J.** 1984. Regulation of sugar metabolism in relation to "feast and famine" existence of plaque, p. 205–211. *In* B. Guggenheim (ed.), *Cariology.* Karger, Basel, Switzerland.

11. **Clancy, A., and R. A. Burne.** 1997. Construction and characterization of a recombinant ureolytic *Streptococcus mutans* and its use to demonstrate the relationship of urease activity to pH modulating capacity. *FEMS Microbiol. Lett.* **151:**205–211.

12. **Davies, D. G., A. M. Charkrabarty, and G. G. Geesey.** 1993. Exopolysaccharide production in biofilms: substratum activation of alginate gene expression by *Pseudomonas aeruginosa. Appl. Environ. Microbiol.* **58:**1181–1186.

13. **Davies, D. G., M. R. Parsek, J. P. Pearson, B. H. Iglewski, J. W. Costerton, and E. P. Greenberg.** 1998. The involvement of cell to cell signaling in the development of a bacterial biofilm. *Science* **280:**295–298.

14. **de Stoppelaar, J. D., J. van Houte, and O. B. Dirks.** 1970. The effect of carbohydrate restriction on the presence of *Streptococcus mutans, Streptococcus sanguis* and iodophilic polysaccharide-producing bacteria in human dental plaque. *Caries Res.* **4:**114–123.

15. **Edwardsson, S.** 1968. Characteristics of caries-inducing human streptococci resembling *Streptococcus mutans. Arch. Oral Biol.* **13:**637–646.

16. **Ellen, R. P.** 1982. Oral colonization by gram-positive bacteria significant to periodontal disease, p. 98–111. *In* R. J. Genco and S. E. Mergenhagen

(ed.), *Host-Parasite Interactions in Periodontal Diseases.* American Society for Microbiology, Washington, D.C.

17. **Ellen, R. P., D. W. Banning, and E. D. Fillery.** 1985. Longitudinal microbiological investigation of a hospitalized population of older adults with a high root surface caries risk. *J. Dent. Res.* **64:**1377–1381.

18. **Fitzgerald, R. J., H. V. Jordan, and H. R. Stanley.** 1960. Experimental caries and gingival pathologic changes in the gnotobiotic rat. *J. Dent. Res.* **39:**923–935.

19. **Fitzgerald, R. J., and P. H. Keyes.** 1960. Demonstration of the etiologic role of streptococci in experimental caries in the hamster. *J. Am. Dent. Assoc.* **61:**9–19.

20. **Fives-Taylor, P. M., F. L. Macrina, T. J. Pritchard, and S. S. Peene.** 1987. Expression of *Streptococcus sanguis* antigens in *Escherichia coli:* cloning of a structural gene for adhesion fimbriae. *Infect. Immun.* **55:**123–128.

21. **Gibbons, R. J.** 1964. Bacteriology of dental caries. *J. Dent. Res.* **43:**1021–1028.

22. **Gibbons, R. J.** 1989. Bacterial adhesion to oral tissues: a model for infectious diseases. *J. Dent. Res.* **68:**750–760.

23. **Gibbons, R. J., and J. van Houte.** 1980. Bacterial adherence and the formation of dental plaques, p. 61–104. *In* E. H. Beachey (ed.), *Bacterial Adherence.* (Receptors and Recognition, Series B, vol. 6). Chapman Hall, London, United Kingdom.

24. **Hillman, J. D., J. van Houte, and R. J. Gibbons.** 1970. Sorption of bacteria to human enamel powder. *Arch. Oral Biol.* **15:**899–903.

25. **Hiroi, T., K. Fukushima, I. Kantake, Y. Namiki, and T. Ikeda.** 1992. De novo glucan synthesis by mutans streptococcal glucosyltransferases present in pellicle promoted firm binding of *Streptococcus gordonii* to tooth surfaces. *FEMS Microbiol Lett.* **96:**193–198.

26. **Jordan, H. V., R. J. Fitzgerald, and J. R. Faber, Jr.** 1959. A survey of the lactobacilli including pigmented strains from the oral cavity of the white rat. *J. Dent. Res.* **38:**611–617.

27. **Keyes, P. H.** 1958. Dental caries in the molar teeth of rats. I. Distribution of lesions induced by high-carbohydrate low-fat diets. *J. Dent. Res.* **37:** 1077–1087.

28. **Krasse, B., S. Edwardsson, I. Svensson, and L. Trell.** 1967. Implantation of caries-inducing streptococci in the human oral cavity. *Arch. Oral Biol.* **12:**231–236.

29. **Levine, M. J., L. A. Tabak, M. Reddy, and I. D. Mandel.** 1985. Nature of salivary pellicles in microbial adherence: role of salivary mucins, p. 125–130. *In* S. Mergenhagen and B. Rosan (ed.),

Molecular Basis of Oral Microbial Adhesion. American Society for Microbiology, Washington, D.C.

30. **Liljemark, W. F., and S. V. Schauer.** 1977. Competitive binding among oral streptococci to hydroxyapatite. *J. Dent. Res.* **56:**157–165.

31. **Liljemark, W. F., C. G. Bloomquist, L. A. Uhl, E. M. Schaffer, L. F. Wolff, B. L. Pihlstrom, and C. L. Bandt.** 1984. Distribution of oral *Haemophilus* species in dental plaque from a large adult population. *Infect. Immun.* **46:**778–786.

32. **Liljemark, W. F., and C. G. Bloomquist.** 1994. Normal microbial flora of the human body. p. 135–144. *In* R. J. Nisengard and M. G. Newman (ed.), *Oral Microbiology and Immunology*, 2nd ed. W. B. Saunders, Philadelphia, Pa.

33. **Liljemark, W. F., and C. Bloomquist.** 1996. Human oral microbial ecology and dental caries and periodontal diseases. *Crit. Rev. Oral Biol. Med.* **7:**180–198.

34. **Listgarten, M. A.** 1976. Structure of the microbial flora associated with periodontal health and disease in man. A light and electron microscopic study. *J. Periodontol.* **47:**1–18.

35. **Loesche, W. J.** 1986. Role of *Streptococcus mutans* in human dental decay. *Microbiol. Rev.* **50:**353–380.

36. **Loesche, W. J.** 1988. Ecology of the oral flora, p. 307–319. *In* R. J. Nisengard and M. G. Newman (ed.), *Oral Microbiology and Immunology*. W. B. Saunders Co., Philadelphia, Pa.

37. **Marsh, P. D.** 1991. Microbiological aspects of the chemical control of plaque and gingivitis. *J. Dent. Res.* **71:**1431–1438.

38. **McCabe, R. M., and J. A. Donkersloot.** 1977. Adherence of *Veillonella* species mediated by extracellular glucosyltransferase from *Streptococcus salivarius. Infect. Immun.* **18:**726–734.

39. **Minah, G. E., E. S. Soloman, and K. Chu.** 1985. The association between dietary sucrose consumption and microbial population shifts at six oral sites. *Arch. Oral Biol.* **30:**397–401.

40. **Moore, L. V. H., W. E. C. Moore, E. P. Cato, R. M. Smibert, J. A. Burmeister, A. M. Best, and R. R. Ranney.** 1987. Bacteriology of human gingivitis. *J. Dent. Res.* **66:**989–995.

41. **Moore, W. E. C., R. R. Ranney, and L. V. Holdeman.** 1982. Subgingival microflora in periodontal disease: cultural studies, p. 13–26. *In* R. J. Genco and S. E. Mergenhagen (ed.), *Host-Parasite Interactions in Periodontal Disease.* American Society for Microbiology, Washington D.C.

42. **Orland, F. J., J. R. Blayney, R. W. Harrison, J. A. Reyniers, P. C. Trexler, and M. Wagner.** 1954. Use of the germfree animal technique in the study of experimental dental caries. I. Basic observations on rats reared free of all microorganisms. *J. Dent. Res.* **33:**147–174.

43. **O'Toole, G. A., and R. Kolter.** 1998. Flagellar and twitching motility are necessary for *Pseudomonas aeruginosa* biofilm development. *Mol. Microbiol.* **30:**295–304.

44. **Palmer, J., and D. E. Caldwell.** 1995. A flow-cell for the study of plaque removal and regrowth. *J. Microbiol. Methods* **24:**171–182.

45. **Rosebury, T.** 1962. Microorganisms indigenous to man. McGraw-Hill, New York, N.Y.

46. **Rykke, M., and G. Rölla.** 1990. Effect of two organic phosphonates on protein adsorption in vitro and on pellicle formation in vivo. *Scand. J. Dent. Res.* **98:**486–496.

47. **Sansone, C., J. van Houte, K. Joshipura, R. Kent, and H. C. Margolis.** 1993. The association of mutans streptococci and non-mutans streptococci capable of acidogenesis at a low pH with dental caries on enamel and root surfaces. *J. Dent. Res.* **72:**508–516.

48. **Scheie, A. A., K. H. Eggen, and G. Rölla.** 1987. Glucosyltransferase activity in human in vivo formed enamel pellicle and in whole saliva. *Scand. J. Dent. Res.* **95:**212–215.

49. **Schilling, K. M., and W. H. Bowen.** 1992. Glucans synthesized in situ in experimental salivary pellicle function as specific binding sites for *Streptococcus mutans. Infect. Immun.* **60:**284–295.

50. **Shapiro, J. A.** 1992. Differential action and differential expression of DNA polymerase I during *Escherichia coli* colony development. *J. Bacteriol.* **174:**7262–7272.

51. **Shimkets, L. J., and M. Dworkin.** 1981. Excreted adenosine is a cell density signal for the initiation of fruiting body formation in Myxococcus xanthus. *Dev. Biol.* **84:**51–60.

52. **Skopek, R. J., and W. F. Liljemark.** 1994. The influence of saliva on interbacterial adherence. *Oral Microbiol. Immunol.* **9:**19–24.

53. **Socransky, S. S., and A. D. Haffajee.** 1992. The bacterial etiology of destructive periodontal disease: current concepts. *J. Periodontol.* **63:**322–331.

54. **Sönju, T., and P.-O. Glantz.** 1975. Chemical composition of salivary integuments formed in vivo on solids with some established surface characteristics. *Arch. Oral. Biol.* **20:**687–691.

55. **Tabak, L. A., M. J. Levine, N. K. Jain, A. R. Bryan, R. E. Cohen, L. D. Monte, et al.** 1985. Adsorption of human salivary mucins to hydroxyapatite. *Arch. Oral Biol.* **30:**423–427.

56. **J. M. Tanzer.** 1979. Essential dependence of smooth surface caries on, and augmentation of fissure caries by, sucrose and *Streptococcus mutans* infection. *Infect. Immun.* **25:**526–531.

57. **van der Hoeven, J. S., M. H. deJong, and P. E. Kolenbrander.** 1985. In vivo studies of microbial adherence in dental plaque, p. 220–227.

In S. E. Mergenhagen and B. Rosan (ed.), *Molecular Basis of Oral Microbial Adhesion.* American Society for Microbiology, Washington, D.C.

58. **van der Hoeven, J. S., and M. J. M. Schaeken.** 1995. Streptococci and actinomyces inhibit regrowth of *Streptococcus mutans* on gnotobiotic rat molar teeth after chlorhexidine varnish treatment. *Caries Res.* **29:**159–162.

59. **van Houte, J., R. J. Gibbons, and S. B. Banghart.** 1970. Adherence as a determinant of the presence of *Streptococcus salivarius* and *Streptococcus sanguis* on the human tooth surface. *Arch. Oral Biol.* **15:**1025–1034.

60. **van Houte, J., R. J. Gibbons, and A. J. Pulkkinen.** 1971. Adherence as an ecological determinant for streptococci in the human mouth. *Arch. Oral Biol.* **16:**1131–1141.

61. **van Houte, J., and D. B. Green.** 1974. Relationship between the concentration of bacteria in saliva and the colonization of teeth in humans. *Infect. Immun.* **9:**624–630.

62. **van Houte, J., J. Russo, and K. S. Prostak.** 1989. Increased pH-lowering ability of *Streptococcus mutans* cell masses associated with extracellular glucan-rich matrix material and the mechanisms involved. *J. Dent. Res.* **68:**451–459.

63. **van Houte, J., C. Sansone, K. Joshipura, and R. Kent.** 1991. In vitro acidogenic potential and mutans streptococci of human smooth-surface plaque associated with initial caries lesions and sound enamel. *J. Dent. Res.* **70:**1497–1502.

64. **van Houte, J.** 1994. Role of micro-organisms in caries etiology. *J. Dent. Res.* **73:**672–681.

65. **Vassilakos, N., J. Rundegren, T. Arnebrant, and P.-O. Glantz.** 1992. Adsorption from salivary fractions at solid/liquid and air/liquid interfaces. *Arch. Oral Biol.* **37:**549–557.

BIOFILMS AND DEVICE-RELATED INFECTIONS

J. William Costerton and Philip S. Stewart

22

With the benefit of hindsight, it is possible to detect a very gradual but profound shift in the nature of the diseases that affect patients in the developed world. Many acute diseases caused by specialized pathogens with specific pathogenic mechanisms, such as typhoid and diphtheria, have been largely eradicated by the use of effective vaccines and modern antibiotics. Their places among the "Horsemen of the Apocalypse" have been taken by a different type of infection, caused by organisms that were previously thought to be saprophytic or environmental, whose sole pathogenic mechanism is often the ability to persist in spite of host defenses and antibiotic chemotherapy. These low-grade infections often develop very slowly, with only a few symptoms, and they usually affect individuals who are compromised by some physiological defect (e.g., cystic fibrosis or diabetes) or by the implantation of a foreign body, such as a medical device. Direct observations of infected tissues from compromised individuals, and of the surfaces of medical devices that have become foci of chronic infections, have shown that the causative organisms actually grow in biofilms in which they are embedded in copious amounts of exopolysaccharide matrix material. The study of bacterial biofilms is more advanced in the engineering field than in the medical field, but the simple realization that biofilms are involved in chronic infections opens the way for a massive transfer of valuable information from the engineering realm to the medical realm and for its application to the treatment of infectious diseases.

INSIGHTS FROM BIOFILM MICROBIOLOGY

Serendipitously, the organism that predominates in virtually all cold-water systems (*Pseudomonas aeruginosa*) is also responsible for many device-related and other chronic infections, and biofilm microbiologists who study environmental and industrial systems are very familiar with biofilms formed by this species. Even the most anthropocentric among us cannot attribute mental processes to prokaryotic cells, so we must assume that they follow the same growth and survival strategies in the human body that have made them so very successful in the environment and in industrial systems. *P. aeruginosa* first came to the attention of biofilm microbiologists because it predominates in cold alpine streams (8) and grows predominantly (99.99%) in biofilms in this natural

J. William Costerton and Philip S. Stewart, Center for Biofilm Engineering, Montana State University, Bozeman, MT 59717.

Persistent Bacterial Infections, Edited by J. P. Nataro, M. J. Blaser, and S. Cunningham-Rundles, © 2000 ASM Press, Washington, D.C.

habitat. We know that bacteria have inhabited freshwater streams for much longer than eukaryotic organisms have existed on earth, so the pronounced tendency of this ubiquitous bacterium to grow in biofilms in its real habitat sends us a clear message of importance to medical microbiology. In the original observations, two parallel teams of microbial ecologists found the rocks along the streams coated with thick biofilms ($>10^8$ cells/cm^2), while the bulk water phase of the alpine stream ecosystem contained only 8 to 10 cells/ml. This predominance of the biofilm mode of growth has been confirmed in literally hundreds of stream environments, in industrial water systems, and in hospital water and air conditioning systems (7). Basic observations of the predominance of biofilms in natural habitats have now been extended to almost all bacterial species, including gram-positive bacteria, and the only exceptions seem to be among organisms that live in mucus layers (e.g., *Campylobacter*) and among intercellular pathogens. In environmental and industrial microbiology, as in medical microbiology, bacteria that are removed from their natural ecosystems and grown in monospecies cultures in liquid media quickly adapt to this very artificial system and adopt the planktonic mode of growth almost exclusively. Two reasons for this adaptation to growth in pure culture appear to be the higher growth rate of planktonic cells, in the absence of antagonists, and the fact that biofilm cells are left behind on the walls of test tubes when liquid cultures are propagated by the traditional methods of subculture. Liquid monospecies cultures are certainly necessary for studies of the genetics or the physiology of individual species, but it is very sobering to realize that this almost universal culture method induces a mode of growth that differs profoundly from that adopted by almost all organisms in nature and in most modern infections.

Engineers in the Center for Biofilm Engineering (CBE) have defined bacterial biofilms in terms of their structures, their remarkable physiological heterogeneity, and their phenomenal resistance to antibacterial agents. Engineers favor direct observation over extrapola-

tion, and the main weapon in their arsenal for the structural examination of biofilms is the confocal scanning laser microscope (CSLM). The CSLM allows us to visualize biofilms on opaque surfaces, without fixation or dehydration, so that we can obtain clear images of living biofilms in real time. CSLM observations of living biofilms, including some formed by one to three species in vitro and some formed in natural ecosystems, showed unequivocally that biofilms are composed of discrete microcolonies interspersed between open water channels that communicate with the bulk fluid (Fig. 1). Some of these microcolonies are shaped like mushrooms, and some assume different shapes described as "stacks" or "towers," but all contain sessile bacterial cells embedded in a hydrated exopolysaccharide matrix whose viscoelastic properties become evident under high-shear conditions (31). The CBE has established the fact that most biofilms assume this microcolony and water channel structure, including all biofilms formed by the few gram-positive species examined to date, and the most significant consequence of this new observation is that we must now explain how these elaborate structures are established and maintained. Kolter and colleagues have shown (22) that planktonic cells of *P. aeruginosa* maneuver on a surface, following initial association, and form aggregates that develop into microcolonies when matrix formation is "switched on" (12). It is clear that these initial stages of biofilm formation are controlled by signals, analogous to the hormones and pheromones that control morphogenesis and behavior in higher organisms. The subsequent structural developments that lead to the microcolony and water channel structures of mature biofilms are even more complex, and we must invoke an even more complex set of signals to control this morphogenesis and to explain the persistence of open water channels when random growth would rapidly occlude them. Mature biofilms obviously constitute primitive multicellular organisms (7), and their signaling systems may constitute a new target for manipulation as we

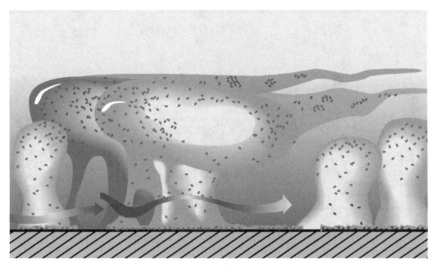

FIGURE 1 Diagrammatic representation of the cellular structure of a microbial biofilm showing the directly observed shapes of matrix-enclosed microcolonies and intervening water channels, in which convective flow occurs.

think about methods to control their formation in infections.

The tendency of engineers to make direct observations, and their skill with miniature instruments, has shown that the complex structures of bacterial biofilms produce equally complex physiological patterns within these sessile populations. Lewandowski and his team of engineers and microbiologists have used very fine (<10-μm) microelectrodes to map characteristics such as dissolved oxygen and pH within biofilms (25), and the data are at once fascinating and disturbing. A map of dissolved oxygen concentrations in a biofilm produced by cells of *P. aeruginosa* (Fig. 2) shows that some of the sessile cells that compose this sessile community grow aerobically while some experience a completely anaerobic environment. Direct observations of the rates of metabolic activity of sessile cells at various locations within biofilms, using chemical probes that measure reducing power, show an equally heterogeneous pattern (38–40). The consequence of this remarkable physiological heterogeneity within biofilms is that there are sessile cells in any mature biofilm that are growing in a huge variety of physiological states and at an equally variety of rates. This physiological heterogeneity is a powerful survival mechanism for sessile communities, because any antibacterial agent must kill all of the cells growing in all of the different physiological states or the cells that survive in any given microcolony will simply propagate and reestablish the biofilm in a matter of hours.

Engineers are accustomed to thinking in terms of mass transfer when they consider the penetration of any molecule through a matrix. These concepts, and the methods that are used to support them, have been very useful in the examination of the penetration of antibacterial agents through the matrices of biofilms with the objective of killing sessile organisms. Stewart and his team of engineers and microbiologists have examined the penetration of both biocides and antibiotics through biofilms (4, 13; P. S. Stewart, F. Roe, J. Rayner, J. G. Elkins, Z. Lewandowski, U. A. Ochsner, and D. J. Hassett, submitted for publication; J. A. Anderl, P. S. Stewart, and M. J. Franklin, submitted for publication); they have concluded that the biofilm matrix presents only a minor barrier to penetration except in cases in which the agent reacts chemically with the matrix mate-

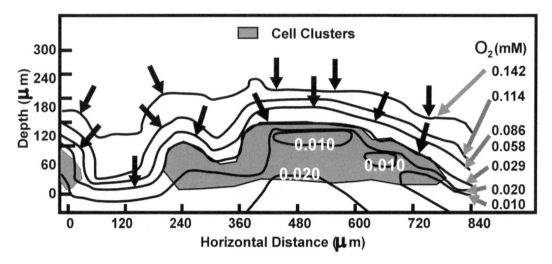

FIGURE 2 Isobar map of dissolved oxygen concentration as measured directly in a living biofilm by the use of a microelectrode, showing that the centers of microcolonies can be essentially anoxic, even when the biofilm is growing in ambient air.

rial. The penetration of an antibacterial agent can be monitored by using the exquisitely sensitive noninvasive technique of attenuated total reflectance-Fourier transform infrared spectroscopy (ATR-FTIR) (35, 38) to determine when the molecule in question reaches the colonized substratum. The CBE team can also monitor penetration by mapping the positions of the surviving sessile cells (19). The biofilm matrix may act as a barrier to the penetration of antibacterial agents if these molecules react with or bind to the matrix material (which is usually an anionic exopolysaccharide), but this barrier can be overcome by simply increasing the concentration of the agent until it exceeds that lost to reaction or binding (30). Limitations in mass transfer are sufficient to explain some low levels of resistance of biofilms to antibiotics, but they are not sufficient to account for the 1,000- to 1,500-fold increases in resistance seen when cells of most species form these sessile populations (28). Most antibiotics affect individual bacterial cells differently, depending on the bacterial growth rate, and many authors (1, 2) have suggested that the low growth rates seen in some sessile cells may make them inherently less susceptible to the

antibiotics that penetrate the matrix of the biofilm. However, the growth rate is only one of many physiological parameters that vary significantly in the different microcolonies that constitute a biofilm, and such parameters as local oxygen tension, pH, and local expression of *rpoS* (16) may affect susceptibility to antibacterial agents equally profoundly. To grasp the clinical consequences of this physiological heterogeneity of biofilms, it is essential to remember that any sessile cell that survives the onslaught of an antibiotic finds itself embedded in a matrix containing the remnants of all of its dead neighbors, and the biofilm reforms very quickly when therapy is finished.

A recent discovery that the cells of *P. aeruginosa* assume a radically different phenotype when they form biofilms may provide a more complete explanation of the phenomenal resistance of sessile populations to antibiotics. We expected that the synthesis of alginate (the matrix material of *Pseudomonas* biofilms) would be triggered by the adhesion of these cells to a surface; we have shown that one of these genes (*algC*) is upregulated within minutes of adhesion (12), and we assume that the whole alginate cassette is expressed in this initial phase of

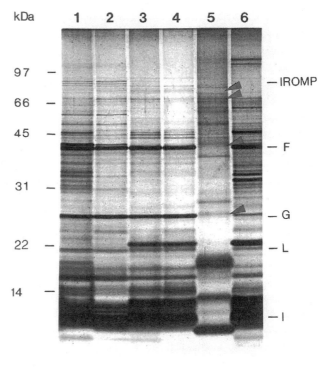

FIGURE 3 Polyacrylamide gel electrophoresis gel showing the pattern of production of OMPs by cells of *P. aeruginosa* in the biofilm mode of growth (lane 5) versus production by cells in the planktonic mode of growth (lanes 1 to 4 and 6). The differences in OMP production between these cells indicate that the biofilm phenotype differs profoundly from the planktonic phenotype (H. Yu and J. W. Costerton, unpublished data).

biofilm formation. However, we were recently surprised to note that the outer membrane proteins (OMPs) of *P. aeruginosa* differ very radically (Fig. 3) between planktonic cells and biofilm cells, indicating the existence of different planktonic and biofilm phenotypes in the organism. The biofilm phenotype appears to include the expression of the *rpoS* gene (K. D. Xu, unpublished data), which is normally expressed only in the stationary growth phase by planktonic cells, and it is very significant that this gene is expressed in bacterial cells recovered directly from the infected lungs of patients with cystic fibrosis (16). If bacterial cells of other species also express a completely different set of genes when they are growing in biofilms, we must reexamine much of the work in medical microbiology that has been based on studies of planktonic cells growing in monospecies cultures. Antibiotics have been screened for their ability to kill planktonic cells, and vaccines have been produced that include the surface antigens expressed by planktonic

cells, but some pathogens actually growing in the body may express a profoundly different phenotype with different permeabilities and different surface proteins. Perhaps, then, it is not surprising that these antibiotics and vaccines have been effective against acute bacterial diseases in which the pathogens grow in the planktonic phenotype but much less effective in the control of biofilm diseases (6).

If we try to imagine the bacterial survival strategies that would have been effective in the earliest stages of the development of life on this planet, growth in stationary biofilms that were protected from unfavorable conditions would prevent bacteria from being swept into acid or boiling downstream pools and from surges of threatening water from upstream sources. Biofilms predominate in modern hot spring areas for exactly these reasons. Later in the development of life, sessile bacteria would be protected from the depredations of bacteriophage viruses and primitive amoebae when they were in the biofilm mode of growth. When we study natural mixed-species biofilms taken directly from rivers and streams, we can watch amoebae cruise over the surfaces of biofilms and even penetrate the water channels of these sessile populations, but these phagocytic eukaryotes capture and ingest only the few planktonic cells that cannot enjoy the protection afforded by the biofilm. We can, therefore, speculate that bacteria adopted the essentially defensive biofilm phenotype long before multicellular animals evolved and that they reverted to this strategy when, as pathogens in the human body, they were faced with the armamentarium of antibodies and antibiotics thrown at them by modern medicine. The large-scale use of medical devices is a relatively new development in medicine, and this provision of readily colonizable surfaces may have selected for the invasion of the body by a new class of pathogens whose main pathogenic mechanism is their ability to produce well-defended biofilms. This might explain the recent success in the hospital environment of species (e.g., *P. aeruginosa* and *Legionella pneumophila*) that were already notably successful biofilm formers in lakes and rivers or notably successful but innocuous colonizers of the human skin (*Staphylococcus epidermidis*). Medical microbiology has been very successful in the control of acute planktonic pathogens, but now it must employ some of the techniques of microbial ecology in order to deal with the new biofilm pathogens that have "crept out of the swamp" to attack those who are compromised by physiological defects or by the implantation of medical devices.

BIOFILM INFECTIONS OF MEDICAL DEVICES

Our clinical colleagues, notably Marrie and Gristina, have reported that bacterial infections associated with medical devices are generally resistant to host defense mechanisms and refractory to antibiotic chemotherapy (18). Because environmental and industrial biofilms are also resistant to phagocytic cells (amoebae) and refractory to treatment with biocides, we examined the surfaces of devices and associated tissues from these infections to determine

whether the causative organisms grow in biofilms. Even though the morphological methods available at that time (scanning and transmission electron microscopy) depended on radical dehydration of the specimens, it was immediately obvious that the bacterial cells involved in these infections grew in biofilms identical to those seen in our previous studies. The bacterial cells on the surfaces of either urinary catheters (28) or pacemaker leads that had been the foci of device-related infections were clearly seen to be embedded in fibrous material even though this matrix was severely condensed by dehydration (Fig. 4). The pivotal role of biofilms in device-related and other chronic bacterial infections was proposed (8), and subsequent examinations of literally hundreds of implanted medical devices have reinforced this observation (17, 21). Virtually all transcutaneous medical devices acquire microbial biofilms that travel into accessible internal tissues in a matter of weeks, and devices that are simply apposed to tissues (like urinary catheters and intrauterine devices [IUDs]) often acquire biofilms because they carry bacteria from colonized tissues into normally sterile organs. Implanted medical devices may acquire biofilms as a result of bacterial contamination during surgery or subsequent hematogenous spread. In the absence of a medical device, biofilms may form on tissue surfaces because of a physiological compromise (cystic fibrosis) or because of tissue damage, such as the formation of sequestrae of dead bone in the initial stages of osteomyelitis (24). In rarer cases, bacterial biofilms may form on the surfaces of healthy tissues (e.g., prostate or endocardium) as a result of a temporary failure of usually effective host defense mechanisms. A partial list of biofilm diseases that affect patients in developed countries is presented in Table 1, and it has been estimated that as many as 60% of the bacterial diseases treated in this decade are actually biofilm infections.

CHARACTERISTICS OF BIOFILM DISEASES

While a biofilm infection can give rise to an acute planktonic infection at any time, the bio-

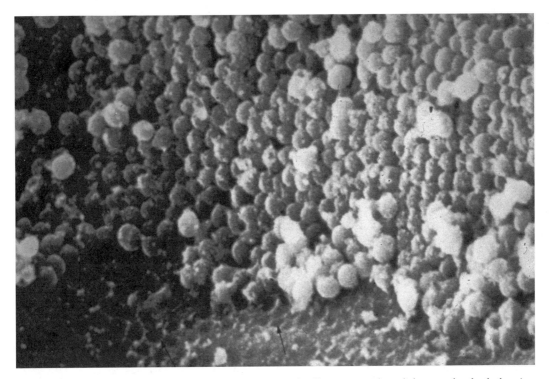

FIGURE 4 Scanning electron micrograph of an *S. aureus* biofilm on an endocardial pacemaker lead, showing spherical bacterial cells embedded in dehydration-condensed matrix material. These biofilm cells were resistant to a 6-week course of very high-dose antibiotic therapy.

film infection itself is not notably aggressive. We have found that all Tenckhoff catheters used in peritoneal dialysis (9) and all of the Hickman catheters used in cancer chemotherapy (33) are completely colonized with microbial biofilms on both their external and lumenal surfaces within 3 weeks of installation. Even though these relatively intrusive devices are completely colonized by bacterial biofilms, most patients are asymptomatic, and acute infections emanating from these sessile bacterial populations occur relatively rarely and appear to depend more on the host defenses than on the presence of the biofilms (10). Some of the most abundant biofilms that we have seen on medical devices occur on the surfaces of the copper wires that form parts of some IUDs (Fig. 5), but endometrial infections associated with these devices are very rare. The amount of surface area colonized by bacterial biofilms

appears to have some bearing on the ability of these smoldering infections to trigger an acute infection, with dissemination of planktonic cells. For example, small pacemaker leads appear to be well tolerated, while the total artificial heart is not (17). The role of host defenses in controlling biofilm infections is discussed below.

The characteristic that distinguishes chronic device-related infections most clearly from acute bacterial infections is the response to antibiotic chemotherapy. While many acute infections can be eradicated by a single brief course of systemic antibiotic therapy, biofilm infections often respond incompletely and then recur. The first detailed examination of a device-related bacterial infection involved a patient who presented with a *Staphylococcus aureus* bacteremia secondary to an olecranon bursitis (26). The patient had been fitted with an endo-

TABLE 1 Partial list of human infections involving biofilms[a]

Infection or disease	Common biofilm bacterial species
Dental caries	Acidogenic gram-positive cocci (e.g., *Streptococcus*)
Periodontitis	Gram-negative anaerobic oral bacteria
Otitis media	Nontypeable strains of *Haemophilus influenzae*
Musculoskeletal infections	Gram-positive cocci (e.g., staphylococci)
Necrotizing fasciitis	Group A streptococci
Biliary tract infection	Enteric bacteria (e.g., *E. coli*)
Osteomyelitis	Various bacterial and fungal species, often mixed
Bacterial prostatitis	*E. coli* and other gram-negative bacteria
Native valve endocarditis	Viridans group streptococci
Cystic fibrosis pneumonia	*P. aeruginosa* and *Burkholderia cepacia*
Meloidosis	*Pseudomonas pseudomallei*
Nosocomial infections	
Intensive-care unit pneumonia	Gram-negative rods
Sutures	*S. epidermidis* and *S. aureus*
Exit sites	*S. epidermidis* and *S. aureus*
Arteriovenous shunts	*S. epidermidis* and *S. aureus*
Schleral buckles	Gram-positive cocci
Contact lens	*P. aeruginosa* and gram-positive cocci
Urinary catheter cystitis	*E. coli* and other gram-negative rods
Peritoneal dialysis (CAPD)[b] peritonitis	A variety of bacteria and fungi
IUDs	*Actinomyces israelli* and many others
Endotracheal tubes	A variety of bacteria and fungi
Hickman catheters	*S. epidermidis* and *Candida albicans*
Central venous catheters	*S. epidermidis* and others
Mechanical heart valves	*S. aureus* and *S. epidermidis*
Vascular grafts	Gram-positive cocci
Biliary stent blockage	A variety of enteric bacteria and fungi
Orthopedic devices	*S. aureus* and *S. epidermidis*
Penile prostheses	*S. aureus* and *S. epidermidis*

[a] Taken from reference 6 with permission.
[b] CAPD, chronic ambulatory peritoneal dialysis.

cardial pacemaker many years previously, and Marrie speculated that the planktonic bacteria that had caused the bacteremia could have colonized the plastic and metal surfaces of the pacemaker lead. Following 6 weeks of therapy with cloxacillin and rifampin, the pacemaker lead was removed and was found to be colonized by a biofilm composed of spherical cells (Fig. 4), and plating of macroscopic biofilm material scraped from these surfaces yielded >10[8] cells of *S. aureus*. From this case study it was clear that sessile cells of this gram-positive pathogen could survive prolonged exposure in vivo to relatively high levels of antibiotics that would readily have killed planktonic cells of the same species.

The exact extent of the inherent resistance of sessile bacteria to antibiotics required in vitro experimentation. *P. aeruginosa* biofilms that had been formed on urinary catheter material in flowing urine were treated with a variety of different antibiotics (28). These experiments, and many subsequent experiments by independent investigators, have now established that sessile bacterial cells are up to 1,000 times as resistant to antibiotics as their planktonic counterparts (7). It is clear that biofilm formation is a common survival strategy that serves prokaryotic organisms well in the human body, just as it serves them very well in environmental and industrial systems. Here, the experience of biofilm microbiologists who work in indus-

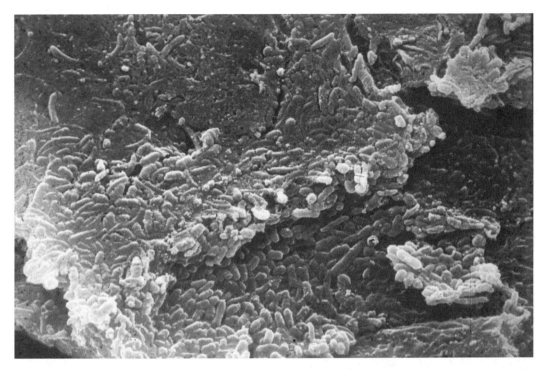

FIGURE 5 Scanning electron micrograph of a mixed-species bacterial biofilm on the copper component of a Copper 7 IUD worn by an asymptomatic patient.

trial systems can be useful in medical microbiology, because these people, who live with biofilm problems every day, have usually resorted to mechanical removal of sessile populations followed by high-dose biocide treatment. Practical clinical wisdom dictates that colonized devices must often be removed before the infections associated with them can be resolved by antibiotic therapy (21, 27).

Just as the inherent antibiotic resistance of biofilm infections correlates well with similar resistance to industrial biocides, the characteristic chronicity of these infections (6) correlates well with observations of biofilms in other ecosystems. Phagocytic white blood cells are as ineffective as wild amoebae in ingesting sessile bacteria (20), and nascent biofilms composed of only a few microcolonies of four to six cells enclosed in matrix material resist phagocytic clearance, even in fiercely defended sites like the peritoneum (36). The humoral immune system is stimulated by the presence of sessile

bacteria growing in biofilms and by the frustrated response of phagocytic cells, and biofilms growing in tissues (like *P. aeruginosa* biofilms in the lung in cystic fibrosis) are seen to be surrounded by masses of immune complex (Fig. 6). Lam et al. (23) have shown that antibodies against *P. aeruginosa* are ineffective in clearing the pathogens in cystic fibrosis, and Cochrane et al. (5) have shown that the formation of immune complexes stimulates damaging cellular responses in which lysosomal enzymes are released. Generally, then, the body's host responses to biofilms are at best ineffective and at worst severely damaging to adjacent tissues. Some clinicians have resorted to immune suppression in order to dampen the body's immune reaction to the presence of sessile bacteria, which may persist for decades in such chronic diseases as cystic fibrosis and prostatitis, and thus to minimize tissue damage by frustrated phagocytosis.

The least understood characteristic of bio-

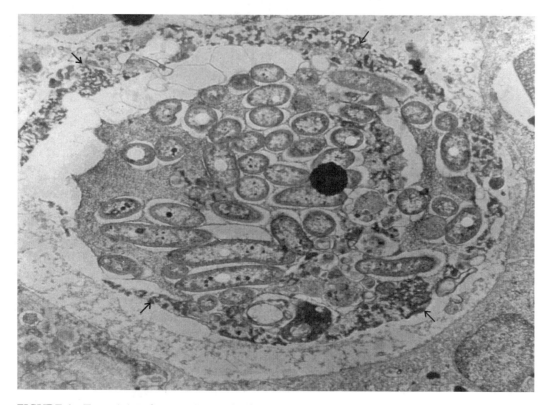

FIGURE 6 Transmission electron micrograph of a matrix-enclosed microcolony of cells of *P. aeruginosa* in the lung of a rat with a model infection designed to mimic cystic fibrosis in human patients. Note the dehydration-related shrinkage of the matrix material and the dark "crust" of immune complex material surrounding the microcolony.

film infections, including those associated with medical devices, is their cryptic, or indolent, nature. Again, this characteristic is explained by recent discoveries in biofilm microbiology. Biofilms are composed of bacterial cells ($\pm 15\%$ by volume) embedded in a voluminous exopolysaccharide matrix ($\pm 85\%$ by volume) in discrete microcolonies. Polysaccharides are generally poorly immunogenic and are not notably inflammatory, so the cellular and humoral immune systems of the body "see" only the lipopolysaccharide and protein molecules that protrude from the immunologically sequestered biofilm. For this reason, large areas of the surfaces of medical devices may be colonized without the patient suffering any detectable symptoms (10). On the other hand, biofilms are programmed to regularly release planktonic

cells from the earliest stages of their formation on a surface, and the total number of planktonic cells that challenge the body's defenses depends on the size of the colonized area that is shedding these highly inflammatory cells. In our studies of transcutaneous medical devices (Tenckhoff and Hickman catheters), we have found that many patients are entirely asymptomatic, even when the total surface areas of their catheters are colonized by thick biofilms, and only a minority of these patients experience bacteremic infection.

Generally, chronic biofilm infections remain very localized, and even patients with cystic fibrosis with massive colonization of the lungs rarely experience infections in other organs. Small medical devices that are completely colonized by sessile bacteria (e.g., stitches and

ing molecules and their analogs will supplement and/or replace the use of conventional antibiotics in the near future. Now that commercial entities connected with the CBE have produced acyl homoserine lactone signal analogs that prevent biofilm formation and promote the detachment of planktonic cells from mature biofilms, the way forward towards their use in the treatment of biofilm infections seems clear. We predict that signals and signal analogs that either block or reinforce signal-controlled behaviors will be used to interdict specific mechanisms by which bacterial pathogens affect their hosts. This interdiction may be as simple as adding molecular blockers of the signals that control toxin production so that a pathogen can occupy its ecological niche, much as *Clostridium difficile* occupies its niche in the large intestine, but cannot produce the toxin that is central to its attack on tissues. Another signal that affected the ability of the pathogen to integrate itself into the ecology of the tissue could then be activated, and the organism would cease to occupy its ecological niche. The strategy behind this approach is to shut off pathogenesis without putting the pathogen under a toxic frontal attack that stimulates its survival mechanisms and that produces resistant strains.

Biofilm diseases would constitute the ideal targets for the manipulation of bacterial behavior, because they depend on the sessile mode of growth as their central pathogenic mechanism. If cells of a single species (e.g., *S. epidermidis*) formed a biofilm on a medical device (e.g., the sewing cuff of a mechanical heart valve), the simple stimulation of their detachment from this colonized surface would lead to their deaths, if the patient's circulating level of antibiotics was suitably elevated. Alternatively, signal analogs that block biofilm formation or promote detachment even as bacteria start to adhere could be incorporated into the biomaterials used to produce these medical devices, and they would completely escape microbial colonization. Even in non-device-related chronic bacterial infections, such as prostatitis (27), the detachment of planktonic

cells from biofilms formed by cells of *Escherichia coli* would remove the infecting sessile population and allow the clearance of these recalcitrant infections by high-dose antibiotic chemotherapy. Biofilm diseases offer the burgeoning companies that propose to use signals to manipulate bacterial behavior a target that is even more attractive than the lucrative targets offered by industrial systems. While the bacterial populations that cause fouling and corrosion in industrial water systems are composed of many species, and some universal signal analogs are already in use (14), biofilm infections often involve only one species, and the selection of suitable signals may be facilitated. There can be little doubt that Kolter and Losick (22) are correct in their predictions, and infectious-disease practitioners will soon have therapeutics at their disposal whose activities are predicated on natural signaling mechanisms.

ACKNOWLEDGMENT

This work was supported by cooperative agreement ECD-8907039 with the National Science Foundation.

REFERENCES

1. **Brown, M. R. W., D. G. Allison, and P. Gilbert.** 1988. Resistance of bacterial biofilms to antibiotics: a growth-rate related effect. *J. Antimicrob. Chemother.* **22:**777–783.
2. **Brown, M. R. W., and P. Williams.** 1985. The influence of environment on envelope properties affecting survival of bacteria in infections. *Annu. Rev. Microbiol.* **39:**527–556.
3. **Ceri, H., M. E. Olson, C. Stremick, R. R. Read, D. Morck, and A. Buret.** 1999. The Calgary biofilm device: new technology for rapid determination of antibiotic susceptibilities of bacterial biofilms. *J. Clin. Microbiol.* **37:**1771–1776.
4. **Chen, X., and P. S. Stewart.** 1996. Chlorine penetration into artificial biofilm is limited by a reaction-diffusion interaction. *Environ. Sci. Technol.* **30:**2078–2083.
5. **Cochrane, D. M. G., M. R. W. Brown, H. Anwar, P. H. Weller, K. Lam, and J. W. Costerton.** 1988. Antibody response to *Pseudomonas aeruginosa* surface protein antigens in a rat model of chronic lung infection. *J. Med. Microbiol.* **27:**255–261.
6. **Costerton, J. W., P. S. Stewart, and E. P. Greenberg.** 1999. Bacterial biofilms: a common cause of persistent infections. *Science* **284:**1318–1322.

7. Costerton, J. W., Z. Lewandowski, D. E. Caldwell, D. R. Korber, and H. M. Lappin-Scott. 1995. Microbial biofilms. *Annu. Rev. Microbiol.* **49:**711–745.

8. Costerton, J. W., G. G. Geesey, and G. K. Cheng. 1978. How bacteria stick. *Sci. Am.* **238:**86–95.

9. Dasgupta, M. K., K. B. Bettcher, R. A. Ulan, V. Burns, K. Lam, J. B. Dossetor, and J. W. Costerton. 1987. Relationship of adherent bacterial biofilms to peritonitis in chronic ambulatory peritoneal dialysis. *Peritoneal Dialysis Bull.* **7:**168–173.

10. Dasgupta, M. K., and J. W. Costerton. 1989. Significance of biofilm-adherent bacterial microcolonies on Tenckhoff catheters in CAPD patients. *Blood Purif.* **7:**144–155.

11. Davies, D. G., M. R. Parsek, J. P. Pearson, B. H. Iglewski, J. W. Costerton, and E. P. Greenberg. 1998. The involvement of cell-to-cell signals in the development of a bacterial biofilm. *Science* **280:**295–298.

12. Davies, D. G., and G. G. Geesey. 1995. Regulation of the alginate biosynthesis gene *algC* in *Pseudomonas aeruginosa* during biofilm development in continuous culture. *Appl. Environ. Microbiol.* **61:**860–867.

13. de Beer, D., R. Srinivasan, and P. S. Stewart. 1994. Direct measurement of chlorine penetration into biofilms during disinfection. *Appl. Environ. Microbiol.* **60:**4339–4344.

14. De Nys, R., P. D. Steinberg, P. Willemsen, S. A. Dworjanyn, C. L. Gabelish, and R. J. King. 1995. Broad spectrum effects of secondary metabolites from the red alga *Delisea pulchra* in antifouling assays. *Biofouling* **8:**259–271.

15. Dunny, G. M., and B. A. Leonard. 1997. Cell-cell communication in Gram-positive bacteria. *Annu. Rev. Microbiol.* **51:**527–564.

16. Foley, I., P. Marsh, E. M. H. Wellington, A. W. Smith, and M. R. W. Brown. 1999. General stress response master regulator *rpoS* is expressed in human infection: a possible role in chronicity. *J. Antimicrob. Chemother.* **43:**164–165.

17. Cristina, A. G., J. J. Dobbins, B. Giamara, J. C. Lewis, and W. C. DeVries. 1988. Biomaterial-centered sepsis and the total artificial heart: microbial adhesion versus tissue integration. *J. Am. Med. Assoc.* **259:**870–877.

18. Gristina, A. G., and J. W. Costerton. 1984. Bacteria-laden biofilms: a hazard to orthopedic prostheses. *Infect. Surg.* **3:**655–662.

19. Huang, C.-T., F. Yu, G. A. McFeters, and P. S. Stewart. 1995. Nonuniform spatial patterns of respiratory activity within biofilms during disinfection. *Appl. Environ. Microbiol.* **61:**2252–2256.

20. Jensen, E. T., A. Kharazmi, K. Lam, J. W. Costerton, and N. Hoiby. 1990. Human polymorphonuclear leukocyte response to *Pseudomonas aeruginosa* biofilms. *Infect. Immun.* **58:**2383–2385.

21. Khoury, A. E., K. Lam, B. Ellis, and J. W. Costerton. 1992. Prevention and control of bacterial infections associated with medical devices. *ASAIO J.* **38:**M174–M178.

22. Kolter, R., and R. Losick. 1998. All for one and one for all. *Science* **280:**226–227.

23. Lam, J., R. Chan, K. Lam, and J. W. Costerton. 1980. Production of mucoid microcolonies by *Pseudomonas aeruginosa* within infected lungs in cystic fibrosis. *Infect. Immun.* **28:**546–556.

24. Lambe, D. W., Jr., K. P. Ferguson, K. J. Mayberry-Carson, B. Tober-Meyer, and J. W. Costerton. 1991. Foreign-body-associated experimental osteomyelitis induced with *Bacteroides fragilis* and *Staphylococcus epidermidis* in rabbits. *Clin. Orthop.* **266:**285–294.

25. Lewandowski, Z., W. Lee, W. G. Characklis, and B. Little. 1989. Dissolved oxygen and pH microelectrode measurements at water immersed metal surfaces. *Corrosion* **45:**92–98.

26. Marrie, T. J., and J. W. Costerton. 1984. Scanning and transmission electron microscopy of in situ bacterial colonization of intravenous and intraarterial catheters. *J. Clin. Microbiol.* **19:**687–693.

27. Nickel, J. C., J. W. Costerton, R. J. C. McLean, and M. Olson. 1994. Bacterial biofilms: influence on the pathogenesis, diagnosis and treatment of urinary-tract infections. *J. Antimicrob. Chemother.* **33:**31–41.

28. Nickel, J. C., I. Ruseska, J. B. Wright, and J. W. Costerton. 1985. Tobramycin resistance of *Pseudomonas aeruginosa* cells growing as a biofilm on urinary catheter material. *Antimicrob. Agents Chemother.* **27:**619–624.

29. Pitt, W. G., M. O. McBride, J. K. Lunceford, R. J. Roper, and R. D. Sagers. 1994. Ultrasonic enhancement of antibiotic action on gram-negative bacteria. *Antimicrob. Agents Chemother.* **38:**2577–2582.

30. Stewart, P. S. 1996. Theoretical aspects of antibiotic diffusion into microbial biofilms. *Antimicrob. Agents Chemother* **40:**2517–2522.

31. Stoodley, P., I. Dodds, Z. Lewandowski, A. B. Cunningham, J. D. Boyle, and H. M. Lappin-Scott. 1999. Influence of hydrodynamics and nutrients on biofilm structure. *J. Appl. Microbiol.* **85:**19S–28S.

32. Suci, P., M. W. Mittelman, F. P. Yu, and G. G. Geesey. 1994. Investigation of ciprofloxacin penetration into *Pseudomonas aeruginosa* biofilms. *Antimicrob. Agents Chemother.* **38:**2125–2133.

33. Tenney, J. H., M. R. Moody, K. A. Newman,

S. C. Schimpff, J. C. Wade, J. W. Costerton, and W. P. Reed. 1986. Adherent microorganisms on lumenal surfaces of long-term intravenous catheters: importance of *Staphylococcus epidermidis* in patients with cancer. *Arch. Intern. Med.* **146:**1949–1954.

34. Terzieva, S., J. Donnelly, V. Ulevicius, S. A. Grinshpun, K. Willeke, G. N. Selma, and K. P. Brenner. 1996. Comparison of methods for detection and enumeration of airborne microorganisms collected by liquid impingement. *Appl. Environ. Microbiol.* **62:**2264–2272.

35. Vrany, J. D., P. S. Stewart, and P. A. Suci. 1997. Comparison of recalcitrance to ciprofloxacin and levofloxacin exhibited by *Pseudomonas aeruginosa* biofilms displaying rapid-transport characteristics. *Antimicrob. Agents Chemother.* **41:**1352–1358.

36. Ward, K. H., M. E. Olson, K. Lam, and J. W. Costerton. 1992. Mechanism of persistent infection associated with peritoneal implants. *J. Med. Microbiol.* **36:**406–413.

37. Wellman, N., S. M. Fortun, and B. R. McLeod. 1996. Bacterial biofilms and the bioelectric effect. *Antimicrob. Agents Chemother.* **40:** 2012–2014.

38. Wentland, E., P. S. Stewart, C.-T. Huang, and G. A. McFeters. 1996. Spatial variations in growth rate within *Klebsiella pneumoniae* colonies and biofilm. *Biotechnol. Prog.* **12:**316–321.

39. Xu, K. D., P. S. Stewart, F. Xia, C.-T. Huang, and G. A. McFeters. 1998. Spatial physiological heterogeneity in *Pseudomonas aeruginosa* biofilm is determined by oxygen availability. *Appl. Environ. Microbiol.* **64:**4035–4039.

40. Yu, F. P., and G. A. McFeters. 1994. Rapid *in situ* assessment of physiological activities in biofilms using fluorescent probes. *J. Microbiol. Methods* **20:**1–10.

INDEX